S0-EJV-411

EICOSANOIDS AND OTHER BIOACTIVE LIPIDS IN CANCER AND RADIATION INJURY

DEVELOPMENTS IN ONCOLOGY

36. D.E. Peterson, G.E. Elias and S.T. Sonis, eds.: Head and Neck Management of the Cancer Patient. 0-89838-747-7.
37. D.M. Green: Diagnosis and Management of Malignant Solid Tumors in Infants and Children. 0-89838-750-7.
38. K.A. Foon and A.C. Morgan, Jr., eds.: Monoclonal Antibody Therapy of Human Cancer. 0-89838-754-X.
39. J.G. McVie, W. Bakker, Sj.Sc. Wagenaar and D. Carney, eds.: Clinical and Experimental Pathology of Lung Cancer. 0-89838-764-7.
40. K.V. Honn, W.E. Powers and B.F. Sloane, eds.: Mechanisms of Cancer Metastasis. 0-89838-765-5.
41. K. Lapis, L.A. Liotta and A.S. Rabson, eds.: Biochemistry and Molecular Genetics of Cancer Metastasis. 0-89838-785-X.
42. A.J. Mastromarino, ed.: Biology and Treatment of Colorectal Cancer Metastasis. 0-89838-786-8.
43. M.A. Rich, J.C. Hager and J. Taylor-Papadimitriou, eds.: Breast Cancer: Origins, Detection and Treatment. 0-89838-792-2.
44. D.G. Poplack, L. Massimo and P. Cornaglia-Ferraris, eds.: The Role of Pharmacology in Pediatric Oncology. 0-89838-795-7.
45. A. Hagenbeek and B. Löwenberg, eds.: Minimal Residual Disease in Acute Leukemia. 0-89838-799-X.
46. F.M. Muggia and M. Rozencweig, eds.: Clinical Evaluation of Antitumor Therapy. 0-89838-803-1.
47. F.A. Valeriote and L. Baker, eds.: Biochemical Modulation of Anticancer Agents: Experimental and Clinical Approaches. 0-89838-827-9.
48. B.A. Stoll, ed.: Pointers to Cancer Prognosis. 0-89838-841-4; Pb. 0-89838-876-7.
49. K.H. Hollmann and J.M. Verley, eds.: New Frontiers in Mammary Pathology. 0-89838-852-X.
50. D.J. Ruiter, G.J. Fleuren and S.O. Warnaar, eds.: Application of Monoclonal Antibodies in Tumor Pathology. 0-89838-853-8.
51. A.H.G. Paterson and A.W. Lees, eds.: Fundamental Problems in Breast Cancer. 0-89838-863-5.
52. M. Chatel, F. Darcel and J. Pecker, eds.: Brain Oncology. Biology, Diagnosis and Therapy. 0-89838-954-2.
53. M.P. Hacker, J.S. Lazo and T.R. Tritton, eds.: Organ Directed Toxicities of Anticancer Drugs. 0-89838-356-0.
54. M. Nicolini, ed.: Platinum and Other Metal Coordination Compounds in Cancer Chemotherapy. 0-89838-358-7.
55. J.R. Ryan and L.O. Baker, eds.: Recent Concepts in Sarcoma Treatment. 0-89838-376-5.
56. M.A. Rich, J.C. Hager and D.M. Lopez, eds.: Breast Cancer: Scientific and Clinical Progress. 0-89838-387-0.
57. B.A. Stoll, ed.: Women at High Risk to Breast Cancer. 0-89838-416-8.
58. M.A. Rich, J.C. Hager and I. Keydar, eds.: Breast Cancer. Progress in Biology, Clinical Management and Prevention. 0-7923-0507-8.
59. P.I. Reed, M. Carboni, B.J. Johnston and S. Guadagni, eds.: New Trends in Gastric Cancer. Background and Videosurgery. 0-7923-8917-4.
60. H.K. Awwad: Radiation Oncology: Radiobiological and Physiological Perspectives. The Boundary-Zone between Clinical Radiotherapy and Fundamental Radiobiology and Physiology. 0-7923-0783-6.
61. J.L. Evelhoch, W. Negendank, F.A. Valeriote and L.H. Baker, eds.: Magnetic Resonance in Experimental and Clinical Oncology. 0-7923-0935-9.
62. B.A. Stoll, ed.: Approaches to Breast Cancer Prevention. 0-7923-0995-2.
63. M.J. Hill and A. Giacosa, eds.: Causation and Prevention of Human Cancer. 0-7923-1084-5.
64. J.R.W. Masters, ed.: Human Cancer in Primary Culture. A Handbook. 0-7923-1088-8.
65. N. Kobayashi, T. Akera and S. Mizutani, eds.: Childhood Leukemia. Present Problems and Future Prospects. 0-7923-1138-8.
66. P. Padetti, K. Takakura, M.D. Walker, G. Butti and S. Pezzota, eds.: Neuro-Oncology. 0-7923-1215-5.

EICOSANOIDS AND OTHER BIOACTIVE LIPIDS IN CANCER AND RADIATION INJURY

Proceedings of the 1st International Conference
October 11–14, 1989
Detroit, Michigan USA

edited by

Kenneth V. Honn
Department of Radiation Oncology
Wayne State University
Detroit, MI USA

Lawrence J. Marnett
Department of Biochemistry
Vanderbilt University
Nashville, TN USA

Santosh Nigam
Department of Gynecological Endocrinology
Klinikum Steglitz, Free University Berlin
Berlin, Germany

Thomas L. Walden, Jr.
Department of Radiation Biochemistry
Armed Forces Radiobiology Research Institute
Bethesda, MD USA

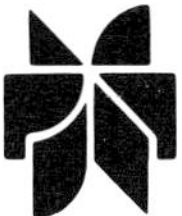

Kluwer Academic Publishers
Boston/Dordrecht/London

Distributors for North America:
Kluwer Academic Publishers
101 Philip Drive
Assinippi Park
Norwell, Massachusetts 02061 USA

Distributors for all other countries:
Kluwer Academic Publishers Group
Distribution Centre
Post Office Box 322
3300 AH Dordrecht, THE NETHERLANDS

Library of Congress Cataloging-in-Publication Data

Eicosanoids and other bioactive lipids in cancer and radiation injury
: proceedings of the 1st international conference, October 11-14,
1989, Detroit, Michigan, USA / edited by Kenneth V. Honn ... [et
al.].
p. cm. — (Developments in oncology ; 67)
"Proceedings of the First International Conference on Eicosanoids
and Other Bioactive Lipids in Cancer and Radiation Injury held in
Detroit, Michigan on October 11-14, 1989"—Pref.
Includes bibliographical references and index.
ISBN 0-7923-1303-8
1. Carcinogenesis—Congresses. 2. Radiation injuries-
-Pathophysiology—Congresses. 3. Eicosanoic acid—Derivatives-
-Physiological effect—Congresses. 4. Lipids—Physiological effect-
-Congresses. 5. Cancer cells—Growth—Regulation—Congresses.
I. Honn, Kenneth V. II. International Conference on Eicosanoids and
Other Bioactive Lipids in Cancer and Radiation Injury (1st : 1989 :
Detroit, Mich.) III. Series.
[DNLM: 1. Eicosanoids—metabolism—congresses. 2. Lipids-
-metabolism—congresses. 3. Neoplasms—chemically induced-
-congresses. 4. Radiation Injuries—congresses. QZ 202 E337 1989]
RC268.5.E32 1991
616.99'4071—dc20
DNLM/DLC
for Library of Congress 91-20794
CIP

Printed on acid-free paper.

Printed in the United States of America

Table of Contents

LIPID PEROXIDATION, EICOSANOID BIOSYNTHESIS, AND RADIATION INDUCED TISSUE INJURY

IMMUNOMODULATION

RECEPTOR MODULATION OF LIPID METABOLISM

EICOSANOID MODULATION OF RECEPTOR EXPRESSION

TUMOR GROWTH INVASION AND DIFFERENTIATION

EFFECTS OF EICOSANOID ANALOGS ON TUMOR GROWTH AND METASTASIS

Preface

This volume contains the proceedings of the First International Conference on Eicosanoids and Other Bioactive Lipids in Cancer and Radiation Injury held in Detroit, Michigan on October 11-14, 1989. The program consisted of 83 oral and 29 poster presentations, 74 of which are included in these proceedings. The major sponsors of the conference were the Armed Forces Radiobiology Research Institute, located in Bethesda, Maryland, the Radiation Oncology Research and Development Center of the Gershenson Radiation Oncology Center, Harper Hospital in Detroit, Michigan, and Schering AG of West Germany. Eighteen other organizations provided additional support.

The conference was unique in its attempt to link the eicosanoid and lipid researchers in the radiobiology and cancer disciplines. The diverse roles that eicosanoids and other bioactive lipids play in these biological phenomena including the participation of lipid oxidation in conversion of procarcinogens, positive and negative modulation of tumor growth, immunomodulation, tissue injury, and yet protection and enhancement of cancer therapy, necessitated scientific interaction to sort out and understand these complex and sometimes contradictory observations. The success of this effort is reflected not only through these proceedings, but also through the decision to continue the conference series with a second meeting to be held in Berlin between September 17-21, 1991.

The proceedings have been divided into 12 sections reflecting the organization of the major symposia at the meeting. These include phospholipid turnover, oxygenases and fatty acid metabolism, radiation and chemical carcinogenesis; lipid peroxidation, eicosanoid biosynthesis, and radiation-induced tissue injury; antioxidant enzyme action; dietary lipid actions, immunomodulation; receptor modulation of lipid metabolism; eicosanoid modulation of receptor expression; tumor growth, invasion, and differentiation; effects of eicosanoid analogs on tumor growth and metastasis; PAF and ether lipids - role in radiation injury and tumor growth; and clinical implications.

The scope of this volume encompasses the complete range of eicosanoid studies in these two fields, beginning with discussions of improved means of detecting eicosanoids using radioimmunoassays, high performance liquid chromatography, and GC-mass spectrometry and including specialized assays of the enzyme systems involved in the metabolism of the bioactive lipids. Studies on the mechanistic basis of bioactive lipids in carcinogenesis and radiation injury have been conducted *in vitro* in biochemical assays and cell culture, culminating in observations *in vivo* including applications in the treatment of cancer patients.

Particular attention has been devoted to addressing the roles and mechanisms of action of bioactive lipids and their analogs in the inhibition of tumor growth. Several of these processes, including changes in immunocompetence, membrane-targeted biochemical effects, release of cathepsin B and cysteine protease inhibitors, modulation of intracellular communication, and alteration of growth regulation are discussed in detail. Further studies expand on the observations that modification of dietary lipids affects carcinogenic expression with related changes in eicosanoid synthesis and in protein kinase C distribution.

The eicosanoids are one of three major groups of radioprotective agents, including the thiols and the biological/immunomodulators, that are currently receiving world-wide attention. The present volume contains the most comprehensive evaluations of the roles of eicosanoids in radiation injury and in protection from radiation injury. This conference and the proceedings have extended the understandings of the eicosanoids with respect to possible receptor mediated mechanisms versus systemic contributions. If prostaglandins are mediators of radiation injury, then blocking their synthesis should induce radiosensitivity. Yet another paradox is presented in one of the chapters illustrating that treatment with indomethacin may radiosensitize some tumors while protecting hemopoietic tissue and lung. Included with this section is the first summary of the behavioral effects of the radioprotective eicosanoids.

The most important end goal of any biomedical research is to provide a basis for scientific understanding of pathological processes through which to prevent disease and improve medical treatment. The last section in this volume describes those investigations with implications for radiotherapy and chemotherapy. These sections provide the latest information on the use of nonsteroidal antiinflammatory agents in the treatment of patients with advanced lung and colon cancer, as well as the diagnostic and prognostic indications of prostacyclin and thromboxane metabolites in the body fluids of breast cancer patients. It has been observed that patients with chronic myelogenous leukemia have decreased leukotriene C_4 activities which may affect the pathogenesis of the disease. Perhaps this was the final, rewarding aspect of the conference, to see the clinical implications that are evolving as a result of the improved understanding.

While our overall understanding of the processes involved have increased, many perplexing observations and unanswered questions remain. Among these are unraveling the paradox surrounding the protective and yet damaging and carcinogenic responses of the eicosanoids. This mystery has been further complicated by the increasing numbers of biological metabolites which are formed, many of which have opposing activities. In addition, some biological properties are elicited by combinations of eicosanoids that cannot be elicited by either of the agents individually. As if this was not difficult enough for the cyclooxygenase and lipoxygenase pathways, we must now integrate and reformulate our thoughts to include the new roles being identified for the hydroxy fatty acids and lipoxins, and for eicosanoid metabolites through the cytochrome P_{450} pathway. One must take into account receptor activity, specificity, agonists, antagonists, up-regulation and down-regulation, not to mention cross-reactivity. Once these factors are considered, the next step is to determine which biological processes are mediated by direct receptor interaction on the cell membrane, those mediated by cell-cell communication, and to what degree to systemic events modulate bioactive lipid activity. How well do those observations made in controlled *in vitro* situations translate to the *in vivo* situation. Finally, it is necessary to reduce this to simple concepts that can be used to maximize therapeutic potential.

On a cautionary note, there is little information available on the long term consequences of bioactive lipid modulation or treatments in radiation injury and cancer. Although the immediate goal is to protect the tissue from radiation injury or to inhibit the tumor, we must have the information available to treat the secondary effects. We already know that eicosanoids have paradoxical roles: stimulation/inhibition, injury/protection. Most of the investigations to date on the roles of eicosanoids in radiation injury or in cell treatments have only examined the first hours or days. We need to examine the long term effects. We need to understand how to maximize receptor interactions and sustain the beneficial second and third messenger systems. Mutation of the *ras* oncogene produces a G-protein in the "on" position. What are the consequences of mutations in enzymes responsible for eicosanoid synthesis? Why do some tumors have elevations in eicosanoid production while others, such as the chronic myelogenous leukemia reported in this volume are lacking? What are the roles for other bioactive lipids? Justifiably, additional conferences like the one in Detroit, and the one in Berlin are needed to focus attention on these issues.

The editors would like to thank all of those who participated in the first conference, and to the authors for their contributions. We gratefully acknowledge the support and assistance of Monika R. Cleveland and Brigette G. Neal for their untiring efforts in producing this volume. On behalf of the participants, we extend deepest appreciation for those organizations whose financial support made the conference and these proceedings possible. We look forward to the participation of our contributors and readers in the future conferences.

Kenneth V. Honn
Lawrence J. Marnett
Santosh Nigam
Thomas L. Walden, Jr.

Acknowledgements

The Organizing Committee along with the participants of this Symposium gratefully acknowledge the primary support provided by the following organizations:

Armed Forces RadiobiologyResearch Institute
Radiation Oncology Research & Development Center
Schering AG West Germany

Additional support was provided by the following organizations:

Advanced Magnetics, Inc.
Bayer AG
BIOMOL
Berlex, Inc.
Cayman Chemical Company, Inc.
Daiichi Seiyaku Co., Ltd.
Harper/Grace Hospitals
Institut Henri Beaufour
Merck Frosst Canada, Inc.
Meyer L. Prentis Comprehensive Cancer Center of Metropolitan Detroit
Michigan Cancer Foundation
Miles, Inc.
Oxford Biomedical Inc.
Ono Pharmaceutical Co., Ltd.
E. R. Squibb & Sons, Inc.
Stuart Pharmaceuticals
The Upjohn Company
Wayne State University

The Organizing Committee wishes to thank the International Advisory Committee for their help in planning this conference.

<u>International Advisory Committee</u>

Contributors

Abou-El-Ela, S.H.
University of Georgia
College of Pharmacy
Dept. of Pharmacology and Toxicology
Athens, GA 30602 USA

Adler, S.H.
Laboratory of Developmental Biology
and Anomalies
NIDR
NIH
Bethesda, MD 20892 USA

Agnelli, G.
Istituto di Semeiotica Medica ed
Universita' di Perugia
06100 Perugia, Italy

Allegrucci, M.
Istituto di Farmacologia
Universita' di Perugia
06100 Perugia, Italy

Alley, M.C.
Program Development Research Grp.
Division of Cancer Treatment
National Cancer Institute
Bldg. 560, Room 32-60
Frederick, MD 21701-1013 USA

Baker, Margaret A.
University of Pennsylvania
195 John Morgan Blvd.
Philadelphia, PA
19104-6072 USA

Barletta, E.
Institute of General Pathology
School of Medicine
University of Florence
1-50134 Florence
Italy

Barrett, J.C.
NIEHS
Laboratory of Molecular Carcinogenesis
P.O. Box 12233 (MD 14-03)
Research Triangle Park, NC
27709 USA

Bastida, E.
Hospital Clinico
Universidad de Barcelona
Barcelona, Spain

Basu, Amaresh
Dept. of Biochemistry and
Molecular Biology
UMDNJ - New Jersey Medical School
Newark, NJ 07103-2757 USA

Becker, David
Department of Chemistry
Oakland University
Rochester, MI 48309 USA

Benedetto, Chiara
Universita Di Torino
Department of Gynecology
Via Ventimiglia 3
10126 Torino
Italy

Bennett, Alan
Dept. Surgery
King's College School of Medicine
and Dentistry
123 Coldharbour Lane
London SE5 9NU England

Bennett, Leslie R.
University of California Los Angeles
Center for Health Sciences
Division of Nuclear Medicine
Los Angeles, CA 90024 USA

Berk, Laurence
Dept. of Radiation Oncology
University of Pennsylvania
3508 Market St.
Philadelphia, PA 19104 USA

Bertomeu, Maria C.
McMaster University
Dept. of Pathology 3N10
1200 Main St. West
Hamilton, Ontario L8N 3Z5
Canada

Bienkowski, Michael J.
Upjohn Company
Cell Biology Department
Kalamazoo, MI 49008 USA

Blank, Merle L.
Medical Sciences Div.
Oak Ridge Assoc. Universities
P.O. Box 117
Oak Ridge, TN 37830-0117 USA

Boaziz, Catherine
Oncology Unit
Centre Hospitalier Universitaire Avicenne
125, route de Stalingrad
9300 Bobigny France

Boggs, S.
Department of Radiation Oncology
University of Pittsburgh School
of Medicine
University of Pittsburgh
Pittsburgh, PA 25216 USA

Borek, Carmia
Div. of Radiation Oncology/Cancer Biology
New England Med. Ctr./Tuffs University
Box 824
750 Washington Street
Boston, MA 02111 USA

Boyd, M.R.
Program Development Research Grp.
Division of Cancer Treatment
National Cancer Institute
Bldg. 560, Room 32-60
Frederick, MD 21701-1013 USA

Bradlow, H. Leon
Institute for Hormone Research
55 E. 34th Street
New York, NY 10016 USA

Braquet, Pierre
Institut Henri Beaufour
Research Labs.
17, Avenue Descartes
92350 Le Plessis-Robinson
France

Breau, Jean-Luc
Oncology Unit
Centre Hospitalier Universitaire Avicenne
125, route de Stalingrad
9300 Bobigny
France

Buchanan, Michael R.
McMaster University
Department of Pathology 3N10
1200 Main St. West
Hamilton, Ontario L8N3Z5
Canada

Bull, Arthur W.
Oakland University
Dept. of Chemistry
Rochester, MI 48309 USA

Bunce, Opal R.
University of Georgia
College of Pharmacy
Dept. of Pharmacology and Toxicology
Athens, GA 30602 USA

Burghardt, Robert C.
Dept. Vet. Anat.
College of Vet. Med.
Texas A&M University
College Station, TX 77843 USA

Calorini, L.
Institute of General Pathology
School of Medicine
University of Florence
1-50134 Florence
Italy

Cameron, G.S.
University of Texas
Cancer Center
Science Park
P.O. Box 389
Smithville, TX 78957 USA

Cashman, John R.
Dept. of Pharmaceutical Chemistry
University of California
P.O. Box 0446
San Francisco, CA 94143-0446 USA

Casini, Alessandro F.
v. Laterino 8
Istituto Patologia Generale
Universita di Siena
53100 Siena
Italy

Cathapermal, Sam
Georgetown University Medical Center
Department of Physiology and Biophysics
Reservoir Road, N.W.
Washington, D.C. 20007 USA

Cecconi, O.
Institute of General Pathology
School of Medicine
University of Florence
1-50134 Florence
Italy

Chan, P.M.
Depts. of Pharmaceutical Chem.
Neurology, Pathology, Rad. Onc.
University of California
P.O. Box 0446
San Francisco, CA 94143-0446 USA

Chang, C.C.
Dept. Pediatrics/Human Devel.
Michigan State University
East Lansing, MI 48824 USA

Chang, Young Sook
Center for Molecular Biology
Wayne State University
2309 Scott Hall
Detroit, MI 48202 USA

Chen, Yong Q.
Department of Radiation Oncology
Wayne State University
431 Chemistry Building
Detroit, MI 48202 USA

Chopra, Hemi
Dept. of Biological Chemistry
503 Woods Basic Science Bldg.
The John Hopkins University
725 N. Wolfe Street
Baltimore, MD 21205 USA

Chung, M.-H.
Biology Division
National Cancer Ctr. Research Inst.
Tsukiji 5-1-1, Chuo-ku
Tokyo, Japan

Claesson, Hans-Erik
Departments of Toxicology and
Physiological Chemistry
Karolinska Institut
Stockholm, Sweden S104-01

Cochrane, C.G.
IMM 12
Scripps Clin. & Research Fdn.
10666 N. Torrey Pines Road
LaJolla, CA 92037 USA

Comporti, M.
v. Laterino 8
Istituto Patologia Generale
Universita di Siena
53100 Siena
Italy

Costantini, Vincenzo
Istituto di Semeiotica Medica ed
Universita' di Perugia
06100 Perugia, Italy

Cunard, C.M.
Wayne State University
School of Medicine
Elliman Building Room 2222
421 East Canfield
Detroit, MI 48201 USA

Datta, Rakesh
Laboratory of Clinical Pharmacology
Dana-Farber Cancer Institute
and Department of Medicine
Harvard Medical School
44 Binney St.
Boston, MA 02115 USA

Davis, Hirsch D.
Department of Behavioral Sciences
AFRRI
Bethesda, MD 20814-5145 USA

Davis, Richard L.
Dept. of Pathology
University of California
School of Medicine
501 HSW
San Francisco, CA 94143-0506 USA

Del Bello, B.
v. Laterino 8
Istituto Patologia Generale
Universita di Siena
53100 Siena
Italy

Diglio, Clement A.
Wayne State University
Department of Pathology
8112 Scott Hall
Detroit, MI 48202 USA

Doupnick, Craig A.
Departments of Toxicology and
Physiological Chemistry
Karolinska Institut
Stockholm, Sweden S104-01

Drab, E.A.
Rush-Presb. St. Luke's
Medical Center
Depts. of Medicine and Therapeautic
Radiology
1653 W. Congress Parkway
Chicago, IL 60612 USA

Dray, F.
Unite de Radioimmunologie Analytique
Institut Pasteur
75724 Paris, France

Duniec, Zofia M.
Wayne State University
Dept. of Radiation Oncology
431 Chemistry Building
Detroit, MI 48202 USA

Edenius, Charlotte
Dept. of Physiological Chemistry
Karolinska Institutet
Box 60400
S-104 01 Stockholm
Sweden

Elford, Howard
Molecules for Health Inc.
Cancer Drug Research Development
3313 Gloucester Road
Richmond, VA 23227 USA

Eling, Thomas
NIEHS
Laboratory of Molecular Biophysics
P.O. Box 12233
Research Triangle Park, NC 27709 USA

Elkousy, Hussein A.
University of Cincinnati
Medical Center
Division of Molecular Toxicology
Dept. of Environmental Health
231 Bethesda Ave.
ML-182
Cincinnati, OH 45267 USA

Fain, John N.
Dept. of Biochemistry
University of Tennessee
Center for the Health Sciences
800 Madison Ave.
Memphis, TN 38163 USA

Fallani, A.
Institute of General Pathology
School of Medicine
University of Florence
1-50134 Florence
Italy

Farkas, Walter R.
Dept. of Environmental Practive
College of Veterinary Med.
University of Tennessee
P.O. Box 1074
Knoxville, TN 37901-1074 USA

Farzaneh, Nushin K.
Radiation Biochemistry Dept.
Bldg. 42
Armed Forces Radiobiology Res. Inst.
Navy Medical Center
Bethesda, MD 20814-5415 USA

Favalli, Cartesio
Dip.Med. Sper. Sc. Bioch.
II Universita di Roma
Via O. Raimondo, 00173 Roma Italy

Fiore, Stefano
Hematology Division
Department of Medicine
Brigham & Women's Hospital
Harvard Medical School
75 Francis St.
Boston, MA 02115 USA

Fioretti, M.C.
Istituto di Farmacologia
Universita' di Perugia
06100 Perugia, Italy

Fischer, Susan M.
University of Texas
Cancer Center
Science Park
P.O. Box 389
Smithville, TX 78957 USA

Fitz, Tony A.
Dept. of OB/GYN
Uniformed Services University of
the Health Sciences
4301 Jones Bridge Rd.
Bethesda, MD 20814 USA

Flem, Kimberly A.
University of Cincinnati
Medical Center
Division of Molecular Toxicology
Dept. of Environmental Health
231 Bethesda Ave.
ML-182
Cincinnati, OH 45267 USA

Fletcher, Clayton
Bowman Gray School of Medicine
of Wake Forest University
Departs. of Radiology and Biochemistry
300 S. Hawthorne
Winston-Salem, NC 27103 USA

Foegh, Marie L.
Georgetown University Medical Center
Department of Surgery
Reservoir Road, N.W.
Washington, D.C. 20007 USA

Fridman, Rafael
NIDR, NIH
Laboratory of Developmental Biol. and
Anomalies
Bldg. 30, Rm. 630
Bethesda, MD 20892 USA

Fujiwara, Keiichi
Bowman Gray School of Medicine
of Wake Forest University
Departs. of Radiology and Biochemistry
300 S. Hawthorne
Winston-Salem, NC 27103 USA

Fukushima, M.
Department of Internal Medicine
Aichi Cancer Center
Chikusa-ku, Nagoya 464
Japan

Fuschiotti, P.
Istituto di Farmacologia
Universita' di Perugia
06100 Perugia, Italy

Gallo, S.
McMaster University
Department of Pathology 3N10
1200 Main St. West
Hamilton, Ontario L8N3Z5
Canada

Garaci, E.
Department of Experimental Medicine
and Biochemical Sciences
II University of Rome
Via O. Raimondo 00173 Italy

Gerozissis, K.
Unite de Radioimmunologie Analytique
Institut Pasteur
75724 Paris, France

Giampietri, A.
Istituto di Farmacologia
Universita' di Perugia
06100 Perugia, Italy

Gillich, Stephen
Department of Chemistry
Oakland University
Rochester, MI 48309 USA

Giraldi, Tullio
Institute of Pharmacology
University of Trieste
I-34100 Trieste
Italy

Glasgow, Wayne C.
NIEHS
Laboratory of Molecular Biophysics
P.O. Box 12233 (MD 14-03)
Research Triangle Park, NC
27709 USA

Gomez, Angel P.
Wayne State University
Dept. of Pharmacology
School of Medicine
6269 Scott Hall
Detroit, MI 48202 USA

Gonzalez, Frank J.
Laboratory of Molecular Carcinogenesis
National Cancer Institute
NIH
Bethesda, MD 20892 USA

Gorman, Robert R.
Upjohn Company
Cell Biology Department
Kalamazoo, MI 49008 USA

Grafstrom, Roland G.
Departments of Toxicology and
Physiological Chemistry
Karolinska Institut
Stockholm, Sweden S104-01

Grelli, S.
1st. Med. Sper. CNR
Rome, Italy

Grossi, Irma
Wayne State University
Radiation Oncology
431 Chemistry Bldg.
5101 Cass Ave.
Detroit, MI 48202 USA

Gudat, F.
Institute of Pathology
University of Basel
Switzerland

Gutin, Philip H.
Depts. of Neurosurgery and Rad. Onc.
M786
University of California, San Francisco
San Francisco, CA 94143 USA

Haakenson, C.M.
Veterans Administration Medical School
White River Jct., Vermont 05001 USA

Hajdu, J.
California State University
Northridge
Northridge, CA 91330 USA

Hajibeigi, A.
Department of Biology
Texas Woman's University
P.O. Box 23971
Denton, TX 75068 USA

Hamilton, Tom
Med. Oncology
Fox Chase Cancer Center
Philadelphia, PA 19111 USA

Hannun, Yusuf A.
Duke University
Depts. of Medicine and Cell Biology
Jones Blvd. Research Drive
Durham, NC 27710 USA

Hanson, Wayne R.
Loyola-Hines Department
of Radiotherapy 114B
Bldg. 1, Rm. F340
Hines VA Medical Center
5th. Ave. & Roosevelt Rd.
Hines, IL 60141 USA

Hardwick, James P.
Argonne Natl. Lab
Biological and Medical Div.
9700 S. Cass Ave.
BEM 202, R. 233b
Argonne, IL 60439 USA

Hardcastle, J.E.
Department of Chemistry
Texas Woman's University
P.O. Box 23971
Denton, TX 75068 USA

Hasler, C.
Dept. Pediatrics/Human Devel.
Michigan State University
East Lansing, MI 48824 USA

Henson, Peter M.
National Jewish Ctr. for Immunology
and Respiratory Medicine
4200 E. 9th. Ave.
Denver, CO 80206 USA

Hiroshima, A.
Dept. of Biochemistry
Tokushima University
School of Medicine
Kuramoto-cho
Tokushima 770, Japan

Holian, Oksana
University of Illinois
College of Medicine
Department of Surgery
Box 6998
Chicago, IL 60680 USA

Holliday, Scott A.
University of Cincinnati
Medical Center
Division of Molecular Toxicology
Dept. of Environmental Health
231 Bethesda Ave.
ML-182
Cincinnati, OH 45267 USA

Honn, Kenneth V.
Wayne State University
Radiation Oncology
431 Chemistry Building
5101 Cass Ave.
Detroit, MI 48202 USA

Hooper, Nigel I.
University of California
School of Public Health
230 Warren Hall
Berkeley, CA 94720 USA

Hosford, David
Institut Henri Beaufour
Research Labs.
AZ de Courtaboeuf 1
ave des Tropiques
91952 Les Ulis Cedex
France

Hubbard, Walter C.
Division of Clinical Immunology
The Good Samaritan Hospital-3N
5601 Loch Raven Blvd.
Baltimore, MD 21239 USA

Huberman, Elizer
Argonne Natl. Lab
Biological and Medical Div.
9700 S. Cass Ave.
BEM 202, R. 233b
Argonne, IL 60439 USA

Hunt, W.A.
Behavioral Sciences Dept.
Armed Forces Radio. Biol.
Research Institute
Bethesda, MD 20814-5145 USA

Hupp, E.W.
Department of Biology
Texas Woman's University
P.O. Box 23971
Denton, TX 75068 USA

Hutson, C.A.
University of California, Los Angeles
Laboratory of Biomedical and
Environmental Sciences
900 Veteran Avenue
Los Angeles, California 90024 USA

Ii, K.
Dept. of Pathology
Tokushima University
School of Medicine
Kuramoto-cho
Tokushima 770, Japan

Inoue, H.
Faculty of Pharmaceutical Sciences
Hokkaido University
Sapporo 060, Japan

Ip, Clement
Roswell Park Memorial Institute
666 Elm St.
Buffalo, NY 14263 USA

Ip, Margot M.
Roswell Park Memorial Institute
666 Elm St.
Buffalo, NY 14263 USA

Ishikawa, H.
Faculty of Pharmaceutical Sciences
Hokkaido University
Sapporo 060, Japan

Ishiwata, I.
Department of Obstetrics and
Gynecology
Teikyo University
School of Medicine
Ishiwata Hospital
Ichihara-city, Chiba 299-01
Japan

Israel, Lucien
Oncology Unit
Centre Hospitalier Universitaire Avicenne
125, route de Stalingrad, 9300 Bobigny
France

Iwamoto, Keisuke S.
University of California, Los Angeles
Laboratory of Biomedical and
Environmental Sciences
900 Veteran Avenue
Los Angeles, California 90024 USA

Jackson, J.H.
Scripps Clin. & Research Fdn.
10666 N. Torrey Pines Road IMM 12
LaJolla, CA 92037 USA

Jamieson, Gordon A.
University of Cincinnati
Medical Center
Division of Molecular Toxicology
Dept. of Environmental Health
231 Bethesda Ave.
ML-182
Cincinnati, OH 45267 USA

Jones, D.S.
Biology Division
National Cancer Ctr. Research Inst.
Tsukiji 5-1-1, Chuo-ku
Tokyo, Japan

Kaibara, Manabu
Department of Obstetrics and
Gynecology
Teikyo University
School of Medicine
Ichihara Hospital
3426-3 Anesaki
Ichihara-city, Chiba 299-01
Japan

Kamiya, H.
Faculty of Pharmaceutical Sciences
Hokkaido University
Sapporo 060, Japan

Kandasamy S. B.
Behavioral Sciences Dept.
Armed Forces Radio. Biol.
Research Institute
Bethesda, MD 20814-5145 USA

Kanemoto, Tomoko
NIDR, NIH
Laboratory of Developmental Biol. and
Anomalies
Bldg. 30, Rm. 630
Bethesda, MD 20892 USA

Kasai, H.
Biology Division
National Cancer Ctr. Research Inst.
Tsukiji 5-1-1, Chuo-ku
Tokyo, Japan

Kennedy, Ann R.
University of Pennsylvania
Dept. of Radiation Oncology
3508 Market Street
Philadelphia, PA 19104-3357 USA

Kimura, Shioko
Laboratory of Molecular Carcinogenesis
National Cancer Institute, NIH
Bethesda, MD 20892 USA

Komatsu, N.
Dept. of Pathology
Tokai University
School of Medicine
Isehara 259-11, Japan

Kot, Peter A.
Dept. Physiol. and Biophys.
Georgetown University
School of Medicine
3900 Reservoir Road, N.W.
Washington D.C. 20007 USA

Kufe, Donald W.
Laboratory of Clinical Pharmacology
Dana-Farber Cancer Institute
and Department of Medicine
Harvard Medical School
44 Binney St.
Boston, MA 02115 USA

Kulmacz, Richard
Dept. of Biochem., M/C 536
Univ. of Illinois at Chicago
1853 W. Polk St.
Chicago, IL 60612 USA

Kuo, J.F.
Emory University
School of Medicine
Department of Pharmacology
Division of Hematology Oncology
PO Box AE
Atlanta, GA 30322 USA

Lafrenie, R.
McMaster University
Department of Pathology 3N10
1200 Main St. West
Hamilton, Ontario L8N3Z5 Canada

Landauer, Micahel R.
Department of Behavioral Sciences
AFRRI
Bethesda, MD 20814-5145 USA

Lands, William
University of Illinois at Chicago
1853 W. Polk, Rm A312
Chicago, IL 60612 USA

Laudicina, Donald
A.B. Hancock, Jr. Memorial Laboratory
for Cancer Research
Depts. of Biochemistry and Chemistry
Center in Molecular Toxicology
Vanderbilt University
School of Medicine, 854 MRB
Nashville, TN 37232 USA

Leikauf, George D.
University of Cincinnati
Medical Center
Division of Molecular Toxicology
Dept. of Environmental Health
231 Bethesda Ave.
ML-182
Cincinnati, OH 45267 USA

Levin, Kenneth J.
Department of Radiation Oncology, L-75
University of California, San Francisco
San Francisco, CA 94143 USA

Levine, Lawrence
Dept. of Biochemistry,
Brandeis University
Waltham, MA 02254 USA

Leyton, J.
University of Texas
Cancer Center, Science Park
P.O. Box 389
Smithville, TX 78957 USA

Lin, Alice H.
Upjohn Company
Cell Biology Department
Kalamazoo, MI 49008 USA

Lindgren, Jan Åke
Dept. of Physiological Chemistry
Karolinska Institutet
Box 60400
S-104 01 Stockholm
Sweden

Lubbert, Horst
Eicosanoid Research
Dept. of Gynecological Endocrinology
FU Berlin, Klinikum Steglitz
Hindenburgdamm 30
D-1000 Berlin 45, FRG

Maclouf, J.
INSERM Unite 150
UA 334 CNRS
Hopital Lariboisiere
75475 Paris
Cedex 10, France

Madhukar, B.V.
Dept. Pediatrics/Human Devel.
Michigan State University
East Lansing, MI 48824 USA

Maellaro, E.
v. Laterino 8
Istituto Patologia Generale
Universita di Siena
53100 Siena
Italy

Mannori, G.
Institute of General Pathology
School of Medicine
University of Florence
1-50134 Florence
Italy

Marr, M.M.
Dept. of OB/GYN
Uniformed Services University of
the Health Sciences
4301 Jones Bridge Rd.
Bethesda, MD 20814 USA

Martin, George R.
Gerontology Research Center
NIA, NIH
Baltimore, MD 21224 USA

Maruyama, T.
Dept. of Biochemistry
Tokushima University
School of Medicine
Kuramoto-cho
Tokushima 770, Japan

Marnett, Lawrence
A.B. Hancock, Jr. Memorial Laboratory
for Cancer Research
Depts. of Biochemistry and Chemistry
Center in Molecular Toxicology
Vanderbilt University
School of Medicine
854 MRB
Nashville, TN 37232 USA

Martin, G.R.
Gerontology Research Center
NIA, NIH
Baltimore, MD 21224 USA

Mastino, A.
Department of Experimental Medicine
and Biochemical Sciences
II University of Rome
Via O. Raimondo 00173 Italy

McBride, William H.
Dept. Radiation Oncology
UCLA Medical Center
10833 LeConte Avenue
Los Angeles, CA 90024-1714 USA

McDermott, M.W.
Depts. of Neurosurgery and Rad. Onc.
M786
University of California, San Francisco
San Francisco, CA 94143 USA

McLemore, T.L.
Program Development Research Grp.
Division of Cancer Treatment
National Cancer Institute
Bldg. 560, Room 32-60
Frederick, MD 21701-1013 USA

Melhuish, P.B.
Dept. Surgery
King's College School of Medicine
and Dentistry
123 Coldharbour Lane
London SE5 9NU
England

Mencia-Huerta, Jean-Michel
Institut Henri Beaufour
Research Labs.
AZ de Courtaboeuf 1
ave des Tropiques
91952 Les Ulis Cedex
France

Mihatsch, M.J.
Institute of Pathology
University of Basel
Switzerland

Milas, Luka
M.D. Anderson Cancer Center
Dept. of Experimental Radiotherapy
1515 Holcombe Blvd.
Houston, TX 77030 USA

Modak, Mukund J.
Dept. of Biochemistry and
Molecular Biology
UMDNJ - New Jersey Medical School
Newark, NJ 07103-2757 USA

Modest, Edward J.
Bowman Gray School of Medicine
of Wake Forest University
Departs. of Radiology and Biochemistry
300 S. Hawthorne
Winston-Salem, NC 27103 USA

Morere, Jean-Francois
Oncology Unit
Centre Hospitalier Universitaire Avicenne
125, route de Stalingrad
9300 Bobigny
France

Moritz, T.E.
Veterans Administration Medical School
White River Jct., Vermont 05001 USA

Morris, R.J.
University of Texas
Cancer Center
Science Park
P.O. Box 389
Smithville, TX 78957 USA

Mueller, Richard A.
Molecular and Cellular Biology Department
G.D. Searle Co.
Skokie, IL 60077 USA

Mugnai, G.
Institute of General Pathology
School of Medicine
University of Florence
1-50134 Florence
Italy

Murphy, Robert C.
National Jewish Ctr. for Immunology
and Respiratory Medicine
4200 E. 9th. Ave.
Denver, CO 80206 USA

Narumiya, Shuh
Dept. of Pharmacology
Kyoto University Faculty of Medicine
Yoshida, Sakyo-ku
Kyoto 606
Japan

Natsui, K.
Dept. of Biochemistry
Tokushima University
School of Medicine
Kuramoto-cho
Tokushima 770, Japan

Nelson, Richard L.
University of Illinois
College of Medicine
Department of Surgery
Box 6998
Chicago, IL 60680 USA

Nenci, G.G.
Istituto di Semeiotica Medica ed
Universita' di Perugia
06100 Perugia, Italy

Nettesheim, P.
LMB & LPP
National Institute of Environmental
Health Sciences
Research Triangle Park, NC 27709 USA

Nigam, Santosh
Eicosanoid Research
Dept. of Gynecological Endocrinology
FU Berlin, Klinikum Steglitz
Hindenburgdamm 30
D-1000 Berlin 45, FRG

Nishimura Susumu
Biology Division
National Cancer Ctr. Res. Inst.
Tsukiji, 5-1-1, Chuo-ku
Tokyo 104, Japan

Norman, A.
Deps. of Radiological Sciences and
Radiation Oncology and Jonsson
Comprehensive Cancer Ctr.
University of CA, Los Angeles
Animal Cancer Ctr.
Hermosa Beach, CA USA

Nüsing, R.
Fakultat fur Biologie
Universitat Kronstanz
775 Kronstanz, West Germany

Ogino, Mitsuhara
Department of Obstetrics and
Gynecology
Teikyo University
School of Medicine
Ichihara Hospital
3426-3 Anesaki
Ichihara-city, Chiba 299-01
Japan

Ohtsuka, E.
Faculty of Pharmaceutical Sciences
Hokkaido University
Sapporo 060, Japan

Okinaga, Shoichi
Department of Obstetrics and
Gynecology
Teikyo University
School of Medicine
Ichihara Hospital
3426-3 Anesaki
Ichihara-city, Chiba 299-01
Japan

Olson, A.C.
Emory University
School of Medicine
Department of Medicine
Division of Hematology Oncology
PO Box AE
Atlanta, GA 30322 USA

Onoda, James M.
Wayne State University
Radiation Oncology
431 Chemistry Building
5101 Cass Ave.
Detroit, MI 48202 USA

Orr, F.W.
McMaster University
Department of Pathology 3N10
1200 Main St. West
Hamilton, Ontario L8N3Z5
Canada

Osborne, Michael P.
Breast Cancer Research Laboratory
Dept. of Surgery
Memorial Sloan-Kettering Cancer Ctr.
1275 York Ave.
New York, NY 10021 USA

Partis, Richard A.
Molecular and Cellular Biology Department
G.D. Searle Co.
Skokie, IL 60077 USA

Patrene, K.
Department of Radiation Oncology
University of Pittsburgh School
of Medicine
University of Pittsburgh
Pittsburgh, PA 25216 USA

Patrick, K.E.
University of Texas
Cancer Center
Science Park
P.O. Box 389
Smithville, TX 78957 USA

Pendleton, Robert B.
University of Illinois at Chicago
1853 W. Polk, Rm A312
Chicago, IL 60612 USA

Peraino, Carl
Argonne Natl. Lab
Biological and Medical Div.
9700 S. Cass Ave.
BEM 202, R. 233b
Argonne, IL 60439 USA

Perissin, L.
Institute of Pharmacology
University of Trieste
I-34100 Trieste
Italy

Phillips, Theodore L.
Dept. of Radiation Oncology
University of California
Medical Center
Room L-75, Box 0226
San Francisco, CA 94143 USA

Piechocki, Marie P.
Wayne State University
Radiation Oncology
431 Chemistry Building
5101 Cass Ave.
Detroit, MI 48202 USA

Pirotzky, Eduardo
Institut Henri Beaufour
Research Labs.
AZ de Courtaboeuf 1
ave des Tropiques
91952 Les Ulis Cedex
France

Quehenberger, O
IMM 12
Scripps Clin. & Research Fdn.
10666 N. Torrey Pines Road
LaJolla, CA 92037 USA

Ramwell, Peter W.
Dept. Physiol and Biophys
Georgetown University
Medical Center
Reservoir Rd. N.W.
Washington, DC 20007 USA

Rapozzi, V.
Institute of Pharmacology
University of Trieste
I-34100 Trieste
Italy

Reddy, Janardan K.
Dept. of Pathology
Northwestern University
Medical School
303 E. Chicago Avenue
Chicago, IL 60611 USA

Reich, Reuven
The Hebrew University of Jerusalem
Dept. of Pharmacology
The Adolph Weinberger Bldg.
P.O.B. 12065
Jerusalem, 91120
Israel

Ross, B.A.
Depts. of Neurosurgery/Rad. Onc. M786
University of California, San Francisco
San Francisco, CA 94143 USA

Royce, L.
Laboratory of Developmental Biology
and Anomalies
NIDR
NIH
Bethesda, MD 20892 USA

Rozhin, Jurij
Wayne State University
Dept. of Pharmacology
School of Medicine
6269 Scott Hall
Detroit, MI 48202 USA

Rubin, David
Rush-Presb. St. Luke's
Medical Center
Depts. of Medicine and Therapeautic
Radiology
1653 W. Congress Parkway
Chicago, IL 60612 USA

Ruggieri, Salvatore
Inst. General Pathology
School of Medicine
University of Florence
50 50134 Firenze
Italy

Russell, John J.
Argonne Natl. Lab
Biological and Medical Div.
9700 S. Cass Ave.
BEM 202, R. 233b
Argonne, IL 60439 USA

Samokyszyn, Victor
A.B. Hancock, Jr. Memorial Laboratory
for Cancer Research
Depts. of Biochemistry and Chemistry
Center in Molecular Toxicology
Vanderbilt University
School of Medicine
854 MRB
Nashville, TN 37232 USA

Schneidkraut, M.J.
Wayne State University
School of Medicine
Elliman Building Room 2222
421 East Canfield
Detroit, MI 48201 USA

Schraufstatter, Ingrid
IMM 12
Scripps Clin. & Research Fdn.
10666 N. Torrey Pines Road
LaJolla, CA 92037 USA

Serhan, Charles N.
Hematology Division
Department of Medicine
Brigham & Women's Hospital
Harvard Medical School
75 Francis St.
Boston, MA 02115 USA

Sevilla, Michael D.
Department of Chemistry
Oakland University
Rochester, MI 48309 USA

Shaughnessy, S.G.
McMaster University
Department of Pathology 3N10
1200 Main St. West
Hamilton, Ontario L8N3Z5
Canada

Sheppard, Kelly-Ann
Hematology Division
Department of Medicine
Brigham & Women's Hospital
Harvard Medical School
75 Francis St.
Boston, MA 02115 USA

Sherman, Matthew L.
Laboratory of Clinical Pharmacology
Dana-Farber Cancer Institute
and Department of Medicine
Harvard Medical School
44 Binney St.
Boston, MA 02115 USA

Shinjo, F.
Dept. of Biochemistry
Tokushima University
School of Medicine
Kuramoto-cho
Tokushima 770, Japan

Shoji, M.
Emory University
School of Medicine
Department of Medicine
Division of Hematology Oncology
PO Box AE
Atlanta, GA 30322 USA

Sloane, Bonnie F.
Wayne State University
Dept. of Pharmacology
School of Medicine
6269 Scott Hall
Detroit, MI 48202 USA

Smith, Martyn T.
University of California
School of Public Health
318 Warren Hall
Berkeley, CA 94720 USA

Smith, Zigrida L.
Medical Sciences Div.
Oak Ridge Assoc. Universities
P.O. Box 117
Oak Ridge, TN 37830-0117 USA

Snyder, Fred
Medical Sciences Div.
Oak Ridge Assoc. Universities
P.O. Box 117
Oak Ridge, TN 37830-0117 USA

Speicher, James M.
Radiation Biochemistry Dept.
Bldg. 42
Armed Forces Radiobiology Res. Inst.
Navy Medical Center
Bethesda, MD 20814-5415 USA

Stamford, I.F.
Dept. Surgery
King's College School of Medicine
and Dentistry
123 Coldharbour Lane
London SE5 9NU
England

Stenke, Leif
Dept. of Physiological Chemistry
Division of Hematology
Karolinska Institutet
Box 60400
S-104 01 Stockholm, Sweden

Stincarelli, G.
Istituto di Farmacologia
Universita' di Perugia
06100 Perugia, Italy

Suzuki, H.
Dept. of Biochemistry
Tokushima University
School of Medicine
Kuramoto-cho
Tokushima 770, Japan

Szabo, Laszio
Dept. of Environmental Practive
College of Veterinary Med.
University of Tennessee
P.O. Box 1074
Knoxville, TN 37901-1074 USA

Takahashi, Y.
Dept. of Biochemistry
Tokushima University
School of Medicine
Kuramoto-cho
Tokushima 770, Japan

Takai, T.
Dept. of Pharmacology
National Cardiovascular Center
Research Institute
Suita, Osaka 565, Japan

Tanabe, T.
Dept. of Pharmacology
National Cardiovascular Center
Research Institute
Suita, Osaka 565, Japan

Taylor, John D.
Department of Biological Sciences
Wayne State University
455 Life Sciences Building
Detroit, MI 48202 USA

Telang, Nitin T.
Breast Cancer Research Laboratory
Dept. of Surgery
Memorial Sloan-Kettering Cancer Ctr.
1275 York Ave.
New York, NY 10021 USA

Tombaccini, D.
Institute of General Pathology
School of Medicine
University of Florence
1-50134 Florence Italy

Timar, Jozsef
Wayne State University
Department of Radiation Oncology
431 Chemistry Building
Detroit, MI 48202 USA

Trosko, James E.
Dept. Pediatrics/Human Devel.
Michigan State University
East Lansing, MI 48824 USA

Trudell, James R.
Department of Anesthesia
Stanford University School of Medicine
Stanford, CA 94305-5117 USA

Ueda, N.
Dept. of Biochemistry
Tokushima University
School of Medicine
Kuramoto-cho
Tokushima 770, Japan

Ullrich, Volker
Fakultat fur Biologie
Universitat Kronstanz
775 Kronstanz, West Germany

Vallari, David S.
Medical Sciences Div.
Oak Ridge Assoc. Universities
P.O. Box 117
Oak Ridge, TN 37830-0117 USA

Van Vunakis, H.
Dept. of Biochemistry,
Brandeis University
Waltham, MA 02254 USA

Van't Riet, B.
Molecules for Health Inc.
Cancer Drug Research Development
3313 Gloucester Road
Richmond, VA 23227 USA

Vargas, Roberto
Georgetown University Medical Center
Department of Physiology and Biophysics
Reservoir Road, N.W.
Washington, D.C. 20007 USA

Villalobos, A.E.
University of California, Los Angeles
Laboratory of Biomedical and
Environmental Sciences
900 Veteran Avenue
Los Angeles, California 90024 USA

Vogler, Ralph
Emory University/School of Medicine
Department of Medicine
Division of Hematology Oncology
PO Box AE
Atlanta, GA 30322 USA

Wade, A.E.
University of Georgia/College of Pharmacy
Dept. of Pharmacology and Toxicology
Athens, GA 30602 USA

Walden, Jr., Thomas
Radiation Biochemistry Dept.
Bldg. 42, Navy Medical Center
Armed Forces Radiobiology Res. Inst.
Bethesda, MD 20814-5415 USA

Wallen, C. Anne
Bowman Gray School of Medicine
of Wake Forest University
Departs. of Radiology and Biochemistry
300 S. Hawthorne
Winston-Salem, NC 27103 USA

Watanabe, K.
Dept. of Pathology
Tokai University
School of Medicine
Isehara 259-11, Japan

Warfield, M.E.
Wayne State University
School of Medicine
Elliman Building Room 2222
421 East Canfield
Detroit, MI 48201 USA

Warner D.
McMaster University
Department of Pathology 3N10
1200 Main St. West
Hamilton, Ontario L8N3Z5
Canada

Weber, Barbara L.
Laboratory of Clinical Pharmacology
Dana-Farber Cancer Institute
and Department of Medicine
Harvard Medical School
44 Binney St.
Boston, MA 02115 USA

Welsch, Clifford
Depts. of Pharmacology and Toxicology
Michigan State University
East Lansing, MI 48824 USA

Winkel, Craig A.
Dept. of Ob/Gyn
Jefferson Medical College
1025 Walnut Street Room 300
Philadelphia, PA 19107 USA

Yamamoto, Shozo
Dept. of Biochemistry
Tokushima University
School of Medicine
Kuramoto-cho
Tokushima 770, Japan

Yan, Mengyao
Department of Chemistry
Oakland University
Rochester, MI 48309 USA

Yokoyama, C.
Dept. of Pharmacology
National Cardiovascular Center
Research Institute
Suita, Osaka 565, Japan

Yoshimoto, T.
Dept. of Biochemistry
Tokushima University
School of Medicine
Kuramoto-cho
Tokushima 770, Japan

Zacharski, Leo R.
Dartmough Medical School
White River Junction, VT
05001 USA

Zakrezewicz, Andreas
Eicosanoid Research
Dept. of Gynecological Endocrinology
FU Berlin, Klinikum Steglitz
Hindenburgdamm 30
D-1000 Berlin 45, FRG

Zorzet, S.
Institute of Pharmacology
University of Trieste
I-34100 Trieste
Italy

PHOSPHOLIPID TURNOVER OXYGENASES AND FATTY ACID METABOLISM

IMMUNOBIOCHEMICAL AND MOLECULAR BIOLOGICAL STUDIES ON ARACHIDONATE 12-LIPOXYGENASE OF PORCINE LEUKOCYTES

S. YAMAMOTO[1], T. YOSHIMOTO[1], H. SUZUKI[1], N. UEDA[1], K. NATSUI[1], Y. TAKAHASHI[1], T. MARUYAMA[1], A. HIROSHIMA[1], F. SHINJO[1], K. II[2], N. KOMATSU[3], K. WATANABE[3], K. GEROZISSIS[4], F. DRAY[4], C. YOKOYAMA[5], T. TAKAI[5], and T. TANABE[5]

Departments of [1]Biochemistry and [2]Pathology, Tokushima University, School of Medicine, Kuramoto-cho, Tokushima 770, Japan, [3]Department of Pathology, Tokai University, School of Medicine, Isehara 259-11, Japan, [4]Unite de Radioimmunologie Analytique, Institut Pasteur, 75724 Paris, France, and [5]Department of Pharmacology, National Cardiovascular Center, Research Institute, Suita, Osaka 565, Japan

Arachidonate 12-lipoxygenase is a dioxygenase which incorporates one molecule of oxygen into arachidonic acid regiospecifically and stereospecifically, and produces 12S-hydroperoxy-5,8,10,14-eicosatetraenoic acid (Figure 1). Since the enzyme was found in platelets as the first mammalian lipoxygenase (1,2), the 12-lipoxygenase has been found in a variety of tissues of a number of animal species (3,4). In addition to 12-lipoxygenase, several more lipoxygenases have been found in mammalian tissues. It is well known that the leukotriene synthesis is initiated by 5-lipoxygenase and the biosynthesis of prostaglandin and thromboxane by cyclooxygenase. These compounds have specific biological activities which regulate the functions of various animal tissues, and their biological functions have been generalized for a variety of animal species and tissues. However, no bioactive compound with such a general function has so far been found in the 12-lipoxygenase pathway of arachidonate metabolism (5).

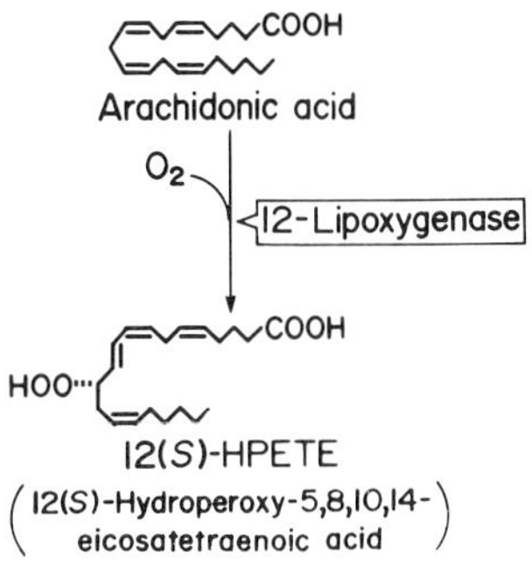

Figure 1. Reaction of arachidonate 12-lipoxygenase.

Several papers reported the biological functions of the 12-lipoxygenase metabolites of arachidonic acid. Goetzl and others reported a chemotactic activity of various HETEs, but considerably high concentrations were required to stimulate leukocyte chemotaxis (6). Later Murota and coworkers demonstrated a potent activity of 12-HETE to stimulate the migration of cultured smooth muscle cells of rat aorta. The activity was shown with 10 fM 12-HETE, and was specific for 12-HETE rather than 5-HETE and 15-HETE (7). However, such a potent activity of the 12-HETE has not been generalized with different cells of other animal species, and the mechanism of the chemotactic activity has not been elucidated. Secondly, a role of the 12-lipoxygenase metabolites in the neurotransmission was discovered with Aplysia ganglion by Feinmark and Schwartz and their colleagues (8). This function of a 12-HPETE metabolite was demonstrated in rat hippocampal neuron (9). Thirdly, Honn and associates reported that the cancer cells had a glycoprotein receptor like platelet GpIIb/IIIa, which was involved in the cancer cell adhesion to vascular endothelial cells. 12-HETE mediates either the expression or the activation of the GpIIb/IIIa-like receptor of the cancer cell (10).

When we were looking for the source of 5-lipoxygenase which was physiologically more important and apparently more interesting, we found a high activity of 12-lipoxygenase in porcine leukocytes (11). Furthermore, we did not detect the 12-lipoxygenase activity in porcine platelets in contrast to other mammalian platelets which were known to contain 12-lipoxygenase as well as cyclooxygenase (11). When we tried to purify the 12-lipoxygenase from porcine leukocytes, we found that the enzyme was readily inactivated by conventional purification methods. Then, we changed our strategy, and a crude enzyme preparation was given to a mouse as antigen to prepare a monoclonal anti-12-lipoxygenase antibody by the hybridoma technique (12). An antibody thus prepared was utilized for immunoaffinity purification of the 12-lipoxygenase. By this step the enzyme could be purified to near homogeneity (13).

Studies on the catalytic properties of the purified enzyme brought about a finding that 15-HPETE as substrate was as active as arachidonic acid. The enzymatic products from 15-HPETE were identified with collaboration with Alan R. Brash. To make a long story short, we found that the purified 12-lipoxygenase was a multifunctional enzyme. In addition to the arachidonate 12-oxygenation, the enzyme catalyzed 15-HPETE oxygenation at positions other than C-12, producing 8S,15S-diHPETE and 14R,15S-diHPETE. Moreover, the enzyme produced a 14,15-epoxy compound of leukotriene nature by an overall dehydration from 15-HPETE (13). Such a multifunctional nature of the enzyme with the allosteric oxygenase activities and the leukotriene A synthase activity was also reported for 5-lipoxygenase and 15-lipoxygenase, and is now considered as a general feature of lipoxygenase catalysis (4).

The substrate specificity studies demonstrated another interesting catalytic property of 12-lipoxygenase. Our group (13) and Nugteren's group (14) reported that the 12-lipoxygenase of porcine leukocytes were active with octadecapolyenoic acids as well as eicosapolyenoic acids. This broad substrate specificity was in contrast to that of platelet 12-lipoxygenase as earlier described by Nugteren (2). According to a recent report from Vliegenthart's group, 12-lipoxygenase of bovine platelets was inactive with linoleic acid while the enzyme of bovine leukocytes was active with linoleic acid as well as arachidonic acid (15).

We had two useful antibodies to precisely analyze this interesting subject of substrate specificity; namely, a monoclonal antibody against the porcine leukocyte enzyme and a monoclonal antibody against the human platelet enzyme. These antibodies cross-reacted with the enzymes of bovine leukocytes and platelets, respectively, and were utilized for immunoaffinity purification of the bovine enzymes. The enzymes were purified by the use of corresponding antibodies (16). We investigated the substrate specificities of the two distinct bovine 12-lipoxygenases thus purified by immunoaffinity chromatography. The platelet enzyme was specific for eicosapolyenoic acids whereas the leukocyte enzyme had a broad substrate specificity for docosa-, eicosa- and octadeca-polyenoic acids (16). Thus, the two 12-lipoxygenases of the same animal species are distinguishable each other not only immunologically but also catalytically.

On the basis of these findings, as shown in Table 1, we conclude that there are two types of 12-lipoxygenases in mammalian tissues, leukocyte-type and platelet-type. The former has a broad substrate specificity in terms of substrate chain length. The latter is specific for eicosapolyenoic acids. The two types of the enzyme are present in bovine tissues. However, 12-lipoxygenase is present in porcine leukocytes but undetectable in porcine platelets, while the enzyme is present in human platelets but undetectable so far in human leukocytes.

Table 1. Two types of 12-lipoxygenases.

Type	Leukocyte-type	Platelet-type
Substrate specificity	C_{18}, C_{20}, C_{22}	C_{20}
Occurence in		
bovine	+	+
porcine	+	-
human	-	+

Another application of our monoclonal anti-12-lipoxygenase antibodies was an enzyme immunoassay of 12-lipoxygenase, which allowed a quantitative determination of 12-lipoxygenase in various porcine tissues (12). One of the two antibodies, which recognized different sites of 12-lipoxygenase, was digested to a Fab fragment. Peroxidase as a label was conjugated to the Fab fragment. The other antibody was linked to protein A-containing Staphylococcus aureus. The two conjugates were incubated with 12-lipoxygenase, and the peroxidase activity of the immunoprecipitate was assayed. The peroxidase-linked immunoassay of 12-lipoxygenase was applied to various porcine tissues. The highest enzyme content was found in leukocytes, followed by small intestine, thymus and lymph node (12). It should be noted that no significant amount of 12-lipoxygenase was detected in platelets by the enzyme immunoassay (12). The sensitivity of the assay was too low to detect 12-lipoxygenase in porcine brain tissues. Recently we improved the sensitivity of the assay by introducing the solid phase method and the avidin-biotin method (17). The new method was about 10 times more sensitive than the previous method, and applied to various parts of porcine brain. Anterior pituitary showed the highest content of 12-lipoxygenase. This value was about 5% of the enzyme content of leukocyte which was the richest source of 12-lipoxygenase. Posterior pituitary had about one-tenth of the enzyme in anterior pituitary. When a high-speed supernatant of porcine anterior pituitary was incubated with arachidonic acid, HPLC analysis demonstrated the production of 12-HETE. An equivalent amount of cerebellum cytosol did not produce a detectable amount of 12-HETE. Furthermore, when the substrate specificity was examined, the 12-lipoxygenase of porcine pituitary was found to be of the leukocyte-type (17).

As mentioned above, significant amounts of 12-lipoxygenase were found by the enzyme immunoassay in several organs in addition to leukocytes. We examined these organs immunohistochemically by the use of a polyclonal antibody, which was raised against porcine leukocyte 12-lipoxygenase purified by immunoaffinity chromatography using a monoclonal anti-12-lipoxygenase antibody. In these organs, parenchymal cells were not stained significantly, and the positively stained cells were resident mast cells or infiltrating leukocytes (18). Therefore, we subjected anterior pituitary to immunohistological examination to find out whether or not the 12-lipoxygenase detected by the enzyme immunoassay was attributed to the leukocytes. When porcine anterior pituitary was stained by the avidin-biotin method, certain parenchymal cells rather than infiltrating leukocytes were positively stained. Electron microscopic observation showed that certain parenchymal cells with granules were positively stained, and the enzyme was located in the cytosol of these cells. The positively stained cells have not yet been identified (17).

Another method to screen 12-lipoxygenase is the measurement of mRNA for 12-lipoxygenase. Poly A-containing mRNAs for 12-lipoxygenase were isolated from porcine leukocytes, and double-stranded cDNA was prepared by the use of oligo(dT) primer. The resultant cDNA mixture was inserted into pBluescript. For screening the 12-lipoxygenase cDNA, two oligonucleotide probes were prepared on the basis of the amino acid sequence of a peptide obtained by digestion of the purified 12-lipoxygenase. Transformed E. coli cells were screened by the use of the two oligonucleotide probes.

The nucleotide sequence of the 12-lipoxygenase cDNA was determined by the dideoxynucleotide chain termination method of Sanger. The amino acid sequence deduced from the nucleotide sequence indicated that the enzyme protein was presumably composed of 662 amino acid residues. The deduced amino acid sequence included the N terminal region of the enzyme and the sequences of the proteolytic fragments which were determined by automated Edman degradation. The amino acid sequence of 12-lipoxygenase of porcine leukocytes was compared with that of human leukocyte 5-lipoxygenase (19) and that of human reticulocyte 15-lipoxygenase (20). In terms of the primary structure, porcine leukocyte 12-lipoxygenase exhibited 86% identity with human reticulocyte 15-lipoxygenase and 41% identity with human leukocyte 5-lipoxygenase.

The cDNA clone thus prepared was utilized for screening 12-lipoxygenase mRNA by Northern blotting. A 3.4-kb mRNA was detected not only in leukocytes but also in pituitary, lung, jejunum, spleen and so on. The results were consistent with those observed by the enzyme immunoassay (12,17).

Several previous papers reported the transformation of exogenous arachidonic acid to 12-HETE by rat pituitary (21-23). Our work now confirmed these earlier observations biochemically and immunohistochemically, ruling out a possibility that the 12-lipoxygenase was derived from infiltrating or contaminating leukocytes. Our work may be relevant to the previous findings that LH-RH excretion from rat median eminence (24) and melatonin excretion from rat pineal gland (25) are stimulated by 12-lipoxygenase product. We still do not know a general theory for the physiological and pathological function of 12-lipoxygenase. Our screening of 12-lipoxygenase by the enzyme immunoassay in various tissues revealed a relatively high content of the enzyme in porcine-pituitary. This finding was supported by the measurement of the 12-lipoxygenase mRNA. These results suggest a neuroendocrine role of the 12-lipoxygenase pathway, which, however, has not yet been established.

REFERENCES

1. Hamberg, M. and Samuelsson, B. Proc. Natl. Acad. Sci. USA. 71:3400-3404, 1974.
2. Nugteren, D.H. Biochim. Biophys. Acta. 380:299-307, 1975.
3. Yamamoto, S. In: Prostaglandins and Related Substances (Eds. C. Pace-Asciak, and E. Granstrom), Elsevier, Amsterdam, 1983, pp. 171-202.
4. Yamamoto, S. Prostaglandins Leukotrienes and Essential Fatty Acids Review 35:219-229, 1989.
5. Brash, A.R. Circulation 72:702-707, 1985.
6. Goetzl, E.J., Woods, J.M., and Gorman, R.R. J. Clin. Invest. 59:179-183, 1977.
7. Nakao, J., Ooyama, T., Ito, H., Chang, W.-C. and Murota, S. Atherosclerosis 44:339-342, 1982.
8. Piomelli, D., Volterra, A., Dale, N., Siegelbaum, S.A., Kandel, E.R., Schwartz, J.H. and Belardetti, F. Nature 328:38-43, 1987.
9. Carlen, P.L., Gurevich, N., Wu, P.H., Su, W.-G., Corey, E.J. and PaceAsciak. C.R. Brain Res. 497:171-176, 1989.
10. Grossi, I.M., Fitzgerald, L.A., Umbarger, L.A., Nelson, K.K., Diglio, C.A., Taylor, J.D. and Honn, K.V. Cancer Res. 49:1029-1037, 1989.
11. Yoshimoto, T., Miyamoto, Y., Ochi, K. and Yamamoto, S. Biochim. Biophys. Acta 713:638-646, 1982.
12. Shinjo, F., Yoshimoto, T., Yokoyama, C., Yamamoto, S., Izumi, S., Komatsu, N. and Watanabe, K. J. Biol. Chem. 261:3377-3381, 1986.
13. Yokoyama, C., Shinjo, F., Yoshimoto, T., Yamamoto, S., Oates, J.A. and Brash, A.R. J. Biol. Chem. 261:16714-16721, 1986.
14. Claeys, M., Kivits, G.A.A., Christ-Hazelhof, E. and Nugteren, D.H. Biochim. Biophys. Acta 837:35-51, 1985.
15. Walstra, P., Verhagen, J., Vermeer, M.A., Veldink, G.A. and Vliegenthart, J.F.G. Biochim. Biophys. Acta 921:312-319, 1987.
16. Takahashi, Y., Ueda, N. and Yamamoto, S. Arch. Biochem. Biophys. 266: 613-621, 1988.
17. Ueda, N., Hiroshima, A., Natsui, K., Shinjo, F., Yoshimoto, T., Yamamoto, S., Ii, K., Gerozissis, K. and Dray, F. J. Biol. Chem. in press.
18. Maruyama, T., Ueda, N., Yoshimoto, T., Yamamoto, S., Komatsu, N. and Watanabe, K. J. Histochem. Cytochem. 37:1125-1131, 1989.
19 Dixon, R.A.F., Jones, R.E., Diehl, R.E., Bennett, C.D., Kargman, S. and Rouzer, C.A. Proc. Natl. Acad. Sci. USA 85:416-420, 1988.
20. Sigal, E., Craik, C.S., Highland, E., Grunberger, D., Costello, L.L., Dixon, R.A.F. and Nadel, J.A.

Biochem. Biophys. Res. Commun. 157: 457-464, 1988.
21. Pilote, S., Vallerand, P. and Borgeat, P. Biochem. Biophys. Res. Commun. 104:867-873, 1982.
22. Yoshimoto, T., Kusaka, M., Shinjo, F., Yamamoto, S. and Dray, F. Prostaglandins 28:279-285, 1984.
23. Vanderhoek, J.Y., Kiesel, L., Naor, Z., Bailey, J.M. and Catt, K.J. Prostaglandin Leukotriene and Medicine 15:375-385, 1984.
24. Gerozissis, K., Vulliez, B., Saavedra, J.M., Murphy, R.C. and Dray, F. Neuroendocrinology 40:272-276, 1985.
25. Sakai, K., Fafeur, V., Vulliez-le Normand, B. and Dray, F. Prostaglandins 35:969-976, 1988.

TRANSCELLULAR BIOSYNTHESIS OF LEUKOTRIENES: IS LEUKOTRIENE A_4 A MEDIATOR?

R.C. MURPHY, J. MACLOUF, and P.M. HENSON

National Jewish Center for Immunology and Respiratory Medicine, Denver, CO 80206 USA and INSERM Unite 150, UA 334 CNRS, Hopital Lariboisiere, 75475 Paris Cedex 10, France

INTRODUCTION

The enzymatic steps involved in the synthesis of prostaglandins, thromboxanes, and leukotrienes have been elucidated in substantial detail in numerous biochemical studies (1,2). In most cases, these studies involved the addition of radiolabeled arachidonic acid to homogenous cell suspensions with characterization of the resultant radiolabeled metabolites. Thus, most of the studies during the 1960s and 1970s were designed to establish those oxidative pathways of arachidonic acid within a single cell type. As a result, the metabolic patterns of eicosanoids generated by a given cell type has been fairly well established, for example, those cells which are found in the blood have been studied in great detail and their primary cyclooxygenase and lipoxygenase metabolites are known (Table 1). While most cells in the blood do metabolize arachidonic acid by one or more cascades, there are some cells which do not participate in the oxidative conversion of arachidonic acid into reactive intermediates. Table 1 indicates that the red blood cell and the lymphocyte (3) cannot metabolize arachidonic acid by either the cyclooxygenase or lipoxygenase pathways. Normally, one considers most cells in the blood to have a

Table 1. Arachidonic Acid Metabolites Generated by Stimulation of Isolated Blood Cells

Cells	Eicosanoid	Oxidase	Intermediate	Secondary Enzyme
Platelet	TxB_2	C.O.	PGH_2	Thromboxane Synthase
	HHT	C.O.	PGH_2	Thromboxane Synthase
	12-HETE	12-LO	12-HPETE	---
Polymorphonuclear Leukocyte	LTB_4	5-LO	LTA_4	LTA_4-Hydrolase
Eosinophil	LTC_4	5-LO	LTA_4	LTC_4-Synthase
	5-HETE	15-LO	15-HPETE	---
Basophil	LTC_4	5-LO	LTA_4	LTC_4-Synthase
Monocyte Macrophage	TxA_2	C.O.	PGH_2	Thromboxane Synthase
	LTB_4	5-LO	LTA_4	LTA_4-Hydrolase
	LTC_4	5-LO	LTA_4	LTC_4-Synthase
Lymphocyte	None	None	---	---
RBC	None	None	---	---

substantial capacity for the production of active eicosanoids. For example, platelets are known to produce thromboxane A_2, a pro-aggregatory substance in response to stimulation and that this eicosanoid plays an important role in thrombus formation (4). The neutrophil on the other hand appears only to have a 5-lipoxygenase pathway for metabolism of arachidonic acid and stimulation of this cell leads to the formation of LTB_4, a chemotactic factor (5). The eosinophil and basophil also metabolize arachidonate by the 5-lipoxygenase pathway and convert the reactive LTA_4 into the sulfidopeptide leukotriene LTC_4, the potent smooth muscle contracting agent and substance which enhances capillary permeability (6). The studies in this manner have greatly expanded our understanding of the complexity of arachidonic acid metabolism and the role which the eicosanoid metabolites may play in health and disease. However, it appears that the synthesis of eicosanoids may be more complex than only occurring within one cell and may involve cell-cell interactions.

Transcellular biosynthesis.

In 1982 Marcus and co-workers (7) provided evidence to suggest that PGH_2 synthesized by the platelet could be transformed into PGI_2 after transfer to endothelial cells. In these experiments, platelets were co-incubated with aspirin treated endothelial cells and the cell suspension was stimulated with calcium ionophore. The metabolite 6-keto-$PGF_{1\alpha}$ was observed which could only arise from platelet derived PGH_2. This introduced the concept that a reactive intermediate in the arachidonic acid cascade, via PGH_2, could be transported from the cell of synthesis (in this case the platelet) to another cell for processing. Later, Fitzpatrick and Samuelsson (8) discovered that even though the red blood cell does not contain any of the oxidative enzymes involved in arachidonic acid metabolism, nonetheless, has the capacity to convert the reactive leukotriene intermediate, LTA_4, into LTB_4. Thus, the RBC contained LTA_4-hydrolase. This was quite a surprise since the red blood cell was thought to be totally inert to metabolism of metabolites of arachidonic acid. Feinmark and Cannon (9) found that stimulating co-incubations of human polymorphonuclear leukocytes with endothelial cells with the calcium ionophore resulted in the production of LTC_4. The synthesis of this sulfidopeptide leukotriene was related to the presence of endothelial cells rather than the presence of basophils or eosinophils in the preparation of the human polymorphonuclear leukocytes. In 1988, Maclouf and Murphy (10) demonstrated that human platelets could efficiently convert exogenous LTA_4 into LTC_4; thus platelets possess LTC_4 synthase and high levels of intracellular glutathione necessary for this conversion. Furthermore, when neutrophils were activated with the calcium ionophore in the presence of platelets, significant quantities of sulfidopeptide leukotrienes could be observed.

From the experiments described above, transcellular biosynthesis of biologically active eicosanoids appears to be a feasible process. However, some questions do remain. First, most experiments were carried out by stimulating cell co-incubations with the calcium ionophore which bypasses many of the receptor-mediated regulatory events of eicosanoid biosynthesis. Secondly, the entire concept of transcellular biosynthesis relies on the fact that the LTA_4 or PGH_2 must be sufficiently stable to shuttle from one cell to another. Both of these intermediates are chemically reactive and have short half-lifes. The question is whether or not they have sufficient stability to carry out such a process at a tissue level. Thirdly, because of the difficulties inherent in demonstrating transcellular biosynthesis, simple cell co-incubations have been studied. It would be helpful to demonstrate transcellular biosynthesis at the tissue level to support the idea that this is an important process *in vivo* leading to eicosanoid biosynthesis.

Phagocytosis and receptor mediated cell stimulation.

Receptor-mediated stimulation of the human neutrophil is a complex process. Recent investigations have suggested that it takes at least two stimuli to fully activate the neutrophil in formation of eicosanoids (11). As seen in Figure 1, when neutrophils are treated with cytochalasin B (5 μ g/mL), very little eicosanoid production from exogenous [^{3}H]-arachidonate is evident as seen in Panel A. However, when additional stimuli of platelet activating factor (10^{-8} M) and fMLP (10^{-7} M) are added, the production of 20-hydroxy-LTB_4, and LTB_4 became quite evident. Using the same concentrations of stimulating agents, neutrophils were then co-incubated with platelets, and an abundant production of LTC_4 by transcellular biosynthesis resulted. These results support the hypothesis that transcellular biosynthesis can occur following physiologically relevant stimuli of neutrophil-platelet mixtures.

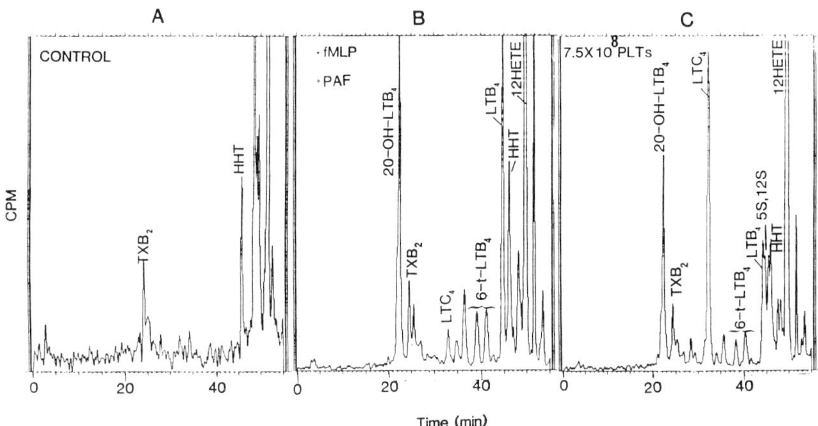

Figure 1. Neutrophils (5 x 10^6/ml) were incubated with cytochalasin B (5 μg/mL) and [^{3}H]-arachidonate (11 μ M, 5 μ Ci). ***A*** Control incubation of cells for 5 min; ***B*** addition of PAF (10^{-8} M) and fMLP (10^{-7} M); ***C*** incubation of neutrophils using identical stimuli in Panel B with co-incubation of 7 x 5 x 10^8 platelets (aspirin treated). After a 5 min incubation period, the reaction was stopped by the addition of two volumes of cold methanol. The methanol supernatant was extracted with hexane to remove excess unreacted free arachidonate and then subjected to reverse phase HPLC separation using a linear gradient system (methanol/water/acetic acid; 40:60:0.05%) to 100% methanol over 40 min. The effluent from the HPLC was directed into an HPLC scintillation detector after mixing with scintillation cocktail.

Phagocytosis has also been employed to stimulate eicosanoid biosynthesis in neutrophils. When neutrophils were treated with opsonized zymosan to induce phagocytosis, very little LTC_4 was produced in the absence of platelets. Furthermore, when neutrophils were treated with fMLP (10^{-6} M), very little LTC was evident. However, when both stimuli were employed, there was a dose-dependent increase of LTC_4 observed in platelet-neutrophil co-incubations when fMLP was increased from 10^{-8} to 10^{-6}M (12). Thus, it is clear that physiologically relevant stimuli can result in transcellular biosynthesis of sulfidopeptide leukotrienes in platelet-neutrophil co-incubations.

Stability of LTA_4.

LTA_4 has been considered to be a reactive intermediate with a very short half-life, t 1/2 30 sec (13). However, when albumin is present in the buffer, it protects this allylic epoxide from aqueous hydrolysis. Thus, the apparent half-life of LTA_4 in albumin containing solutions is significantly enhanced (13).

Experiments have also been carried out where neutrophils were stimulated with the calcium ionophore (5 μ M) for various times from 4 min to 55 min followed by centrifugation and removal of the supernatant (10). As seen in Figure 2, the supernatant was either transferred to buffer, transferred to a platelet suspension (1.5 x 10^9/ml) or acidified then neutralized before being transferred to the platelet suspension. Only when platelets were present was there a substantial production of LTC_4 which was maximal at 8 min after initiation of ionophore stimulation. Thus, even after 8 min there was abundant LTA_4 in the supernatant which could be taken up by the platelet following transfer and converted into LTC_4. These results suggest that LTA_4 is sufficiently stable to exist in the extracellular environment and be available for transcellular biosynthetic events.

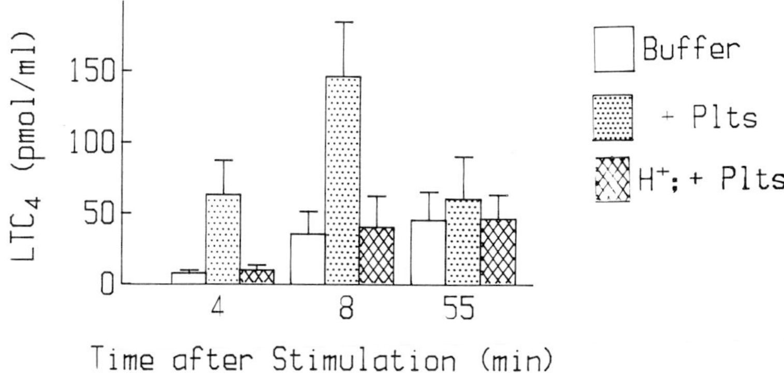

Figure 2. Neutrophils (2 x 10^7/ml) were stimulated with calcium ionophore (5 μM) for the time indicated. Following incubation, tubes were centrifuged at an aliquot of the supernatant was diluted either in buffer containing 4 mg/L BSA, transferred to a platelet suspension (1.5 x 10^9/ml), or acidified to pH 3, then neutralized and transferred to an identical platelet suspension. After 30 min additional incubation, the tubes are analyzed for LTC_4 by enzyme immunoassay. The results represent the mean ± S.E.M. before 4-5 experiments (10).

Tissue transcellular biosynthesis.

Transcellular biosynthesis of eicosanoids is difficult to demonstrate in a complex tissue system. This is due to the numerous cell types which are present, multiple metabolic pathways for degradation of eicosanoids, and the difficulty in obtaining stimulation of specific cells within a tissue or organ system. Experiments have been carried out using blood as a model tissue system with phagocytosis of zymosan particles to initiate LTA_4 biosynthesis by the phagocytic cells present in whole blood (14). Using such a model system, numerous eicosanoids were synthesized in a time-dependent manner. For example, LTB_4 and 20-hydroxy-LTB_4 were found to increase in concentration up to 30 min of stimulation with a plateau at approximately 5 - 10 ng/ml. LTE_4 follows a similar time course with a plateau approximately 0.5 to 1 ng/ml of whole blood. In contrast, the production of thromboxane B_2, which no doubt arises from platelets, increased almost linearly up to 1 hr. Platelet activating factor, had a peak level approximately 20 to 30 min following initial addition of zymosan which rapidly fell after 30 min to very low levels. Peak levels for PAF were approximately 10 ng/ml. When cells are isolated from whole blood and reconstituted in different mixture ratios, it was found that the production of LTB_4 was approximately 2-fold higher in whole blood compared to neutrophils incubated alone or with platelets. No doubt this is due to the fact that red blood cells participate in LTB_4 biosynthesis by a transcellular route. Sulfidopeptide leukotriene production were almost unmeasurable where neutrophils were incubated in the buffer and treated with opsonized zymosan. Yet a substantial amount of sulfidopeptide leukotriene was synthesized when platelets were added and a very similar amount was observed during phagocytosis of zymosan particles in whole blood. These results support the concept that transcellular biosynthesis may be a significant process occurring at the tissue level through the release of LTA_4 as a mediator of the stimulation event.

Much of the earlier biochemical studies had focused on a single cell carrying out the multiple events of leukotriene biosynthesis. It is clear that LTA_4, even though a reactive substance, can nonetheless travel from a cellular site of synthesis to a different cellular site of transformation. In such instances, LTA_4 should be considered to be a mediator of this stimulatory event since it carries the information of cell activation to an adjacent cell. The acceptor cell then processes LTA_4 into another substance which can be recognized by cells containing appropriate receptors. Little is known about the direct biological activities of LTA_4, nonetheless, it is clear that the products of further chemical processing, namely LTB_4 and LTC_4, possess profound biological properties.

ACKNOWLEDGEMENT

This work is supported, in part, by a grant from the National Institutes of Health (HL34303). Partial support for collaboration between the French and U.S. laboratories was made possible by a grant from NATO.

REFERENCES

1. Samuelsson, B., Goldyne, M., Granstrom, E., Hamberg, M., Hammarstrom, S., and Malmsten, C.

Ann. Rev. Biochem. 42:997-1029, 1978.
2. Lewis, R.A. and Austen, K. F. J. Clin. Invest. 73:889 (1984).
3. Goldyne, M.E. Pharmacol. Res. 21:241-145, 1989.
4. Hamberg, M., Svensson, J., and Samuelsson, B. Proc. Natl. Acad. Sci. USA 71:345, 1975.
5. Ford-Hutchinson, A.W., Bray, M.A., and Doig, M.W. Nature. 286:264, 1981.
6. Barnes, P.J., Chung, K.F., and Page, C.P. Pharmacol. Rev. 40:49, 1989.
7. Marcus, A. J., Broekman, M.J., Safier, L.B., Ullman, H.L., and Islam, N. Biochem. Biophys. Res. Commun. 109:130, 1982.
8. McGee, J. E. and Fitzpatrick, F.A. Proc. Natl. Acad. Sci. USA 83:1349, 1986.
9. Feinmark, S. J. and Cannon, P.J.: J. Biol. Chem. 261:16466, 1986.
10. Maclouf, J. and Murphy, R.C. J. Biol. Chem. 263:174-181, 1988.
11. Dewald, B., Thelen, M., and Baggiolini, M. J. Biol. Chem. 263:16179-16184, 1988.
12. Maclouf, J., Murphy, R.C., and Henson, P.M. Blood 74:703-707, 1989.
13. Fitzpatrick, F., Morton, D., and Wynalda, M.J.. Biol. Chem. 257:4680-4683, 1982.
14. Fradin, A., Zirrolli, J.A., Maclouf, J., Vausbinder, L., Henson, P.M., and Murphy, R.C. J. Immunol., 143:3680-3685,1989.

THE OCCURENCE OF THROMBOXANE SYNTHASE IN TUMOR CELLS

[1]R. NÜSING, [1]V. ULLRICH, [2]F. GUDAT,and [2]M.J. MIHATSCH

[1]Faculty of Biology , University of Konstanz, FRG, [2]Institute of Pathology, University of Basel, CH

INTRODUCTION

Different studies have shown, that human tumors are able to synthesize prostanoids (1-3) with significant increases in production during tumor development (4,5). An influence of cyclooxygenase metabolites of arachidonic acid on processes such as cell proliferation, migration, adherence, and hemostatic mechanisms were suggested.

During metastasis tumor cells first invade the microvasculature and then disseminate to distant organs under possible interaction with host platelets. The mechanisms by which platelets may promote metastasis relate to formation of platelet-tumor cell aggregates and adhesion of the aggregates to the vascular endothelium. Also the tumor cell itself may express prostanoid receptors coupled to the PI-response and become adherent to endothelial cells. In contrast PGI_2 or PGE_2 which are linked to adenylyl cyclase may counteract this process. In this regard the endogenous balance of antiaggregatory PGI_2 and its antagonist TXA_2 may be of interest. This has led to the hypothesis that a dominance of TXA_2 in the circulation could promote the potential of cancer cells to spread (6).

Several lines of evidence suggest that tumor cells can induce platelet aggregation which may play a role in their hematogenous dissemination. In agreement with the assumption that the platelet-tumor cell interaction is a crucial step in metastasis formation Honn et al. (7) have shown, that PGI_2 could reduce lung colony formation by injected tumor cells. But the above hypothesis is conflicted by results obtained from Karpatkin et al. (8), who found no effect of PGI_2 on the prevention of pulmonary metastasis.

In a study with different human intracranial tumors Castelli et al. (9) reported about a correlation in the increase of prostanoid production with anaplastic grade, from normal brain to glioblastomas. The arachidonic acid metabolism profile of normal brain and glioma were strikingly similar and exhibited a net prevalence of TXB_2 and low levels of 6-keto-$PGF_{1\alpha}$. Nevertheless, average prostanoid production was significantly higher in pathological tissue. It is interesting to note, that gliomas synthesize higher relative proportions of TXB_2 and lower relative amounts of 6-keto-$PGF_{1\alpha}$ than meningiomas.

The synthesis of abnormal amounts of selected prostanoids might facilitate or impair the growth and dissemination of the tumor or affect the host's defense mechanisms. In metastatic compared to benign ovarian cancer tissue TXB_2 but not 6-keto-$PGF_{1\alpha}$ were significantly higher (10).

TXA_2 has been shown in some experimental studies to favor tumor growth and spread (11,12), while the opposite has been reported for PGI_2 (12). Studies using exogenous PGI_2 or PGI_2-analogs resulted in an inhibition of colony formation by various tumor lines. Prostacyclin also inhibits tumor-platelet adhesion (13,14) and tumor cell-tumor cell adhesion (15) .

TXA_2 is the major cyclooxygenase metabolite of arachidonic acid in platelets. This potent vasocontrictive and proaggregatory substance has a very short half time of 30 s in aqueous solutions and hydrolyzes spontaneously to the biological less active compound TXB_2 . It is of interest that the stable metabolite TXB_2 increases tumor cell adhesion to nylon fibers (16). In contrast a study by Spagnuolo et al. (17) supported a primary role of TXA_2 as the mediator of increases of leukocyte adherence, whereas exogenous TXB_2 did not enhance PMN adherence. McGillen et al. (18) have recently shown that PGI_2 inhibits PMN adhesiveness to nylon. Overall the available data indicate an important function of the PGI_2:TXA_2-ratio for tumor cell adhesion to host cells in a tissue.

Whereas many studies have focused on hematogenous dissemination with possible interraction between circulating host platelets, endothelial cell, and tumor cell, only a few reports were dealing with the arachidonic acid metabolism of tumor tissue and the significance of prostanoids for growth and proliferation.

The role of prostaglandins and thromboxane (Tx) in the control of tumor cell proliferation and neoplasia is currently being widely investigated. Chiabrando et al. (4) examined arachidonic acid metabolites in lungs of control and Lewis lung carcinoma-bearing mice. Compared to control lung they found an increase of TXB_2 and a decrease of 6-keto-$PGF_{1\alpha}$ in tumor-bearing lungs. Analysis of prostanoid profile in M5076 ovarian reticulosarcoma homogenates at various time points during tumor growth revealed TXB_2 as by far the most abundant product. In contrast 6-keto-$PGF_{1\alpha}$ decreased. Since the metabolism of AA was studied in whole homogenates it was not clear wether the major sources of arachidonic acid metabolites are the neoplastic cells themselves or whether infiltrating macrophages or other cells contribute.

RESULTS & DISCUSSION

After the purification of human platelet Tx-synthase by our group (19) an antiserum and monoclonal antibodies become available (20). Immunohistochemical staining revealed the presence of this enzyme in monocytic cells of many tissues (21) but also of some epithelial structures (21). Since carcinomas are derived from such cells we were interested whether tumor cells can express Tx-synthase protein. We were sucessful in most tumors but not in all. In cryosections of adenocarcinomas antigenicity to anti-Tx-synthase antibody is only expressed by stroma cells, whereas tumor cells were negative. The same distribution of Tx-synthase were found in sections of Ewing's sarcoma. Again only the stroma cells were stained by our antibody.

As demonstrated by us recently, in normal connective tissue stroma primarily monocytic cells show capacity for Tx-production (21). But invasion of macrophages into pathological tissue can not account for the intense staining of the stroma in neoplasia.

Interestingly in cryosections of an amelanotic melanoma or of leiomyosarcoma we found a specific staining of tumor cells with anti-Tx-synthase antibody. No kind of stroma cell exhibited antigenicity to the antibody. From this we suggest that tumor cells may have a dramatic modulative function on prostanoid enzyme regulation of surrounding cells.

There is a considerable amount of evidence that TXA_2 may function as immunomodulator. Whereas the suggestion that TXA_2 probably enhance lymphocyte proliferation in response to mitogens was conflicted by contradictive results (22,23), Rola-Pleszczcynski et al. (24) found the TXA_2 analog U-44069 to markedly depress natural cytotoxicity. The use of Tx-synthase inhibitors and Tx-receptor blockers gave evidence that TXA_2 could exert a negative feedback on natural cytotoxicity function through its receptor.

Possibly tumor cells use Tx as a immunsuppressive agent on host defense elements, enhancing viability and thus the ability of cells to leave the primary tumor mass and to successfully grow at a metastatic site.

Attention has also focused on the possibility that the constitutive activation of protein kinase C (PKC) is one way for a continuous proliferative response. For example, a strong correlation was found between basal levels of membrane-bound PKC and the lung colonizing capacity of a series of variants of the B16 melanoma (25). Protein phosphorylation may be one mechanism for signals reaching the nucleus and modulating changes in gene expression. The central consequence of TXA_2 action is the activation of the PI-response with stimulation of PKC. From this, a mechanistic model might be thought of as an autocrine model where tumor-TXA_2 have direct effects on tumor cell behavior.

REFERENCES

1. Honn, K.V., Bockman, R.S. and Marnett, L.J. Prostaglandins 21: 833-864, 1981.
2. Levine, L. Adv. Cancer Res. 35: 49-79, 1981.
3. Bockman, R.S. Cancer Invest. 1: 485-493, 1983.
4. Chiabrando, C., Broggini, M., Castagnoli, M.N., Donelli, M.G., Noseda, A., Visintainer, M., Garattini, S. and Fanelli, R. Cancer Res. 45: 3605-3608, l985.
5. Chiabrando, C., Broggini, M., Castelli, M.G., Cozzi, E., Castagnoli, M.N., Donelli, M.G., Garattini, S., Giavazzi, R. and Fanelli, R. Cancer Res. 47: 988-991, 1987.
6. Honn, K.V., Busse, W.D. and Sloane, B.F. Biochem. Pharmacol. 32: 1-11, 1983.
7. Honn, K.V., Cicone, B. and Skoff A. Science 212: 1270 -1272, 1981.
8. Karpatkin, S., Ambrogio, C. and Pearlstein, E. Cancer Res. 44: 3880-3883, 1984.
9. Castelli, M.G., Chiabrando, C., Fanelli, R., Martelli, L., Butti, G., Gaetani, P. and Paoletti, P. Cancer Res. 49: 1505-1508, 1989.
10. Heinoneu, P.K. and Metsa-Ketela, T. Gynecol. Obstet. Invest. 18: 225-229, 1984.
11. Honn, K.V. In: Prostaglandins and Cancer: First International Conference (Eds. T.J. Powles, R.S. Bockman, K.V. Honn and P. Ramwell), Alan R. Liss, New York, 1982, pp. 733-752.
12. Drago, J.R. and Al-Mondhiry, H.A.B. Anticancer Res. 4: 391-394, 1984.
13. Menter, D.G., Harkins, C., Onoda, J.M., Riordem, W., Sloane, B.F., Taylor, J.D. and Honn, K.V. Invasion Metastasis 7: 109-128, 1987.
14. Menter, D.G., Steinert, B.W., Sloane, B.F., Taylor, J.D. and Honn, K.V. Cancer Res. 47: 2425-2432, 1987.
15. Honn, K.V., Menter, D.G., Onoda, J.M., Taylor, J.D. and Sloane, B.F. In: Cancer Invasion and Metastasis: Biologic and Therapeutic Aspects (Eds. G.L. Nicolson and L. Milas), Raven Press, New York, 1984, pp. 361-388.
16. Varani, J. and McCoy, I.P. In: Mechanisms of Cancer Metastasis: Potential Therapeutic Implications for Therapy (Eds. K.V. Honn, W.E. Powers and B.F. Sloane), Martinus Nijhoff, Boston, 1985, pp. 259-274.

17. Spagnuolo, P.J., Ellner J.J., Hassid, A. and Dunn, M. J. Clin. Invest. 66: 406-414, 1980.
18. McGillen, J., Patterson, R. and Phair, J. J. Infect. Dis. 141: 382-388, 1980.
19. Haurand, M. and Ullrich, V. J. Biol. Chem. 260: 15059 -15067, 1985.
20. Nusing, R., Wernet, M.P. and Ullrich, V. Blood, submitted.
21. Nusing, R., Lesch, R. and Ullrich, V. Eicosanoids, submitted.
22. Kelly, J.P., Johnson, M.P. and Parker, C.W. J. Immunol. 122: 1563-1571, 1979.
23. Gordon, D., Nouri, A.M.E. and Thomas, R.V. Br. J. Pharmacol. 74: 469-475, 1981.
24. Rola-Pleszczynski, M., Gagnon, L., Bolduc, D. and LeBreton G. J. Immunol. 135: 4114-4119.
25. Gopalakrishna R. and Barsky, S.H. Proc. Natl. Acad. Sci. USA 85: 612-616, 1988.

STIMULATION AND INHIBITION OF OXYGEN RADICAL FORMATION BY ASCORBIC ACID AND 13-*CIS*-RETINOIC ACID

L. J. MARNETT, V. SAMOKYSZYN, and D. LAUDICINA

A.B. Hancock, Jr. Memorial Laboratory for Cancer Research, Departments of Biochemistry and Chemistry, Center in Molecular Toxicology, Vanderbilt University School of Medicine, Nashville TN 37232

INTRODUCTION

Oxygen radicals are implicated in various stages of carcinogenesis and radical scavengers inhibit tumorigenesis in some models (1-4). However, many presumed radical scavengers exhibit radical generating activity under certain conditions. For example, vitamin C (L-(+)-ascorbic acid) is well known to act as an antioxidant and a prooxidant (5-10). Its antioxidant activity derives from its ability to reduce peroxyl radicals that propagate lipid peroxidation or to reduce the oxidized form (tocopheryl oxyl radical) of the naturally-occuring antioxidant vitamin E (6,7,11). Its prooxidant activity is a result of its ability to reduce metals (especially Fe^{+3}-complexes) to forms that react with O_2 to initiate lipid peroxidation (5).

Another example of a molecule with dual effects on oxygen radical generation is 13-*cis*-retinoic acid,a vitamin A analog with differentiation-inducing, anti-acne, and cancer chemopreventive activities (12-16). Its *trans* isomer is the active component of Retin-A® (tretinoin) which has recently been reported to reverse photoaging (17). The extended polyene chain of retinoids is sensitive to oxidation and several oxygenated metabolites as well as the enzyme systems that form them have been characterized (18-21). Its prooxidant activity results from its ability to donate a H atom from the 4 position to form a carbon-centered radical that couples to O_2 to produce a peroxyl radical. Its antioxidant activity may result from its ability to scavenge peroxyl radicals by addition to its extended polyene chain.

The enzymes cyclooxygenase and lipoxygenase are among the few enzymes in nature that generate hydroperoxides as stable reaction products. These polyunsaturated fatty acid hydroperoxides are usually reduced by peroxidases but occasionally escape enzymatic reduction and react with metal complexes and metalloproteins (22,23). This produces strong oxidizing agents that can trigger lipid peroxidation *inter alia*. Ascorbate and 13-*cis*-retinoic acid are weak reducing substrates for the peroxidase activity associated with cyclooxygenase so they should inhibit hydroperoxide-dependent lipid peroxidation at high concentrations (24). However, at low concentrations they are not effective peroxidase reductants and their effect on hydroperoxide-dependent lipid peroxidation is not known. Therefore, we conducted experiments to evaluate the effects of ascorbic acid on hydroperoxide-dependent lipid peroxidation in rat liver microsomes. In subsequent experiments, we investigated the effects of 13-*cis*-retinoic acid on ascorbate-dependent lipid peroxidation. The results of these experiments are summarized here.

MATERIALS AND METHODS

Preparation of Microsomes.

Liver microsomes were prepared from male Fischer 344 rats from Charles River weighing between 200 to 225 g according to the procedure of Tunek *et al* with modifications (25). Rats were sacrificed by CO_2 esphyxiation and livers homogenized in a sodium phosphate buffer (100 mM) pH 7.4, containing 250 mM sucrose. The microsomal pellet obtained by ultracentrifugation was washed once in 100 mM phosphate to remove any remaining sucrose, since it has been shown to interfere with thiobarbituric acid (TBA) assay values (26). The microsomes were then resuspended in this buffer, frozen immediately with liquid N_2, and stored at -80° C until use.

Lipid peroxidation assays.

To evaluate the effect of ascorbic acid on hydroperoxide-dependnet lipid peroxidation, microsomes (0.5 mg protein/mL) were preincubated in a 100 mM phosphate buffer pH 7.4 for two min at 37°C in a shaking water bath under an air atmosphere. Simultaneous addition of ascorbate and linoleic acid hydroperoxide (LAHP) initiated the reactions. The hydroperoxide was added in methanol to a final concentration of 0.1%. Incubations were performed at 37°C for time periods up to one hour during which time 1.0 mL aliquots were removed and added to 2 mL of TBA-TCA-HCl reagent (0.375% TBA, 15% TCA, dissolved in 0.25 N HCl) to terminate the reaction. The samples were mixed thoroughly and placed in a boiling water bath for 15 min. The TBA reagent described above contained 0.01% butylated hydroxytoluene to prevent autoxidation of microsomal lipids during heating (27). After cooling, tubes were centrifuged in a table top centrifuge for 10 min to pellet the microsomal material and the absorbance of the supernatant read at 535 nm. Malondialdehyde (MDA) formation was quantitated using a molar extinction coefficient of $1.49 \times 10^5\ M^{-1}cm^{-1}$ (28).

To assess the effect of 13-*cis*-retinoic acid, peroxidation was initiated with ADP-chelated iron and ascorbate (29,30). Microsomes (0.5 mg protein/mL) and 13-*cis*-retinoic acid or vehicle alone (0.8 % DMSO) were preincubated for 1 min at 37°C in 0.1 M Tris·HCl (pH 7.5) containing Fe^{3+} (15 μM) and ADP (4 mM) followed by the addition of ascorbate (1 mM). After 20 min, an equal volume of TBA reagent was added and the mixture was heated in a boiling water bath for 15 min, centrifuged at 1000 x g, and the absorbance of the supernatant determined at 535 nm.

RESULTS

Ascorbate.

The effect of ascorbate on microsomal lipid peroxidation was tested with the naturally occuring fatty acid hydroperoxide LAHP. LAHP is a major endogenous hydroperoxide in phospholipids from animal tissue and induces lipid peroxidation by a combination of non-enzymatic and cytochrome P-450-dependent reactions (31). Rat liver microsomes were incubated with 100 μM LAHP at 37°C with concentrations of ascorbate ranging from 0 to 1 mM. Lipid peroxidation was measured as MDA equivalents by the TBA assay on aliquots removed at regular time intervals. LAHP induced rapid lipid peroxidation whereas ascorbate (1.0 mM) induced no lipid peroxidation at times up to 60 min (32). Microsomes treated with ascorbate plus LAHP displayed higher MDA formation than microsomes treated with LAHP alone at incubation times beyond 10 min. Inclusion of Fe^{3+}- ADP (15 μM Fe^{3+}/4.6 mM ADP) with ascorbate plus LAHP did not significantly increase MDA generation over that observed with ascorbate plus LAHP.

The magnitude of ascorbate stimulation of LAHP-dependent lipid peroxidation increased with increasing incubation times (Figure 1). LAHP/ascorbate treatment yielded MDA values at 60 min in excess of three-fold those obtained using LAHP alone. Minimal differences in the extent of stimulation were observed when the initial concentration of ascorbate was varied from 0.25-1.0 mM. This suggests the linear region of the ascorbate dose-response is at much lower concentrations. Addition of as little as 1 μM LAHP to microsomes plus ascorbate caused an increase in peroxidation above that observed in incubations of microsomes plus ascorbate. The extent of peroxidation appeared to correlate with the square root of hydroperoxide concentration which is typical of radical initiators (33).

Experiments performed with ascorbate and LAHP using Chelex 100-treated buffers to minimize iron contamination exhibited identical time courses to those in Figure 1. Likewise, EDTA only inhibited

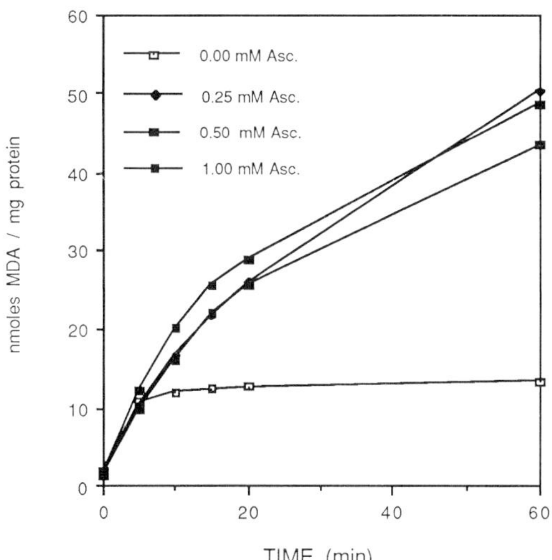

Figure 1. Effect of ascorbate on the time course of LAHP-dependent lipid peroxidation.

LAHP-dependent peroxidation slightly. In contrast, EDTA exhibited a marked inhibitory effect on ascorbate-stimulated microsomal peroxidation by LAHP. The I_{50} for inhibition by EDTA was approximately 1 μM for each hydroperoxide (32).

13-*Cis*-Retinoic Acid.

Preincubation of 13-*cis*-retinoic acid (150 μM) with microsomes virtually abolished ascorbate-dependent lipid peroxidation as measured by the extent of MDA generation (98% reduction). Incubations containing the vehicle DMSO (0.8 %, v/v) were identical to control incubations indicating that the retinoid, and not DMSO, inhibited peroxidation. 13-*Cis*-retinoic acid completely abolished lipid peroxidation at concentrations as low as 25 μM and exhibited an IC_{50} of ~10 μM. By comparison, 10 μM butylated hydroxyanisole inhibited lipid peroxidation completely.

The effect of 13-*cis*-retinoic acid on O_2 uptake associated with lipid peroxidation was determined under conditions that inhibit MDA generation to confirm that the retinoid was actually inhibiting lipid peroxidation and not interfering with the TBA assay. In control incubations, all of the O_2 was depleted after ~ 40 sec. Preincubating 13-*cis*-retinoic acid with microsomes completely inhibited O_2 uptake associated with lipid peroxidation. The absence of O_2 uptake in systems containing retinoid, Fe^{3+}, ADP, and ascorbate but devoid of microsomes indicated that the iron-oxo intermediate responsible for initiation of lipid peroxidation does not react with retinoid allylic C-H bonds via hydrogen atom abstraction.

These results suggested that 13-*cis*-retinoic acid may be inhibiting lipid peroxidation by scavenging chain-propagating peroxyl radicals. Evidence that 13-*cis*-retinoic acid reacts with microsomal unsaturated fatty acid-derived peroxyl radicals was obtained by HPLC analysis of incubation mixtures. Incubating the retinoid with microsomes, ADP-Fe^{3+}, and ascorbate resulted in the generation of several metabolites not observed when 13-*cis*-retinoic acid was incubated with microsomes alone. One of the oxidation products was identified as 5,8-oxy-13-*cis*-retinoic acid. This metabolite cochromatographed with an authentic standard and its uv spectrum exhibited a l_{max} at 303 nm characteristic of the 5,8-oxy metabolite (20,34). The mass spectrum (chemical ionization) of its methyl ester exhibited an M+1 ion of m/e 331 and the parent ion (m/e 330) was the base peak. These as well as fragmentation ions at 315 $(M-CH_3)^+$, 299 $(M-OCH_3)^+$, 271 $(M-CO_2CH_3)^+$, 217, 177, 165, 164, and 135 are characteristic of 5,8-oxy-13-*cis*-methylretinoate (20,34). Generation of this metabolite during lipid peroxidation is consistent with our previous observations that peroxyl radicals epoxidize the 5,6-double bond of 13-*cis*-retinoic acid and that the epoxide readily rearranges to the 5,8-oxy metabolite under the conditions employed in the workup (34,35). Epoxidation of all *trans*-retinoic at the 5,6 position has previously been observed in tissue homogenates under conditions that favor lipid peroxidation (30).

DISCUSSION

Ascorbate-Stimulation of LAHP-Dependent Lipid Peroxidation.

The present study demonstrates that ascorbate exerts a significant prooxidant effect on LAHP-induced lipid peroxidation in rat liver microsomes. The synergistic effect of ascorbate is only evident at times longer than those at which peroxidation by hydroperoxide alone has ceased (10-20 min). At short times, ascorbate appears to have no effect on LAHP-dependent peroxidation. Cytochrome P-450 contributes to LAHP reduction but there appears to be a significant non-enzymatic component that is not inhibited by boiling but is inhibited by EDTA (36).

A likely explanation for the stimulatory effect of ascorbate is that it reacts with metal ions (presumably iron) released during the incubation of hydroperoxide with microsomes. Ascorbate-dependent lipid peroxidation of untreated microsomes at pH < 7 or microsomes supplemented with iron chleates at pH > 7 is known to result from reduction of Fe^{3+} to Fe^{2+}, which then reacts with O_2 to initiate peroxidation (5). In the present experiments, no MDA was produced when intact microsomes were treated with ascorbate in the absence of hydroperoxide. This implies the level of ascorbate-reducible iron (particularly non-heme iron) in microsomes isolated by the present method was too low to initiate peroxidation. Addition of LAHP to liver microsomes is known to partially destroy the heme of cytochrome P-450 (36-38). Heme destruction probably results in iron release into the medium from which it is taken up and complexed to electron-rich sites in the microsomes. At these sites, it can be reduced by ascorbate. Thus, the synergy between hydroperoxides and ascorbate would be the result of hydroperoxide-dependent iron mobilization followed by ascorbate-dependent initiation. Indeed, Wills demonstrated in 1966 that addition of H_2O_2 to rat liver microsomes destroyed their ability to support NADPH-dependent lipid peroxidation but subsequent addition of ascorbate could trigger peroxidation (5). Apparently, a similar mobilization or reorientation of iron can be accomplished by boiling the microsomes prior to treatment with ascorbate. The fact that extremely low EDTA concentrations are sufficient to significantly inhibit MDA formation appears to be an indication of the minute amounts of iron responsible for catalysis. The identity of the iron pool is unknown although recent results point to a possible involvement of cytochrome P-450 or ferritin (36,39).

Figure 2 summarizes our model to explain the synergistic stimulation of peroxidation by ascorbate. Hydroperoxide dependent oxidation of microsomal components renders an undefined pool of microsomal iron reducible by ascorbate. Reduction triggers additional peroxidation of membrane lipids. This model requires hydroperoxide generation to trigger iron mobilization. Although relatively low levels of hydroperoxide trigger peroxidation, non-enzymatic production of lipid hydroperoxides is inhibited by cellular antioxidants (primarily, ascorbate and vitamin E). Thus, one anticipates severe oxidative stress, capable of overwhelming antioxidant defense systems, would be required to generate the hydroperoxide. Adequate levels of hydroperoxide to support peroxidation and iron mobilization are more likely to be produced enzymatically. The enzymes cyclooxygenase and lipoxygenase oxygenate polyunsaturated fatty acids to hydroperoxides in response to a variety of cell stimuli. In contrast to non-enzymatic pathways of hydroperoxide generation, cyclooxygenase and lipoxygenase are not inhibited by ascorbate and vitamin E. In fact, hydroperoxide generation by both enzymes has been shown to result in iron mobilization either from the enzyme (by cyclooxygenase) or cellular respiratory pigments (by lipoxygenase) (40,41). This fulfills the precondition for ascorbate enhancement of lipid peroxidation.

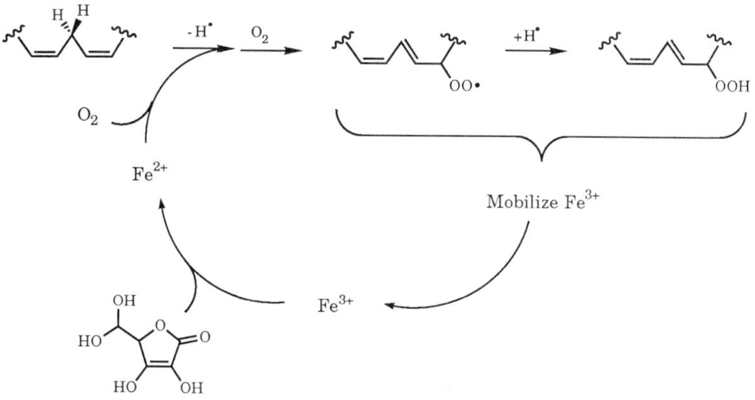

Figure 2. Mechanism of ascorbate stimulation of hydroperoxide-dependent lipid peroxidation

Inhibition of Lipid Peroxidation by 13-*Cis*-Retinoic Acid.

13-*Cis*-retinoic acid appears to be an effective inhibitor of ascorbate-dependent microsomal lipid peroxidation *in vitro* as determined by its effects on MDA generation and O_2 uptake. Evidence for the reaction of the retinoid with unsaturated fatty acid-derived peroxyl radicals is demonstrated by the detection of several retinoid metabolites generated during lipid peroxidation, including 5,8-oxy-13-*cis*-retinoic acid, that were not observed in microsomes alone. Peroxyl radical addition reactions result in formation of the 5,8-oxy metabolite through formation of the 5,6-epoxide (34). Peroxyl radicals may also add to other double bonds of the polyene to generate unidentified metabolites.

If a significant amount of hydrogen atom abstraction by iron-oxo derivatives of iron-ADP or chain-carrying peroxyl radicals had occurred in the present case, the subsequent reaction of the retinoid carbon-centered radical with O_2 to form peroxyl radicals would have enhanced O_2 consumption (prooxidant effect). Its extended polyene chain makes retinoic acid much more reactive to peroxyl radical addition than the isolated double bonds of unsaturated fatty acids (42). This enables lower concentrations of retinoids to deplete the levels of peroxyl radicals which are quantitatively the most significant oxidants present during the propagation phase of lipid peroxidation. The inability of retinoic acid to donate H to peroxyl radicals is consistent with previous observations and suggests its allylic methylene group is less reactive than the bisallylic methylene group of polyunsaturated fatty acids (34).

It is clear that a delicate balance exists between the prooxidant and antioxidant activity of ascorbic acid and 13-*cis*-retinoic acid. Factors such as oxidant nature, membrane composition, iron content, and oxygen tension may determine whether these molecules inhibit or stimulate cellular peroxidation. Their complex pharmacological and toxicological properties may reflect this ambivalence.

ACKNOWLEDGEMENT

This work was supported by a research grant from the National Institutes of Health (CA47479).

REFERENCES

1. Troll, W., and Weisner, R. (1985) Annu. Rev. Pharmacol. Toxicol. 25, 509-528
2. Cerutti, P. (1985) Science 227, 375-381
3. Kensler, T.W., and Taffe, B.G. (1986) Adv. Free Rad. Biol. 2, 347-387
4. Perchellet, J.-P., and Perchellet, E.M. (1988) ISI Atlas of Science: Pharmacology 325-333
5. Wills, E.D. (1966) Biochem. J. 99, 667-676
6. Bendich, A., Machlin, L.J., Scandura, O., Burton, G.W., and Wayner, D.D.M. (1986) Adv. Free Rad. Biol. 2, 419-444
7. Doba, T., Burton, G.W., and Ingold, K.U. (1985) Biochim. Biophys. Acta 835, 298-303
8. Niki, E., Kawakami, A., Yamamoto, Y., and Yamiya, Y. (1985) Bull. Chem. Soc. Jpn. 58, 1971-1975
9. Sadrzadeh, S.M.H., and Eaton, J.W. (1988) J. Clin. Invest. 82, 1510-1515
10. Frei, B., Stocker, R., and Ames, B.N. (1988) Proc. Natl. Acad. Sci. USA 85, 9748-9752
11. Packer, J.E., Slater, T.F., and Willson, R.L. (1979) Nature 278, 737-738
12. Roberts, A.B., and Sporn, M.B. (1984) in The retinoids (Sporn, M.B., Roberts, A.B., and Goodman, D.S., eds) pp. 210-286, Academic Press, New York
13. Peck, G.L., Olsen, T.G., Yoder, F.W., Strauss, J.S., Downing, D.T., Pandya, M., Butkus, D., and Arnaud-Battandier, J. (1979) N. Engl. J. Med. 300, 329-333
14. Bollag, W. (1972) Eur. J. Cancer 8, 689-693
15. Verma, A.K., Rice, H.M., Shapas, B.G., and Boutwell, R.K. (1978) Cancer Res. 38, 793-801
16. Verma, A.K., Shapas, B.G., Rice, H.M., and Boutwell, R.K. (1979) Cancer Res. 39, 419-425
17. Weiss, J.S., Ellis, C.N., Headington, J.T., Tincoff, T., Hamilton, T.A., and Voorhees, J.J. (1988) J. Am. Med. Assn. 259, 527-532
18. Frolik, C.A., Roller, P.P., Roberts, A.B., and Sporn, M.B. (1980) J. Biol. Chem. 255, 8057-8062
19. Vane, F.M., Bugge, J.L., and Williams, T.H. (1982) Drug Metab. Dispos. 253, 7319-7324
20. McCormick, A.M., Napoli, J.L., Schnoes, H.K., and DeLuca, H.F. (1979) Arch. Biochem. Biophys. 192, 577-583
21. Sietsma, W.K., and DeLuca, H.F. (1982) J. Biol. Chem. 257, 4265-4270
22. Marnett, L.J. (1984) in Free Radicals in Biology, Vol 6 (Pryor, W.A., ed) pp. 63-94, Academic Press, New York
23. Eling, T.E., Thompson, D.C., Foureman, G.L., Curtis, J.F., and Hughes, M.F. (1990) Annu. Rev. Pharmacol. Toxicol. 30, 1-45
24. Markey, C.M., Alward, A., Weller, P.E., and Marnett, L.J. (1987) J. Biol. Chem. 262, 6266-6279
25. Tunek, A., Platt, K.L., Bentley, P., and Oesch, F. (1978) Mol. Pharmacol. 14, 920-929
26. Baumgartner, W.A., Baker, N., Hill, V.A., and Wright, E.T. (1975) Lipids 10, 309-311
27. Beuge, J.A., and Aust, S.D. (1978) Methods. Enzymol. 105, 302-311
28. Bull, A.W., and Marnett, L.J. (1985) Anal. Biochem. 149, 284-290
29. Orrenius, S., Dallner, G., and Ernster, L. (1964) Biochem. Biophys. Res. Comm. 14, 329-334
30. Buege, J.A., and Aust, S.D. (1978) Methods. Enzymol. 52, 302-310
31. Hrycay, E., and O'Brien, P.J. (1971) Arch. Biochem. Biophys. 147, 14-27
32. Laudicina, D.C., and Marnett, L.J. (1990) Arch. Biochem. Biophys. 278, 73-80
33. Pryor, W.A. (1966) Free radicals, McGraw-Hill, New York
34. Samokyszyn, V.M., and Marnett, L.J. (1987) J. Biol. Chem. 262, 14119-14133
35. Jungalwala, F.B., and Cama, H.R. (1965) Biochem. J. 95, 17-26
36. O'Brien, P.J., and Rahimtula, A. (1975) J. Agr. Food Chem. 23, 154-158
37. Masuda, Y., and Murano, T. (1978) Jap. J. Pharmacol. 29, 179-186
38. Iba, M.M., and Mannering, G.J. (1987) Mol. Pharmacol. 36, 1447-1455
39. Minotti, G. (1988) Arch. Biochem. Biophys. 268, 398-403
40. Egan, R.W., Paxton, J., and Kuehl, F.A. (1976) J. Biol. Chem. 251, 7329-7335
41. Schewe, T., Albracht, S.P.J., and Ludwig, P. (1981) Biochim. Biophys. Acta 636, 210-217
42. Ingold, K. (1969) Acc. Chem. Res. 2, 1-9

FATTY ACID CYCLOOXYGENASE METABOLISM OF ARACHIDONIC ACID IN HUMAN TUMOR CELLS

W.C. HUBBARD, M.C. ALLEY, T.L. MCLEMORE and M.R. BOYD

Program Development Research Group, Division of Cancer Treatment, National Cancer Institute, Bldg. 560, Rm. 32-60, Frederick, MD 21701-1013

INTRODUCTION

The prostaglandins, leukotrienes and related eicosanoids have been implicated as mediators in human malignant disease, particularly in cellular events related to tumor metastasis, cell proliferation, tumor promotion and host immunoregulation (1-23). There is substantial evidence that human tumor cells may synthesize significant quantities of prostaglandins. Elevated production of prostaglandin E_2 (PGE_2) has been demonstrated in lung cancer patients in vivo (24,25). Other studies have shown that prostanoid biosynthesis is elevated in human tumor tissues in comparison with production in normal human tissues (26-28) and that cultured human tumor cells synthesize significant quantities of prostanoids (29-32). In the present studies, the profiles of prostanoid biosynthesis from endogenous arachidonic acid in 55 established cell lines derived from human tumors of the colon, lung, prostate, ovary, kidney, and the central nervous system were determined. The objective of these studies was the determination of PGH synthase activity in diverse histological classes of human tumor cells in order to discern whether fatty acid cyclooxygenase metabolism of arachidonic acid may be uniquely characteristic of certain histological classes of human tumors.

MATERIALS AND METHODS

The sources of established cell lines derived from human tumors employed in these studies and details of assignment of histological classification of tumors of origin are summarized in a published report (33). Methods for adaptations of established cell lines for culture in a standard culture medium, cell cultivation procedures, experimental protocols, prostanoid identification and quantitation by combined capillary gas chromatography mass spectrometry and sources of reagents and eicosanoid standards are also detailed in published reports (27-31,33).

RESULTS

Prostaglandin H (PGH) synthase activity was determined via summation of the cumulative levels of prostaglandin $F_{2\alpha}$ ($PGF_{2\alpha}$), 9α, 11β-prostaglandin F_2 ($9\alpha,11\beta,PGF_2$), prostaglandin D_2 (PGD_2) prostaglandin E_2 (PGE_2), thromboxane B_2 (TxB_2) and 6-keto-prostaglandin $F_{1\alpha}$ ($6KPGF_{1\alpha}$) synthesized from endogenous arachidonic acid in calcium ionophore A23187-stimulated human tumor cells. Cumulative levels of $PGF_{2\alpha}$, PGE_2 and TXB_2 in 55 human tumor cell lines are summarized in Table 1.

TABLE 1. Prostanoid Biosynthesis From Endogenous Arachidonic Acid In Calcium Ionophore-Stimulated Human Tumor Cells

Histological Classification/ cell line	Prostanoid (pmol/10^6 cells)[a,b]		
	$PGF_{2\alpha}$	PGE_2	TxB_2
LUNG:			
Small cell carcinoma			
NCI-H69 (8)[c]	ND[d]	ND	ND
NCI-H82 (8)	ND	ND	ND
NCI-H128 (6)	ND	ND	ND
NCI-H146 (6)	ND	ND	ND
NCI-H524 (4)	ND	ND	ND
DMS-114 (8)	ND	ND	ND
DMS-187 (7)	ND	ND	ND
DMS-273 (8)	1.3±0.3	0.3±0.1	ND
SHP-77 (4)	ND	ND	ND
Squamous cell carcinoma			
NCI-H520 (4)	ND	ND	ND
SK-MES-1 (6)	ND	ND	ND
Adenosquamous carcinoma			
NCI-H125 (4)	ND	ND	ND
NCI-H647 (4)	9.7±2.4	96.8±11.1	0.4±0.1
Bronchioloalveolar cell carcinoma			
NCI-H322 (8)	0.6±0.2	9.5±3.4	ND
NCI-H358 (8)	0.4±0.1	8.7±2.6	ND
Adenocarcinoma			
EKVX (8)	2.2±0.3	26.2±6.4	ND
NCI-H23 (6)	ND	ND	ND
NCI-H324 (8)	8.3±3.6	24.7±6.7	ND
NCI-H522 (4)	0.4±0.1	0.3±0.1	ND
Calu-3 (8)[e,f,g]	57.3±5.9	26.1±6.2	18.4±5.1
Calu-6 (8)[e]	1.8±0.6	21.1±5.4	1.3±0.4
A549 (8)	16.7±5.7	44.3±6.1	18.8±4.1
A549/Asc-1 (8)	7.1±3.1	31.7±6.2	1.8±0.5
HOP-19 (6)	ND	5.4±1.2	ND
HOP-62 (4)	2.1±0.2	6.7±1.8	ND
Lg. cell undifferentiated carcinoma			
A427 (6)	12.6±4.1	13.3±3.1	ND
NCI-H460 (8)	2.0±0.4	42.2±9.0	ND
HOP-18 (4)	0.8±0.2	13.6±2.4	ND
COLON:			
Colorectal adenocarcinoma			
DLD-1 (4)	ND[d]	ND	ND
SW-620 (4)	ND	ND	ND
COLO 205 (4)	ND	ND	ND
COLO 320 DM (4)	ND	ND	ND
HCT-15 (4)	ND	ND	ND
WiDr (10)[e]	4.1±1.3	4.0±1.1	1.6±0.7

TABLE 1. Continued

Histological Classification/ cell line	Prostanoid (pmol/10^6 cells)[a,b]		
	$PGF_{2\alpha}$	PGE_2	TxB_2
Colorectal carcinoma			
HCC 2998 (4)	ND	ND	ND
HCT 116 (4)	ND	ND	ND
LoVo (4)	0.3±0.1	0.4±0.1	ND
Adenocarcinoma			
HT29 (7)	0.9±0.3	8.6±2.1	ND
OVARY:			
Ovarian adenocarcinoma			
A2780	ND	1.3±0.3	ND
OVCAR4 (4)	ND	ND	ND
OVCAR8 (4)	ND	ND	ND
OVCAR3 (4)	2.3±0.8	1.3±0.5	ND
OVCAR5 (4)	ND	1.1±0.3	ND
PROSTATE:			
Prostate adenocarcinoma			
PC-3 (4)	ND	ND	ND
PC-3M (4)	ND	ND	ND
CNS:			
Glioblastoma			
SNB7 (4)	ND	ND	ND
Glioblastoma astrocytoma			
SNB78 (4)	ND	ND	ND
Medulloblastoma			
TE671 (4)	ND	ND	ND
KIDNEY:			
Renal call carcinoma			
SN12C (4)	ND	ND	ND
SN12S1 (4)	ND	ND	ND
SN12K1 (4)	0.3±0.1	5.3±1.7	ND
CaKi-1 (4)	ND	ND	ND
A498 (4)	ND	ND	ND
UO-31 (4)	ND	ND	ND
Hypernephroma			
RXF 393 (4)	ND	ND	ND

[a]Data are expressed as mean ± SD.
[b]Fifteen-min incubation period.
[c]Numbers in parentheses, number of observations.
[d]ND, not detectable.
[e]Detectable quantities of PGD_2
[f]Detectable quantities of $9\alpha,11\beta\text{-}PGF_2$
[g]Detectable quantities of $6KPGF_{1\alpha}$

Detectable levels of one or more prostanoid species were present in the culture medium of representative cell lines as follows: one of seven cell lines from tumors of renal origin; three of five cell lines from ovarian tumors; three of ten cell lines originating from colon tumors and sixteen of twenty-eight cell lines derived from lung tumors. Detectable levels of prostanoids were not evident in cell lines derived from malignancies of the central nervous system (three cell lines) and the prostate (two cell lines). Prostanoid biosynthesis from endogenous arachidonic acid exceeding 5 pmol/10^6 cells was distributed among the established cell lines as follows: colon tumors (2 of 10 cell lines), renal tumors (1 of 7 cell lines), and lung tumors (14 of 28 cell lines). Incidences of prostanoid biosynthesis > 5 pmol/10^6 cells in cell lines derived from the different histological subclassifications of human lung tumors was as follows: squamous cell carcinoma (0 of 2 cell lines), adenosquamous cell carcinoma (1 of 2 cell lines) large cell undifferentiated carcinoma (3 of 3 cell lines), bronchioloalveolar cell carcinoma (2 of 2 cell lines), adenocarcinoma (8 of 10 cell lines) and small cell carcinoma (0 of 9 cell lines). Thus, prostanoid biosynthesis > 5 pmol/10^6 cells was confined almost exclusively to established cell lines derived from non-small cell carcinomas of the lung.

Significant levels of three different prostanoid species were isolated from human tumor cells exhibiting PGH synthase activity > 5 pmol/10^6 cells. These prostanoids were PGE_2, $PGF_{2\alpha}$ and TxB_2. PGE_2 was the most abundant prostanoid isolated from 13 of 14 cell lines derived from human non-small cell carcinomas of the lung. In addition, PGE_2 levels were higher in HT29 cells (derived from a colon tumor) and in SN12KI cells (derived from a renal tumor). $PGF_{2\alpha}$ levels exceeded PGE_2 levels in one cell line (Calu-3 cells) derived from an adenocarcinoma of the lung. Equal quantities of PGE_2 and $PGF_{2\alpha}$ were isolated from A427 cells (large cell undifferentiated carcinoma of the lung) and WiDr cells (derived from a colon tumor). TxB_2 production > 5 pmol/10^6 cells was evident in two cell lines (Calu-3 and A549; both derived from adenocarcinomas of the lung). Detectable levels of TxB_2 was present in culture medium of three additional cell lines (Calu-6, A549/Asc-1; adenocarcinomas and NCI-H647; adenosquamous carcinoma) derived from lung tumors. TxB_2 was detected in the culture medium of one cell line (WiDr) derived from a colon tumor. $9\alpha,11\beta$-PGF_2, a metabolite of PGD_2, and $6KPGF_{1\alpha}$ reached detectable levels in one cell line (Calu-3). PGD_2 was detected in the culture medium of 3 cell lines, Calu-3, Calu-6 and WiDr.

In summary, studies of fatty acid cyclooxygenase metabolism of arachidonic acid in established cell lines derived from human tumors of the lung, colon, ovary, prostate, kidney and central nervous system indicate that tumor cell lines derived from human non-small carcinomas of the lung exhibit a higher incidence of PGH synthase activity > 5 pmol/10^6 cells. These findings suggest that prostanoid biosynthesis may be characteristic in certain subclassifications of human lung tumors, particularly in non-small carcinomas of the lung.

ACKNOWLEDGEMENTS

The authors wish to express their gratitude to Mr. Glenn Gray for performance of quantitative analysis of prostanoids by combined gas chromatography-mass spectrometry, and to Sheila Testerman and Beverly Bales for preparation and organization of the text of the manuscript.

This project has been funded at least in part with Federal funds from the Department of Health and Human Services under Contract N01-CO-74102. The context of this publication does not necessarily reflect the views or policies of the Department of Health and Human Services, nor does mention of trade names, commercial products, or organizations imply endorsement by the United States Government.

REFERENCES

1. Honn, K.V., Bockmann, R. S. and Marnett, L. J. Prostaglandins, 21: 833-850, 1981 .
2. Rolland, P. H., Martin, P. M., Jacquemier, J., Rolland, A. M. and Toga, M. J. Natl. Cancer Inst., 64: 1061-1070, 1980.
3. Bennett, A., Charlier, E. M., McDonald, E. M., Simpson, J. S., Stanford, I. F. and Zebro, T. Lancet, 2: 624, 1977.
4. Bennett, A. In: Practical Applications of Prostaglandins and Their Synthesis Inhibitors (Ed. S. M. M. Karim), MTP Press, Lancaster, United Kingdom, 1979, pp. 149-188.
5. Bennett, A. In: Endocrinology of Cancer, Vol. 3 (Ed. D. P. Rose), CRC Press, Boca Raton, FL, 1982, pp. 113-126.
6. Honn, K. V., Busse, W. D. and Sloane, B. F. Biochem. Pharmacol ., 32: 1-11, 1983.
7. Sydney, E. and Salmon, M. D. In: Prostaglandins and Cancer: First International Conference (Eds. T. Powles, T. J. Bockman, K. V. Honn and P. Ramwell), Alan R. Liss, New York, 1984, pp. 633-651.
8. Meerpohl, H. G., Bauknecht, T., Tritschler, V. and Lang, H. In: International Workshop: Heterogeneity of Mononuclear Phagocytes (Ed. W. Forster), Academic Press, New York, 1981, pp. 428-461.
9. Walker, C., Kristensen, F., Bettens, F. and DeWeck, A. L. J. Immunol., 130: 1770-1778, 1983.
10. Young, M. R. and Henderson, S. Immunol . Commun., 11: 345-352, 1982.
11. Brunda, M. J., Herberman, R. B. and Holden, H. T. J. Immunol, 124: 2682-2688, 1980.
12. Taffet, S. M. and Russell, S. W. J. Immunol ., 126: 424-432, 1981 .
13. Bresnick, E., Meunier, P. and Lamden, M. Cancer Lett., 7: 121-124, 1979 .
14. Verma, A., Ashendel, C. L. and Boutwell, R. K. Cancer Res., 40: 308-312, 1980.
15. Levine, L. Adv. Cancer Res., 35: 49-52, 1981.
16. Fisher, S. M., Mills, G. D. and Slaga, T. J. Carcinogenesis (Long.), 3: 1243-1250, 1982.
17. Levine, L. In: Prostaglandins and Related Lipids, Vol. 2 (Eds. T. J. Powles, R. S., Bockmann, K. V. Honn and P. W. Ramwell), Alan R. Liss, New York, 1984, pp. 189-205.
18. Furstenberger, G., Gross, M. and Marks, F. In: Prostaglandins and Related Lipids, Vol. 2, (Eds. T. J. Powles, R. S. Bockmann, K. V. Honn and P. W. Ramwell), Alan R. Liss, New York, 1984, pp. 239-251.
19. Fischer, S. M. and Slaga, T. J. In: Prostaglandins and Related Lipids, Vol. 2 (Eds. T. J. Powles, R. S. Bockmann, K. V. Honn and P. W. Ramwell), 1984, pp. 255-261.
20. Fischer, S. M. In: Icosanoids and Cancer (Eds. H. Thaler-Dao, A. Crastes de Paulet and R. Paoletti), Raven Press, New York, 1984, pp. 79-90.
21. Furstenberger, G., Gross, M. and Marks, F. In: Icosanoids and Cancer (Eds. H. Thaler-Dao, A. Crastes de Paulet and R. Paoletti), Raven Press, New York, 1984, pp. 91-100.
22. Kato, R. T., Nakadate, T. and Yamamoto, S. In: Icosanoids and Cancer (Eds. H. Thaler-Dao, A. Crastes de Paulet and R. Paoletti), Raven Press, New York, 1984, pp. 101-114 .
23. Levine, L., Goldstein, S. M., Snoek, G. T. and Rigas, A. In: Icosanoids and Cancer (Eds. H. Thaler-Dao, A. Crastes de Paulet and R. Paoletti (eds.), Raven Press, New York, 1984, pp. 115-121 .
24. Seyberth, H. W., Segre, G. V., Morgan, J. L., Sweetman, B. J., Potts, J. T. and Oates, J. A. N. Engl. J. Med., 293: 1278-1283, 1975.
25. Seyberth, H. W., Segre, B. V., Hamet, P., Sweetman, B. J., Potts, J. T., Jr. and Oates, J. A. Trans. Assoc. Am. Phys., 89: 92-104, 1976.
26. Bennett, A., Carroll, M. A., Stamford, I. F., Whimster, W. F. and Williams, F. Br. J. Cancer, 46: 888-893, 1982.
27. McLemore, T. L., Hubbard, W. C., Litterst, C. L., Liu, M.C., Miller, S., McMahon, N. A., Eggleston, J. C. and Boyd, M. R. Cancer Res., 48: 3140-3147, 1988.

28 . Castelli, M . G ., Ch i abrando, C ., Fanelli, R ., Martelli, Butti, G., Gaetani, P. and Paoletti, P. Cancer Res., 49: 1505-1508, 1989 .
29. Hubbard, W. C., Alley, M. C., McLemore, T. L. and Boyd, M. R. Cancer Res., 48: 2674-2677, 1988.
30 . Hubbard, W . C ., Alley, M . C ., McLemore, T . L . and Boyd, M . R . Cancer Res., 48: 4770-4775, 1988.
31. Hubbard, W. C., Alley, M. C., McLemore, T. L. and Boyd, M. R. Cancer Res., 49: 826-832, 1989.
32. Lau, S. S., McMahon, J. B., McMenamin, M. G. Schuller, H. M. and Boyd, M. R. Cancer Res., 47: 3757-3762, 1987.
33. Alley, M. C., Scudiero, D. A., Monks, A., Hursey, M. L., Czerwinski, M. J., Fine, D. L., Abbott, B. J., Mayo, J. G., Shoemaker, R. H. and Boyd, M. R. Cancer Res., 48: 598-601, 1988 .

IDENTIFICATION OF LINOLEIC ACID METABOLISM AS A COMPONENT OF THE EPIDERMAL GROWTH FACTOR SIGNAL TRANSDUCTION PATHWAY IN BALB/c 3T3 FIBROBLASTS

T. E. ELING and W. C. GLASGOW

Laboratory of Molecular Biophysics, National Institute of Environmental Health Sciences, Research Triangle Park, North Carolina 27709

INTRODUCTION

Polypeptide mitogens like epidermal growth factor (EGF) and platelet-derived growth factor (PDGF) stimulate quiescent cell cultures to initiate DNA synthesis and cell division. The mitogenic signal is activated via binding of the growth factor to specific high affinity cell surface receptors and elicits a variety of biochemical changes in the cell including activation of arachidonic acid metabolism (1-7).

We are interested in examining the role of lipid metabolism in the mitogenic response of BALB/c 3T3 cells to EGF. BALB/c 3T3 fibroblasts arrested at subconfluence by serum-depletion are induced by EGF to initiate cell cycle traversal. Our laboratory recently (7) reported that EGF-stimulated BALB/c 3T3 cells to release and then convert arachidonic acid into metabolites that act as important intracellular mediators of the mitogenic signal (1). PGE_2 was the major arachidonic acid metabolite. Indomethacin inhibited EGF dependent mitogenesis but the addition of prostaglandins restored mitogenesis. In these studies, lipoxygenase inhibitors were particularly effective. However, only low levels of lipoxygenase-derived arachidonate metabolites were detected. Since linoleic acid is often a major lipid component of biological membranes and is an excellent substrate for many lipoxygenases, we decided to study the effects of EGF on linoleic acid metabolism in BALB/c 3T3 fibroblasts.

We report here that EGF treatment of quiescent BALB/c 3T3 cells stimulates lipoxygenase-mediated oxygenation of linoleic acid 13-hydroxyoctadecadienoic acid (See Figure 1) and these mono-hydroxy linoleate derivatives are very active in potentiating EGF-induced DNA synthesis.

RESULTS and DISCUSSION

EGF stimulated metabolism of linoleic acid.

Quiescent BALB/c 3T3 fibroblasts were incubated with exogenous [^{14}C] linoleic acid (10 μM) and epidermal growth factor (10 ng/ml) for 4 hours. Reverse-phase HPLC analysis of incubation mixture extracts revealed that EGF stimulated the conversion of [^{14}C]-linoleic acid to product(s) which coeluted with authentic standards of 13-hydroxyoctadecadienoic acid (13-HODD) and 9-hydroxyoctadecadienoic acid (9-HODD). However, in the absence of EGF, no metabolites of linoleic acid were detected.

The formation of hydroxy linoleic acid products in EGF-stimulated BALB/c 3T3 cells was suppressed > 95% by the lipoxygenase inhibitors ETYA and NDGA. The cyclooxygenase inhibitor indomethacin (10 μM) did not block EGF-induced linoleate metabolism. These results suggest that the product(s) are formed via lipoxygenase-like reactions.

Identification of linoleic acid metabolites.

To further characterize the linoleate compound(s) formed in EGF-stimulated BALB/c 3T3 cells, the material eluting as the HODD fraction was collected for further analysis. On straight phase HPLC, the cellular product eluted as a major peak of radioactivity which co-chromatographed with 13-HODD standard and a minor fraction (10-15%) coeluting with a standard of 9-HODD. Ultraviolet spectrophotometric analysis of the material isolated from SP-HPLC showed an absorption band with λ_{max} 235 nm in methanol. Each purified compound and its corresponding reduced analogue was derivatized as the methyl ester trimethylsilyl ether and subsequently analyzed by electron impact (EI) gas chromatography-mass spectrometry (GC-MS). The combined information obtained from chromatographic, UV, and GC-MS analyses provide rigorous evidence that the isolated linoleic oxygenation products of BALB/c 3T3 cells are 13-hydroxyoctadeca-9, 11-(Z,E)-dienoic acid and 9-hydroxyoctadeca-10, 12-(E-Z)-dienoic acid, with the 13-HODD being the major product.

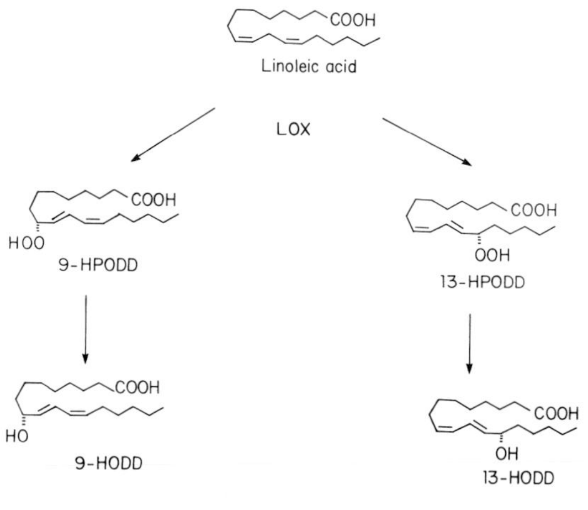

COOH
Linoleic acid
LOX
COOH
HOO
9-HPODD
COOH
OOH
13-HPODD
COOH
HO
9-HODD
COOH
OH
13-HODD

Figure 1. Linoleic acid metabolism in BALB/c 3T3 cells.

Compound + EGF (10 ng/ml)		$[^3H]$ Thymidine Incorporation (expressed as % of EGF response)
9-HPODD	10^{-8} M	160 ± 15
9-HPODD	10^{-7}M	150 ± 7
9-HPODD	10^{-6}M	185 ± 6
9 HODD	10^{-8}M	130 ± 4
9-HODD	10^{-7}M	135 ± 2
9-HODD	10^{-6}M	195 ± 5
13-HPODD	10^{-8} M	255 ± 5
13-HPODD	10^{-7}M	275 ± 15
13-HPODD	10^{-6}M	330 ± 10
13-HODD	10^{-8} M	280 ± 3
13-HODD	10^{-7}M	330 ± 4
13-HODD	10^{-6}M	300 ± 10
PGG_2	10^{-8} M	100 ± 8
PGG_2	10^{-7}M	110 ± 5
PGG_2	10^{-6}M	275 ± 10
PGH_2	10^{-8} M	100 ± 5
PGH_2	10^{-7}M	100 ± 5
PGH_2	10^{-6}M	275 ± 10
$PGF_{2\alpha}$	10^{-8} M	300 ± 10
$PGF_{2\alpha}$	10^{-7}M	370 ± 40
$PGF_{2\alpha}$	10^{-6}M	450 ± 30
PGE_2	10^{-8} M	95 ± 4
PGE_2	10^{-7}M	98 ± 3
PGE_2	10^{-6}M	140 ± 5
PGD_2	10^{-8} M	96 ± 3
PGD_2	10^{-7}M	95 ± 3
PGD_2	10^{-6}M	100 ± 8

Table I.

Effects of Linoleic and Arachidonic Acid Metabolites on EGF-induced DNA Synthesis in BALB/c 3T3 Cells. Cells were grown to near confluence in 96-well plates and then were serum-depleted for 16 hours. Test compounds and EGF were added simultaneously and DNA synthesis was measured by $[^3H]$ thymidine incorporation after 24 hours. Data (mean ± standard deviation, five determinations) are expressed relative to stimulation by EGF alone (designated 100% = 30,000 DPM).

Effects of linoleic acid and arachidonic acid metabolites on mitogensis in BALB/c 3T3 cells.

The effects of EGF and linoleic acid and arachidonic acid metabolites on DNA synthesis in BALB/c 3T3 fibroblasts were assessed by measuring incorporation of radioactive thymidine into trichloroacetic acid-insoluble material after 24 hrs.

After identifying lipoxygenase metabolites of linoleic acid as products of EGF-stimulated BALB/c 3T3 cells, we were interested in testing the activity of these compounds (both the alcohols and their hydroperoxy precursors) in promoting EGF-dependent-DNA synthesis. When the linoleate metabolites and prostaglindins were added alone to quiescent BALB/c 3T3 cells, they stimulated [^{3}H] thymidine incorporation to a very small extent. However, when added in the presence of EGF, these compounds greatly potentiated the growth factor induced cellular response. 9-HPODD and 9-HODD were able to act synergistically with EGF and double the amount of [^{3}H] thymidine incorporated at a concentration of 10^{-6}M (Table 1). The primary linoleate metabolites, 13-HPODD and 13-HODD, displayed an even more dramatic response. The hydroperoxy compound, 13-HPODD, stimulated a 3-fold increase in EGF-dependent DNA synthesis at concentrations as low as 10^{-10}M. Likewise, 13-HODD at 10^{-7}M produced a 3-4 fold potentiation of the EGF response. With the exception of $PGF_{2\alpha}$, prostaglandins were less potent than the linoleic acid metabolites in stimulating EGF dependent DNA synthesis.

These studies indicate that the oxidation of linoleic acid to 9- and 13-H(P)ODD is required for the stimulation of DNA synthesis in BALB/c 3T3 cells in response to the growth factor EGF.

Future studies will focus on the mechanism involved in the EGF-stimulation of linoleic acid metabolism and the biochemical processes involved in the stimulation of DNA synthesis by these lipids.

REFERENCES

1. Carpenter,G., King,L.,Jr., and Cohen,S. (1979) J. Biol. Chem. 254, 4884-4891.
2. Shier,W.T. (1980) Proc. Natl. Acad. Sci. U.S.A. 77, 137-141.
3. Habenicht,A.J.R., Glomset,J.A., King,W.C., Nist,C., Mitchell,C.D., and Ross,R. (1981) J. Biol. Chem. 256, 12329-12335.
4. Shier,W.T., and Durkin,J.P. (1982) J. Cell Physiol. 112, 171-181.
5. Habenicht,A.J.R., Georig,M., Grulich,J., Roth,D., Gronwald,R., Loth,U., Schettler,G., Kommerell,B., and Ross,R. (1985) J. Clin. Invest. 75, 1381-1387.
6. Habenicht,A.J.R., Glomset,J.A., Goerig,M., Gronwald,R., Grulich,J., Loth,U., and Schettler,G. (1985) J. Biol. Chem. 260, 1370-1373.
7. Nolan,R.D., Danilowicz,R.M., and Eling,T.E. (1988) Mol. Pharm. 33, 650-656.

LOCALIZATION AND EXPRESSION OF THE EICOSANOID METABOLIZING P4501VA GENE FAMILY IN RAT TISSUES AND HEPATIC TUMORS

J. P. HARDWICK[1,2], J. J. RUSSELL[1], S. KIMURA[3], F. J. GONZALEZ[3], J. K. REDDY[4], C. PERAINO[1], and E. HUBERMAN[1]

[1]Biological and Medical Division, Argonne National Laboratories, Argonne, IL, 60439; [2]Northeastern Ohio Universities College of Medicine, 4209 S.R. 44, Rootstown, Ohio 44272; [3]Laboratory of Molecular Carcinogenesis, National Cancer Institute, NIH, Bethesda, MD 20892; [4]Dept. of Pathology, Northwestern University Medical School, 303 E. Chicago Avenue, Chicago, IL 60611

INTRODUCTION

The ω-P450 hydroxylase (1VA1-CYP4A) is an eukaryotic gene family(1,2) whose members hydroxylate physiological compounds such as saturated fatty acids, cholesterol, arachidonic acid, leukotrienes and prostaglandins (2,3). Three genes of the rat 1VA gene family have been characterized and shown to be induced by tumor-promoting hypolipidemic drugs (2,3). The physiological function of the ω-oxidized products remains largely undefined. However, the existence of specific P450 isozymes to metabolize these substrates suggests that their induction by tumor promotors may be instrumental in altering the level of autocrine and paracrine mediators of cell growth and differentiation during the development of neoplasia.

Hepotocarcinogenesis induced by various carcinogens results in the development of cellular nodules (CN), resistant to carcinogen cytotoxicity, and eventually the development of heptocellular carcinoma (HCC)(4,5). These lesions display a number of functional, morphological, and biochemical abnormalities (5). A decrease in the amount of carcinogen activating enzymes (phase I), such as, cytochrome P450, have been demonstrated in HCC and CN lesions whereas the detoxification enzymes are significantly elevated (5,6). The mechanism of resistance of hepatocyte nodules to hepatocarcinogens and hepatotoxins appears to be due to a repression in the carcino-gene activating cytochrome P450 isozymes, an increase in the detoxification conjugation enzymes, and a decreased uptake of the carcinogen (4,5,7).

In the present study, we examined the localization and expression of the P4501VA genes in liver and kidney of rats, that were given the hypolipidemic tumor promotor, clofibrate. We also determined the expression of these P450 isozymes in rat tumors produced with complete carcinogen or by a two stage initiation promotor protocol (4). The results of this study indicated that the 1VA gene family members were localized in all zones of the hepatic lobule and induced in the periportal region in rats that were given clofibrate. These genes were also expressed in the proximal and convoluted tubules of the kidney. Both P4501VA1 and 1VA3 are isozymes of the liver while P4501VA2 is a constitutive P450 of the kidney. In hepatic tumors, the expression of the 1VA genes was depressed. Northern and Western immunoblot analysis indicated that a fetal P450 ω-hydroxylase was expressed in these tumors.

MATERIALS AND METHODS

Induction of liver tumors.

Hepatocellular carcinomas were induced in F-344 rats by feeding 0.025% ciprofibrate (RLC), 2-acetylaminofluorene (2-AAF), or 2ppm of aflatoxin (AF) for a period of 30-50 weeks as described (6). The diethylnitrosamine (DEN), phenobarbital (PB), hepatocellular tumors were developed by the two-stage Peraino neonatal induction protocol (7). Transplantable tumors were serially transplanted in weanling F-344 rats every 4-5 weeks (6).

Immunohistochemistry and In Situ hybridization.

Portions of primary and transplantable tumors were frozen at -70°C, and 5μm cryostatic sections were placed on silanized slides then fixed for 1 h with 4% paraformaldehyde and 5mM $MgCl_2$ containing phosphate buffered saline. Sections were incubated with P4501VA antibodies (2). The tissue P4501VA levels were determined by the streptavidin-biotin peroxidase complex. In situ hybridization was performed with a 5' Taq1 200bp fragment of 1VA1, and 14 mer oligonucleotides to 1VA2 and 1VA3 (2,3). DNA probes were tailed with [^{35}S] dATP and hybridized to proteinase K digested tissue sections.

Northern RNA and Western Immunoblot Analysis.

Total RNA isolated by the quanidinium thiocyanate extraction was analyzed by Northern blot analysis as described previously (2). Western immunoblots were performed with microsomes from tumor and liver as described (2), except that the antibody-antigen complexes were visualized by the streptavidin-biotin immunoperoxidase method with 4-chloro-1-napthol used as the chromogenic reagent.

RESULTS

Localization of P4501VA gene family members in liver and kidney.

By immunohistochemical methods, we determined that the P4501VA gene family members were found throughout all zones of the hepatic lobule with a greater concentration at the portal triad. The periportal location of the IVA antigen is apparent in liver of clofibrate-treated rats (Figure 1A-arrow).

P4501VA is localized at the brush border of the proximal tubules of the kidney. Clofibrate treatment results in an intense staining of both the proximal and distal convoluted tubules with P4501VA antibody in the kidney (Figure 1B-arrow). Because of their 70-80% amino acid similarity, the antibody used in this study cross-reacts with all members of the 1VA gene family, therefore, it was necessary to use sequence specific oligonucleotides to determine whether there is a differential expression of these genes in the liver. Both 1VA1 and 1VA3 mRNA is found in all zones of the hepatic lobule, but similar to the immunochemical data, an increased expression of these genes were found in the periportal region (Figure 2A). P4501VA2 mRNA was not found in control liver but was present in liver of clofibrate treated rats. All three 1VA mRNAs were induced in the periportal region of the liver upon clofibrate

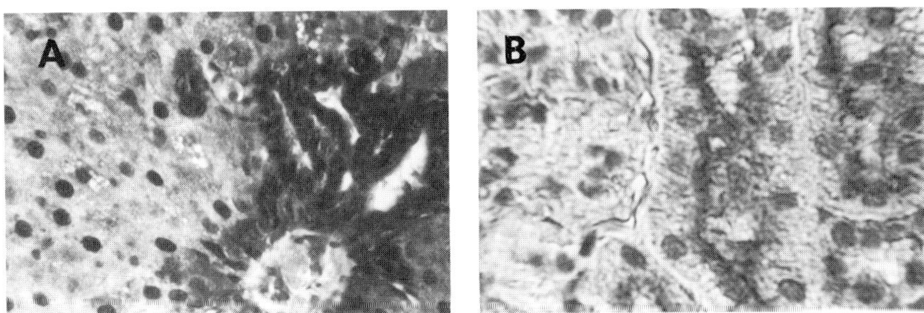

Figure 1. Immunohistochemical localization of P4501VA in liver (A) and kidney (B) of clofibrate treated rats.

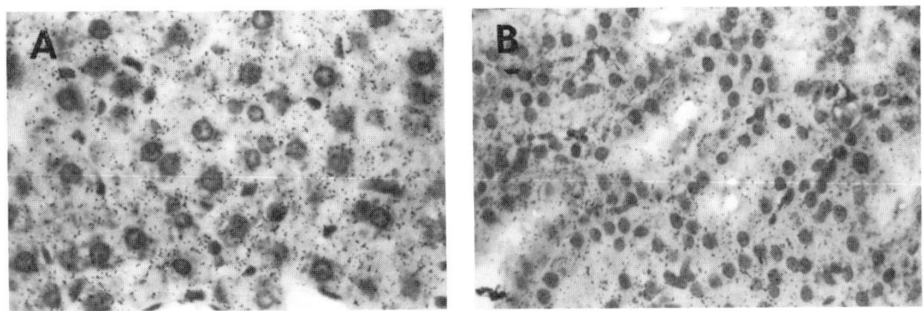

Figure 2. Localization of P4501VA1 mRNA in (A) Liver and (B) Kidney of Clofibrate Administered Rats.

administration. Hybridization of kidney sections revealed that 1VA2 is a constitutive P450 isozyme localized in the medullary tubules. After clofibrate administration, the level of both 1VA1 and 1VA3 mRNA, are mainly localized in the proximal and convoluted tubules (Figure 2B).

Expression of P4501VA genes in hepatocellular tumors.

In hepatocellular tumors, the cellular expression of the P4501VA gene family members was determined by in situ hybridization. P4501VA1 was detected in 2-AAF induced HCC and localized in fibroid and oval cells, as well as in the membranous connective tissue (Figure 3). Both P4501VA1 and

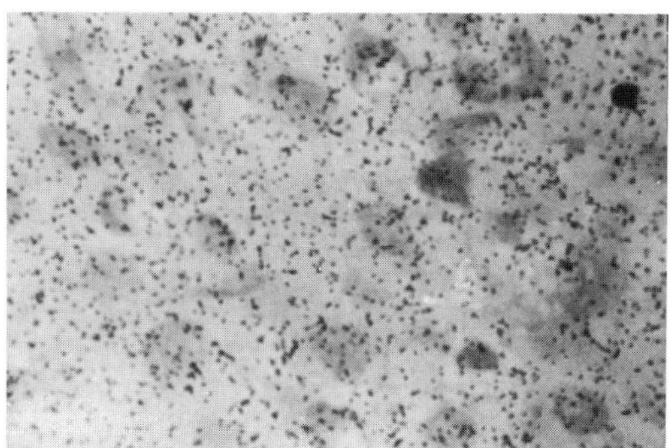

Figure 3. P4501VA1 Expression of 2-AAF Induced Tumors

1VA3 mRNA was detected in all tumors, while 1VA2 mRNA was a minor species. Because most of the probe's activity is associated with the connective tissue of the tumors, it is uncertain whether these species are differentially expressed in these tumors. Northern blot analysis of the total RNA extracted from tumors with 1VA2 and 1VA3 oligonucleotide probes hybridized under high stringency indicates that the expression of these genes was not induced (Figure 4). Hybridizations performed with the complete cDNA of P4501VA1 under high stringency show that the expression of this gene was also reduced. However, under relaxed hybridization conditions, a RNA sequence similar to the P4501VA gene family was expressed (Figure 4). The molecular weight of the mRNA expressed in these tumors is similar to that of other P4501VA gene family members. To determine whether a related P450 is expressed in these tumors, Western immunoblot analysis was performed on the microsomes. A new immunochemically reactive band was detected in tumor and fetal liver microsome. This fetal P450 ω-

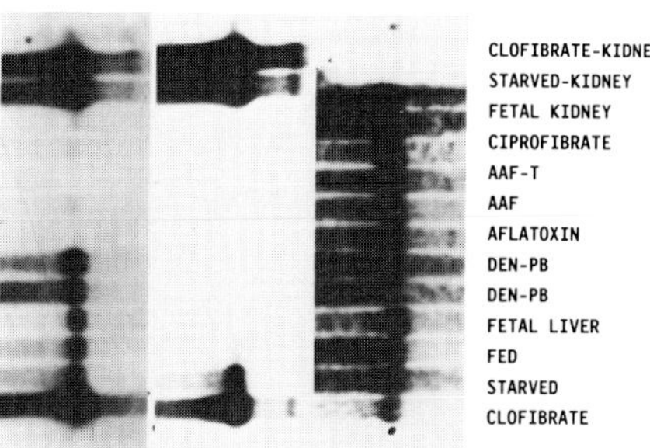

Figure 4. Northern Blot Analysis of Tumors

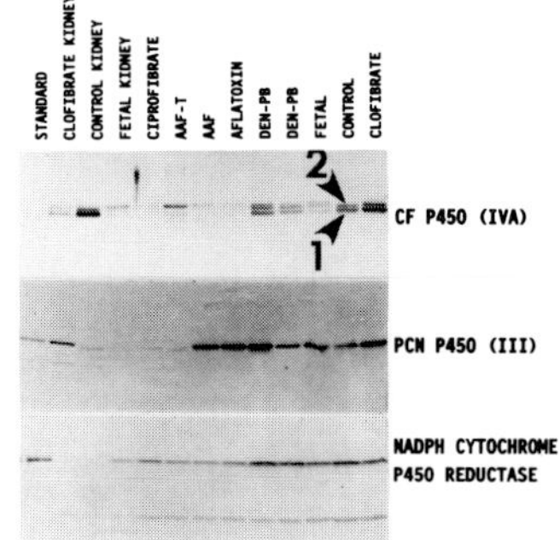

Figure 5. Western Immunoblot Analysis of Tumors

hydroxylase was not detected in microsomes from control rats, nor from those treated with clofibrate for less than one week. However, this P450 was found in microsomes from rats given clofibrate for one week (Figure 5) and in tumors produced with 2-AAF, AF clofibrate, AF, ciprofibrate or DEN-PB. The reduced expression of P4501VA1 (Figure 5, arrow one) and P4501VA3 (Figure 5, arrow two) supports the hypothesis that many P450 isozymes are depressed in HCC (5,8). The expression of the fetal ω-hydroxylase in tumors produced by 2-AAF, AF, ciprofibrate, or the DEN-PB protocol implies that this P450 plays a role in the development of hepatic tumors. The substrate specificity of this fetal P450 is not known at present. However, we believe that this species may play a role in cell growth because its level of expression in transplantable 2-AAF tumors is elevated (Figure 5). We assumed that this P450 is the eicosanoid metabolizing prostaglandin omega hydroxylase. Alterations in the level of eicosanoids by specific cytochrome P450 isozymes may function in the control of growth and differentiation in normal and malignant cells.

ACKNOWLEDGMENT

This work was supported in part by the United States Department of Energy, Office of Health and Environmental Research, under Contract W-31-109-ENG-38 and a grant to James P. Hardwick from the ILSI Research Foundation.

REFERENCES

1. Gonzales, F.J., Pharmacol. Rev. 40:243-288, 1989.
2. Hardwick, J.P., Song, B.J., Huberman, E., and Gonzalez, F.J. J. Biol. Chem. 262:801-810, 1987.
3. Kimura, S., Hardwick, J.P., Kozak, C.A., and Gonzalez, F.J., DNA. 8: 517-525, 1989.
4. Peraino, C. and Jones, C.A. In: The Pathobiology of Neoplasia (Eds. A.E. Sirica), Plenum Press, N.Y., 1989, pp. 131-148.
5. Roomi, M.W., Ho, R.K., Sarma, D.S.R. and Farber, E. Cancer Res. 45:564-571, 1985.
6. Rao, M.S., Nemali, M.R., Usuda, N., Scarpelli, D.G., Makino, T., Pitot, H., and Reddy, J.K. Cancer Res. 48:4919-4925, 1988.
7. Peraino, C., Richards, W.L., and Stevens, F.J. In: Mechanisms of Tumor Promotion, Vol. 1 (Eds. T.J. Slaga), CRC Press, Boca Raton, Florida. 1983. pp. 91-105.
8. Roomi, M.W., Bacher, M.A., Gibson, G.G., Parke, D.V., and Farber, E. Biochem. Biophys. Res. Comm. 152:921-925, 1987.

DEFICIENT LIPOXIN FORMATION IN CHRONIC MYELOGENOUS LEUKEMIA

J. Å. LINDGREN, C. EDENIUS and L. STENKE

Department of Physiological Chemistry, Karolinska Institutet, Box 60400, S-104 01 Stockholm, Sweden

INTRODUCTION

Recently, we reported formation of lipoxins from endogenous substrate, via platelet-dependent lipoxygenation of granulocyte-derived leukotriene (LT)A_4 (1). Furthermore, human platelet suspensions transformed synthetic LTA_4 to lipoxins. The platelets also efficiently converted LTA_4 to cysteinyl-containing leukotrienes (2).

The lipoxins are biologically active trihydroxylated derivatives of arachidonic acid (3). Lipoxin (LX)A_4 (5(S),6(R),15(S)-trihydroxy-7,9,13-*trans*-11-*cis*-eicosa-tetraenoic acid) and LXB_4 (5(S),14(R),15(S)-trihydroxy-6,10,12-*trans*-8-*cis*-eicosatetraenoic acid) possess biological activities such as bronchoconstriction, vasodilation and stimulation of protein kinase C, and inhibit natural killer cell cytotoxicity and chemokinesis of human neutrophils (3-7). Furthermore, LXA_4 induce prostacyclin synthesis and formation of thromboxane A_2 (8,9). Lipoxin B_4 was recently reported to stimulate colony-forming ability of human peripheral mononuclear cells (10).

Since human platelets possess only one major lipoxygenase activity, a role of the 12-lipoxygenase in platelet-dependent lipoxin formation was suspected. Platelet 12-lipoxygenase deficiency has been reported in patients with chronic myelogenous leukemia (CML) and other myelo-proliferative disorders (11-13). It was therefore of interest to investigate transcellular lipoxin formation in granulocytes and platelets from patients with CML. The present findings demonstrate, that 12-lipoxygenase deficient platelets from three different patients with this neoplastic disorder were unable to convert exogenous or granulocyte-derived LTA_4 to lipoxins (14) .

METHODS

Preparation of platelet and granulocyte suspensions from peripheral human blood, incubation of cell suspensions, sample purification, lipoxygenase product determination using reversed-phase high-performance liquid chromatography (RP-HPLC), gas chromatography-mass spectrometry (GC/MS) and radioimmunological determination of thromboxane B_2 were carried out as described (1,2,14) .

RESULTS

Platelet suspensions from three different CML-patients did not produce measurable amounts of 12-HETE after stimulation with arachidonic acid (75-150 μM), while the cyclooxygenase product hydroxyheptadecatrienoic acid (HHT) was formed in amounts comparable to those detected in control incubations (Figure 1). Furthermore, platelets from these patients also produced thromboxane B_2 upon arachidonic acid stimulation. The results indicated a deficient 12-lipoxygenase but an intact cyclooxygenase activity.

Pure granulocyte suspensions from one of the 12-lipoxygenase deficient patients produced both 5- and 15-HETE (6.9 nmol/ml and 692 pmol/ml, respectively) as well as leukotrienes B_4 and C_4 after stimulation with ionophore (1 μM) and arachidonic acid (50 μM) (results not shown).

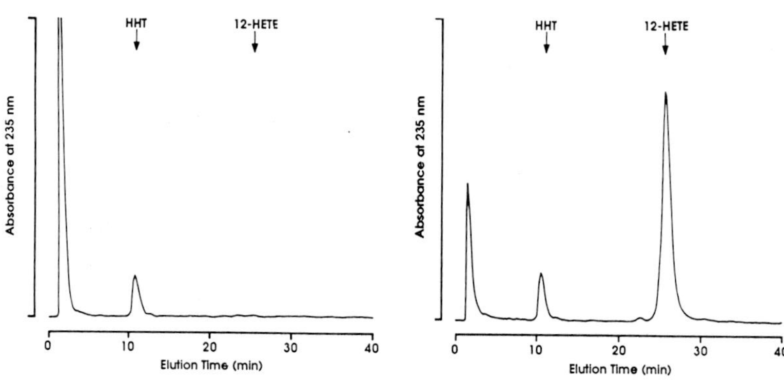

Figure 1. RP-HPLC chromatogram of HETEs formed after arachidonic acid stimulation (150 μM, 30 min, 37°C) of platelet suspensions from a CML patient (left panel) and a normal healthy donor (right panel).

Suspensions of mixed platelets/granulocytes (30:1) from the patients did not form significant amounts of lipoxins after stimulation with ionophore A23187 (1 μM; Figure 2B). In addition, no 5(S),12(S)-DHETE production could be observed (results not shown), further supporting the lack of 12-lipoxygenase activity. In comparison, mixed platelet/granulocyte suspensions from healthy donors stimulated with ionophore A23187 produced lipoxin A_4, lipoxin B_4 and several lipoxin isomers including two compounds coeluting with 11-trans-LXA_4 and 8-trans-LXB_4 (Figure 2A). All compounds showed typical UV-spectra of conjugated tetraenes. The amounts formed were 134 ± 45 and 88 ± 26 pmol/ml of LXA_4 and LXB_4 (mean ± S.D.; n=5), respectively. When granulocytes from one of the three patients were mixed with platelets from a normal healthy donor and stimulated with ionophore A23187, lipoxin formation was restored (Figure 2C). Neither cell type alone, derived from patients or healthy donors produced detectable amounts of lipoxins after ionophore A23187-stimulation.

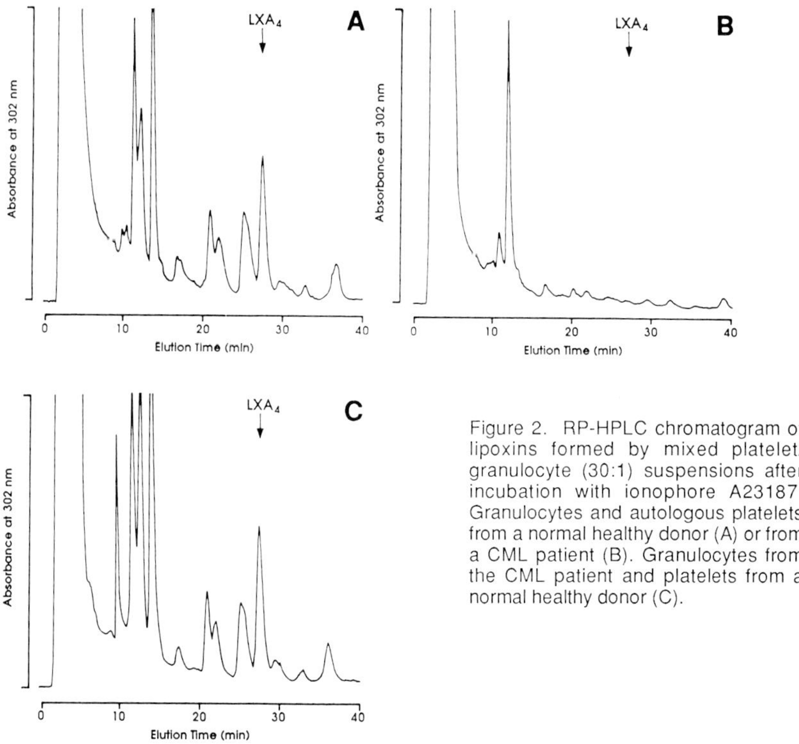

Figure 2. RP-HPLC chromatogram of lipoxins formed by mixed platelet/ granulocyte (30:1) suspensions after incubation with ionophore A23187. Granulocytes and autologous platelets from a normal healthy donor (A) or from a CML patient (B). Granulocytes from the CML patient and platelets from a normal healthy donor (C).

No detectable amounts of lipoxins were formed when pure platelet suspensions from the CML patients were incubated with exogenous LTA_4 (4 or 20 μM) in the presence of ionophore A23187 (1 μM). In parallell control incubations with platelets from healthy volunteers, normal levels of LXA_4 were formed (cf 1).

DISCUSSION

Certain patients with chronic myelogeneous leukemia (CML) lack or have a decreased platelet 12-lipoxygenase activity (11-13). However, the pathophysiological relevance of these findings has been questioned, since the biological role of the 12-lipoxygenase is uncertain. This enzyme efficiently transform arachidonic acid to 12-hydroperoxy-eicosatetraenoic acid (12-HPETE), which is enzymatically or non-enzymatically reduced to 12-hydroxy-eicosatetraenoic acid (12-HETE) (15). Furthermore, human platelets produce leukotriene-like dihydroxy-eicosatetraenoic acids via the 12-lipoxygenase pathway (16). This lipoxygenase is also involved in interactions between platelets and neutrophils leading to formation of unique lipoxygenase products, such as 5(S),12(S)-DHETE (17,18) and 5(S),20-DHETE (19). Although 12-HPETE has been reported to stimulate leukotriene formation in leukocytes (20), the biological significance of the 12-lipoxygenase products is unclear.

A novel role for the 12-lipoxygenase was suggested by our findings of platelet-dependent lipoxygenation of granulocyte-derived LTA_4 leading to formation of the biologically active lipoxins from endogenous pools of arachidonic acid (1). Involvement of 12-lipoxygenase in lipoxin formation was further indicated by the present results obtained with 12-lipoxygenase deficient platelets derived from chronic myelogenous leukemia patients. These platelets were unable to produce 12-HETE after stimulation with arachidonic acid, confirming the 12-lipoxygenase deficiency. In contrast, CML-granulocytes possessed 5- and 15-lipoxygenase activities, indicated by the formation of 5-HETE and 15-HETE as well as leukotrienes C_4 and B_4. Mixed platelet/granulocyte suspensions from the patients did not produce measurable amounts of lipoxins nor was the double dioxygenation product 5(S),12(S)-DHETE formed after ionophore stimulation. However, when CML-granulocytes were mixed with normal platelets from a healthy donor the formation of lipoxins was normalized, demonstrating a normal release of LTA_4 from these granulocytes (1). The abnormality of the 12-lipoxygenase deficient platelets was further indicated by the inability of these cells to transform exogenous LTA_4 to lipoxins.

White blood cells and platelets from CML patients have been reported to be functionally defect in many respects (12,13,21-23). We have recently reported increased leukotriene C_4 production in leukocytes from these patients (24). The present findings demonstrate an inability of CML platelets to participate in lipoxin formation. Since this dysfunction parallells a deficient 12-lipoxygenase activity, the results further indicates a role of the 12-lipoxygenase in lipoxin synthesis. Although lipoxins have been reported to influence myelopoiesis (10), the pathophysiological relevance of the present findings needs to be further elucidated.

ACKNOWLEDGEMENTS

We thank Ms. Inger Forsberg and Ms. Barbro Nasman-Glaser for excellent technical assistance. This project was supported by the Swedish Cancer Society, the Swedish National Association against Heart and Lung Diseases, the Swedish Medical Research Council and the Reseach Funds of the Karolinska Institute.

REFERENCES

1. Edenius, C., Haeggstrom, J. and Lindgren, J.Å (1988) Biochem. Biophys. Res. Commun. 157, 801-807.
2. Edenius, C., Heidvall, K. and Lindgren, J.Å (1988) Eur. J. Biochem. 178, 81-86.
3. Serhan, C.N., Hamberg, M. and Samuelsson, B. (1984) Proc. Natl. Acad. Sci. 81, 5335-5339.
4. Samuelsson, B., Dahlen, S.-E., Lindgren, J.Å, Rouzer, C.A. and Serhan, C.N. (1987) Science 220, 568-575.
5. Dahlen, S.-E., Franzen, L., Raud, J., Serhan, C.N., Westlund, P., Wikstrom, E., Bjork, T., Matsuda,

5. H. Webber, S.E., Veale, C.A., Puustinen, T. and Samuelsson, B. (1988) In Adv. in Exp. Med. and Biol.: Lipoxins (P. Y.-K. Wong and C. N. Serhan, Eds), Vol. 229, pp. 107-130. Plenum Press, New York.
6. Lefer, A.M., Stahl, G.L., Lefer, D.J., Brezinski, M., Nicolaou, K.C., Veale, C.A., Abe, Y. and Smith, J. (1988) Proc. Natl. Acad. Sci.(USA) 85, 8340-8344.
7. Busija, D.W., Armstead, W., Leffler, C.W. and Mirro, R. (1989) Am. J. Physiol. 256, 468-471.
8. Brezinski, M.E., Gimbrone Jr, M.A., Nicolaou, K.C. and Serhan, C.N. (1989) FEBS Lett, 245, 67-172.
9. Wikstrom, E., Westlund, P., Nicolaou, K. C. and Dahlen, S.-E.(1989) Agents and Actions, 26, 90-92.
10. Popov, G.K., Nekrasov, A.S., Khshivo, A.L., Pochinskii, A.G., Lankin, V.Z. and Vikhert, A.M. (1989) Bull. Exp. Biol. Med. 107, 93-96.
11. Okuma, M. and Uchino, H. (1979) Blood 54, 1258-1271.
12. Schafer, A.(1982) N. Engl. J. Med. 306, 381-386.
13. Stenke, L., Lauren, L., Reizenstein, P. and Lindgren. J.Å. (1987) Exp. Hematol. 15, 203-207.
14. Edenius, C., Stenke, L. and Lindgren, J.Å (1989) Submitted.
15. Hamberg, M. and Samuelsson, B. (1974) Proc. Natl. Acad. Sci.(USA) 71, 3400-3404.
16. Westlund, P., Edenius, C. and Lindgren, J.Å (1988) Biochim. Biophys. Acta. 962, 105-115.
17. Lindgren, J.Å, Hansson, G. and Samuelsson, B. (1981) FEBS Lett. 128, 329-335.
18. Borgeat, P., Fruteau de Laclos, B., Picard, S., Drapeau, J., Valler, P. and Corey, E.J. (1982) Prostaglandins 23, 713-724.
19. Marcus, A.J., Safier, L.B., Ullman, H.L., Broeckman, M.J., Islam, N.,Oglesby, T.D. and Gorman, R.R. (1984) Proc. Natl. Acad. Sci. (USA) 81, 903-907.
20. Maclouf, J., Fruteau de Laclos, B. and Borgeat, P. (1982) Proc. Natl. Acad. Sci. (USA) 79, 6042-6046.
21. El Hallem, H., Fletcher, J. (1979) Br. J. Hematol. 41, 49-55.
22. Anklesaria, P.N., Advani, S.H., Bhisey, A.N. (1985) Leuk. Res. 9, 641-648.
23. Okuma, M., Takayama, H. and Uchino, H. (1982) Br. J. Haematol. 51, 469-474.
24. Stenke, L., Samuelsson, J., Palmblad, J. Reizenstein, P. and Lindgren, J.Å (1989) Br. J. Haematol. In press.

RADIATION AND CHEMICAL CARCINOGENESIS

RADIATION INJURY AND CARCINOGENESIS

A. R. KENNEDY

Department of Radiation Oncology, University of Pennsylvania School of Medicine, Philadelphia, PA 19104

General Characteristics-Radiation Carcinogenesis.

Radiation is known to be a universal carcinogen, capable of causing cancer in most mammalian tissues (1). The specific type of radiation injury which leads to cancer, however, is still unknown; many hypotheses for the mechanism of radiation induced cancer are discussed elsewhere (1).

It is widely believed that it is a change in the cellular DNA which gives rise to the malignant transformation of a cell. Radiation is known to produce several different types of characteristic DNA lesions, such as single and double-strand breaks (at the phosphodiester bond) in the DNA, apurinic and apyrimidinic sites, and specific products such as 5,6 dihydroxydihydrothymine (from ionizing radiation) or pyrimidine dimers (from UV light), etc. The biologic consequences of these DNA lesions are unknown.

It is generally recognized that carcinogenesis is a multi-step process which involves two or more intracellular events to transform a normal cell into a cancer cell. There are three major hypotheses concerning the mechanism(s) by which radiation induces these changes: a) mutations, including changes in single genes or alterations in chromosome structure, b) changes in the gene expression patterns of cells and c) induction of an oncogenic virus which in turn causes cancer. Although there continues to be controversy among investigators as to which of these mechanisms plays the major role in radiation carcinogenesis, the hypotheses are not mutually exclusive; carcinogenesis may involve different mechanisms at different stages in the multi-step process.

The somatic mutation theory of carcinogenesis, originally proposed by Theodor Boveri in 1914 (2), still receives widespread support, as has been discussed in detail elsewhere (1). According to this theory, a change in the DNA sequence results in cancer. Specific mutations which have been observed in DNA in radiation induced carcinogenesis are shown in Figure 1 (3-10).

The major alternative to the somatic mutation theory is the "epigenetic" theory of carcinogenesis, i.e., that malignant cells do not result from changes in the genetic code, but instead result from changes in the expression patterns of the cellular genes. According to this theory, a carcinogen alters the expression pattern of a normal cell and thereby changes it into a pre-neoplastic or a cancer cell. Of importance to this theory is the fact that nuclei transplanted from cancer cells to enucleated cells or ova can produce normal cells and even complete normal organisms of several species, including mice (reviewed in ref.11). Evidence that an epigenetic change is involved in radiation carcinogenesis is discussed below.

Figure 1. Oncogene Alterations Observed in Radiation Induced Carcinogenesis

1. Ras Alterations

   Mouse Lymphomas [Guerrero et al. (3,4)]
   Dog lung tumors and leukemia cells [Frazier et al.(5)]
   Rat skin tumors [Sawey et al. (6)]

2. Alterations in c-myc

   Rat skin tumors [Sawey et al. (6)]
   In vitro-Mouse C3H10T1/2 cells [Sawey and Kennedy (7)]

3. Non-ras Genes Which Cause Transformation in the NIH3T3 Transfection Assay System

   In vitro-mouse C3H10T1/2 cells [Borek et al. (8)]
   In vitro-mouse C3H10T1/2 cells [Sawey and Kennedy(7)]
   In vitro-human W1-38 cells. [Mizuki et al. (9)]
   Mouse skin tumors [Jaffe and Bowden (10)]

The theory that radiation induces a virus which ultimately causes cancer has been discussed at length in radiation biology. In one strain of mouse, radiation induces the "radiation leukemia virus," which has been thought to play a role in the induction of thymic lymphoma/leukemia (12). The evidence for the virus playing a causative role in the genesis of this disease has recently been challenged, however (13, 14).

It is now widely accepted that initiation, the first step in malignant transformation, begins the carcinogenic process, while promotion is often required to complete it (15). The "two-stage" model of carcinogenesis was originally developed from studies on mouse skin which involved administration of a low dose of an initiating carcinogen followed by repeated treatment with a promoting agent (16,17). The concept of two-stage carcinogenesis is now widely believed to be applicable to many different organ systems in vivo and many in vitro transformation systems. Many different initiating and promoting agents have been studied in both in vivo (18,19) and in vitro systems (20). At high doses, most initiating agents are carcinogenic by themselves, with only one exposure being necessary for carcinogenesis to occur (21). Promoting agents, however, must be given over a long period of time (22). Several different phases of promotion can be distinguished in in vivo promotion systems, with different compounds being able to promote or suppress the various specific stages involved in promotion (19). Promoting agents often shorten the latent period for cancer development (22). Another stage in carcinogenesis is referred to as tumor progression, which refers to the conversion of a benign tumor into a malignant tumor.

Radiation is likely to play a role in all of the phases of carcinogenesis which have been studied experimentally. Radiation has been shown to work as an "initiating agent" for several types of carcinogenesis in vivo (23), including two-stage carcinogenesis with croton oil (24) or TPA (25,26) as the promoting agents, and with several different promoting agents in in vitro transformation systems (20). Although the mechanisms of promotion are unknown, many promoting agents induce free radicals in cells (27,28). Free-radical generating agents can act as tumor promoters in vivo and in vitro (29), and inhibitors of free radical reactions suppress tumor promotion (30). There is currently much research aimed at defining the role of free radicals in promotion. As the biological effects of radiation are thought to be produced by free radicals (31), and promoting agents may bring about their effects through free radicals (15), it is believed that sequential radiation exposures may bring about tumor promotion. Radiation is known to be capable of inducing tumor progression (10).

The mechanisms of tumor promotion has been widely thought to involve epigenetic phenomena, primarily due to the major effects of promoters on gene expression (17). Many other effects have been shown to occur following promoter treatment, however, such as the inhibition of intercellular communication (32) and genetic changes such as chromosome aberrations (33), aneuploidy (34), sister chromatid exchanges (35,36) and single strand DNA breaks (37). Although it is now recognized that promoters may cause several types of genetic changes, they have not been shown to cause single base mutations in DNA (21). Although many hypotheses exist about the mechanism of action of tumor promoters, it is known that proliferation is essential for tumor promotion to occur (38). In fact, promoters have their effect in vitro only when applied to proliferating cells (39).

Cell proliferation after exposure to radiation (and other carcinogens) is clearly essential for the malignant transformation of a cell (40). It was recognized during the early years of cancer research that tissue irritation, which increased cell division, increased the probability of tumor development. Following carcinogen treatment, such actions as wounding a rabbit's ear or partial hepatectomy resulted in tumors in the ear or liver, respectively, where they would otherwise not have occurred (41). Bleeding an animal which had been exposed to x-rays resulted in leukemia in animals which otherwise would not have developed it (42). While a low dose of ^{210}Po alpha radiation did not induce lung cancer by itself, lung cancer did arise in animals who received a series of saline instillations into the lung (at 5 months after the single 210po treatment), which caused increased epithelial cell proliferation. Twenty to 40% of the animals exposed to the saline instillations developed tumors (43,44). The evidence for cell proliferation, and promotional factors in general, playing a role in human cancer has been discussed elsewhere (4 5).

Our own studies have suggested that the first event in radiation induced carcinogenesis is a high frequency event occurring in a large fraction of the irradiated cells (40,46-49). Several studies involving in vivo/in vitro carcinogenesis have led to a similar conclusion (50-53; reviewed in reference 49). The in vitro phase of these studies has allowed a determination of the number of carcinogen-treated cells with the capability of giving rise to cancer in animals. The results of such studies have shown that a very small number of carcinogen-treated cells give rise to cancer in animals (50-53); thus, a high frequency initiating event must be occurring in these systems. The fact that such a small number of carcinogen-exposed cells can give rise to transformed foci in vitro or carcinomas in vivo is not consistent with the notion that specific locus mutations initiate the malignant process. Mutations at specific loci are known to occur at frequencies many orders of magnitude lower than those observed for malignantly transformed cells observed in these experiments. Although these results challenge the notion that the initiating event in carcinogenesis is a mutagenic event, they do not exclude mutagenesis as a later event in carcinogenesis. In fact, our own results suggest that a mutagenic event, such as those shown in Figure 1, occurs as a later event in radiation induced malignant transformation (40,54).

The hypothesized high frequency initiating event is likely to be a change in gene expression, as it is known that carcinogens are capable of bringing about such changes (55) and that such changes occur in a high proportion of the carcinogen treated cells (56). There is also evidence that radiation is capable of inducing cellular processes at a high frequency which at a later time result in rare genetic events. For example, radiation is known to induce the SOS system, an error-prone DNA repair system, in E. coli in a widespread fashion: SOS repair then results in mutations that are rare genetic changes (57). SOS functions are activated for only a short period of time, but other radiation induced systems are known to be activated for long periods of time. Recombinational events continue to occur for many generations after irradiation in yeast (58). A process similar to radiation induced recombination in yeast could be induced by radiation in mammalian cells and then lead to a recombinational event which results in malignant transformation. There is evidence suggesting the existence of similar radiation induced processes which lead to cell killing (59, 60) and mutagenesis (61).

Modifiers of Radiation Carcinogenesis.

In addition to the promotional factors discussed above, many other factors can affect the induction of cancer by radiation. Notable among these are the agents which have been shown to inhibit promotional factors, such as the retinoids (Vitamin A derivatives), anti-inflammatory steroidal agents, anti-oxidants, vitamins, protease inhibitors, etc. (62). Many of these same classes of agents also suppress carcinogenesis induced by a high carcinogen dose (19,20,63). Such modifying factors for carcinogenesis are equally effective in many in vivo and in vitro transformation assay systems and with many different carcinogens, including radiation, as the cancer-causing agents (20). It is likely that all carcinogens switch on carcinogenesis via a common pathway, as the modifying agents for carcinogenesis affect the process in a similar fashion even though agents with very different characteristics have been utilized as the initiating carcinogens.

Compounds capable of affecting tumor promotion include eicosanoids, as discussed elsewhere (see, for example, ref. 64) and in this volume. Components of the arachidonic acid cascade may also affect radiation induced carcinogenesis, although no causative role for any specific compound has yet been defined. In our studies, we have observed that several compounds known to affect specific pathways in the arachidonic acid cascade have significant effects on the induction of radiation induced transformation in C3H10T1/2 cells, as shown in Figure 2. For example, radiation transformation is suppressed by aspirin (65) and indomethacin (66), both of which inhibit cyclooxygenase. Adding exogenous lipoxygenase to irradiated cultures also suppresses radiation induced transformation (Kennedy, unpublished data) as does the addition of the bee venom toxin melittin, a stimulator of

Fig. 2 Modifiers of Radiation Carcinogenesis Which Affect the Arachidonic Acid Cascade from Membrane Phospholipids

(Abbreviations-see below)

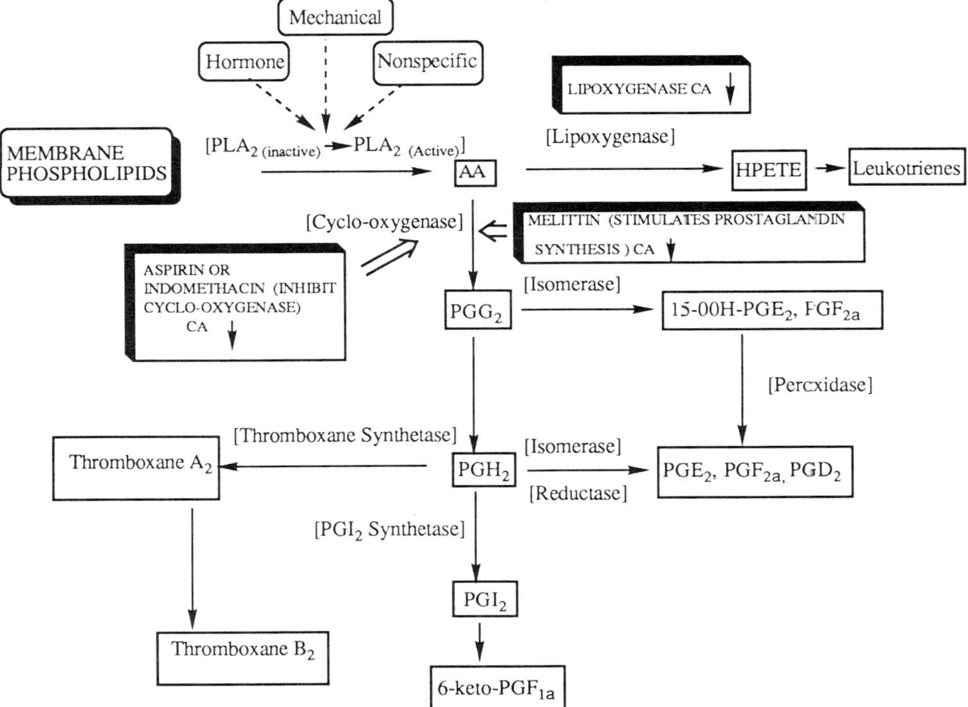

Abbreviations used: PLA_2-phospholipase A_2; AA-arachidonic acid; HPETE-hydroperoxyeicosatetraenoic acid; PGG, PGH, PGE, PGF, PGD, PGI-prostaglandin G, H, E, F, D, I, respectively; TXA, TXB-thromboxane A and B, respectively; PG-synthase includes the cyclo-oxygenase, peroxidase, and isomerase activites. (Modified from reference 75; Ca-carcinogenesis.)

prostaglandin synthesis (66). Other inhibitors of radiation transformation, such as vitamin E (67,68) affect components of the arachidonic acid cascade at several different points, as has been reviewed recently (69). While vitamin E has major effects on arachidonic acid metabolism, primarily related to its properties as an antioxidant, it is also a surfactant (70-74) and, at high concentrations, functions as a detergent (66). High concentrations (nearly toxic levels) of vitamin E are necessary to inhibit radiation transformation in vitro (67).

Hormones are also known to have major effects on arachidonic acid metabolism (75), and have been shown to have significant effects on radiation carcinogenesis and transformation in vitro, as has been reviewed (20). Several steroid hormones have been studied in our laboratory and have had both inhibiting and enhancing effects on radiation transformation (76-81). It is of interest that glucocorticord hormones can have opposite effects on radiation transformation in the presence and absence of the phorbol ester tumor promoting agent, 12-0-tetradecanoyl-phorbol-13-acetate (TPA), as illustrated in Figure 3.

Figure 3. Effects of Glucocorticoid Hormones on Radiation Transformation and Radiation Transformation Enhanced by TPA Treatment

Glucocorticoid Hormone	Modification of Radiation Transformation	TPA Enhancement of Radiation Transformation	References
Dexamethasone	-	inhibits	77,80
Cortisone	enhances	inhibits	77,80
Cortisol	inhibits	inhibits	66,80

Glucocorticoid hormones such as cortisone are highly anti-promotional, both in vivo and in vitro, while being able to enhance radiation and chemical carcinogenesis in the absence of promotion (discussed in references 77 and 80). Steroid hormones such as cortisone are known to block phospholipase and thus, inhibit the release of arachidonic acid from phospholipids (75); it is clear their effects on radiation transformation cannot be explained totally by the inhibition of phospholipase.

We have observed that many agents which affect arachidonic acid metabolism have highly significant effects on radiation carcinogenesis; their precise mechanism(s) of action, however, remain to be elucidated.

ACKNOWLEDGEMENTS

Research in the author's laboratory is supported by NIH Grants CA22704, CA46496, and CA34680.

REFERENCES

1. National Academy of Sciences, Advisory Committee on the Biological Effects of Ionizing Radiation (BEIR V): The Effects on Populations of Exposure to Low Levels of Ionizing Radiation. Washington, D.C. National Academy of Sciences, National Research Council.
2. Boveri, T.H. Fischer, Jena., 1914.
3. Guerrero, I., Calzava, P., Mayer, A. and Pellicer, A. Proc. Natl. Acad. Sci. 181: 202-205, 1984.
4. Guerrero, I., Villasante, A., Corces, V. and Pellicer, A. Science 225: 11591162, 1984.
5. Frazier, M.E., Lindberg, R.A., Mueller, D.M., Gee, A. and Seed, T.M. Int. J. Rad. Biol. 49: 542-543, 1986.
6. Sawey, M.J., Hood, A.T., Burns, F.J. and Garte, S.J. Molec. Cell. Biol. 7: 932-935, 1987.
7. Sawey, M.J. and Kennedy, A.R. In: Proceedings of the 14th Gray Conference, Oxford, England, pp. 433-438, 1989.
8. Borek, C., Ong, A. and Mason, H. Proc. Natl. Acad. Sci. USA 84: 794-798, 1987.
9. Mizuki, K., Nose, K., Okamoto, H., Tschida, N. and Hayasi, K. Biochem. Biophys. Res. Comm. 128: 1037-1043, 1985.
10. Jaffe, D.R. and Bowden, G.T. Proceedings of the 8th International Congress of Radiation Research, Edinburgh, July, 1987. Volume 1, edited by Fielden, E.SM., Fowler, J.F., Hendry, J.H. and Loh, D. Taylor & Francis, Philadelphia, PA p. 188, 1987.
11. Braun, A. The Story of Cancer: On its Nature. Causes and Control (Wesley, Reading, MA), 1977.
12. Lieberman, M. and Kaplan, H.S. Science 130: 387-388, 1959.
13. Duplan, J.F., Guillemain, B. and Astier, T. In: Radiation Carcinogenesis (Eds. A.C. Upton, R.E. Albert, F.J. Burns and R.E. Shore), Elsevier, pp. 73-84, 1986.
14. Lieberman, M., Hansteen, G.A., McCune J.M., Scott, M.L., White, J.H. and Weissman, I.L. J. Exp. Med. 166:1883-1893, 1987.
15. Copeland, E.S. (ed.). Cancer Res. 43: 5631-5637,1983.
16. Berenblum, I. In: F.F. Becker (ed.), Cancer: A Comprehensive Treatise, Vol. 1, pp. 323-344, New York: Plenum Publishing Co. 1975.
17. Boutwell, R.K. Toxicol. 2: 419-443, 1974.
18. Farber, E. Arch. Pathol. Lab. Med. 104: 499,1980.
19. Pelling, J.C. and Slaga, T.J. In: M.J. Mass, et al (ed.), In: Carcinogenesis, Vol. 8, Raven Press, New York, pp. 369-393, 1985.
20. Kennedy, A.R. In: Mechanisms of Tumor Promotion, Vol. III, "Tumor Promotion and Carcinogenesis In Vitro" edited by Slaga, T.J. Chapter 2, pp. 13-55, CRC Press, Boca Raton, 1984.
21. Weinstein, I.B., Lee, L.S., Fisher, P.B., Mufson, A. and Yamasaki, H. In: E.C. Miller et al. (eds.), Naturally Occurring Carcinogens. Mutagens and Modulators of Carcinogenesis, University Park Press, Baltimore, p. 301, 1979.
22. Ryser, H.J.P. N. Engl. J. Med. 285: 721-734, 1971.
23. Mole, R.H. Natl. Cancer Inst. Monogr. 14: 217-290, 1964.
24. Shubik, P., Goldfarb, A.R., Ritchie, A.C. and Lisco, H. Nature 171:934-935, 1953.
25. Jaffe, D.R. and Bowden, G.T. Radiation Res. 106: 156-165,1986.
26. Fry, R.J.M., Ley, R.D., Grube, D. and Staffeldt, E. In: Carcinogenesis, vol. 7, edited by E. Hecker et al. pp. 155-165, Raven Press, New York, 1982.
27. Goldstein, B.O., Witz, G., Amoruso, M., Stone, D.S. and Troll, W. Cancer Lett. 11: 257, 262, 1981.
28. Fischer, S.M. and Adams, L.M. Cancer Res. 45: 3130-3136,1985.
29. Kennedy, A.R., In: Oxygen and Sulfur Radicals in Chemistrv and Medicine, (Ed., A. Breccia, M.A.J. Rodgers, and G. Semerano.). Edizioni Scientifiche, "Lo Scarabeo", (Bologna, Italy), pp. 201-209, 1986.
30. Slaga, T.J., Solanki, V. and Logani, M. In: Radioprotectors and Anticarcinogens. O.F. Nyggard and M.G. Simic, eds., Academic Press, New York, pp. 471-485, 1983.
31. Little, J.B. and Williams, J.R. In: Handbook of Physiology, S.R. Geiger, H.L. Falk, S.D. Murphy and P.H.K. Lee (eds.), pp. 127-155, Bethesda, Maryland, American Physiological Society, 1977.
32. Trosko, J.E., Yotti, L.P., Warren, S.T., Tsushimoto, G. and C.C. Chang. In: Carcinogenesis, vol. 7,

edited by E. Hecker et al., pp. 565-585,1982.
33. Emirit, I. and Cerutti, P.A. Nature 293: 144-146, 1981.
34. Parry, J.M., Parry, E.M. and Barrett, J.C. Nature 294: 263-265, 1981.
35. Kinsella, A. and Radman, M. Proc. Natl. Acad. Sci. USA 75:6149-6153, 1978.
36. Nagasawa, H. and Little, J.B. Proc. Natl. Acad. Sci. USA 76:1943-1947, 1979.
37. Birnboim, H.C. Science 215: 1247-1249, 1982.
38. Scribner, J.D. and Suss, R. In: International Review of Experimental Pathology, G.W. Richter and M.A. Epstein, Eds., volume 18, pp. 138-198, Academic Press, New York, 1978.
39. Kennedy, A.R., Murphy, G. and Little, J.B. Cancer Res. 40: 1915-20, 1980.
40. Kennedy, A.R., Cairns, J. and Little, J.B. Nature 307:85-86, 1984.
41. Suss, R., Kinzel, V. and Scribner, J.D. Cancer-Experiments and Concepts. New York, Springer-Verlag, 1973.
42. Gong, J.K. Science 174: 833-835, 1971.
43. Little, J.B., McGandy, R.B. and Kennedy, A.R. Cancer Res. 38: 1929-1935, 1978.
44. Shami, S., Thibideau, L., Kennedy, A.R. and Little, J.B. Cancer Res. 42: 1405-1411, 1982.
45. Kennedy, A.R. In: Cancer of the Respiratory Tract: Predisposing Factors. Carcinogenesis-A Comprehensive Survey, Volume 8, Edited by Mass, M.J., Kaufman, D.G., Siegfried, J.M., Steele, V.E., and Nesnow, S. Raven Press, New York, pp. 431-436, 1985.
46. Kennedy, A.R., Fox, M., Murphy, G. and Little, J.B. Proc. Natl. Acad. Sci. USA 77: 7262-66, 1980.
47. Kennedy, A.R. and Little, J.B. Carcinogenesis 1:1039-1047, 1980.
48. Kennedy, A.R. and Little, J.B. In: Cancer: Achievements. Challenges and Prospects for the 1980's. Edited by J.H. Burchenal and J.F. Oettgen, Vol.1, pp.491-500, Grune and Stratton Inc., 1981.
49. Kennedy, A.R. In: Carcinogenesis: A Comprehensive Survey, Volume 9 Ammalian Cell Transformation: Mechanisms of Carcinogenesis and Assay for Carcinogens, edited by J.C. Barrett and R.W. Tennant, Raven Press, New York, pp. 355-364, 1985.
50. Mulcahy, R.T., Gould, M.N. and Clifton, K.H. Int. J. Radiat. Bio. 45: 419- 426, 1984.
51. Terzaghi, M., and Nettesheim, P. Cancer Res. 39: 4003-4010,1979.
52. Clifton, K.H., Tanner, M.A. and Gould, M.N. Cancer Res. 46: 2390, 2395,1986.
53. Clifton, K.H., Kamiya, K. Mulcahy, R.T. and Gould, M.N. In: Assessment of Risk from Low-Level Exposure to Radiation and Chemicals, pp. 329- 344, A.D. Woodhead, C.J. Shellabarger, V. Pond and A. Hollaender (eds.), New York, Plenum Publishing Corp., 1985 .
54. Kennedy, A.R. and Little, J.B. Radiation Res. 99: 228-248, 1984.
55. Fahmy, M.J. and Fahmy, O.G. Cancer Res. 40: 3374-3382, 1980.
56. Scott, R.E. and Maercklein, P.B. Proc. Natl. Acad. Sci. USA 82: 2995-2999, 1985.
57. Witkin, E.M. Bacteriol. Rev. 40: 869-907, 1976.
58. Fabre, F. and Roman, H. Proc. Natl. Acad. Sci. USA 74: 1667-1671, 1977.
59. Gorgojo and J.B. Little, Int. J. Radiat. Biol. 55: 619-630, 1989.
60. Seymour, C.B., Mothersill, C. and Alper, T. Int. J. Radiat. Biol. 50: 167-179, 1986.
61. Stamato, T., Weinstein, R., Peters, B., Hu, J. Doherty, B. and Giaccia, A.Somatic Cell Molec. Genetics 13: 57-66, 1987.
62 . Slaga, T.J. (ed.) Carcinogenesis: A Comprehensive Survey, Vol. 5., Modifiers of Chemical Carcinogenesis, Raven Press, New York, 1980.
63. Wattenberg, L.W. Cancer Res. 45: 1-8,1985.
64. Fischer, S.M. In: Icosanoids and Cancer, edited by H. Thaler-Dao et al., Raven Press, New York, pp. 79-89, 1984.
65. Radner, B.S. and A.R Kennedy: Suppression of x-ray induced transformation by valium and aspirin in mouse C3H10T1/2 cells. Cancer Letters, 51:49-57, 1990.
66. Little, J.B. and Kennedy, A.R. In: Carcinogenesis, Vol. 7, edited by E. Hecker et al., pp. 243-257, Raven Press, New York, 1982 .
67. Radnor, B.S. and Kennedy, A.R. Cancer Letters 32: 25-32, 1986.
68. Borek, C., Ong., A., Mason, H., Donahue, L. and Biaglow, J. Proc. Nat. Acad. Sci. USA 83: 1490-1494, 1986.
69. Panganamala, R.U., and Cornwell, D.G. In: Part V, Protective Effect of Vitamin E Against Drugs and Air Pollutants. Annals New York Academy of Sciences, pp. 376-390, 1982.
70. Path, G.S. and D.G. Cornwall, J. Lipid Res. 19: 416-422, 1978.
71. Maggio, B., Diplock, A.T. and J.A. Lucy. Biochem J. 161: 111-121,1977.
72. Fukuzawa, K., Hayashi, K. and Suzuki, A. Chem. Phys. Lipids 18: 39-48, 1977.
73. Fukuzawa, K., Ikeno, H., Tokumura, A. and Tsukatani, H. Chem. Phys. Lipids 23:13-22, 1979.
74. Fukuzawa, K., Chida, H. and Suzuki, A. J. Nutri. Sci. Vitaminol. 26: 427- 434, 1980.
75. Bockman, R.S. Cancer Investigation 1(6): 485-493, 1983.

76. Kennedy, A.R., and Weichselbaum, R.R. Carcinogenesis 2: 67-69,1981.
77. Kennedy, A.R., and Weichselbaum, R.R. Nature 294: 97-98,1981.
78. Kennedy, A.R. Cancer Letters 29: 289-292, 1985.
79. Umans, R.S. and Kennedy, A.R. Eur. J. Cancer Clin. Oncol. 23: 339-342, 1987.
80. Kennedy, A.R. and Umans, R.S. Cancer Letters 40: 177-183,1988.
81. Umans, R.S. and Kennedy, A.R. Cancer Letters 40: 177-183, 1988.

TUMOR PROMOTION AND THE ARACHIDONATE CASCADE

S.M. FISCHER, G.S. CAMERON, K.E. PATRICK, J. LEYTON, and R.J. MORRIS

University of Texas Cancer Center, Science Park, Smithville, Texas 78957

INTRODUCTION

Experimental chemical carcinogenesis studies in animals, particularly the multistage model in mouse skin (1-3) are valuable in identifying those biological events or agents that play either an essential or modulatory role in the development of tumors. The promotion stage is most often accomplished by using 12-O-tetradecanoyl phorbol-13-acetate (TPA), although a variety of agents have been identified as skin-tumor promoters (3,4). Among the many morphological and biochemical responses of the skin to promoters, the induction of inflammation followed by increased epidermal cell proliferation (hyperplasia) are events common to all promoters and appear to be required events (5).

There is now substantial evidence that TPA induces eicosanoid synthesis in epidermal cells *in vivo* and *in vitro* (6). Since it is well established that eicosanoids are one of the major mediators of inflammation, questions have arisen as to the role and/or requirement for these metabolites in the tumor process. Using several approaches, the conclusion of studies by several different laboratories indicate that (i) exogenous application of prostaglandins with TPA can modify tumor development (7), (ii) use of inhibitors of various parts of the arachidonate cascade causes an inhibition in tumor development (8) and (iii) reduction of arachidonic acid levels in epidermal membranes by altering dietary fatty acid intake results in a reduction in tumor number (9).

Current work in our laboratory is now aimed at addressing three questions concerning the relationship of TPA to eicosanoid synthesis and subsequent alterations in skin function. First, what is the mechanism by which TPA causes arachidonate release from the membrane? Second, are there differences between basal and differentiated cells with regard to arachidonate metabolism? Third, what is the relationship of inflammation to proliferation of the overlying epidermis.

METHODS AND MATERIALS

Cell culture.

Primary cultures of epidemmal cells from newbom SSIN mice were established as previously described and labelled ovemight with ^{14}C-arachidonic acid (10). These prelabelled cultures were then treated with TPA or other agents for 3 hr after which the media was removed and extracted. Eicosanoid release was measured as amount of released radiolabel; prostaglandin E_2 was likewise measured following TLC of the extracted media (10).

Separation of epidemlal cells.

Epidermal cells isolated from trypsinized adult SSIN mouse skins were layered on a 50% Percoll gradient as previously described (11). Separation into three fractions, based on their state of differentiation, were obtained following centrifugation. The cells in these fractions were incubated with ^{14}C-arachidonic acid and the synthesis of radiolabelled prostaglandins and HETEs measured.

Induced Inflammation/Hvperplasia Studies.

The epidemlis of the inside of the ear of SSIN mice was removed by abrasion with fine emery paper. At various times following the procedure, histological cross-sections of the ear were made and the extent of hyperplasia of the outer ear epidermis evaluated. In another experiment, 10 μ1 of 2% carragheenan was injected subcutaneously into the dorsal skin. Histological sections were evaluated for hyperplasia of the overlying epidermis.

RESULTS

In order to determine whether protein kinase C (PKC) mediates the TPA induced release of arachidonic acid, several approaches were taken. First, as shown in Figure 1, the PKC inhibitor H-7 (from Seikagaku America) was found to inhibit both the TPA response and the response to the diacyclyglycerol (DAG) 1,2-dioctanoyl-sn-glycerol. DAG is believed to be the natural ligand or activator of PKC; TPA performs this function with even greater efficacy (12). The observation (data not shown) that 4αTPA, a nonpromoting analog of TPA (13) also causes arachidonic acid release (at a level comparable to TPA if used at a l0-fold higher dose) that is not inhibited by H-7, further supports PKC involvement.

Additionally, prior treatment with TPA or DAG suppresses the release of arachidonate upon subsequent treatment 15 to 18 hr later, as shown in Figure 2. This is interpreted as being due to the down-regulation of PKC (12). If the treatment protocol is TPA first, followed by 4αTPA, such down-regulation of arachidonic acid release is not observed (data not shown). Collectively, these results support a conclusion that TPA induces arachidonic release *via* PKC activation.

To better understand the cellular source and function of specific eicosanoids in the skin, it is of value to know if all or only specific populations of epidermal cells synthesize and/or respond to eicosanoids. To address the first question, epidermal cells were separated on the basis of their state of differentiation, with fraction 1 denoting the most differentiated, fraction 2 those committed to differentiation and fraction 3 having the most basal, least differentiated characteristics. When these populations of cells, used either as viable preparations or freeze-thawed (this eliminates the competing reaction of incorporation of arachidonate into lipids) were analyzed for their ability to metabolize exogenous arachidonate, the most differentiated cells were found to have the greatest synthetic activity with respect to both prostaglandins and HETEs (Figure 3). The basal cells have relatively very little synthetic activity, suggesting that the expression of prostaglandin synthetase and the lipoxygenases are a function of commitment to differentiation.

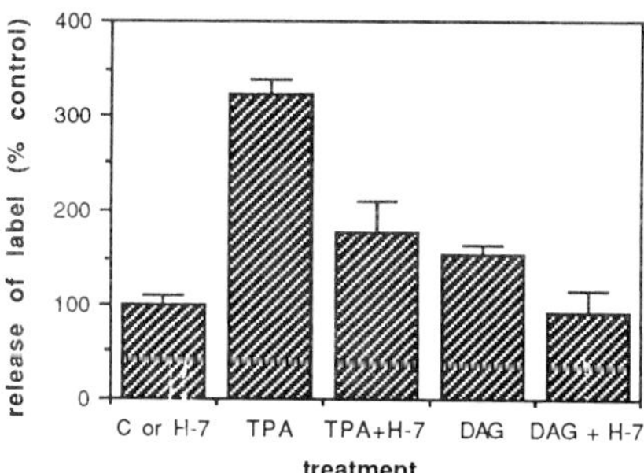

Figure 1. Inhibition of TPA or DAG-induced release of ^{14}C-arachidonic acid by the protein kinase C inhibitor (H-7) in cultured murine epidermal cells. Confluent cultures of murine epidermal cells, grown in a completely defined, serum-free medium were labelled overnight (15 hr) with 0.1 μCi/ml of ^{14}C-arachidonic acid. The cultures were then washed and fresh medium added containing 1 μg/ml TPA, 100 μg/ml H-7, both or solvent only (acetone). The media was collected at 3 hr and used to measure total release of labelled eicosanoids. Values represent the mean ± std. dev.

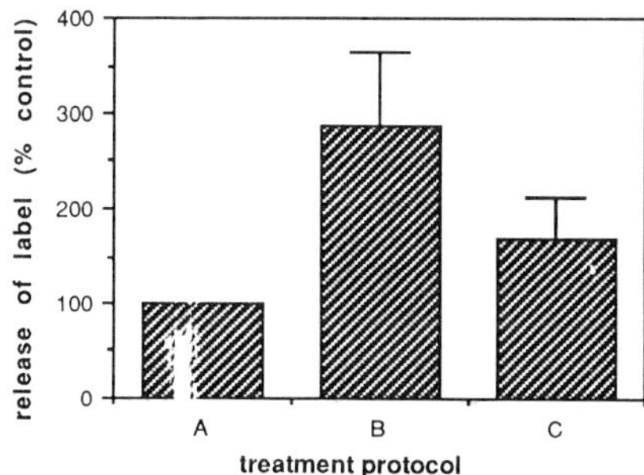

Figure 2. Inhibition of TPA-induced release of eicosanoids by prior TPA treatment: Apparent down-regulation of responsiveness. Confluent cultures of murine epidermal cells, grown in a completely defined, serum-free medium were treated for 2 hr with the first agent, washed, labelled overnight (15 hr) with 0.1 μCi/ml of ^{14}C-arachidonic acid, washed and then treated for 3 hr with the second agent. TPA was used at a concentration of 1 μg/ml. The collected media was used to measure total release of labelled eicosanoids. The treatment protocols were: A, acetone --> acetone; B, acetone --> TPA; C, TPA --> TPA. Values represent the mean of the difference from the control (group A) ± SEM from 4 experiments of 3 to 4 cultures each.

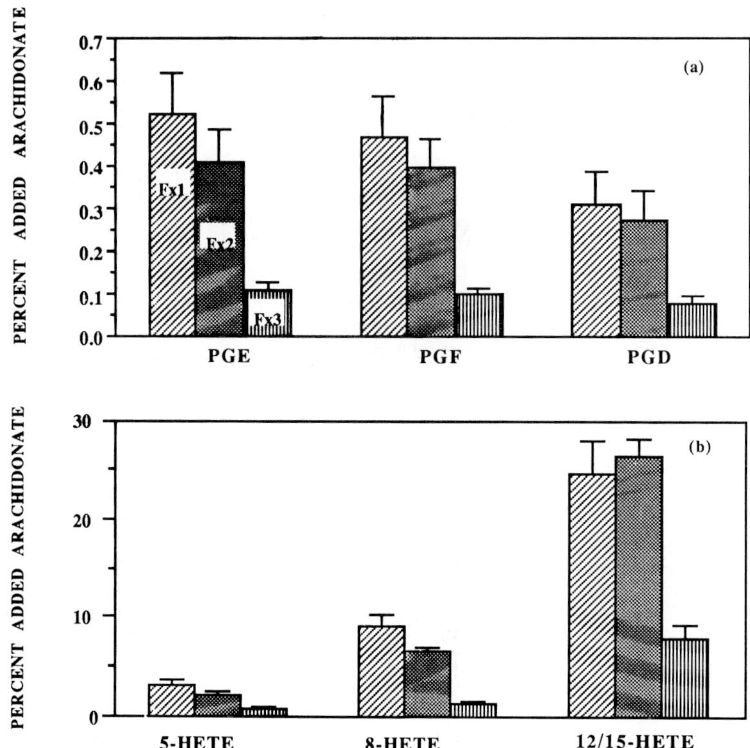

Figure 3. Prostaglandin and HETE synthesis in epidermal cells of varying states of differentiation. Murine epidermal cells were isolated by trypsinization and separated according to state of differentiation by Percoll density gradient centrifugation. Fraction 1 (Fx I) represents the most differentiated, Fx 3 the least differentiated. Cells or homogenates from each fraction were incubated with radiolabelled arachidonic acid, followed by extraction and TLC for (panel A) prostaglandins (PGs) or (panel B) HETEs. Data are expressed as percentage of added arachidonate recovered as each of the metabolites; values are the mean ± SEM.

An effort is being made to determine whether the hyperplasia that occurs as a result of promoter treatment is due to the direct mitogenic action of TPA on the epidermis or whether it is indirect, i.e., that inflammation induces hyperplasia. To this end, two types of inflammatory conditions were established in which no soluble promoters were applied. In the first, an injury-induced inflammation, the inner ear was abraded lightly. This results in hyperplasia of the epidermis of the outer ear (Figure 4). Likewise, dermal inflammation induced by injection of carragheenan was associated with hyperplasia of the overlying epidermis (data not shown). It therefore appears that inflammation induced by a variety of chemical or physical means can cause enhanced epidermal cell proliferation.

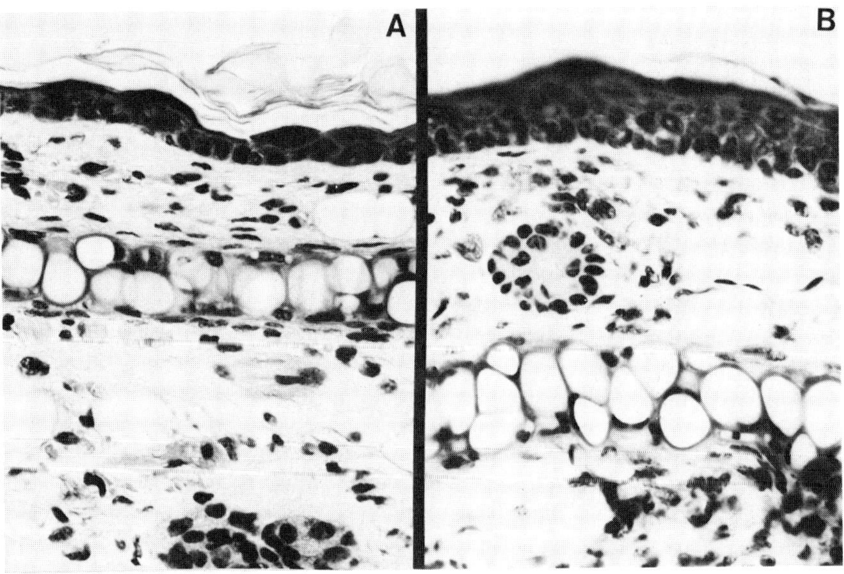

Figure 4. Hyperplasia induced by abrasion of opposing side of ear. The ventral side of the ear was lightly abraded with 15 strokes of fine emory paper. At one day intervals ears were excised, fixed in formalin, embedded in parafin and sectioned. The epidermis on the dorsal or opposite side of the ear responded with hyperplasia that was maximal at 48 hr. Panel A, untreated control ear; panel B, 48 hr after abrasion.

DISCUSSION

There is substantial evidence suggesting that PKC mediates most, if not all, the actions of TPA (14). However, the biological responses of the skin to other types of promoters, including the non-PKC types benzoyl peroxide, chrysarobin and ethyl phenylpropriolate (4,15,16) and notably, wounding (17) are strikingly similar. These responses include the development of inflammation, induction of ornithine decarboxylase and the later formation of histologically the same types of tumors. It is, therefore, important to understand where in the sequence of events PKC type and non-PKC type promoters converge in their action. We propose that is at the level of arachidonic acid release, metabolism and subsequent inflammation We have evidence (data not shown) that non-PKC promoters also cause arachidonate release. We currently hypothesize that the major difference between TPA and non-PKC promoters is the mechanism by which this release occurs. TPA is able to use PKC as an amplification system to enhance its signal (and thus TPA elicits responses at hormone-like doses) while other promoters, which generally are efficacious only at doses orders of magnitude greater than TPA, work more through a non-specific phospholipase A_2 activation due to physical membrane perturbations.

The majority of the arachidonic acid released by promoter treatment is from the epidermal cells, primarily because they are in direct contact with topically applied agents and because they represent the majority of the cellularity of the skin. Because the epidermis is made up of keratinocytes in varying states of differentiation, with the more basal, least differentiated resting on the basement membrane, it is of interest to determine whether it is the basal or the more differentiated cells that are the major responders with regard to synthesis of eicosanoids. Our work indicates that the majority of the synthetic enzymes are found in the differentiated cells. The functional significance of this may lie in considering the outer, differentiated epidermal cells as the first line of defense. The subsequent edema, influx of inflammatory cells into the skin and hyperplasia may provide dilution, degradative enzymes and removal of debris. What is still unknown is whether the increased eicosanoids directly affect keratinocyte function and if so, whether this is of an autocrine or paracrine nature.

The inflammatory component of the response to tumor promoters appears to be necessary for tumor development, based on the antitumor properties of anti-inflammatory agents. Because this inflammation is linked to subsequent hyperplasia, which is also required for promotion of tumors, and because it occurs with all types of promoters, the question arises as to whether chronic inflammation/hyperplasia, regardless of its etiology, is the real biological promoter, i.e., whether it is sufficient in itself to cause tumor promotion. This question remains to be answered but is certainly testable, using any of a number of inflammatory conditions.

CONCLUSIONS

1. The development of skin tumors can be modified by altering the eicosanoid levels, either through application of eicosanoids, use of inhibitors or dietary modification of substrate levels.
2. The basal keratinocytes contain little prostaglandin synthetase while the most differentiated keratinocytes contain the most.
3. All mouse skin tumor promoters cause the release of arachidonic acid; for the phorbol esters, protein kinase C may serve as a signal amplification pathway.
4. Our current hypothesis is that the eicosanoids cause or contribute to the inflammation seen with all types of promoters and that this inflammation drives the observed hyperplasia.

ACKNOWLEDGEMENTS

This work was supported by NIH Grants CA-34443 and CA-46886 (S.M.F.)

REFERENCES

1. Slaga, T.J., Fischer, S.M., Nelson, K., and Gleason, G.L. Proc. Natl. Acad. Sci., USA, 77:3659-3663, 1980.
2. Slaga, T.J., Fischer, S.M., Weeks, C.E., and Klein-Szanto, A.J.P. In: Rev. Biochem. Tox. (Elsevier/North Holland Publishing, NY.) pp. 231-282,1981.
3. Slaga, T.J. In: Mechanisms of Tumor Promotion (CRC Press, Boca Raton, FL) pp. 1-16, 1984.
4. DiGiovanni, J., Decina, P.C., Pritchett, W.P., Canton, J., Aalfs, K.K., and Coombs, M.M. Cancer Res. 45:2584-2589, 1985.
5. Gschwendt, M., Kittstein, W., Furstenberger, G. and Marks, G. Cancer Lett. 25:177-185, 1984.

6. Arachidonic Acid Metabolism and Tumor Promotion, eds. S.M. Fischer and T.J. Slaga, Martinus Nijhoff Publ., Boston, 1985.
7. Fischer, S.M., Gleason, G.L., Bohrman, J.S., and Slaga, T.J. Carcinogensis. 1:245-248, 1980.
8. Fischer, S.M., Cameron, G.S., Baldwin, J.K., Jasheway, D.W., Patrick, K.E., and Belury, M.A. In: Skin Carcinogenesis: Mechanisms and Human Relevance, Alan R. Liss, Inc., N.Y. 1989, pp 249-264.
9. Leyton, J., Lee, M., Locniskar, M., Fischer, S. (in preparation).
10. Fischer, S.M., Baldwin, J.K., Jasheway, D.W., Patrick, K.E., Cameron, G.S. Cancer Res. 48: 658-664,1988.
11. Fischer, S.M., Nelson, KDG, Reiners, J.J. Jr., Viaje, A., Pelling, J.C., Slaga, T.J. J. Cutaneous Pathol. 9:43-49,1982.
12. Nishizuka,Y. Science 233:305-312, 1986.
13. Van Duuren, B.L., Tseng, S.S., Segal, A., Smith, A.C., Melchionne, S., Seidman, I. Cancer Res. 39:2644-2646, 1979.
14. Nishizuka, Y. Cancer, 63:1892-1903,1989.
15. Klein-Szanto, A.J.P. and Slaga, T.J. J. Invest. Dermatol. 79:30-34,1982.
16. Cameron, G.S., Patrick, K.E. and Fischer, S.M. (in preparation).
17. Argyris, T.S. In: Carcinogenesis. Vol. 7, Raven Press, N.Y., 1982, pp 43-48.

EICOSANOIDS AND BIOACTIVE LIPIDS AS MODIFIERS OF MULTISTAGE CARCINOGENESIS IN VITRO

C. BOREK

Center for Radiological Research, Department of Radiation Oncology and Department of Pathology/Cancer Center, Columbia University, New York, NY 10032

INTRODUCTION

Every cancer arises through a multistep process involving a series of genetic events. While one or more of the steps requires activation of normal cellular genes into oncogenes (1) the ultimate course and frequency of the neoplastic process are largely determined by an interplay of exogenous and endogenous factors (1,2). Permissive factors such as hormones act as co-transforming agents and potentiate carcinogenesis (1). These are balanced under normal conditions by cellular protective factors which suppress the neoplastic process.

The role of bioactive lipids and eicosanoids in the neoplastic process has become a focus of interest in recent years (3).

FREE RADICALS, ANTIOXIDANTS, AND LIPID PEROXIDATION

Lipids act as primary targets for oxidation by environmental carcinogens such as radiation, chemicals and ozone thereby generating reactive oxygen species and free radical intermediates such as malonaldehyde which play a role in initiation and promotion of carcinogenesis (4,5).

A number of cellular inherent defensive mechanisms prevail which either prevent peroxidation of lipids and oxidation of protein thereby suppressing the propagation of cascade reactions that generate a wide range of species which cause molecular damage (6). These include enzymes such as SOD, catalase, glutathione peroxidase and thiols. Also included are a variety of dietary factors such as vitamins E, C, A, β-carotene and selenium. These antioxidants have proved to be potent anticarcinogens (6-9) and act in different ways.

For example, Selenium and vitamin E act alone and in additive fashion as radio-protecting and chemopreventng agents inhibiting radiation and chemically induced transformation as well as ozone. Selenium confers protection in part by inducing or activating cellular free-radical scavening systems and by doubling peroxide breakdown, thus enhancing the capacity of the cell to cope with oxidant stress. Vitamin E acts by an alternate complementary mechanism. Vitamin E acts as a chain-breaking antioxidant inhibiting the lipid peroxidation and the formation of malonaldeyde, a compound with oncogenic potential (5-8).

An important determinant in the efficiency of cellular protection by inherent antioxidants lies in the interaction among various factors. The metabolic functions of vitamin E and selenium are interrelated, and selenium plays a role in the storage of vitamin E. Vitamin E action is also closely related to that of vitamin C, which appears to increase its antioxidant (9) and anticarcinogenic effects (6).

HORMONES AND EICOSANOIDS AS PERMISSIVE FACTORS

Thyroid hormones act as permissive co-transforming factors in carcinogenesis. The hormone is involved in oxygen metabolism in the cells and may modify free radical reactions thus exacerbating the effects of physical and chemical carcinogens (10, 11).

Our work has shown that the hormone is required for cell transformation by radiation as well as direct and indirectly acting chemical carcinogens (10). In addition, the hormone is critical for cellular transformation by cellular onogenes (11) as well as for gene expression. More recently we are finding that thyroid hormone enhances the production of eicosanoids in radiation exposed cells (Borek and Levine, in preparation) in a dose related manner similar to the hormone dose related response of transformation (10). The work suggested that eicosanoids can serve as permissive factors in radiation transformation.

LIPIDS AS PROTECTIVE FACTORS

Bioactive lipids can act as protective factors in neoplastic transformation.

In earlier work we showed that the membrane composition of sphingolipids in hepatoma cells (12) as well as in radiation transformed hamster embryo cells (13) differs from the composition and synthesis in the normal cells (12) (Figure 1). The distinct differences between the normal and neoplastic cells indicated a preponderance of GM_1 and GM_3 gangliosides. A striking decrease in GD_{1a} was observed in the transformed cells as compared to the normal.

The repression of synthesis or accelerated catabolism of GD_{1a} could have contributed to the effects observed. Regardless of the mechanism which altered the ganglioside patterns the phenotypic change could play a role in the loss of contact inhibition and cell-cell communication which were present in the normal cells and absent in the neoplastic cells (14).

More recently we extended our work on the role of sphingolipids in carcinogenesis. Our findings indicate that sphinganine and sphingosine act as powerful inhibitors of multistage carcinogenesis in C3H/10T-1/2 cells and suggest that these membrane components may act as protective factors (15). We found that the free long-chain bases suppressed cell transformation by x-irradiation and blocked the ability of the phorbol ester tumor promoter phorbol-12-myristate-13-acetate (PMA) to increase the transformation frequency.

The inhibitory effect of promotion in the cells was associated with an inhibition of protein kinase C, the receptor for PMA which plays a control role in signal transduction and growth control.

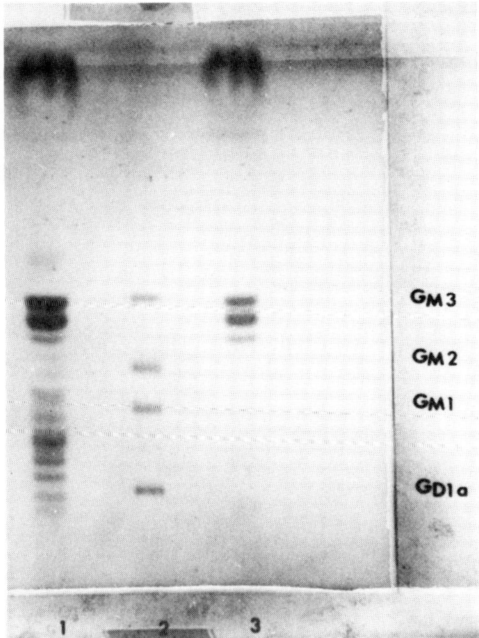

Figure 1. Thin-layer chromatogram of gangliosides from normal hamster embryo cells and X-ray transformed LSH 5 cells. Lane 1 gangliosides in control cells, lane 2 ganglioside standards, and lane 3 gangliosides in X-ray transformed cells. Note that in the transformed cells gangliosides higher than GM3 are absent. (From reference 13)

CONCLUSION

The role of cellular lipids as membrane targets for oxidation by carcinogens makes them prime candidates for the initiation of cascades of free radical reactions and the formation of intermediates, which damage DNA, cross link proteins and modify structural and functional parameters in the cell which can lead to genetic changes and carcinogenesis.

The process of lipid peroxidation and production of eicosanoids appear to be influenced by thyroid hormone, and may be in part responsible for the action of thyroid hormone as a permissive and co-transforming factor in radiation chemical and gene mediated carcinogenesis.

Cellular lipids such as sphingolipids play a role as endogenous protectors in the cell modulating and cellular membrane structure and susceptibility to transformation and modifying signal transduction via inhibition of protein kinase C.

ACKNOWLEDGEMENTS

The work was supported by Grant No. CA-12536 from the National Cancer Institute/NIH, and by a contract from the National Foundation of Cancer Research

REFERENCES

1. Borek, C. In: Mechanisms of Cellular Transformation by Carcinogenic Agents (Eds. D. Grunberger and S. Goff), Pergamon Press, New York, 1987, pp. 155-195.
2. Weinstein, I.B. Cancer Res. 4135-4142, 1988.
3. Levine, L. In: Eicosanoids, Lipid Peroxidation and Cancer (Heidleberger) Springer-Verlag, 1988, pp. 11-20.
4. Borek, C., Zaider, M., Ong, A., Mason, H. and Witz, G. Carcinogenesis 7:1611-1613, 1986.
5. Borek, C., Ong, A., Mason, H., Donahue, L. and Biaglow, J.E. Proc. Natl. Academy of Sciences 83:1490-1494, 1986.
6. Borek, C. In: Medical, Biochemical and Chemical Aaspects of Free Radicals (Eds. Hayaishi, O., Niki, E., Kondo, M., and Yoshikawa, T.) Elsevier Science Publishers, The Netherlands, 1989, pp. 1461-1469.
7. Borek, C. Br. J. Cancer 55:74-86, 1987.
8. Hayaishi, O., Niki, E., Kondo, M. and Yoshikawa, T. (Eds.) Medical and Chemical Aspects of Free Radicals Elsevier Science Publishers, The Netherlands, Vols. 1 and 2, 1989.
9. Niki, E., Saito, T., Kawakami, A. and Kamiya, Y. J. Biol. Chem. 259:4177-4182, 1984.
10. Borek, C., Guernsey, D.L., Ong, A. and Edelman, I.S. Proc. Natl. Acad. Sci. USA 80:5749-5752,1983.
11. Borek, C. Ann. N.Y. Acad. of Sci. 551:95-102,1988.
12. Brady, R.O., Borek, C. and Bradley, R.M. J. Biological Chemistry 244:6552-6554, 1969.
13. Borek, C., Pain, C. and Mason, H. Nature. 266:452-454, 1977.
14. Borek, C., Higashino, S. and Loewenstein, W.R. J. Membrane Biol. 1:274-293, 1969.
15. Borek, C., Ong, A., Stevens, V. and Merrill, A.H. Abstract #838 in Proc. AACR 30:211, 1988.

PREVENTION OF PEROXIDE PRODUCED DNA STRAND SCISSION IN HUMAN TUMOR CELLS BY LIPOXYGENASE INHIBITORS

M. A. BAKER

Department of Radiation Oncology, University of Pennsylvania, Philadelphia, PA 19104, USA

INTRODUCTION

Hydrogen peroxide, radiation, and many cancer chemotherapy drugs cause oxidative damage to cells including DNA strand breaks. Hydrogen peroxide is several orders of magnitude more toxic to cells at 37° C than at 0° C (1). At low doses, these agents produce mutation and transformation in various cells. The phorbol esters, transforming agents which are structurally unrelated to peroxide have also been reported to produce oxidative damage in cells. Many of the actions of tumor necrosis factor, a peptide with diverse cellular effects, appear to be mediated through "free radical-like" damage. Other cellular events, including protein kinase C translocation, the induction of proto-oncogene *fos*, and intracellular Ca^{2+} increase result from treatment with peroxides, transforming agents and various growth factors (2). It seems likely then that the DNA strand breaks produced by radiation, xenobiotics, or peroxides cannot be exclusively attributed to chemical interactions. That is, the "indirect" action of radiation may be mediated through rapidly initiated cellular mechanisms which lead to DNA scission rather than by hydroxyl radical reactions on the DNA molecule itself. The following experiments support these hypotheses.

Using a human lung adenocarcinoma derived cell line, A549, we tested the toxicity, DNA strand breaking activity and peroxidative damage produced by three hydroperoxides; hydrogen peroxide, tertiary butyl-hydroperoxide (tBH), and cumene hydroperoxide (CuH). Despite different lipophilicities of the peroxides, all three were approximately equitoxic and all produced similar quantities of DNA single strand breaks. Peroxides at 100 - 150 μM produced levels of DNA strand breaks equivalent to 500 - 700 rads of X-rays but with less toxicity. DNA single strand breaks were produced by the peroxides in less than 1 min and were maximal at 15 min after which time the number of breaks decreased. The organic hydroperoxides produced detectable amounts of malondialdehyde in cell suspensions but H_2O_2 did not. H_2O_2 but not tBH or CuH produced extensive single strand breaks in DNA after cell lysis and proteinase K treatment (manuscript in preparation).

These data and a previous report showing that hydroperoxyeicosatetraenoic acids (HPETEs) can be clastogenic to fibroblasts (4) led us to explore whether peroxides induced DNA strand breaks may be mediated through arachidonic acid metabolism. We tested the ability of several lipoxygenase and cyclooxygenase inhibitors to prevent hydroperoxide induced DNA strand breaks and cell death.

MATERIALS AND METHODS

The human adenocarcinoma cell line, A549, in log phase growth in RPMI 1640 medium supplemented with 10% fetal bovine serum was used in all experiments. The cells were harvested by trypsinization, washed and resuspended in Dulbecco's phosphate buffered salts solutions without calcium but with Mg^{2+} increased to a total of 1 mM and with 5 mM glucose added. All treatments were done at 37° C and at a cell concentration of 1 X 10^6 cells/ml. Arachidonic acid metabolism inhibitors; esculetin, quercetin, nordihydroguaiaretic acid (NDGA), BW 755c, or indomethacin when used were dissolved in 95% ethanol and incubated with the cells for 20 min at 37° C before peroxide challenge. Esculetin, quercetin, and BW 755c were kind gifts of Dr. Kenneth Honn. Lipoxygenase products; 5(S)-, 12(S)-, 15(S)-HPETEs and 15(S)HETE and 4-hydroxynonenal were purchased from BioMol, Plymouth Meeting, PA. The eicosanoids were supplied as dilute solutions in ethanol. The ethanol was removed by drying under nitrogen immediately before use. Other chemicals and reagents were purchased from Sigma, St. Louis, MO.

For DNA strand break assays the alkaline filter elution technique was used (3). Qd refers to the -100 X the log of the ratio of the fraction of DNA retained on the filter for treated vs untreated cells after 25 ml of buffer have passed over the filter at a rate of 2 ml/hr.

RESULTS AND DISCUSSION

Our initial studies used esculetin as a potent and specific lipoxygenase inhibitor (5) and indomethacin as a specific cyclooxygenase inhibitor. The results demonstrated that DNA single strand breaks produced by all three hydroperoxides could be attenuated by esculetin or esculetin plus indomethacin. Indomethacin alone either increased or did not effect the number of single strand breaks present after one hour. Later, studies on the time course of DNA single strand break induction and repair showed maximal breaks after 15 minutes incubation at 37° C and that rejoining began thereafter. We subsequently chose to study the effects of various other lipoxygenase and cyclooxygenase inhibitors after 15 min of incubation only. We choose to use the organic hydroperoxide, tBH, at 0.1 mM for these studies as we attained consistent control levels of breaks in each experiment. Table 1 summarizes these results.

Agents with predominantly lipoxygenase inhibitory activity, esculetin and quercetin, prevented 40 -60% of the maximum DNA strand breaks produced by tBH. Agents with combined cyclooxygenase and lipoxygenase inhibitory activity were less effective. Indomethacin, a cyclooxygenase inhibitor, had little effect. NDGA which has lipoxygenase activity and at higher concentrations, cyclooxygenase activity, interestingly inhibited more effectively at 20 than at 50 μM. BW755c also has both lipoxygenase and cyclooxygenase inhibitory activity (6) and had no effect at the concentrations tested. The effect of DMTU was tested to show whether a general free radical scavenger, by virtue of its hydrogen donation capacity, (7) could also prevent DNA strand breaks. DMTU inhibited DNA strand breaks produced by tBH and CuH but not by HOOH (data not shown).

Table 1
Effect of Various Inhibitors on DNA Single Strand Breaks Produced by 0.1 mM t-Butyl hydroperoxide in 15 Minutes

Treatment	Concentration (μM)	Qd	Percent Inhibition
tert-Butyl-OOH	100	186 ± 8	±4%, n=4
+ Esculetin	20	122	34%
+Indomethacin	20	165	11%
+Esc. + Indo.	20@	124	33%
+Quercetin	50	96	48%
+ "	100	80	57%
+NDGA	20	129	31%
+ "	50	164	12%
+BW755c	50	197	0%
+ "	100	179	4%
+DMTU	10 mM	104	44%

To ascertain whether these results translate into downstream protection, clonogenic survival of cells challenged with peroxides was tested in the presence and absence 20 μM esculetin (Figure 1). In each case, esculetin reversed the peroxide effect on survival. That is, that the peroxides were found to be growth stimulatory at 10 to 50 μM and toxic at higher concentrations. Thus, the complex effect of peroxides on cell processes may include an adaptive or hormetic response at low concentrations which may also involve lipoxygenase activity (Figure 1).

The lipoxygenase products 5-, 12-, and 15-(S)-HPETEs produced detectable DNA strand breaks at 50 μM or below after 15 min (Figure 2). A reportedly toxic lipid peroxidation product, 4-hydroxynonenal (4-HNA), was tested only at 5 and 10 μM with little effect. The reduced metabolite of 15(S)-HPETE, 15(S)-HETE was ineffective at causing DNA breaks. At 50 μM the 5(S)-HPETE was twice as clastogenic as 15(S)- and four times more than the 12(S)-HPETE. At 50 μM after 15 min, tBH produced strand breaks equivalent to the 15(S)-HPETE (Qd = 20).

These results indicate that peroxide induced DNA strand breaks do not result purely from hydroxyl radical generation from the peroxyl moiety of the agent. The efficiency of DNA strand break induction by HPETEs compared to other unphysiological but lipophilic peroxides and the inhibition of DNA strand break elaboration by lipoxygenase inhibitors imply that the lipoxygenase pathway has a role in clastogenic activity and toxicity of peroxides. Membrane damage produced by peroxide generating drugs or radiation, thus, may act synergistically to that produced by direct damage to the DNA. These factors may contribute to the inherent radiation sensitivity or promotability of various cell types.

The demonstration that a hydrogen donor, DMTU, inhibited hydroperoxide induced DNA strand breaks raises the question as to the specificity of the effects on arachidonic acid metabolism. DMTU was tested at 500 fold higher concentrations than esculetin and produced an equivalent degree of inhibition. Esculetin was reported as a 5- and 12-lipoxygenase inhibitor (5) and the 5(S)-HPETE was the most po-

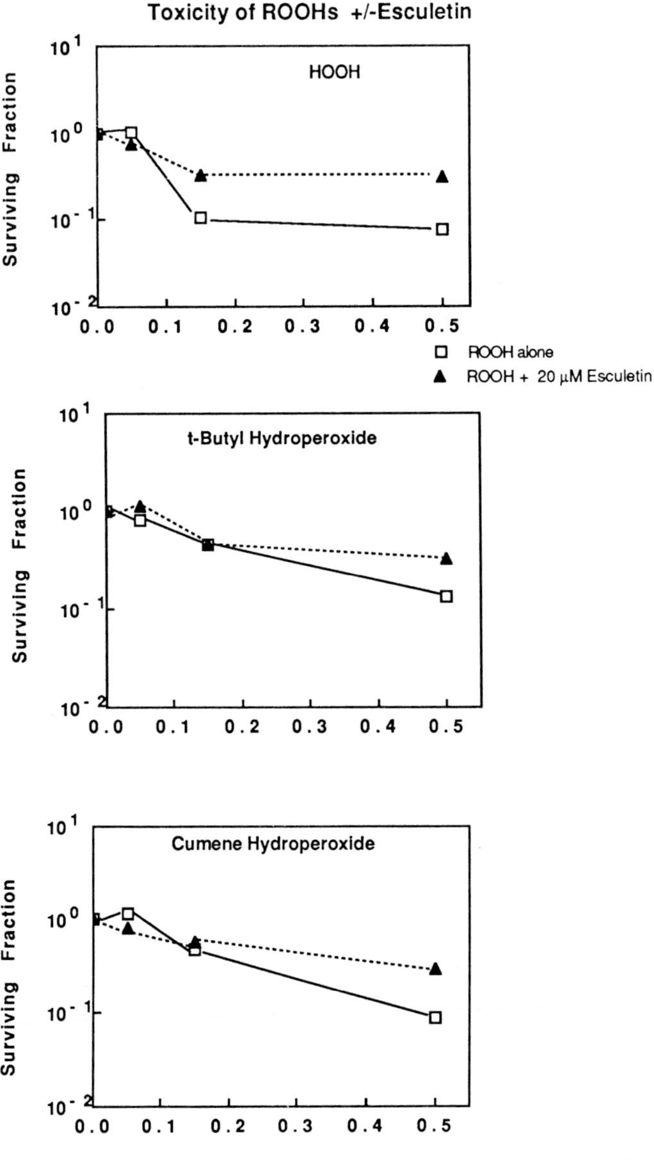
Toxicity of ROOHs +/-Esculetin
HOOH
t-Butyl Hydroperoxide
Cumene Hydroperoxide
Surviving Fraction
10^{1}
10^{0}
10^{-1}
10^{-2}
0.0
0.1
0.2
0.3
0.4
0.5
ROOH alone
ROOH + 20 μM Esculetin
ROOH (mM)

Figure 1.

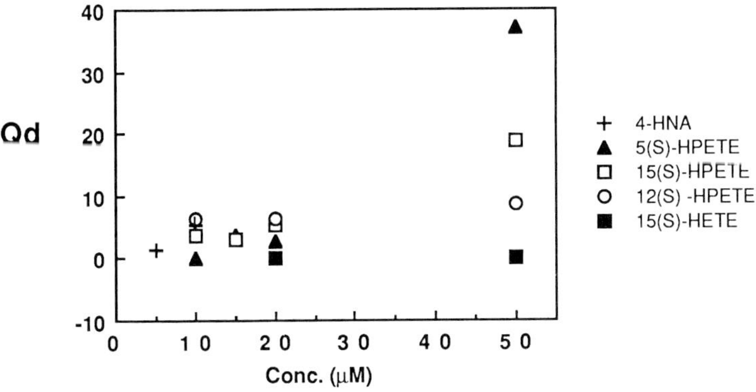

Figure 2. Single Strand Breaks Produced by Lipoxygenase Products

tent strand break induce of the 3 HPETEs tested. It may be that the lung adenocarcinoma cell used, A549, has this pathway. Experiments showing actual release of arachidonic acid and metabolites will be required to confirm these speculations.

REFERENCES

1. Ward, J.F., Evans, J.W., Limoli, C.L., and Calabro-Jones, P.M. Br. J. Cancer 55 (Suppl 8): 205-112, 1987.
2. Cerutti, P.A. Science 227: 375-381,1985.
3. Ochi, T. and Cerutti, P.A. Proc. Nat. Acad. Science 84:990-994,1987.
4. Kohn, K.W., Ewig, R.A.G. Erickson, L.C., and Zwelling, L.A. in DNA repair: A laboratory manual of Research Procedures (E. Friedberg and P. Hanawalt, eds) New York, Marcel Dekker, pp. 379-401, 1981.
5. Neichi, T., Koshihara, Y., and Murota, S. Biochim. Biophys. Acta 753:130-132, 1983.
6. Higgs, G.A., Flower, R.J. and Vane, J.R. A new approach to anti-inflammatory drugs. Biochem. Pharm. 28:1959-1961, 1979.
7. Fox, R.B. J. Clin. Invest. 74:1456-1464,1984.

8-HYDROXYDEOXYGUANOSINE, A DNA ADDUCT FORMED BY OXYGEN RADICALS: ITS IMPLICATIONS ON THE MUTAGENIC AND CARCINOGENIC ACTION OF OXYGEN RADICAL-FORMING AGENTS

H. KASAI, M.-H. CHUNG, D.S. JONES, H. INOUE*, H. ISHIKAWA*, H. KAMIYA*, E. OHTSUKA* and S. NISHIMURA

Biology Division, National Cancer Center Research Institute, Tsukiji 5-1-1, Chuo-ku, Tokyo, and *Faculty of Pharmaceutical Sciences, Hokkaido University, Sapporo 060, Japan

INTRODUCTION AND SUMMARY

It has been suggested that oxygen radicals are involved in both initiation and promotion of carcinogenesis (1,2). Oxygen radicals are produced by mutagens/carcinogens in the environment, but are also formed during various kinds of cellular metabolism. We previously observed that the C-8 position of deoxyguanosine residues in DNA is hydroxylated to produce 8-hydroxydeoxyguanosine (8-OH-dG) in DNA *in vitro* by various oxygen radical-producing agents (3). The formation of 8-OH-dG was also observed in cellular DNA when mice or rats were irradiated by ionizing radiation or administrated oxygen radical-forming carcinogens (4-6).

The extent of formation of 8-OH-dG in DNA *in vivo* seems to be equivalent to that of thymine glycol which is known to be a major product formed by oxygen radicals. Analysis of 8-OH-dG in DNA was facilitated by a simple HPLC coupled with an electrochemical detector developed by Floyd *et. al.* (7). Thus, analysis of 8-OH-dG in DNA can be used for monitoring oxidative DNA damage *in vivo*.

An important question is what is the biological effect of 8-OH-dG in DNA. To answer this question, oligodeoxynucleotides containing 8-OH-dG in a specific position were chemically synthesized, and used as a template for DNA synthesis *in vitro*. It was shown that an 8-OH-dG residue in DNA is often misread, not only in the position of 8-OH-dG residue itself, but also at a pyrimidine residue next to the 8-OH-dG (8). To further investigate the involvement of 8-OH-dG in mutagenesis/carcinogenesis, the second position of deoxyguanosine (dG) in codon 12 of a synthetic normal c-Ha-*ras* gene was specifically replaced with 8-OH-dG, and its transforming activity was analysed by DNA transfection using NIH3T3 cells as recipient cells. A small number of transformed foci appeared with the 8-OH-dG containing c-Ha-*ras* gene; the efficiency is approximately the same as that with the c-Ha-*ras* gene having O^6-methyldeoxyguanosine at the same position.

In addition, an attempt has been made to isolate an enzyme which specifically cleaves the site of an 8-OH-dG residue in DNA. For this purpose, double-stranded oligodeoxynucleotides having 8-OH-dG in a specific position were used as substrates. It was possible to detect an activity that cleaves the strand containing the modified base and we have purified the enzyme without contamination of other DNases from *Escherichia coli*. The enzyme may be a new endonuclease which specifically recognizes 8-OH-dG in double-stranded DNA, thus implying that 8-OH-dG present in DNA is not artificially formed, but actually produced *in vivo* by oxygen radicals, and the cells acquire a mechanism to repair it.

MATERIALS AND METHODS

Tissues or leukocytes were frozen at -80°C until the DNA isolation. Defrosted tissues were gently homogenized in a Teflon homogenizer for the minimum time (10 - 20 sec) in the absence of air. To that end, all the apparatus and solutions were saturated with argon gas before the homogenization. DNA was isolated by Marmur's method, except that cells were lysed by 2% sodium dodecylsulfate at 37°C for 30 min. Portions of DNA samples (3 - 5 A_{260} units) were dissolved in 200 µl of 20 mM sodium acetate buffer (pH 4.8), digested completely with 20 µg of nuclease P1 at 37°C for 30 min, and then treated with 1.3 units of *E. coli* alkaline phosphomonoesterase in 0.1 M Tris-HCl buffer (pH 7.5) for 1 hr.

The resulting deoxynucleoside mixture was injected into a HPLC column coupled with an electrochemical (EC) detector (7): apparatus, Toyo Soda HLC-803D; column, Beckman Ultrasphere ODS (0.46x25 cm); eluent, 10% aqueous methanol containing 12.5 mM citric acid, 25 mM sodium acetate, 30 mM NaOH, 10 mM acetic acid; flow rate, 1 ml/min; EC detector, Toyo Soda EC-8000, 600 mV (oxidation). The molar ratio of 8-OH-dG to dG in each DNA sample was determined based on the peak height of authentic 8-OH-dG with the EC detector and the UV absorbance at A_{290} of dG.

MATERIALS

<u>8-OH-dG.</u>

Standard sample of 8-OH-dG was prepared from dG with the Udenfriend system as described previously (3). Briefly dG (1 g) was dissolved in 780 ml of 0.1 M sodium phosphate buffer (pH 6.8), and 140 ml of 0.1 M ascorbic acid, 65 ml of 0.1 M EDTA and 13 ml of 0.1 M $FeSO_4$ were added. Oxygen gas was then bubbled at 37°C. After the reaction for 3 hrs in dark, the solution was adjusted to pH 3.7 by 1 N HCl, and charcoal powder (10 g) was added. The charcoal packed into a column (2x13 cm) was washed with 500 ml H_2O, and the material was eluted with 500 ml of aqueous acetone (1:1, v/v). The eluate was evaporated to dryness, and the residue was fractionated by preparative HPLC [column; TSK-Gel LS-410 ODS SIL (2.15x30 cm) from Toyo Soda, solvent: 15% aqueous MeOH].

<u>8-OH-dG containing oligodeoxynucleotides.</u>

The oligodeoxynucleotides containing 8-OH-dG in a specific position was chemically synthesized as previously reported (8). First, 8-OH-dG containing short oligomers (13-mer and 16-mer) were synthesized by the solid-phase phosphotriester method using protected dimers and a monomer: N^2-Acetyl-5'-monomethoxytrityl-8-methoxydeoxyguanosine-3'-O-chlorophenyl) phosphate was used as a monomer unit for 8-OH-dG. After condensation and cleavage from its support, the product was heated in concentrated ammonia to produce 8-methoxydeoxyguanosine. The oligomer containing 8-methoxydeoxyguanosine was then treated with *N,N'*-dimethylformamide and triethylamine to convert 8-methoxydeoxyguanosine to 8-OH-dG. The product was purified by HPLC and joined to other oligodeoxynucleotide which was separately synthesized by a DNA synthesizer (Applied Biosystems 380A) to make longer oligodeoxynucleotide by using T4 polynucleotide kinase, T4 DNA ligase and a complementary oligomer covering the both fragments as a sprint.

RESULTS

Formation of 8-OH-dG in DNA *in vitro.*

In order to identify mutagens present in broiled food, we previously developed a new method which is based on adduct formation with the fluorescent guanosine derivative, 2'-deoxy-2' (2", 3" - dihydro-2", 4"-diphenyl-2" -hydroxy-3 " -oxo-1" pyrrolyl) guanosine (9). This method was applied to screen heated glucose as a model of broiled food in order to identify the active principle(s) present. Several adduct peaks were detected in the HPLC chromatogram. Consequently, by ucing isopropylideneguanosine (IPG) as the adduct trap, the structure of one of the adducts were determined to be as 8-hydroxy-IPG. This was a rather unexpected and interesting result. Although various oxidation products of DNA components such as thymine glycol and 5-hydroxymethyluracil have been reported, the hydroxylation reaction at the C-8 position of guanine residue in DNA has not been reported at that time. Thus we pursued mechanism of the formation of 8-OH-dG in DNA.

When a solution of dG or DNA (double stranded and single stranded) was shaken with various oxygen radical-forming agents, the formation of 8-OH-dG was always observed. Those oxygen radical-forming agents include reducing agents (3), X-ray (10) asbestos plus hydrogen peroxide (11), and polyphenol with hydrogen peroxide and ferric ion (12). It is interesting to note the 8-OHdG is the only major product produced from purine deoxynucleosides by oxygen radical-producing chemicals, while X-ray produces both 8-OH-dG and 8-hydroxydeoxyadenosine.

Formation of 8-OH-dG in DNA *in vivo.*

The formation of 8-OH-dG in DNA has also been observed *in vivo*. Namely, when the whole body of mice was irradiated with γ-ray, the amount of 8-OH-dG residue in liver DNA of the irradiated mice was increased proportionally to the dose of γ-ray (Figure 1 and Figure 2). It should be noted that the amount of 8-OH-dG in DNA after *in vivo* irradiation were three orders of magnitude lower than those after *in vitro* irradiation of DNA. Therefore the sensitive method to detect 8-OH-dG by using an electro-chemical detector was found to be very useful. It should be noted that extent of formation of 8-OH-dG *in vivo* seems to be almost comparable to that of thymine glycol formation as shown in Table I.

8-OH-dG was also produced in DNA *in vivo* by administration of oxygen radical-producing carcinogens into rats. By oral administration of a renal carcinogen, potassium bromate ($KBrO_3$), to the rat, a significant increase of 8-OH-dG in kidney DNA was observed (5). Amount of 8-OH-dG increased in kidney DNA is approximately 5 8-OH-dG per 10^5 dG molecule. On the contrary to kidney, the increase of 8-OH-dG content in DNA of liver, a non-target tissue was not significant, suggesting that formation of 8-OH-dG in tissue DNA is closely related to $KBrO_3$ carcinogenesis.

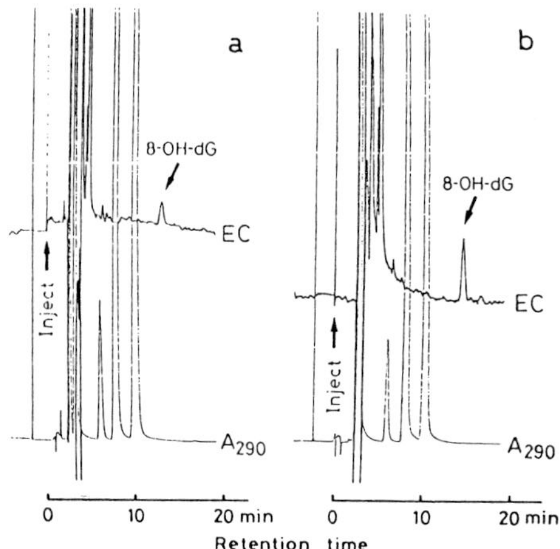

Figure1. Detection of 8-OH-dG in mouse liver DNA by HPLC coupled with an electrochemical detector. (a) Control mouse liver DNA; (b) liver DNA from a mouse irradiated with 173 Krad of γ-rays. (Reprinted with permission from ref. 4).

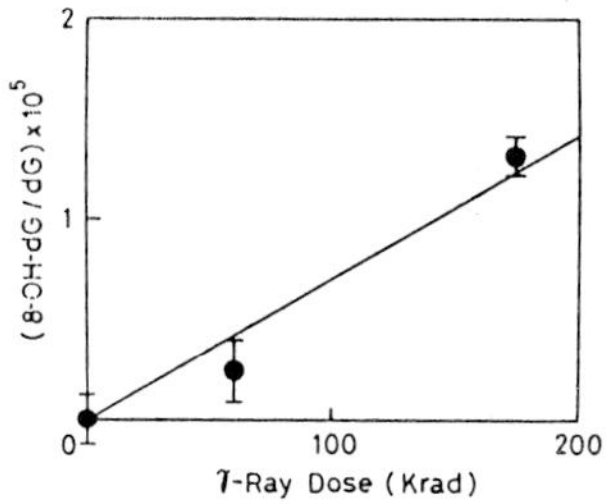

Figure 2. Formation of 8-OH-dG in mouse liver DNA on whole body irradiation with γ-rays. (Reprinted with permission from ref. 4).

Table I. Comparison of yield of 8-OH-dG with that of thymine glycol formed in DNA by X-ray irradiation *in vivo*.

8-OH-dG/10^7 dG/Krad		Thymine glycol/10^7 dG/Krad*	
Mouse liver 0.13 Krad/min	Mouse Liver 14 Krad/min	HeLa cells 0.4 Krad/min	BS-C-1 cells 1.5 Krad/min
0.8	3.2	2.0	3.4

*Taken from the paper by Leadon *et al.* (22).

A similar result was obtained with another chemical carcinogen, ciprofibrate. Ciprofibrate is known to be a peroxisome proliferator that induces hepatocellular carcinoma in rats and mice. It was suggested that the proliferation of peroxisomes and induction of peroxisome-associated enzymes results in oxidative stress which then leads to tumorigenesis. J. K. Reddy and his colleagues, collaborating with us, have shown that administration of ciprofibrate in diet at a concentration of 0.025% for 16, 28, 36, or 40 weeks resulted in progressive increases in the level of 8-OHdG in rat liver DNA (6). The increase of 8-OH-dG level seems to be attributed to persistent peroxisome proliferation resulting from chronic ciprofibrate treatment, since no increase in 8-OH-dG was found in liver DNA of rats that received a single dose of ciprofibrate. Increased lipid peroxidation has been observed in liver of rats chronically treated with peroxisome proliferators (13). In this connection, it is interesting to note that 8-OH-dG was formed when auto-oxidized linolenic acid or linoleic acid were reacted with dG or DNA (14)

Transforming activity of normal c-Ha-*ras* gene by replacing G in the second position of the 12th codon by 8-OH-dG.

An important question is whether the formation of 8-OH-dG can be considered a likely cause of mutation or carcinogenesis by oxygen radicals. To investigate this possibility, we previously examined the effect of an 8-OH-dG residue in DNA on the fidelity of DNA replication using a DNA synthesis system *in vitro* with *E. coli* DNA polymerase I (Klenow fragment) (8). The synthetic oligo-deoxynucleotides, with or without an 8-OH-dG residue in a specified position were used as templates for DNA synthesis under the conditions of the dideoxy chain termination sequencing method. It was shown that an 8-OH-dG residue in DNA is misread to insert A, T, C and G with an almost equal frequency. In addition, pyrimidine residues next to the 8-OH-dG were also misread (Figure 3).

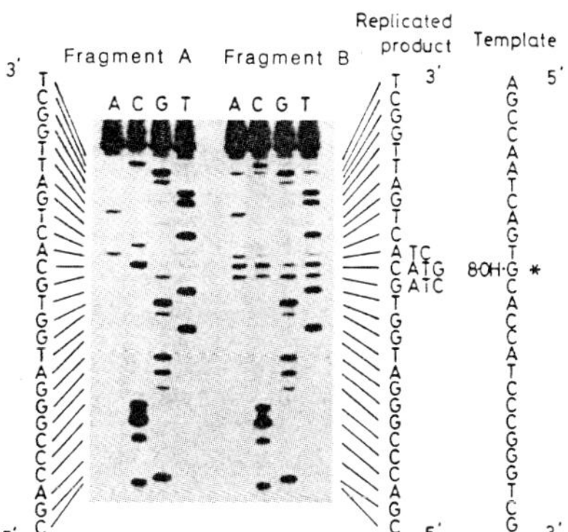

Figure 3. Autoradiographs of 12% polyacrylamide sequencing gel, showing the sequence of the products synthesized under the direction of 8-OH-dG containing DNA template, Fragment B. Fragment A is its counterpart containing normal dG. (Reprinted with permission from ref. 8).

To further examine the effect of 8-OH-dG in DNA in mutation, a synthetic normal c-Ha-*ras* gene having an 8-OH-dG residue only at the second position of the 12th codon in place of G has been constructed and used for transfection of NIH3T3 cells. For this study, synthetic human c-Ha-*ras* genes (15) were ligated to the 3'-end of Rous sarcoma virus long terminal repeat (16). Also a vector containing the normal c-Ha-*ras* gene having GGT at the 12th codon was constructed. In addition, c-Ha-*ras* genes having either 8-OHdG or O^6-methyldeoxyguanine (O^6-Me-dG) at the second position of the 12th codon (GGT) was prepared by cassette mutagenesis. As shown in Table 2, a small number of transformed foci appeared with the 8-OH-dG containing c-Ha-*ras* gene: the efficiency was approximately the same as that with the c-Ha-*ras* gene having O^6-Me-dG. Although the further study is needed to identify the type of mutation present in the c-Ha-*ras* gene isolated from the transformed cells, this preliminary experiment suggests that 8-OH-dG in DNA can induce mutation *in vivo.*

Table 2. Transformation of NIH3T3 cells with synthetic c-Ha-*ras* gene containing 8-OH-dG or O^6-Me-dG at codon 12.

Amount of DNA/plate	Transformant/plate			
	Gly-12	Val-12	8-OH-dG	O^6-Me-dG
20 ng	0	101	0.2	2
50 ng	0	172	4.4	4

Gly-12, 5'-GGT-3' -CCA-; Val-12, 5'-GTT-3' -CCA-;

8-OH-dG or O6-Me-dG, 5'-G$\overset{*}{\text{G}}$T-3', -CCA-

$\overset{*}{\text{G}}$ is modified base.

8-OH-dG specific endonuclease from *E. coli.*

The 8-OH-dG produced in liver DNA by irradiation of mice decreased with time, suggesting the presence of a repair enzyme(s) acting on 8-OH-dG in mouse liver (4). We have also noticed that the mean levels of 8-OH-dG in peripheral blood leukocytes increased immediately after smoking, but rapidly returned to the original level (unpublished results). Thus an attempt has been made to isolate an enzyme from *E. coli* which specifically cleaves the site of an 8-OH-dG residue in DNA. For this purpose, a double-stranded 46-mer having 8-OH-dG was used as a substrate. We were able to detect an activity that cleaves the strand containing 8-OH-dG, and have purified the enzyme without contamination of other DNases by successive purification procedures as ammonium sulfate precipitation, DEAE-cellulose and Sephadex G-100 column chromatography. The cleavage was observed only with double-stranded DNA, but not with single-stranded DNA containing 8-OH-dG. The enzyme cleaves both phosphodiester bonds, 3' and 5' to 8-OH-dG residue, leaving phosphate on the deoxyribose moiety of neighboring bases. This endonuclease showed no activity on DNAs with mismatches G:A and G:T. This enzyme was found to differ from *E. coli* endonuclease III and endonuclease IV. The enzyme may be a new endonuclease which specifically recognizes 8-OH-dG in double-stranded DNA, thus implying that 8-OH-dG present in DNA is not artifically formed, but actually produced *in vivo* by oxygen radicals, and the cells acquire a mechanism to repair it.

DISCUSSION

Oxygen radicals induce to produce various kind of DNA damage such as DNA strand scission and formation of thymine glycol and 5-hydroxymethyluracil in addition to 8-OH-dG formation (17). An important question is what type of DNA damage is relevant to mutagenesis/carcinogenesis caused by oxygen radicals. Much attention was paid previously to DNA strand scission and thymine glycol formation in this context, since those DNA damages were discovered many years ago, and extensively studied since then. However, as described in this article, it can be seen that 8-OH-dG cannot be ignored when one considers the molecular mechanism of mutagenesis/carcinogenesis by oxygen radicals, although further studies are needed in order to get a clearer picture. In this connection, it is noteworthy to mention that point mutation in *E. coli, Neurospora crassa* and mammalian cells caused by γ-ray or X-ray irradiation was found to be GC --> AT and GC --> TA as well as AT --> GC and AT --> TA mutations, indicating that damage in a G:C pair is involved in mutagenesis (18-21).

The amount of 8-OH-dG present in DNA is quite large as compared with formation of DNA adducts by alkylating agents or other chemical carcinogens (approximately $1/10^5$ against $1/10^8$ per dG). One can argue that if 8-OH-dG is really mutagenic, how cells can survive with such a high extent of modification. However, it is possible that the frequency of misreading of 8-OH-dG found in *in vitro* DNA synthesis does not exactly represent the *in vivo* situation, since it is a model system using a single-stranded DNA as a template. The mutation frequency of 8-OH-dG may be much smaller *in vivo.*

Quite a large amount of 8-OH-dG is detected in DNA without treatment by oxygen radial forming agents. This background level of 8-OH-dG cannot be diminished despite many precautions to avoid oxidation of DNA during isolation (approximately one 8-OH-dG per 10^5 dG). A question is raised as to whether these 8-OH-dG residues are endogeneously present in DNA, or produced artificially during the isolation process. Although a final answer has not yet been obtained, it should be mentioned that the amount of 8-OH-dG present in human peripheral blood leukocytes DNA varied almost 10 folds depending upon the individual (1-10 8-OH-dG/10^5 dG). However it can also be argued that generation of H_2O_2 or other oxygen radical forming peroxides are produced metabolically in vitro after the cells are lysed, and such metabolic activities differ with each individual.

Perhaps the most important future approach to elucidate a mechanism of involvement of 8-OH-dG in mutagenesis/carcinogenesis is to further investigate mechanisms of repair of 8-OH-dG in DNA in both bacteria and mammalian cells. Isolation of mutant(s) for repair of 8-OH-dG should give more clear information on this interesting problem. In addition, studies on *in vivo* mutation by using a plasmid vector containing 8-OH-dG in a specific position should be informative.

REFERENCES

1. Ames, A.N. *Science* 221:1256-1264, 1983.
2. Cerutti, P.A. *Science* 227;375-381, 1985.
3. Kasai, H. and Nishimura, S. *Nucleic Acids Res.* 12:2137-2145, 1984.
4. Kasai, H., Crain, P.F., Kuchino, Y., Nishimura, S., Ootsuyama, A. and Tanooka, H. *Carcinogenesis* 7:1849-1851, 1986.
5. Kasai, H., Nishimura, S., Kurokawa, Y. and Hayashi, Y. *Carcinogenesis* 8:1959-1961, 1987.
6. Kasai, H., Okada, Y., Nishimura, S., Rao, M.S. and Reddy, J. K. *Cancer Res.49:* 2603-2605, 1989.
7. Floyd, R.A., Watson, J.J., Wong, P.K., Altmiller, D.H. and Richard, R.C. *Free Radical Res. Commun* 1:153-172, 1986.
8. Kuchino, Y., Mori, F., Kasai, H., Inoue, H., Iwai, S., Miura, K., Ohtsuka, E. and Nishimura, S. *Nature* 327:77-79, 1987.
9. Kasai, H., Hayami, H., Yamaizumi, Z., Saito, H. and Nishimura, S. *Nucleic Acids Res.* 12:2127-2136, 1984.
10. Kasai, H., Tanooka, H., and Nishimura, S. *Gann* 75:1037-1039, 1984.
11. Kasai, H. and Nishimura, S. *Gann* 75:841-844, 1984.
12. Kasai, H. and Nishimura, S. *Gann* 75:565-566, 1984.
13. Goel, S.K., Lalwani, N.D., and Reddy, J.K. *Cancer Res.* 46:1324-1330, 1986.
14. Kasai, H. and Nishimura, S. Proceeding of the 4th Biennial General Meeting of the Society for Free Radical Research, Kyoto, Japan, 9-10 April 1988; Hayaishi, O., Niki, E., Kondo, M. and Yoshikawa, T. (Eds), Elsevier Science Publishers, B.V., Amsterdam, pp. 1021-1023, 1989.
15. Miura, K., Inoue, Y., Nakamori, H., Iwai, S., Ohtsuka, E., Ikehara, M., Noguchi, S. and Nishimura, S. *Jpn. J. Cancer Res. (Gann)* 77:45-51, 1986.
16. Kamiya, H., Miura, K., Ohtomo, N., Koda, T., Kakinuma, M., Nishimura, S. and Ohtsuka, E. *Jpn. J. Cancer Res. 80:* 200-203, 1989.
17. Sies, H. *Angew. Chem. Int.,* Ed. Engl. 25:1058-1071, 1986.
18. Glickman, B.W., Rietveld, K. and Aaron, C.S. *Mutation Res.* 69:1-12, 1980.
19. Malling, H.V. and deSerres, F.J. *Radiat. Res.* 53:77-87, 1973.
20. Grosovsky, A.J., deBoer, J.G., deJong, P.J., Drobetsky, E.A. and Glickman, B.W. *Proc. Natl. Acad. Sci. USA* 85:185-188, 1988.
21. Guerrero, I. and Pellicer, A. *Mutation Res.* 185:293-308, 1987.

REACTION OF DNA PEROXYL RADICALS WITH CYSTEAMINE AND GLUTATHIONE: THE FORMATION OF SULFOXYL RADICALS

M. D. SEVILLA, M. YAN, D. BECKER and S. GILLICH

Department of Chemistry, Oakland University, Rochester, MI 48309

INTRODUCTION

The oxygen enhancement effect has been attributed to defect (radical) fixation by oxygen which prevents repair by sulfhydryls (1-4). Actually, in model systems, oxygen in the absence of thiols is a slight radioprotector of DNA and does not act to increase damage (5,6). Indigenous thiols not only account for the radioprotective effects but their radical reactions in the presence of oxygen are also a likely source of the oxygen enhancement effect. Prutz has suggested in recent studies that disulfide anion radicals formed by thiyl radical attack on thiol (reaction 1) are the primary species responsible for the radioprotective effect of thiols (7).

$$DNA(-H)\bullet + RSH \rightarrow RS\bullet + DNA \quad (1)$$

$$DNA\bullet + O_2 \rightarrow DNAOO\bullet \quad (2)$$

$$RS\bullet + RSH \rightarrow RSSR\bullet^- + H^+ \quad (3)$$

$$DNA(-H)\bullet + RSSR\bullet^- + H^+ \rightarrow DNA + RSSR \quad (4)$$

In this work the reactions of thiols with DNA primary radical intermediates formed after γ-irradiation of frozen anoxic and oxic solutions of DNA-thiols are investigated Results are interpreted base on our previous work on the reactions of thiyl radicals with oxygen to form various sulfoxyl radicals (8-11) Evidence is found for each of the intermediates described above and additional species formed by the reaction of peroxyl radicals with thiols.

MATERIALS AND METHODS

Preparation of DNA-thiol samples.

Nitrogen bubbled solutions of thiol (1 to 30 mM) are prepared in distilled water. In a nitrogen purged glove bag, 100 mg calf-thymus DNA (Chemical Dynamics) is added to one mL of this solution. At these high DNA concentrations, the DNA remains in a double helix without added electrolyte. The vial is capped and let stand overnight. Anoxic frozen ice plugs are prepared in a glove bag by drawing the viscous DNA-thiol solution into a 5mm (ID) glass tube and freezing it in liquid nitrogen. By rapidly thawing the outside of the sample and pushing the remaining sample out of the tube with a stainless steel rod into liquid nitrogen an ice plug is formed of the proper dimensions. To prepare oxic samples the DNA-thiol is bubbled with air or oxygen (depending on the concentration of oxygen desired) for a few minutes before freezing. Samples are then irradiated for doses of ca. 5 kGy (0.5 Mrad) and investigated by ESR spectroscopy. The ESR facilities have been described previously (8).

RESULTS

The reaction of radiation-produced DNA radicals with the known radioprotective agent, cysteamine (CyaSH) was investigated. Oxygenated and anoxic solutions of DNA (100 mg/mL) and cysteamine (2 mg/mL) were irradiated and their ESR spectra recorded as the samples were annealed. In Figures 1 and 2 we show an analysis of all spectra collected for these samples as they were annealed from 77K to 210K. Computer analyses of the spectra of DNA samples are based on spectra of the individual DNA radicals and the individual spectra of the thiyl, disulfide anion and sulfoxyl radicals (8-10, 15). In these graphs the conversion of one radical species to another are clearly shown. In Figures 1 (oxic) and 2 (anoxic) the original DNA primary anion (T^{-}• and perhaps C^{-}•) and cation (G^{+}•) radicals begin to react at temperatures near 150K for T^{-}• and 170K for $G^{+•}$. Note that although we will describe the cationic species as G^{+}, this species likely deprotonates from G to C at low temperatures to form G(-H)• and $C(H^{+})$. Annealing also results in the gradual protonation of the anion to form TH•. Under oxygen, Figure 1, the concentration of TH• is reduced by its reaction to form peroxyl radicals and by reaction of its precursor (T^{-}•) to form O_2^{-}

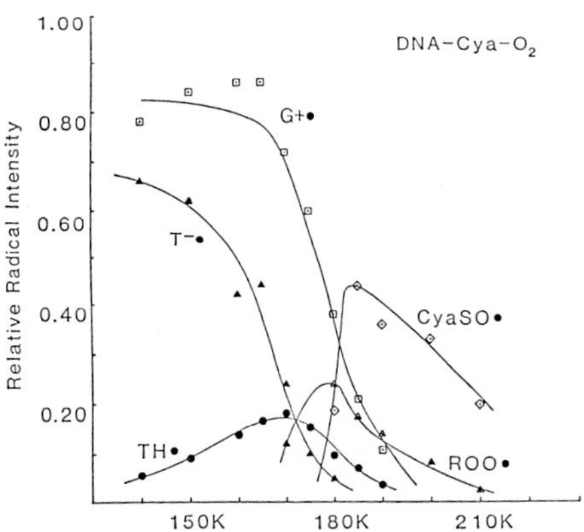

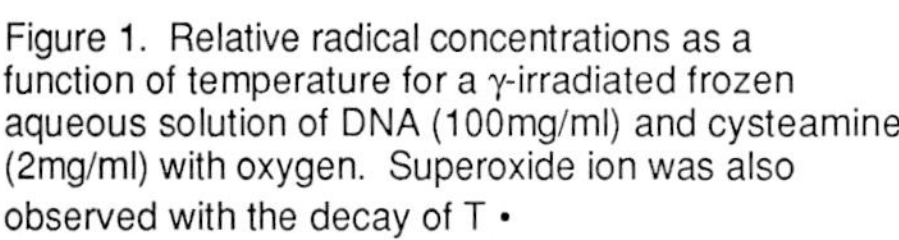
Figure 1. Relative radical concentrations as a function of temperature for a γ-irradiated frozen aqueous solution of DNA (100mg/ml) and cysteamine (2mg/ml) with oxygen. Superoxide ion was also observed with the decay of T •

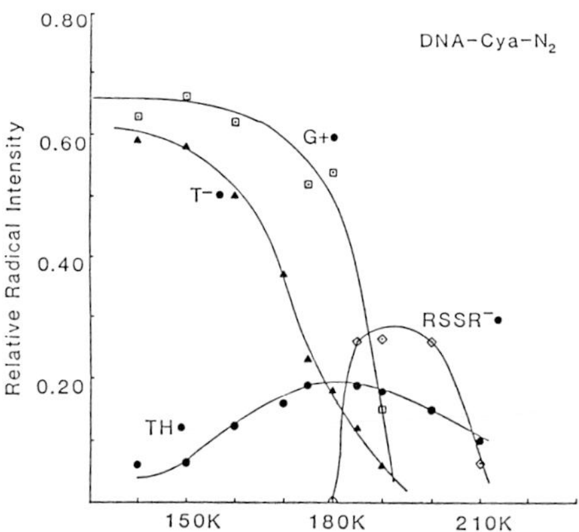

Figure 2. Relative radical concentrations as a function of temperature for an identical sample to that in Figure 1 except under nitrogen. The decay in total signal intensity with temperature is due to ion recombination.

(reactions 5a and 5b). The superoxide ion, $O_2^{-}\cdot$, which is not shown in Figure 1, was found in oxygen samples at levels up to 15% of the total radical yield (at 175K). It increases in intensity with the loss of T (reaction 5b) and decays more rapidly than ROO•. ROO• refers to both peroxyl species, CyaSOO• and DNAOO•. We find that ROO• increases as $G^{+}\cdot$ is lost. This we attribute to the formation of CyaS• by electron transfer to $G^{+}\cdot$ and the subsequent reaction of the thiyl radical with oxygen to form CyaSOO• (reactions 6 and 7) as well as the direct reaction of G(-H)• with oxygen (reaction 5a).

$$\text{DNA}\cdot\ (\text{TH}\cdot,\ \text{G(-H)}\cdot) + O_2 \rightarrow \text{DNAOO}\cdot\ (\text{THOO}\cdot,\ \text{G(-H)OO}\cdot) \quad (5a)$$

$$\text{DNA}^{-}\cdot(\text{T}^{-}\cdot) + O_2 \rightarrow \text{DNA(T)} + O_2^{-}\cdot \quad (5b)$$

$$\text{DNA}^{+}\cdot(\text{G(-H)}\cdot) + \text{CyaSH} \rightarrow \text{CyaS}\cdot + H^{+} + \text{DNA} \quad (6)$$

$$\text{CyaS}\cdot + O_2 \rightarrow \text{CyaSOO}\cdot \quad (7)$$

At 200K in Figure 1 very little peroxyl radical is found. The major species present is the cysteamine sulfinyl radical, CyaSO•. We believe the peroxyl radicals (DNAOO• and CyaSOO•) react with CyaSH to form the sulfinyl radical, CyaSO•, reaction 8 or reaction sequence 9.

$$\text{DNAOO}\cdot + \text{CyaSH} \rightarrow \text{CyaSO}\cdot + \text{DNAOH} \quad (8)$$

or

$$\text{DNAOO}\cdot + \text{CyaSH} \rightarrow \text{CyaS}\cdot + \text{DNAOOH} \quad (9)$$
$$\text{CyaS}\cdot + O_2 \rightarrow \text{CyaSOO}\cdot$$
$$\text{CyaSOO}\cdot + \text{CyaSH} \rightarrow \text{CyaSO}\cdot + \text{CyaOH}$$

The DNA product, DNAOH or DNAOOH, depends on which of the two mechanisms is correct. Thus far our results show good evidence for the production of CyaSOO• as an intermediate, which points to the second mechanism; however, the source of the CyaSOO• could be from reactions 6 and 7 rather than reaction 9. Experiments performed in the absence of oxygen have been very informative regarding reaction 6. For example, on annealing the anoxic sample to 185 K we observe the formation of $\text{CyaSSCya}^{-}\cdot$ (Figure 2). We interpret the formation of the disulfide anion radical as the result of reaction of thiol with the cationic center ($G^{+}\cdot$) to form thiyl radical (reaction 6) followed by the reaction of thiyl radical with parent thiol (reaction 10).

$$\text{CyaS}\cdot + \text{CyaSH} \rightarrow \text{CyaSSCya}^{-}\cdot + H^{+} \quad (10)$$

Preliminary analysis suggests CyaS• is present as an intermediate in these spectra. These anoxic experiments show, for the first time, the repair of a primary DNA ion radical lesion by a thiol, and the subsequent formation of the disulfide anion radical. This anion radical has been proposed as a participant in the radioprotection by thiols (12). There is an early ESR study of irradiated anoxic DNA-10% cysteamine freeze dried samples which also reports radical transfer to thiol from DNA; however, no free radical identifications were made (13).

For DNA-glutathione samples similar results to DNA-CyaSH samples were found in oxygenated samples except that the yield of sulfoxyl radical species were somewhat reduced. Very interesting results have been found in our work with DNA-GSH samples in the absence of oxygen. Here we observe the formation not of the expected disulfide anion radical ($GSSG^{-}\cdot$) as found for CyaSH and other thiols, but the glutathione carbon radical •G(-H)SH. This is a significant result, in keeping with our results with glutathione alone in frozen solutions (8) which suggested that GS• was able to readily abstract the cysteine residue α-carbon hydrogen atom (reaction 11).

$$GS\cdot + GSH \rightarrow GSH + \cdot G(\text{-}H)SH \; [\gamma\text{-glu-NHC}(CH_2SH)\text{CO-gly}] \qquad (11)$$

Abstraction from weak C-H bonds by thiyl radicals is not unexpected since the S-H bond energy is ca. 88 kcal and many C-H bonds have lower bond energies. For example, hydrogen abstraction by the thiyl radical has just recently been suggested as a means of initiation of lipid autoxidation (14). The formation of the carbon-centered species in GSH can occur intramolecularly as well as intermolecularly. Formation of the carbon species may account for the fact that glutathione is not as efficient a radioprotective agent as cysteamine.

In summary, these results show the conversion of DNA primary radicals to sulfhydryl radicals in good yield. Further, they show that formation of disulfide anion radicals are completely suppressed in the oxygenated system. This is in accord with the hypothesis of Prutz (7) that the disulfide anion radical is a radioprotective agent which oxygen removes. However, the fact that sulfoxyl radicals are produced in the presence of oxygen also leaves open the question whether these species are damaging. At present we have observed RSO• and RSOO• in DNA samples; in other work we have shown that $RSO_2\cdot$ and $RSO_2OO\cdot$ result from RSOO• in the presence of light (10, 15). Since we have earlier postulated that the $RSO_2OO\cdot$ radical is likely a highly reactive hydrogen abstraction agent (15), it may play a role in DNA damage.

ACKNOWLEDGMENT

This work is supported by grants from the National Institutes of Health (ROICA45424-03) and the Department of Energy (DEFG0286ER60455).

REFERENCES

1. Howard-Flanders, P., Nature. 186, 485-487, 1960.
2. Hutchinson, F., Radiat. Res. 14, 721-723, 1961
3. Alper, T., Cellular Radiobiology, (Cambridge: Cambridge University Press), 1979, p. 58.
4. Schulte-Frohlinde, D., Free Radical Res. Commun. 6, 181-184, 1989.
5. Held, K.D., Harrop, H.A. and Michael, B.D., Int. J. Radiat. Biol. 45, 615 - 626, 1984.
6. Quintiliani, M., Int. J. Radiat. Biol. 50, 573-594, 1986.
7. Prutz, W.A., Int. J. Radiat. Biol. 56, 21-33, 1989.
8. Becker, D., Swarts, S., Champagne, M. and Sevilla, M.D., Int. J. Radiat. Biol . 53, 767-786, 1988.

9. Sevilla, M.D., Yan, M. and Becker, D., Biochem. Biophys. Res. Commun. 155, 405-410, 1988.
10. Swarts, S.G., Becker, D., DeBolt, S. and Sevilla, M.D., J. Phys. Chem. 93, 155-161, 1989.
11. Sevilla, M.D., Yan, M., Becker, D. and Gillich, S., Free Radical Res. Commun. 6, 99 -102, 1989 .
12. Prutz, W.A. and Monig, H., Int. J. Radiat. Biol. 52, 677-682, 1987.
13. Milvy, P., Radiat. Res. 47, 83-93, 1971.
14. Schoenich, C., Asmus, K. -D., Dillinger, U. and Bruchhausen, F.V., Biochem. Biophys. Res. Commun., 161, 113-120, 1989.
15. Sevilla, M. D., Becker, D., and Yan, M., Int. J. Radiat. Biol., 57:65-81, 1990.

FATTY ACID-INDUCED MODULATION OF CARCINOGENESIS IN HUMAN AND MOUSE MAMMARY EXPLANT CULTURES

N. T. TELANG[1], A. BASU[2], M. J. MODAK[2], H. L. BRADLOW[3], and M. P. OSBORNE[1]

[1]Breast Cancer Research Laboratory, Department of Surgery, Memorial Sloan-Kettering Cancer Center, 1275 York Avenue, New York, NY 10021; [2]Department of Biochemistry and Molecular Biology, UMDNJ - New Jersey Medical School, Newark, N.J. 07103-2757; [3]Institute for Hormone Research, New York, N.Y. 10016

INTRODUCTION

Out of some 140,000 new cases of breast cancer in the United States, one out of 10 (10%) have a lifetime risk of developing breast cancer (1), and only 25% of women developing breast cancer present identifiable risk factors (2). Thus, in majority of women the causative factor(s), and therefore relative risk for developing breast cancer remains unknown.

Several epidemiological and clinical investigations together with laboratory studies on animal models have provided a strong support to the concept that dietary macronutrients, such as fats, are capable of modifying the progression of breast cancer (3-6). However, the evidence for specific components of dietary fat to directly influence the process of initiation, and/or promotion of carcinogenesis in mammary epithelium is equivocal. The lack of definitive identification of causative agent(s) for human breast cancer, and the absence of specific evidence for clinically relevant chemopreventive efficacy of dietary interventions have prompted us to develop **in vitro** models for human breast cancer, wherein initiation and modulation of carcinogenesis can be examined directly on the target tissue. These **in vitro** models utilize explant cultures of non-transformed mammary tissue from reduction mammoplasty or mastectomy samples as well as from inbred strains of mice that possess defined risk for developing mammary cancer. In our newly developed explant culture system mammary tissue can be maintained in a chemically defined, serum free medium for at least 10 to 35 days (7-10). This **in vitro** approach provides a means to examine the response of the target tissue to prototype carcinogens at molecular, metabolic and cellular levels, and then to evaluate modulators of carcinogenesis to positively or negatively regulate the process of initiation and/or promotion of preneoplastic transformation. The application of preneoplastic alterations as the quantitative end points, thus provide a means to evaluate chemopreventive efficacy of dietary components such as selected fatty acids, micronutrients, naturally occuring and synthetic vitamins and endocrine modulators directly on human mammary tissue.

In the present communication, experiments designed to identify specific molecular and metabolic markers that quantify the response of human and murine mammary tissue to prototype carcinogens, are discussed. Furthermore, the two markers are also validated for their ability to measure the molecular and metabolic alterations induced by selected fatty acids. This approach utilizing comparative human and murine experiments provides a model that reduces the need for extrapolation of carcinogenesis and chemopreventive data for their clinical relevance.

EXPERIMENTAL METHODS AND DESIGN

Human Mammary Tissue.

Non-involved mammary tissue was used from premenopausal subjects. All the mastectomy patients presented confirmed evidence of infiltrating and/or **in situ** ductal carcinoma. The non-involved tissue from these patients was therefore considered to be at 'high-risk'. The mammoplasty patients lacked pathological evidence of cancer, and the tissue therefore was considered to be at low risk.

Mouse Mammary Tissue.

The inguinal (#4) mammary glands from 6 to 8 week old virgin female BALB/c mice were used for the experiments. This strain does not produce mature mouse mammary tumor virus (MMTV) particles, and therefore, exhibits a low incidence of naturally occuring mammary tumors (tumor incidence: less than 10% at 24 months, 11). The mammary glands of BALB/c mice are however, highly susceptible to tumorigenic transformation by chemical carcinogens (7,12).

Explant Cultures.

The explant cultures were prepared from non-involved human mammary terminal duct lobular units from high and low risk patients (TDLU-HR and TDLU-LR) or from mouse mammary tissue fragments containing ducts with terminal end buds (TEB) as shown in Figure 1. The methodology used to maintain the mammary tissues as explant cultures was essentially similar to that reported previously (7-10,13,15).

Exposure to Fatty Acids and Carcinogens.

The free fatty acids linoleic acid (LNA, C18:2, n-6) and eicospentaenoic acid (EPA, C20:5, n-3) were complexed to BSA fraction V, and used on the cultures at the final concentrations of 5 ug/ml. The carcinogens Benzo (a) pyrene (BP) and 7,12-dimethylbenz (a) anthracene (DMBA) were used on the cultures at the final concentrations of 1 ug/ml and 2 ug/ml respectively. The cultures were maintained in the presence of the fatty acids for 7 days, and then treated with the carcinogens between the 7th and the 8th day for 24 hours. The treated cultures were then maintained for an additional 48 hours in the presence of the fatty acids and processed for the ras p21 assay (10,13,14). In parallel cultures the extent of estradiol metabolism was measured during the last 48 hours of the culture (15,16).

RESULTS AND DISCUSSION

In this study explant cultures of human and mouse mammary tissues maintained in a chemically defined, serum-free medium are utilized to examine their common and unique responses to carcinogenic insult. The acute, direct effects of the prototype carcinogens BP and DMBA were examined by measuring the carcinogen-induced alteration in the extent of ras proto oncogene product, ras p21

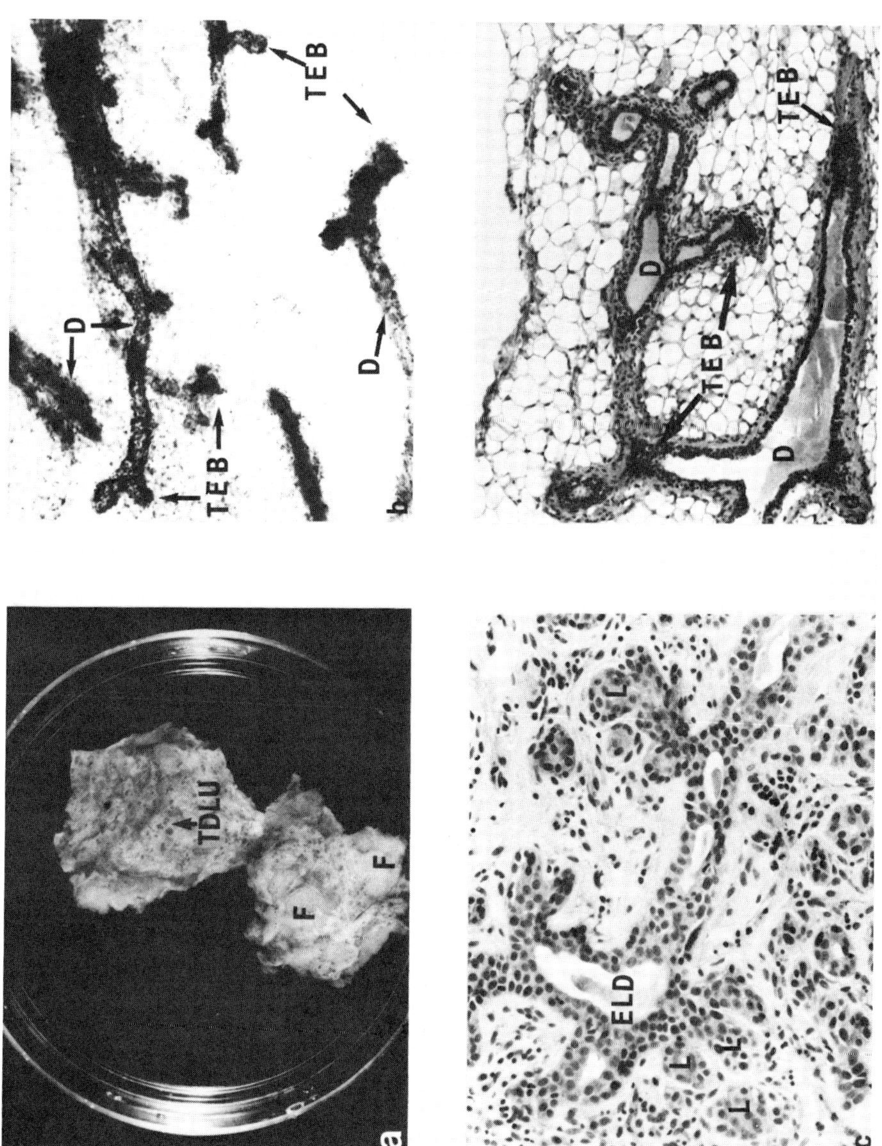

Figure 1.

and in estradiol metabolism via the C16-alpha-hydroxylation pathway. These two markers provided a means to quantitate target tissue responsiveness to carcinogens at molecular and metabolic levels respectively. The same two markers were utilized to evaluate the extent of positive or negative regulation of carcinogenesis, by selected fatty acids.

The experiments designed to examine target tissue specificity of BP on human mammary tissue demonstrated that the carcinogen selectively enhanced both the markers in TDLU, the target tissue for tumor, but not in mammary fat (MF). It was also interesting to note that relative extents of ras p21 levels and of estradiol 16-alpha-hydroxylation in the explant cultures of TDLU exposed to the solvent were substantially higher than those in MF, (Figures 2a,b). These results indicate that TDLU is more susceptible to BP treatment than is MF possibly because of the higher constitutive extents of the two markers. Furthermore, this specific response of TDLU to BP treatment indicates relevance of the two markers in acute, direct effects of a carcinogen on non-involved human mammary tissue. The altered susceptibility of TDLU to BP, that differs depending upon the relative risk for developing breast cancer, is clearly demonstrated from the data presented in Figures 3a,b. TDLU-HR exhibited greater elevation in ras p21 levels and in estradiol 16-alpha-hydroxylation than did TDLU-LR . This observation raises the possibility that differential susceptibility of TDLU-LR and TDLU-HR to carcinogenic insult may, in part, be due to molecular and/or metabolic alterations in non-involved tissue derived from cancerous breast. This contention is further supported by our previous study (17) that showed higher constitutive levels of the two markers in TDLU-HR.

To compare the molecular and metabolic response of TDLU and TEB to carcinogens, human TDLU and mouse TEB were treated with BP and DMBA respectively and relative extent of ras p21 levels and of estradiol 16-alpha-hydroxylation were measured (Figures 4a,b). It was observed that the mammary tissue from both the sources exhibited substantial elevation in the relative extents of ras p21 levels and estradiol 16-alpha-hydroxylation in response to the treatment with prototype carcinogens. Elevated levels of ras oncogene expression has been reported in carcinogen-induced murine mammary tumors (18,19), in human mammary tissues at different stages of cancer progression (20), and in overt human breast cancers (21,22). Similarly, estradiol 16-alpha-hydroxylation has been noted to increase in mice that differ in relative risk for developing breast cancer (23), in breast cancer patients (24) and in human subjects that are at high risk for developing breast cancer (25). These studies however, have not established the significance of ras expression and estradiol metabolism in the initiational events of tumorigenic transformation. The data presented in Figures 4a,b, showing parallel increases of the molecular and metabolic events in mammary tissue exposed to the initiators BP and/or DMBA suggests a common molecular and metabolic response of the non-transformed tissue to carcinogenic insult. The similarity of this response in human and mouse mammary tissue indicates that the two types of tissue may respond similarly to the acute effects of carcinogens.

Clinical as well as laboratory investigations have supported the concept that dietary fat can modulate the development of breast cancer (3-6).It is not known whether fatty acids are able to directly

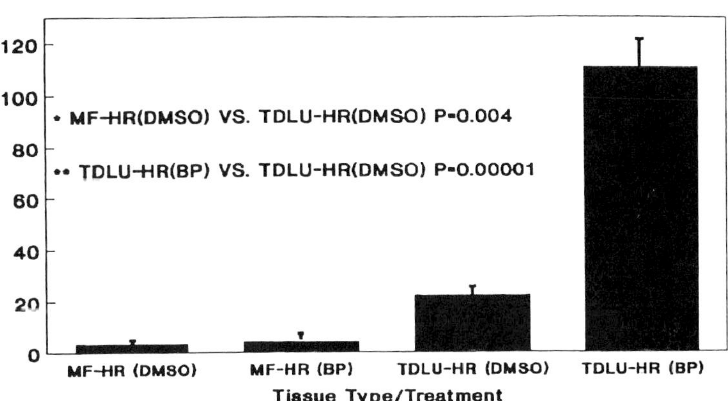
Specificity of the effect of BP
on human mammary tissues
ras p21 levels
120
100
80
60
40
20
0
* MF-HR(DMSO) VS. TDLU-HR(DMSO) P=0.004
** TDLU-HR(BP) VS. TDLU-HR(DMSO) P=0.00001
MF-HR (DMSO)
MF-HR (BP)
TDLU-HR (DMSO)
TDLU-HR (BP)
Tissue Type/Treatment

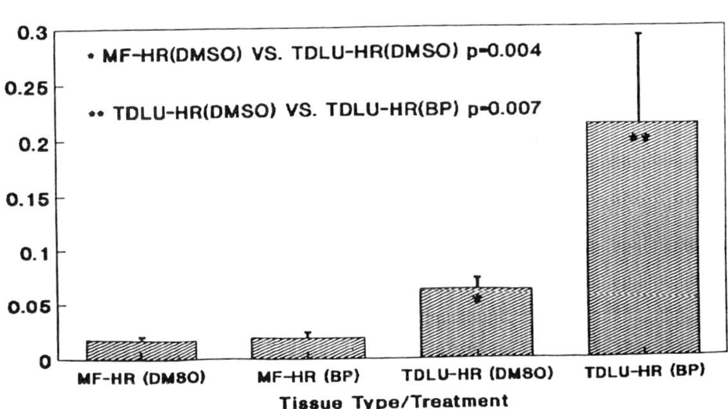
Specificity of the effect of BP
on human mammary tissues
E2 16a-Hydroxylation
0.3
0.25
0.2
0.15
0.1
0.05
0
* MF-HR(DMSO) VS. TDLU-HR(DMSO) p=0.004
** TDLU-HR(DMSO) VS. TDLU-HR(BP) p=0.007
MF-HR (DMSO)
MF-HR (BP)
TDLU-HR (DMSO)
TDLU-HR (BP)
Tissue Type/Treatment

Figure 2.

Cancer Risk-Dependent Increase in ras-oncogene levels

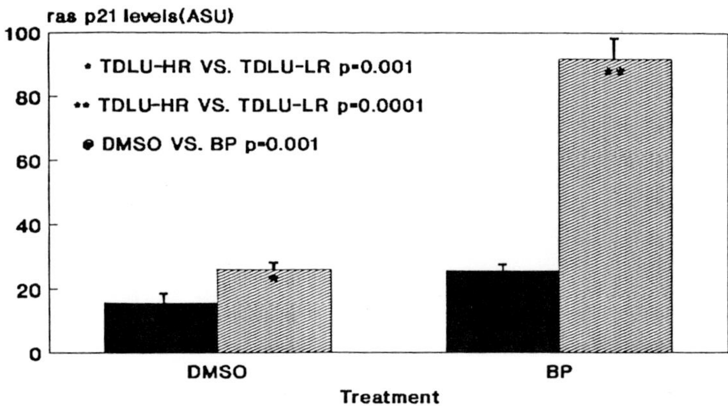

Cancer Risk-Dependent Increase in Estradiol Metabolism

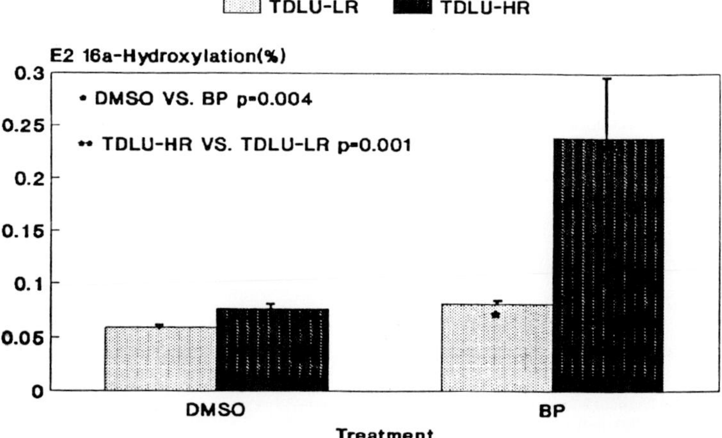

Figure 3.

influence the response of mammary tissue to carcinogenic agents. In the experiment presented in Figures 5a,b the effect of fatty acids LNA and EPA on carcinogenesis was evaluated by determining the changes induced by these agents in relative extents of ras p21 levels and of estradiol 16-alpha-hydroxylation. Pretreatment of the carcinogen-exposed cultures of human TDLU and mouse TEB with LNA resulted in an increase in ras p21 levels and estradiol 16-alpha-hydroxylation. In contrast, pretreatment with EPA either did not alter, or caused suppression in the extent of the two events. This fatty acid-induced modulation of carcinogen action at molecular and metabolic levels is consistent with our previous observations (13,26), and supports the concept that diets rich in n-6 fatty acids enhance, and those rich in n-3 fatty acid suppress mammary tumor development (3-6). The results from the present study thus provide evidence that the prototype dietary modulators, LNA and EPA may also be effective during initiational events of carcinogenesis. In conclusion, the results presented in this communication demonstrate a common response of human and mouse mammary tissue to carcinogens and to dietary modulators of mammary carcinogenesis. The **in vitro** system derived from human mammary tissue therefore could provide a useful model to evaluate clinically relevant chemopreventive interventions for human breast cancer.

SUMMARY

The major obsevations resulting from this study can be summarized as follows:

1. The molecular event (ras expression) and the metabolic event (estradiol 16-alpha-hydroxylation) can be perturbed by prototype chemical carcinogens in human and mouse mammary explant cultures.
2. Both the events exhibit specificity depending upon the cell type and upon the relative risk for developing breast cancer.
3. The two events are responsive to modulation by n-6 and n-3 polyunsaturated fatty acids that are known to modulate experimental mammary cancer.
4. Parallel enhancement of the two events in human and mouse mammary tissue indicates a common response to carcinogenic insult, and suggest a potential utility of these events as markers of carcinogenesis.
5. Fatty acid-induced change in the two markers of carcinogenesis in human mammary tissue provides a means to evaluate clinical relevance of chemopreventive efficacy of dietary interventions.

ACKNOWLEDGMENT

Supported by National Institutes of Health Grant # R29 CA 44741 to NTT and by the fund from Iris and B. Gerald Cantor Foundation to MPO.

Carcinogen-Induced Elevation of
ras expression in mammary tissues

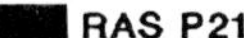
RAS P21

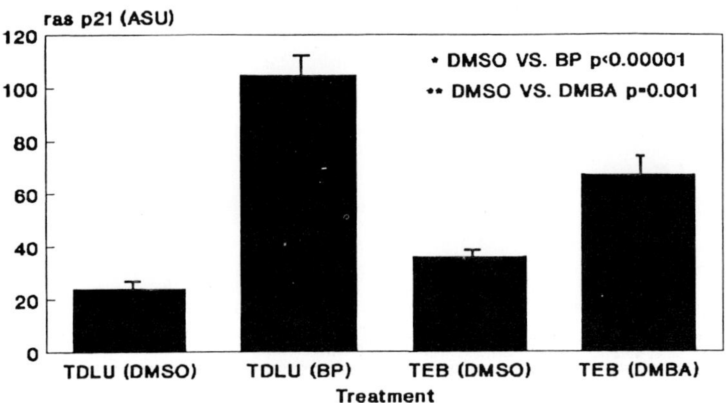

Carcinogen-Induced Elevation of
Estradiol Metabolism in mammary tissues

E2 16a-Hydroxylation

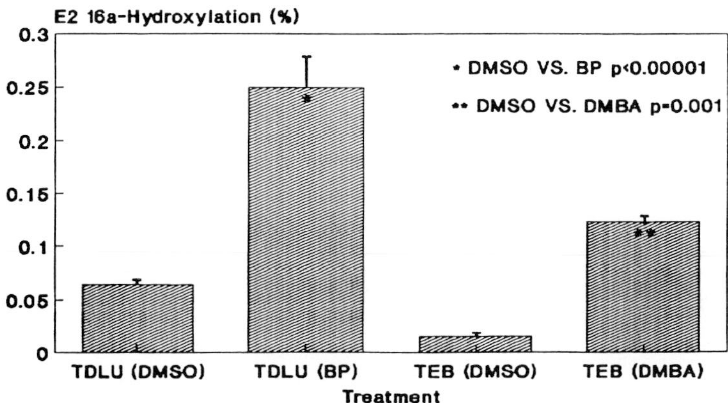

Figure 4.

Effect of FA on Carcinogen-Induced ras Proto-oncogene in Mammary Tissues

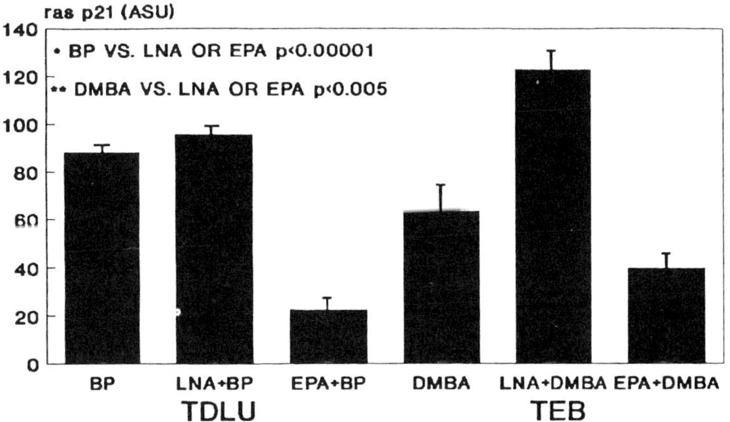

Effect of FA on Carcinogen-Induced Estradiol Metabolism in Mammary Tissues

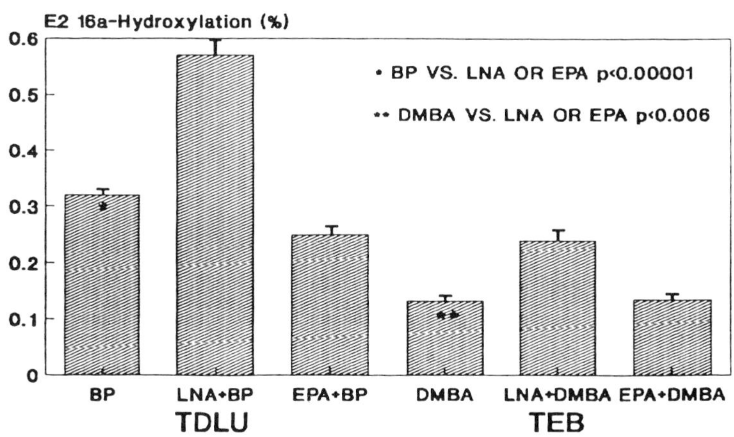

Figure 5.

REFERENCES

1. Cancer Facts and Figures. American Cancer Society, New York.1989.
2. Williams, W.R., and Osborne, M.P. In: Breast Diseases. (Eds). J.R. Harris, S. Hellman, I.C. Henderson, and D.W.Kinne. J.B. Lippincott & Co. Philadelphia, 1987, pp 109-120.
3. Smith, R.E. Cancer Detect. Prevent. 10:193-196, 1987.
4. Kinlen, L.J. Prog. Lipid. Res. 25:527-531, 1986.
5. Gabor, H., Hillyard, L.A., and Abraham, S. J. Nat. Cancer Inst. 74:1299-1305, 1985.
6. Gabor, H., and Abraham, S. J. Nat. Cancer Inst. 76:1223-1229, 1986.
7. Telang, N.T., Banerjee, M.R., Iyer, A.P., and Kundu, A.B. Proc. Nat. Acad. Sci. USA, 76:5886-5890,1979.
8. Telang, N.T.,and Sarkar, N.H. Cancer Res. 43:4891-4900, 1983.
9. Telang, N.T., Bockman, R.S., Modak M.J., and Osborne, M.P. In: Carcinogenesis and Dietary Fat. (Ed) S. Abraham. Kluwer Academic Publishers. Boston, 1989, pp 427-452.
10. Telang, N.T., Basu, A., Modak, M.J., and Osborne, M.P. Ann. NY Acad. Sci. 1990, 586:230-237.
11. Nandi, S. and McGrath, C.M. Adv. Cancer Res. 17:354-414,1973.
12. Iyer, A.P. and Banerjee, M.R. J. Nat. Cancer Inst. 66:893-905. 1981.
13. Telang, N.T., Basu, A., Kurihara, H., Osborne, M.P., and Modak, M.J. Anticancer Res. 8:971-976,1988.
14. Basu, A., and Modak, M.J. J. Biol. Chem. 262:2369-2373,1987.
15. Telang, N.T., Bradlow, H.L., Kurihara, H., and Osborne, M.P. Breast Cancer Res. & Treatment. 13: 173-181,1989.
16. Bradlow, H.L., Hershcopf, R.J., Martucci, C.P., and Fishman, J. Ann. N.Y. Acad. Sci. 464:138-151,1986.
17. Osborne, M.P., Telang, N.T., Kurihara, H., and Bradlow, H.L. Proc. Amer. Assoc. Cancer Res. 28:236 (Abstract), 1988.
18. Dandekar, S., Sukumar, S., Zarbl, H., Young, L.J.T., and Cardiff, R. Mol. Cell Biol. 6:4104-4108, 1986.
19. Zarbl, H., Sukumar, S., Arthur, A.V., Martin-Zanca, D., and Barbacid, M. Nature (London) 315:381-385, 1985.
20. Ohuchi, N., Thor, A., Page, D.L., Hand, P.H., Halter, S.A., and Schlom, J. Cancer Res. 46:2511-2519,1986.
21. Spandidos, D.A., and Agnantis, N.J. Anticancer Res. 4:269-272, 1984.
22. Spandidos, D.A. Anticancer Res. 7:991-996,1987.
23. Bradlow, H.L., Hershcopf, R.J., Martucci, C.P., and Fishman, J. Proc. Nat. Acad. Sci. USA 82:6295-6299, 1985.
24. Schneider, J., Kinne, D.W., Fracchia, A., Pierce,V., Anderson, K.E., Bradlow, H.L., and Fishman, J. Proc. Natl. Acad. Sci. USA, 79:3047-3051, 1982.
25. Osborne, M.P., Karmali, R.A., Hershcopf, R.J., Bradlow, H.L., Kourides, I.A., Williams, W.R., Rosen, P.P., and Fishman, J. Cancer Invest. 6:629-631, 1988.
26. Telang, N.T., Bockman, R.S., and Sarkar, N.H. Carcinogenesis. 5:1123-1127, 1984.

RADIATION PROTECTION AND CANCER THERAPY BY LINOLEATE

K. S. IWAMOTO, L. R. BENNETT, A. E. VILLALOBOS, C. A. HUTSON, W. H. MCBRIDE and A. NORMAN

Departments of Radiological Sciences and Radiation Oncology and Jonsson Comprehensive Cancer Center, University of California, Los Angeles; and Animal Cancer Center, Hermosa Beach, California

INTRODUCTION

Linoleate (LA) injected i.p. into mice one day after the inoculation of Ehrlich ascites tumor cells prevented the growth of the tumor (1). It also protected mouse bone marrow cells against radiation damage even when injected an hour or more after exposure of the mice to gamma rays (2). It seems likely, therefore, that combined radiation and LA therapy may be useful for the control of selected cancers. We have begun an investigation of the combined therapy both by clinical studies of the safety and efficacy of LA therapy in 41 dogs and 12 cats with advanced cancer and by laboratory studies.

MATERIALS AND METHODS

Dogs and cats with a variety of advanced cancers which did not respond to other treatments were entered into this study with the informed consent of their owners. Cancer was confirmed and classified by a pathologist in all animals but one whose meningioma was classified on the basis of CT scans alone. We started the study by injecting sodium LA, but switched to feeding safflower oil (SFO), which is 76% LA, when we found that we could obtain higher plasma levels safely of nonesterified LA by that route.

Sodium LA (Sigma Chemical Company) was used without further purification. It was free of pyrogens and of lipopolysaccaride, and gave a single smooth peak in the gas chromatogram. It was dissolved in physiological saline and sterile filtered for injection. SFO (Hollywood Foods) was mixed with a partial meal of the dog or cat food normally eaten by the animal and given at mealtime.

Animals were injected at weekly intervals with the following doses of sodium LA: 40 mg/kg i.p., 100 mg/kg i.v., or 0.4 mg/g of tumor i.t. Initially the SFO was given once a week at a dose of 3 ml/kg. Later the animals that tolerated the weekly dose were increased to 3 treatments a week on 3 successive days. The animals were treated on an outpatient basis so that in some cases the schedule of treatments had to be altered. Only animals which received at least 2 treatments were included in the study. When it was feasible autopsies were performed on animals which died or were euthanized. Each animal served as its own control in assessing the efficacy and toxicity of LA therapy. Five normal adult dogs were used to test for possible adverse reactions, and to study blood chemistries and cell counts.

Five animals with lymphoma received orthovoltage x-ray therapy with SFO. In addition 40 mice were inoculated with mouse lymphoma cells. They were divided into 4 groups: one received 4 daily 2 Gy doses of gamma rays, the second received the radiation followed by an i.p., injection of 1 mg LA, the third just had the LA injections and the fourth served as the control.

Plasma levels of nonesterified LA and other fatty acids were determined in some animals by gas chromatography (3), and complete blood counts and blood chemistries were also obtained.

RESULTS

Preliminary data analysis indicated a wide spectrum of responses ranging from dramatic remissions to no evident effect on the tumor. In a few cases the SFO may have stimulated growth of the tumor or produced a flu like condition with lassitude and fever. The study period has not been long enough to permit classifying any of the animals as cures. In some cases after a good initial response the animal was withdrawn from the study; in others, accidents or euthanasia prevent follow up. Table 1 summarizes the results.

Table 1
Results of LA therapy

Cancer	No. of dogs			Remarks
	+	+/-	-	
Hemangiosarcoma	1		1	i.p.
Giant splenic hematoma	2			i.p.
Meningioma	1			
Undif. sarcoma		1		
Apocrine gland CA			1	
Mastocytoma			1	
Nasal mucosa CA			2	
Fibro histocytoma			1	
Undif. CA	1			i.p.
Cutaneous T cell lymphoma	3		1*	*Radiation
Insulinoma	1			i.v.
Osteogenic sarcoma	1	1	1	
Fibrosarcoma	3	1	1	3 i.t.
Melanoma	1	2	4	
B cell lymphoma		4*		*Radiation
Squamous cell CA		1		
Plasmocytoma		1		
Totals	14	11	16	
Cancer	**No. of cats**			**Remarks**
	+	+/-	-	
Undif. CA, ascites	1			i.p.
Hepatocellular CA	1			i.p.
Undif. CA, palate		1		
Squamous cell CA, oral	1		5	
Salivary gland CA			1	
Fibrosarcoma, leg			1	
Apocrine gland CA			1	
Totals	3	1	8	

The positive responders include those which showed either a reduction in tumor mass or a marked improvement in general well being usually accompanied by an unexpectedly long survival. For example, the first cat showed a large decrease in ascites tumor cells following i.p. injections of LA, but the solid tumors in the abdomen continued to grow. A dog with meningioma became very weak before the start of therapy, improved greatly and lived unexpectedly for 11 more months. A dog with insulinoma had a partial pancreatectomy. This was followed after a temporary remission of symptoms by a return of elevated insulin levels. The dog showed an excellent clinical improvement following i.v. injections of LA. Therapy was discontinued when the veins were lost due to the LA infusions. Finally, 3 out of 4 dogs with cutaneous T cell tumors (mycosis fungoides) showed excellent response to SFO. On the other hand many cancers including melanoma, osteogenic sarcoma and squamous cell carcinoma of the mouth, a common tumor in cats, failed to respond to therapy.

Combined radiation therapy and SFO failed to halt the downward slide of 4 dogs with B cell and 1 dog with T cell lymphoma. However, Figure 1 shows that in a controlled experiment in mice the combined therapy was effective. The median survival for the control and LA group, curve C, was 24 d, for the radiation group, curve B, 27 d and for the radiation plus LA group, curve A, 35 d.

Figure 2 shows the plasma levels of LA in a dog, the center bar in each group of 3, flanked to the left by oleic and to the right by arachidonic acid, before and 4 h after each feeding of SFO when the maximum is reached. Note that oleic acid rises almost as high as the LA although SFO contains 76% LA and only about one seventh as much oleic acid. The LA levels rise to almost 600 micromolar at day 5, after the last feeding. On day 10 the dog received the normal food without additional SFO; the LA levels did not change.

Figure 1. Survival of mice

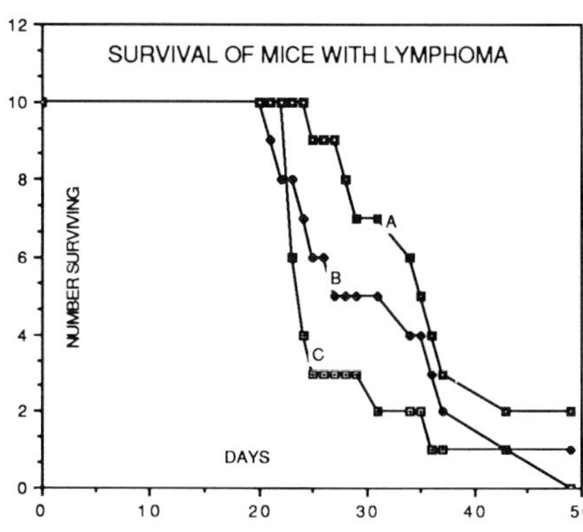

Figure 2. Plasma levels

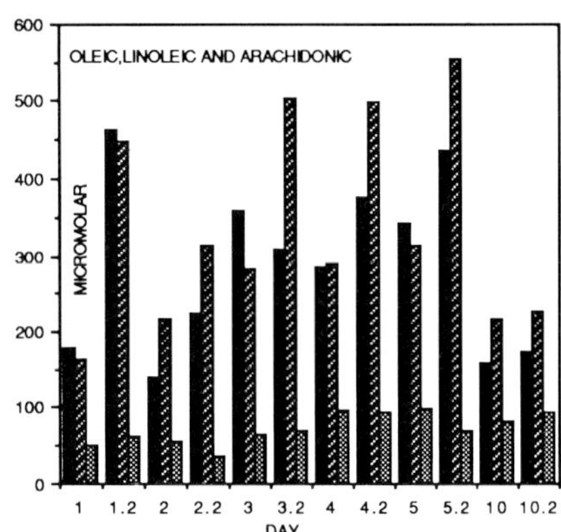

The dog showed no ill effects from the high LA diet. That was the experience with most of the animals treated for cancer; a few with large tumor burdens, however, vomited or refused to eat the oily meal, and a few developed a mild diarrhea. The lack of toxicity is reflected in the blood counts and chemistries shown in Table 2. The only significant effect is the sharp temporary fall in the serum glutamine transaminases.

TABLE 2. BLOOD COUNTS AND CHEMISTRY FROM DAILY SFO

	DAY											
	1		2		3		4		5		10	
	PRE	POST	PRE	POST	PRE	POST	PRE	POST	PRE	POST	PRE	POST
Hgb	17.6	19.3	19.0	19.8	17.3	18.8	18.3	19.5	18.6	16.3	18.1	18.0
PCV	50.5	53.5	54.0	53.5	50.0	55.5	52.5	54.5	55,5	48.0	50.0	50.5
WBC	7900	13000	10400	13100	8900	13900	9700	12600	11100	13300	12600	13700
RBC	8.16	8.81	8.55	8.86	8.10	8.70	8.45	8.60	8.69	7.58	8.17	7.88
BAND	0	0	O	0	0	0	0	0	0	0	0	0
SEG	54	53	61	68	69	59	65	73	69	64	61	65
LYM	35	36	23	18	25	23	20	18	11	23	22	25
MONO	10	7	11	7	1	10	7	5	11	11	10	6
EOS	0	3	5	7	5	8	8	4	9	2	7	4
BASO	0	0	0	0	0	0	0	0	0	0	0	0
ALK PHOS	73	65	69	64	63	62	55	48	49	43	50	48
SGOT	33	0	45	0	39	0	48	0	45	5	31	33
SGPT	21	16	23	32	24	52	26	0	29	0	28	24
CREA TININE	1.2	1.0	1.5	1.4	1.7	1.1	1.7	1.5	1.3	1.3	1.2	1.2
PANC AMYLASE	841	814	875	876	826	836	849	829	832	821	801	846

DISCUSSION

LA or SFO has proven effective in treating a variety of spontaneous dog and cat malignancies. The results with hepatocellular carcinoma in one cat and with a meningioma in a dog are similar to the encouraging results reported for patients treated with daily doses of 12 g LA and 1.4 g linolenic acid (4). The high plasma levels that can be safely attained by feeding SFO are important for controlling tumors. However, penetration into tumors with dense stroma is a problem for LA; this is illustrated by the results of treating a cat with ascites tumor cells of uncertain origin - the first weekly i.p. injections both reduced the number of tumor cells in the ascites fluid and raised the plasma level of LA. But the solid tumors in the abdomen continued to grow and, after the 4th week, i.p. injections failed to raise the plasma levels of LA or to control the ascites tumor.

The SFO dose of 3 ml/kg is not toxic. The temporary drop in serum transaminase levels was not accompanied by any other evidence for liver disease. It suggests that LA may play a role in peptide and amino acid metabolism which may be significant for its antitumor properties. The corresponding SFO dose in an average human adult is about 120 ml, this can be taken easily with some added chocolate or other flavor.

The efficacy of combined LA and radiation therapy is suggested by the experiment on mice with lymphoma; but more experimental work is required before clinical trials can be recommended. The efficacy of SFO treatment for mycosis fungoides, which is clinically very similar to the human disease and for which no effective therapy exists, indicates that it should be explored further. More generally the lack of toxicity of SFO and its efficacy in controlling several spontaneous cancers in dogs and cats indicates that an evaluation in humans is reasonable at this time.

REFERENCES

1. Norman A, Bennett LR, Mead JF, Iwamoto KS. Nutr Cancer, 11:107-115, 1988.
2. Norman A, McBride WH, Bennett LR, et al. Postirradiation Int J Radiat Biol, 54:521-524, 1988.
3. Lepage G, Roy CC. J Lipid Res, 29:227-235, 1988.
4. Van der Merwe CF, et al. Br J Clin Pract, 41: 907- 915, 1987.

LIPID PEROXIDATION, EICOSANOID BIOSYNTHESIS, AND RADIATION INDUCED TISSUE INJURY

AN OVERVIEW OF EICOSANOID-INDUCED RADIATION PROTECTION

W. R. HANSON

Loyola-Hines Dept. of Radiotherapy, Hines VA Medical Center, Hines, IL 60141

INTRODUCIION

The large family of natural eicosanoids and the growing number of synthesized eicosanoid analogues have a wide range and diversified array of biological actions. Many naturally occurring eicosanoids are associated either directly or coincidentally with many pathological disorders. In contrast, several prostaglandins (PGs) and fewer leukotrienes (LTs) have been shown to play some role in protecting tissue from acute or chronic injury. This protective effect of eicosanoids led Collier (1) to suggest that they may be one of the bodies major homeostatic mechanisms.

Cytoprotection.

Cytoprotection was first described by Robert (2) as a PG-induced protective effect from injuries produced in the gastric or intestinal mucosa by high concentrations of ethanol (ETOH), acids, bases, or heat. Robert et al. (3) further showed that this effect was true cytoprotection rather than an antiulcer effect associated with gastric antisecretory compounds like cimetidine. Subsequently, PG-induced cytoprotection was shown in some other tissues such as the small intestine (from stress or nonsteroidal anti-inflammatory-induced ulcers), pancreas (from altered diet-induced injury), liver (from carbon tetrachloride injury or necrosis resulting from D-galactosamine), and kidney (from cyclosporine). [See "Biological Protection by Prostaglandins" (4) for a review]. Evidence showing cytoprotection was the impetus to investigate PGs and LTs in our laboratory as possible protectors from radiation injury.

Radiation Protection.

Prasad (5) reported in 1972 that PGE_1 protected Chinese hamster ovary (CHO) cells from a single dose of photon radiation. Lehnert (6) reported results in 1975 showing that PGE_1 protected V-79 cells on the shoulder portion of the survival curve but increased sensitivity measured after higher doses of radiation. Both authors suggested that the PG-induced increases in adenylate cyclase and cyclic adenosine monophosphate (cAMP) was at least a part of the mechanism of PG-induced effects on cell survival after radiation. In contrast to these early reports, other investigators have failed to show PG-induced protection *in vitro.* Holahan et al.(7) failed to show any change in the radiation sensitivity of V-79 cells treated with 16,16 dimethyl (dm) PGE_2. Similarly, Millar and Jinks (8) did not find PG-induced radiation protection of several cell lines by the A series PGs. Likewise, in our laboratory, we did not find radiation protection of CHO cells by several PGs including E_1, I_2 and 16,16 dm E_2. In an extensive study, Rubin failed to show any protection of cultured bovine aortic cells by wide variety of eicosanoids (see

Rubin et al., this volume).

Unlike the equivocal results found *in vitro, in vivo* PG-induced radiation protection has been consistently found in our laboratory and in others (9-13). Since the first in vivo investigations a number of studies have been conducted in our laboratory, mainly using the intestinal clonogenic assay (14), LD50/$_6$, and animal longevity of irradiated mice, to further explore the details of radiation protection by the eicosanoids. A summary of the results of clonogenic assays of mice treated with several eicosanoids is shown in figure 1.

The PG dose response was nearly the same for all PGs; there was rapid increase in the degree of protection at low PG doses followed by a broad plateau. Although the dose response was nearly the same for all PGs tested, the structure activity relationship was remarkably different. PGE_1 did not protect but PGE_2 increases protection to 200% of controls. The only difference between these two PGs is the number of double bonds in the alpha side chains. Another feature of eicosanoid-induced protection shown in Figure 1 is that the degree of protection was greater for the PG analogues than for the natural compounds. This increase in activity does not appear to be related to metabolic differences since the time-course for protection is about the same for naturally occurring PGs and their analogues (11).

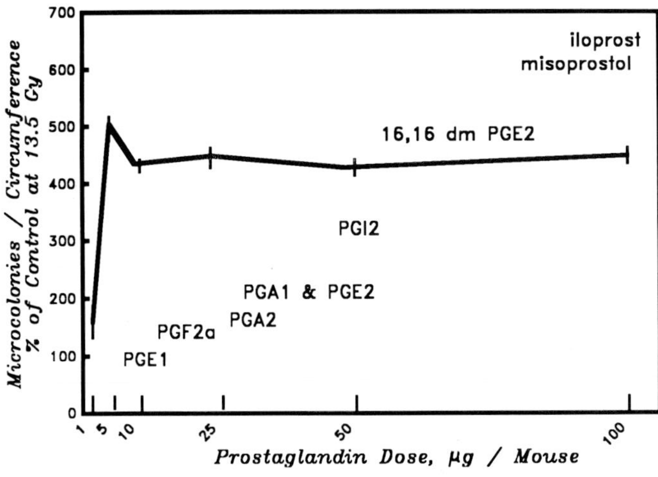

Figure 1. Microcolonies / intestinal circumference as percent of controls at 13.5 Gy versus dose of prostaglandin / average 30 g mouse. The dose response curve was nearly the same for all PGs and is shown for 16,16 dm PGE_2 only. The names of the PGs are placed at their respective levels of protection. Data points for 16,16 dm PGE_2 are the means of 5 mice $\pm$ 1 SEM.

Mechanisms of Eicosanoid-Induced protection.

The mechanisms of eicosanoid-induced protection are not known; however, there are some data to at least unravel part of the puzzle. There is evidence to suggest that PGs affect cells through membrane receptors (15,16). The shape of the PG dose-response curve for radiation protection (Figure l) suggests that the receptor sites are saturated above a certain concentration when PGs are given in a single dose. In addition, radiation protection by misoprostol (a mixture of four isomers) is stereospecific; that is, only one of the isomers is protective (17).

Since PGs protect animals at microgram concentrations, it is unlikely that the PGs exert their protective effect directly. It is more likely that they trigger cellular changes which result in protection. The location of the actual site where protection occurs is also unknown. Alkaline elution studies showed that an aminothiol and widely studied radioprotector, WR-2721, reduced the number of initial single strand breaks in DNA following gamma irradiation. In contrast, 16-16 dm PGE_2 did not reduce the number of DNA breaks (18). The PG-induced radioprotection, therefore, may not be associated directly with DNA strand breaks. Since strand breakage is only one measure of DNA damage by radiation, caution must be exercised in assuming that PGs do not play a role in protection by interacting either directly or indirectly with DNA to protect cells. However, these data suggest that PGs may protect targets other than DNA. Supporting evidence for this contention comes from the data showing cytoprotection from ETOH, acids, bases, and heat which are all associated with cell surface injury. The single common link between the various forms of injury may be oxygen radicals. How PGs may protect from these radicals remains to be discovered.

Although the mechanisms to account for protection are unknown, some direction for future investigations may come from a comparison of the properties of cytoprotection compared to radiation protection. There are many similarities between cytoprotection and radioprotection; some of which are listed in Figure 2.

Common Characteristics of "Cyto" and "Radio" Protection

- Dose response, ligand binding, and stereospecificity suggest that protection is mediated via a ligand–receptor mechanism
- Analogues can be more protective than "natural" eicosanoids
- Eicosanoids are protective given before but not after the injury
- Time course for eicosanoid–induced protection is identical
- Protection by some eicosanoids is dependent upon glucocorticoids
- In vitro protection by eicosanoids is not consistently found

Figure 2. Summary of common characteristics between cytoprotection and radiation protection.

These common features leads to the hypothesis that the mechanisms associated with cytoprotection and radiation protection are the same. Therefore, what is found experimentally for cytoprotection should also be seen for radiation protection. A recent example is based on work done by Szabo et al. (19) showing that cytoprotection was diminished in adrenalectomized animals. Furthermore, glucocorticoids added back cytoprotection. Based upon these studies, we showed that radiation protection by some of the eicosanoids was also dependent upon glucocorticoids (20).

Clinical Significance of PG or LT-induced Radiation Protection.

The abundant evidence that a wide variety and large number of human tumors secrete excessive PGs (21-26) leads to the implication that tumors may be protected from radiation therapy by endogenous products of the arachidonic acid (AA) cascade. Furthermore, blocking the AA cascade with the cyclooxygenase inhibitors, such as the nonsteroidal anti-inflammatory agents (NSAIA), or 5-lipoxygenase inhibitors may increase tumor radiosensitivity. Evidence supporting this contention was presented by Weppelmann and Monkemeier (27) who showed that both 5 and 10 year survival was increased in women given a NSAIA before ^{60}Co gamma treatment compared to those irradiated only. Further supporting evidence that endogenous PGs may predict tumor radiation response comes from the data of Furuta et al. (28) showing that indomethacin increased the radiation response of experimental tumors which secreted large amounts of PGs; however, indomethacin had no effect on tumors which did not produce excessive PGs.

Another potential effect of endogenous PGs or LTs in the radiation treatment of cancer comes from observations that radiation increases PG production *in vivo* (29-32). If increased tissue concentrations of PGs were sufficiently great, they may protect these tissues (or tumors) during a 6 week fractionated course of radiation therapy. In addition to the above considerations of the role of eicosanoids during radiation therapy, exogenously administered AA products or analogues may also be considered as possible adjuncts in the radiation treatment of cancer to protect normal tissue. The realization of a beneficial clinical use of eicosanoids to increase the therapeutic gain would depend upon the availability of the eicosanoid to the tumor. A study of the mechanisms of PG radioprotection may lead to methods of selectively blocking the AA cascade within tumors to sensitize malignant tissue and at the same time, allow the protection of normal tissue with exogenous PG administration alone or with other protective agents. As a result of the array of biologic effects and the observed radiation protection by the family of PGs and LTs, the metabolism, pharmacology, mode of action, stimulation and inhibition of the AA cascade have important implications in cell biology and clinical medicine.

ACKNOWLEDGMENTS

The work outlined in this overview was supported by Contract No. DNA00186-0038 from the Defense Nuclear Agency, Department of Defense, G.D. Searle and Co., The Upjohn Co. and Schering AG, Berlin. The author expresses his appreciation to Ms. K. Houseman, and Ms. N. Pooley for their excellent technical assistance and to Ms. B Kalemba for the preparation of this manuscript.

REFERENCES

1. Collier, H.O.J. In: Prostaglandins and Related Lipids, Volume I (Ed. P. Ramwell,) Alan R. Liss, Inc., New York, 1980, pp. 87-105.
2. Robert, A., Gastoenterology, 69:1045-1047. 1975.
3. Robert, A., Lancaster, C., Davis, J.P., Field S.O. and Nezamis, J.E., Scand. J. Gastroenterol. 19: (Suppl. 101), 69-72, 1984.
4. Cohen, M.M., Editor Biological Protection with Prostaglandins, Volumes I and II, CRC Press, Inc., Boca Raton, Florida, 1986.
5. Prasad, K.N., Int. J. Radiat. Biol. 22:187-189, 1972.
6. Lehnert, S., Radiat. Res. 62:107-116,1975.
7. Holahan, E.V., Blakely, W.F., and Walden, T.L., In: Prostaglandin and Lipid Metabolism in Radiation Injury (Eds. T.L. Walden and H.N. Hughes), Plenum Publishing Corp., New York, 1987, pp. 253-262.
8. Millar, B.C. and Jinks, S., Int. J. Radiat. Biol. 46:367-373, 1984.
9. Hanson, W.R. and Thomas, C., Radiat. Res. 96:393-398,1983.
10. Hanson, W.R. and Ainsworth, E.J. Radiat. Res. 103:196-203,1985.
11. Hanson, W.R. and DeLaruentiis, K., Prostaglandins, 33:93-104,1987.
12. Hanson, W.R., Radiat. Res. 111:361-373, 1987.
13. Walden, Jr., T.L., Patchen, M. and Snyder, S.L., Radiat. Res. 109:540-549, 1987.
14. Withers, H.R. and Elkind, M.M., Int. J. Radiat. Biol. 17:261-267, 1970.
15. Kuehl, Jr., F.A. and Hunes, J.L., Proceedings of the National Academy of Science, U.S.A. 69: 480-491,1972.
16. Gorman, R.R. and Miller, O.V., Biochem. Biophys. Acta 132:560-571,1973.
17. W.R. Hanson, K.A. Houseman, A.K. Nelson, and P.W. Collins, Prostaglandins, Leukotrienes, and Essential Fatty Acids, 32:101-105, 1988.
18. Hanson, W.R. and Grdina, D.J., Internat. J. of Radiat. Biol. 52:67-76,1987.
19. S. Szabo, G.T. Gallagher, H.C. Horner, P.W. Frankel, R.H. Underwood, S.J. Konturek, T. Brzozowski, and J.S. Trier, Gastroenterology, 85:1384-1390, 1983.
20. W.R., Hanson, K.A. Houseman and P.W. Collins, Digestive Diseases and Sciences 34:1314, 1989.
21. Bennett, A., Charlier, E.M., McDonald, A.M., Simpson, J.S., Stamford, I.F. and Zebro, T., Lancet 2:624-626,1977.
22. Bennett, A., Carroll, M.A., Stamford, I.F., Whimster, W.F., and Williams, F. Br. J. Cancer 46:888-893, 1982.
23. Bockman, R.S. Cancer Investigation, 1: (6), 485-493, 1983.
24. Cummings, K.B. and Robertson, R.P., J. Urol. 118:720-723, 1977.
25. Karmali, R.A. 33: (6), 322-332,1983.
26. Prowles, T.J., Coombes, R.C., Neville, A.M., Ford, H.T., Gazet, J.C. and Levine, L., Lancet 2:138-142, 1977.
27. Weppelmann, B. and Monkemeier, D., Gynecologic Oncology 17:196-199, 1984.
28. Y. Furuta, N. Hunter, T. Barkley, Jr., E. Hall, and L. Milas, Cancer Research, 48:3008-3013, 1988.
29. Eisen, V. and Walker, D.I., Br. J. Pharmac. 57: 527-532,1976.
30. Pausescu, E., Chirvasie, R., Teodosiu, T. and Paun, C., Radiat. Res. 65:163-171, 1976.
31. Schneidkraut, M.J., Kot, P.A., Ramwell, P.W. and Rose, J.C., Advances in Prostaglandin, Thromboxane, and Leukotriene Research, 12:107-111,1983.
32. Steel, L.K., Sweedler, I.K. and Catravas, G.N., Radiat. Res. 94:156-165,1983.

VASCULAR MYOINTIMAL PROLIFERATION

S. CATHAPERMAL[1], M. L. FOEGH[2], R. VARGAS[1], and P. W. RAMWELL[1]

Georgetown University Medical Center, Department of Physiology & Biophysics[1] and Department of Surgery[2], Washington, D.C. 20007

INTRODUCTION

Vascular myointimal hyperplasia is a response to injury. The initial injury can be caused by different factors, such as radiation, viral infections, development of immune complexes, and hyperlipidemia. Vascular injuries may also be caused by invasive procedures, such as percutaneous transluminal coronary angioplasty, organ transplantation and vascular bypass surgery. It is thought that injury to the endothelium allows platelets and leukocytes to adhere to the underlying internal elastic lamina and smooth muscle and promote the release of mitogenic and chemo-attractant factors, such as platelet derived growth factors, thromboglobulin, and others. The injury may allow monocytes and leukocytes to pass into the vascular wall. Monocytes also release platelet derived growth factor and other growth factors, such as tumor necrosis factor, and probably fibroblast growth factor, epidermal growth factor, and insulin-like growth factor. The leukocytes which adhere to the injured endothelium also release powerful chemo-attracting factors like leukotriene B4, as well as oxygen free radicals which, in turn, lead to release of growth factors. A great deal of basic research and clinical effort is now focused on inhibiting growth factor expression and chemo-attractants released during vascular injury which all are factors leading to myointimal proliferation. This effort is directed to the unacceptably high restenosis rate (>30%) following coronary angioplasty and organ transplantation, as well as the stenosis present in coronary and peripheral atherosclerosis.

CHRONIC RADIATION INJURY

Vascular injuries caused by irradiation vary according to both the length of exposure and the amount of radiation involved. Vascular responses to radiation fall into three categories: acute, intermediate, and the late or chronic response. The earliest visible effects of radiation on blood vessels are changes in the endothelium (1), with defoliation of endothelial cells from the basal membrane and vacuolization of the cytoplasm (2). The early post radiation reaction resembles an inflammatory response with infiltration of mononuclear cells.

The intermediate responses are characterized by swelling and sloughing of endothelial cells. There is also vascular leakage allowing plasma proteins to seep into the tissues. This extra vascular plasma contains numerous growth factors which may facilitate myointimal proliferation (3).

Chronic radiation injury is characterized by changes in larger vessels. Increased amounts of acellular material, including collagen are deposited in the intima and media of the vessels, causing thickening of the vessel walls and narrowing of the vessel lumen (4). Localized areas of myointimal proliferation may also contribute to the thickening of the vessel walls (5). Other changes in the vessel wall include degeneration of the elastic fibers, atrophy of smooth muscle cells, and replacement of the elastic lamina by fibrous tissue (6). Occlusion of coronary arteries from smooth muscle cell proliferation has also been attributed to radiation (7).

Arteriosclerotic occlusion of large arteries has been observed in patients undergoing radiation therapy for Hodgkin's disease and breast cancer. In some of these patients, the radiation has caused intimal hyperplasia of the coronary arteries, resulting in myocardial infarction and subsequent death. Myocardial infarctions occurring as much as 28 years post-radiation have been reported (8). The arteriosclerosis or intimal hyperplasia caused by radiation injury is stimulated by the same factors as that stimulate general arteriosclerosis, e,g., smoking and hyperlipidemia. In animal models, radiation cause lesions only in the presence of a high cholesterol diet (9). This may, however, simulate the clinical situation, since many patients have high cholesterol levels.

CORONARY & PERIPHERAL ATHEROSCLEROSIS

Cardiovascular diseases, especially myocardial infarction, are among the leading causes of death. Other manifestations of atherosclerosis are cerebral ischemia and peripheral circulatory problems. The theory of the pathogenesis of atherosclerosis is that lesions known as fatty streaks occur early in life (10). In early lesions, macrophages are the predominant part of the fatty streaks and may represent an inflammatory response. In advanced lesions, there is a mixture of proliferating smooth muscle cells, macrophages, lymphocytes, lipids, and calcium deposits.

The incidence of coronary artery disease in the normal population is greater in patients with peripheral atherosclerosis while the incidence in transplant patients is unrelated to the degree of existing atherosclerosis (11). The major contributing factor to atherosclerosis is smoking, which causes additional injury to the vasculature (12). The involvement of platelets in atherosclerosis has been suggested to be important since platelets adhere to atherosclerotic lesions and may release chemo-attractant factors and growth factors, such as platelet derived growth factor. The lipoproteins, especially low density lipoproteins, may play an important role in the injury of the endothelium, as this may be the basis for adherence of leukocytes and platelets.

ACCELERATED TRANSPLANT ARTERIOSCLEROSIS

Accelerated transplant arteriosclerosis was first described in cardiac transplant patients but the high incidence of vascular lesions in coronary arteries of cardiac allografts has led to the study of other transplanted organs.This accelerated graft arteriosclerosis has become the major cause of organ graft failure and no organ allografts appear to be exempt from myointimal thickening. The problem is most spectacularly seen in cardiac allografts where accelerated coronary arteriosclerosis is the major cause of death or retransplantation after the first three months. This occurs in 30 to 40 percent of patients (13,14). The pathophysiology of graft arteriosclerosis has not yet been elucidated, but the general belief is that immunological events linked to the incompatibility of the graft and the host cause vascular lesions. Although the mechanisms are unknown, recent epidemiological data have suggested that infection with cytomegalovirus is associated with coronary arteriosclerosis in transplant patients.

Coronary transplant arteriosclerosis is peritubular and affects the entire length of the arteries, unlike non transplant arteriosclerosis, where the lesions are focal. The graft lesions do not seem to affect arteries outside the suture line of the transplanted organ, indicating that these lesions are probably not caused by circulating factors. The myointimal hyperplasia in the grafts is not very different from lesions seen in atherosclerosis. However, the mechanism of the migration and myointimal proliferation in the graft is unclear. It may be initiated by a release of mitogenic peptide-like platelet derived growth factors, such as insulin-like growth factor, fibroblast growth factor, and many others (15)

Currently, there is no treatment for transplant arteriosclerosis, but some experimental studies indicate that an octapeptide called angiopeptin may inhibit the intimal hyperplasia (16, 17). Recent studies indicate that 17β estradiol is also effective (18).

PERCUTANEOUS TRANSLUMINAL CORONARY ANGIOPLASTY

Transluminal coronary and peripheral artery angioplasty are treatments for atherosclerosis. A balloon catheter is inflated at the site of narrowing, causing dilation of the stenotic site of the artery and restore flow. The major problem following angioplasty is a high restenosis rate (25 to 55%) occurring within the first three to six months after successful dilation (19).

The pathological features of restenosis of arteries following angioplasty have been studied in animal models and in patients. The sequence of events following endothelial cell injury is deposition of platelets in the area of angioplasty followed by migration and proliferation of smooth muscle cells from the medial layer through the internal elastic lamina to the intima. In patients these vascular lesions have been shown to consist of smooth muscle cells and macrophages. Antiplatelet drugs have been unsuccessful in preventing restenosis, implying that factors other than platelet related are important for the smooth muscle cell migration and proliferation. Other drugs like calcium channel blockers have also been disappointing in clinical studies. Recently experimental studies in rats and rabbits have shown that an octapeptide, angiopeptin, inhibits intimal hyperplasia (20).

CORONARY ARTERY BYPASS

Coronary artery bypass is another modality for treatment of coronary atherosclerosis. The saphenous vein or internal mammary artery is used to bypass the stenosed coronary artery. As in balloon angioplasty, graft stenosis occurs at a high rate. The saphenous vein bypass graft seems more prone to intimal hyperplasia than the mammary artery, and occlusion of the saphenous vein is similar to the one seen in arteries following angioplasty. Intimal hyperplasia of the vein grafts has been attributed to endothelial cell injury during harvesting and implantation (21,22), and consists of smooth muscle cells, macrophages, and lymphocytes.

VASCULITIS

Vasculitis is an inflammatory process of the blood vessel walls. Different pathogenic factors are involved in vasculitis. For arteritis perinodosa immune complexes are involved in the vasculitis that leads to inflammation of the blood vessels followed by myointimal proliferation. In animal models, frequent injections of bovine serum albumin or high doses of foreign proteins induce the same vascular changes (23). It is of interest that, in vasculitis, high plasma cholesterol levels promote intimal hyperplasia. This suggests that the immunologically injured intima will accumulate lipids causing proliferative changes (24).

Idiopathic aortitis, also known as African aortitis, Takayasu's disease, non-specific aorto-arteritis, and de Martorell's syndrome, is a disease of unknown origin and usually occurs in young females. Pathologically, it consists of an inflammatory proliferation in the adventitia, progressively evolving to occlusion of the arteries. Distribution of the disease has been categorized into various subtypes; Type I is disease confined to the aortic arch, Type II is confined to the descending aorta, Type III is a combination of disease of the arch and descending aorta, and Type IV is aortic disease associated with pulmonary artery fibrosis (25).

In advanced arteritis the characteristic appearance of the aortic intima is frequently altered by secondary dystrophy, calcification, and arteriosclerosis. An injured intima with focal loss of endothelial integrity predisposes to accelerated arteriosclerosis (26). Occasionally, the arteriosclerotic changes are so severe as to totally obscure the preceding arteritis.

CONCLUSIONS

In conclusion, myointimal proliferation is an inflammatory response to injury. The nature of the injury need not be specific as demonstrated by the availability of a large number of pathophysiological models and the pathology described herein. The mechanism of myointimal proliferation involves a phenotypic change of the smooth muscle to an earlier or more embryonic cell. The phenotypic change and the subsequent rapid proliferation are due to growth factors and cytokines which are presently being identified. Their interaction is likely to be complex and could involve autocrine as well as paracrine mechanisms. The problem is to identify drugs which inhibit the rapid proliferation without serious hemodynamic or other side effects, such as delayed wound healing. Recent studies in different models indicate that a stable long acting somatostatin analogue, angiopeptin, may be effective in preventing angioplasty restenosis (20) and accelerated transplant atherosclerosis (27).

REFERENCES

1. Eassa, E. M., and Casarett, G. W. Effect of Epsilon-Amino-n-Caproic Acid (EACA) on radiation induced increase in capillary permeability. Radiology. 106, (1973) 679-688.

2. Fajardo, L. F., and Stewart, J. R. Capillary injury preceding radiation induced myocardial fibrosis. Radiology. 101, (1971) 429-433.
3. Adamson, I. Y. R., and Bowden, D.H. Endothelial injury and repair in radiation-induced pulmonary fibrosis. Am. J. Pathol. 112, (1983) 224-230.
4. Zollinger, H. U. Radiation Vasculopathy. Pathol. Eur. 5 (2), (1970) 145-163.
5. Hopewell, J. W., and Young, C. M. A. Changes in the microcirculation of normal tissues after irradiation. Int. J. Radiat. Oncol. Biol. Phys. 4, (1978) 53-58.
6. Kwock, L., Davenport, W. C., Clark, R. L., et al. The effects of ionizing radiation on the pulmonary vasculature of intact rats and isolated pulmonary endothelium. Radiation Research. 111, (1987) 276-291.
7. Narayan, K. and Cliff, W. J. Morphology of irradiated microvasculature. Am J. Pathol. 106, (1982) 47-62.
8. Mc Reynolds, R., Gold, G. L., Roberts, C. W. Coronary heart disease after mediastinal irradiation for Hodgkin's disease. Am. J. Med. 60. (1976) 39-45.
9. Fajardo, L. F. Radiation induced coronary artery disease. Chest. 71, (1977) 563-564.
10. Joris, I., Zand, T., Nunnai, J. J., Krolikowski, E. J., and Majno, G. Studies on the pathogenesis of atherosclerosis. 1. Adhesion and emigration of mononuclear cells in the aorta of hypercholesterolemic rats. Am. J. Pathol. 113, (1983) 341-358.
11. Kannel, W. B., Mc Ghee, D. L. Update on some epidemiological features of intermittent claudication: the Framingham study. J. Am. Geriatr. Soc. 33, (1985) 13-18.
12. Serruys, P. W., Luijten, H. E., Beatt, K. J., Geuskens, R., de Feyter P. J., Van de Brand, M., Reiber, J. H. C., Tenkaten, H.J., Van Es, G.A., Hugenholtz, P. G.: Incidence of restenosis after successful coronary angioplasty: A time-related phenomena: A quantitative angiographic follow up study. Circulation. (1988) 77, 361-374.
13. Billingham, M. E., Cardiac transplant atherosclerosis. Transpl. Proc. 19 (Suppl. 5) (1987) 19.
14. Hess, M., Lipid mediators in organ transplantation: does cyclosporine accelerate coronary atherosclerosis. Transpl. Proc. 19 (Suppl. 5) (1987) 71.
15. Ross, R., The pathogenesis of atherosclerosis. An update. N. Engl. J. Med. 314 (1986) 488-500.
16. Lundergan, C., Foegh, M.L., Vargas, R., Eufemio, M., Bormes, G. W., Kot, P. A., and Ramwell, P. W. Inhibition of myointimal proliferation of the rat carotid artery by the peptides, angiopeptin and BIM 23034. Atherosclerosis. 80 (1989) 49-55.
17. Foegh, M. L., Khiribadi, B. S., Chambers, E., Amamoo, S., and Ramwell, P. W. Inhibition of coronary artery transplant atherosclerosis in rabbits with angiopeptin, an octapeptide. Atherosclerosis. 78 (1989) 229-236.
18. Foegh, M. L., Khirabadi, B. S., Nakanishi, T., Vargas, R., and Ramwell, P. W. Estradiol protects against experimental cardiac transplant atherosclerosis. Transpl. Proc. 19 (Suppl. 5) (1987) 90-95.
19. Liu, M. W., Roubin, G. S., King, S. B. Restenosis after coronary angioplasty: potential biologic determinants and role of intimal hyperplasia. Circulation (1989) 77, 1374-1387.
20. Conte, J. V., Foegh, M. L., Calcagno, D., Wallace, R. B., and Ramwell, P. W. Peptide inhibition of myointimal proliferation following angioplasty in rabbits. Transpl Proc. 21 (1989) 3686-3688.
21. Bush, H. L., Graber, J. N., Jackubowski, J. A., et al. Favourable balance of prostacyclin and thromboxane A2 improves early patency of human "in situ" vein grafts. J. Vasc. Surg. 1 (1984) 149-159.
22. Abbott, W. M., Wieland, S., and Austen, W. G. Structural changes during preparation of autogenous venous grafts. Surgery. 76 (1974) 1032-1040.
23. Kawai. S., Okada. R., Fukuda. Y. An experimental study of atherosclerosis as a sequela of coronary arteritis. Japanese Circulation Journal. 51, (1987) 1421-1424.
24. Robbs, J. V., Human, R. R., Rajaruthnam, P. Operative treatment non-specific aorto-arteritis (Takayasu's disease). J. Vasc. Surg. 3, (1980) 605-609.
25. Lande, A., Berkman, M. Y. Aortitis: Pathologic, clinical and ateriographic review. Radiol. Clin. North. Am. 14, (1976) 219-240.
26. Kawai, S., Fukuda, Y., and Okada, R. Atherosclerosis of the coronary arteries in collagen disease and allied disorders, with special reference to vasculitis as a preceding lesion of coronary atherosclerosis. Japanese circulation Journal. 246, (1982) 1208-1221.
27. Foegh, M. L., Khirabadi, B. S., Chambers, E., and Ramwell, P. W. Peptide inhibition of accelerated transplant atherosclerosis. Transpl. Proc. 21 (1989) 3674-3676.

ABSENCE OF PROSTAGLANDIN E_2-INDUCED RADIOPROTECTION IN TWO CELL LINES LACKING SPECIFIC PGE_2-BINDING SITES

T. L. WALDEN, JR., N. K. FARZANEH, J. M. SPEICHER, and T. A. FITZ*

Radiation Biochemistry Department, Armed Forces Radiobiology Research Institute, Bethesda, Maryland 20814-5145 and *Department of Obstetrics and Gnyecology, Uniformed Services University of the Health Sciences, Bethesda, Maryland 20814

ABSTRACT

Prostaglandin E_2 (PGE_2) is an effective radioprotective agent *in vivo* but is not consistently radioprotective *in vitro*. The present study examines the possibility that PGE_2-induced radioprotection is receptor mediated, and therefore, that cell lines lacking PGE_2 receptors will not be protected. Two cell lines were examined: the DC3 transformed rat granulosa cell line which responds to PGE_2 and the $HSDM_1C_1$ mouse fibrosarcoma cell line which produces PGE_2.

Addition of up to 28 μM PGE_2 between two hours prior to or following ^{60}Co γ-irradiation did not modify the radiosensitivity of either cell line. This lack of radioprotection might be associated with an absence of PGE_2 receptors since specific binding of [^{3}H]-PGE_2 was undetectable in both cell lines, although cAMP secretion in DC3 cells was stimulated by PGE_2 treatment. Since $HSDM_1C_1$ cells produce LTC_4 in addition to PGE_2, the use of cyclooxygenase blockers may not have produced radiosensitization because LTC_4 synthesis was simultaneously increased.

INTRODUCTION

Eicosanoid-induced radioprotection has been observed *in vitro* (1) and *in vivo* (2,3) but this is not a universal phenomenon of either eicosanoids (4) or cells (5). Evidence indicates that the radioprotection is mediated through receptor activity (1,3,4). This is illustrated by the fact that LTC_4 induced radioprotection of V79A03 Chinese hamster fibroblasts was eliminated if the cells to be irradiated were harvested by trypsinization instead of by scraping, which would leave cell surface proteins intact (1,4). Treatment with LTC_4 two hours prior to irradiation was effective in enhancing cellular survival in cells harvested by scraping four hours prior to irradiation or in cells harvested by trypsinization 16 hours prior to irradiation (4). The LTC_4 receptor on the cell surface of V79A03 cells has been characterized as a glycoprotein with a molecular weight of 40 kdal (6,7). Studies on misoprostil-induced protection of murine intestinal crypt cells demonstrated that the stereospecificity of the eicosanoids was important for activity, implying a receptor-based activation (3). In addition to action at the cellular level, systemic processes such as hypoxia (5) have also been observed and these processes may contribute to the larger dose reduction factors obtained *in vivo* (2).

Cellular protection induced by eicosanoids has significant implications for cancer therapy since tumors may synthesize increased levels of eicosanoids (8). The increased synthesis may act in an autocrine fashion to directly protect tumors, or indirectly by suppressing the immune system. In some instances, radiosensitivity of the prostaglandin producing tumor can be enhanced by pretreatment with cyclooxygenase inhibitors such as indomethacin. However, this inhibition of cyclooxygenase is not effective for all tumor cell lines (8,9).

The $HSDM_1C_1$ murine sarcoma cell line spontaneously produces PGE_2, although pretreatment with PGA_2 or the use of fluriprofen to inhibit prostaglandin synthesis did not alter the radiosensitivity (9). There are several possible explanations. First, eicosanoid-induced protection could be a receptor mediated event and $HSDM_1C_1$ cells lack the appropriate receptors. With regard to the fluriprofen treatment of $HSDM_1C_1$, arachidonic acid metabolism might be shunted to other radioprotective eicosanoids through the lipoxygenase pathway. Alternatively, the radioprotective mechanism invoked by eicosanoid stimulation may not be present in this cell line. The present investigation was initiated to examine these possibilities. To further extend the receptor-mediated hypothesis, prostaglandin-induced radioprotection was examined in the DC3 cell line which is derived from prostaglandin-responsive rat granulosa cells.

METHODS AND MATERIALS

Cell lines.

Two cell lines were used for these experiments, the DC3 transformed rat granulosa cell line, obtained from W.A. Schmidt (UMV Texas Medical School, Houston, TX), and the $HSDM_1C_1$ mouse fibrosarcoma cell line (American Type Culture Collection, Rockville, MD). The cell lines were grown in plastic dishes in a humidified incubator at 37°C containing an atmosphere of 3% CO_2 in air. All tissue culture medium supplies were obtained from Gibco Laboratories (Grand Island, NY). DC3 cultures were maintained in α-MEM medium supplemented with Earle's salts, 2 mM L-glutamine, 10% fetal bovine serum, and an antibiotic mixture of penicillin-streptomycin. The $HSDM_1C_1$ cells were maintained in Ham's F12 medium supplemented with 15% fetal bovine serum, 5% horse serum, 2 mM L-glutamine, and an antibiotic mixture of penicillin-streptomycin. Cells were harvested for experiments by scraping.

Irradiation.

Cells were irradiated using a 250 kVp Phillips X-ray machine at 13.5 mA. The beam was filtered with 0.26 mm Cu and 1 mm Al, with a target to object distance of 36.9 cm, at a dose rate of 1.7 Gray (Gy)/min. Survival curves were determined for the following radiation doses: 0, 1, 2, 5, 7, 10, 15, and 20 Gy. Drug toxicity and/or radiation sensitivity was determined 7 days later by the conventional survival assay based on colony formation.

Binding Assays.

Binding assays were conducted using a modification of a procedure described earlier (10). Briefly, tubes containing 50,000 to 75,000 DPM $[^3H]$-PGE_2 (specific activity 200 Ci/mmol, DuPont-New England

Nuclear, Boston, MA) and 50,000 to 1,000,000 cells were incubated in 50 μl of Hank's buffered salts solution, and 25 mM HEPES (pH 5.7). The total volume of the reaction mixture including the cells was 100 μl. Incubations were conducted at 30°C in a shaking water bath for 45 minutes. The reactions were stopped by the addition of 1 ml of ice cold buffer and the cells were either collected by centrifugation at 13,000 x gravity or by filtration on a glass fiber filter. The radioactivity remaining in the cell pellet or the cells on the filter paper was quantitated by liquid scintillation counting. All assays were run in triplicate or quadruplicate and non specific binding was assessed in a parallel series of tubes containing 1 μg unlabeled PGE_2. Sheep corpora luteal cells which have PGE_2 receptors were used as a positive control.

Prostaglandin E_2 measurement.

Prostaglandin E_2 and leukotriene C_4 concentrations in the tissue culture media were determined using radioimmunoassay kits obtained from DuPont-New England Nuclear.

cAMP analyses.

Cell cultures were grown to confluence in 60 mm dishes containing 5 mls of medium. The dishes were divided into three groups each containing three dishes: 1) no treatment (Control), 2) 4 μl ethanol, and 3) 4 μl ethanol containing PGE_2 at a final concentration of 28 μM. The dishes were incubated at 37°C, and aliquots of media were removed at 0, 30, 90, and 180 minutes. The concentration of cAMP in the medium was determined in duplicate by radioimmunoassay as described (11).

Statistics.

All experiments described in this paper have been replicated at least once. Statistical analyses were performed using the ANOVA and t-tests (RS/1 Program, BBN Software Products Corp., Cambridge, Mass.; calculations not shown).

RESULTS

Survival curves were determined for both cell lines in the presence and absence of 28 μM PGE2. The time for addition of PGE_2 ranged from 2 hrs prior to 2 hr following irradiation. In addition, the $HSDM_1C_1$ cell line was also incubated in the presence of 0.18 μM ibuprofen added 2 hrs prior to irradiation (Sigma Chemical Co., St. Louis, MO). This concentration of ibuprofen inhibited prostaglandin synthesis (data not shown). Radiation survival curves for untreated DC3 cells and for cells that received a 2 hr pretreatment of 28 μM PGE_2 were not significantly different (Figure 1 and Table 1). The radiation survival parameters of the DC3 cell line have not been previously described. They appear to have considerable resistance to radiation induced reproductive death as indicated by the large n numbers between 100 to 106, and the quasi-threshold dose (D_q) of 7.3 Gy. As mentioned in the legend to Table 1, there was no significant difference between PGE_2-treated and untreated cells (t-test, $\alpha=0.05$). $HSDM_1C_1$ cells used in another radiation study had a D_q of 0.97 Gy, and a *n* number of 1.45 (9). The previous study utilized survival fractions down to 0.01. By continuing the surviving fractions down to 0.0001 in the present studies, the $HSDM_1C_1$ survival curve became sharper and closely resembled that of the DC# cells. Survival curves for the $HSDM_1C_1$ cells are not shown since pretreatment with PGE_2 or

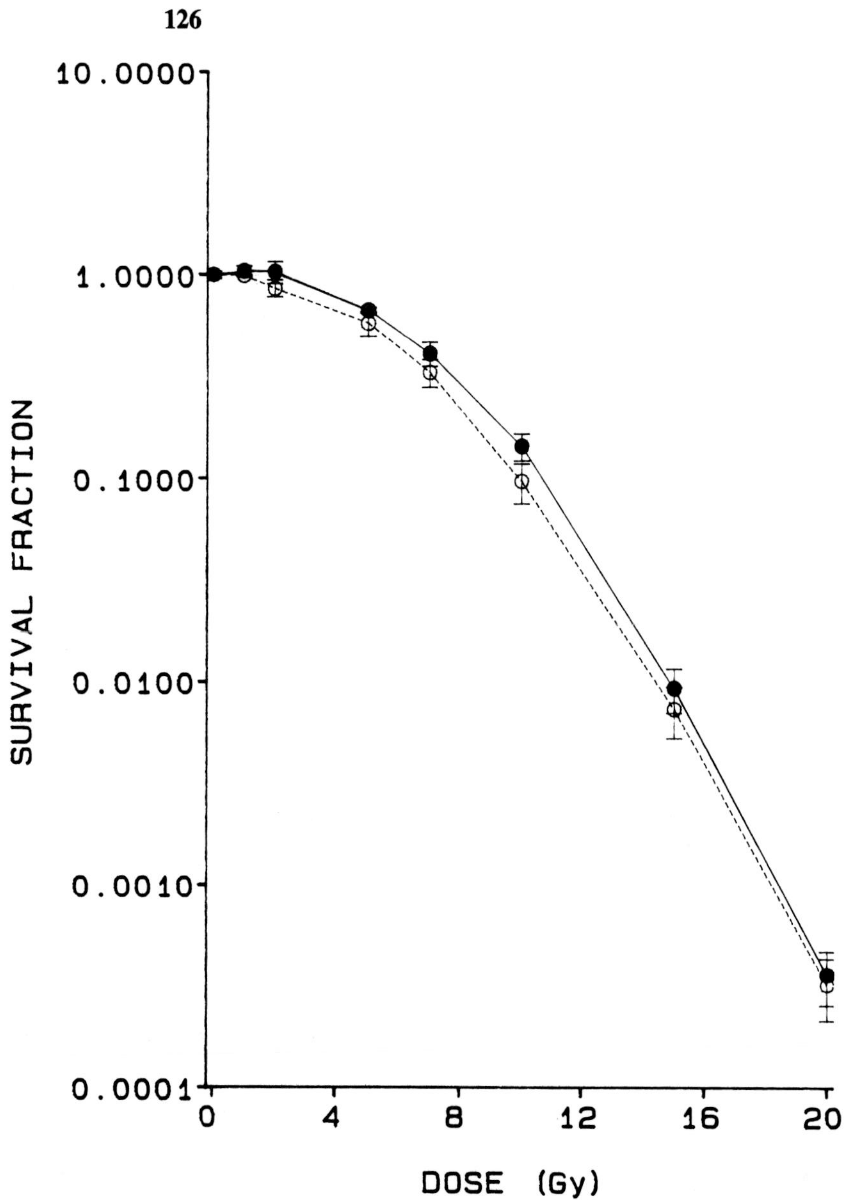

Figure 1. Radiation survival curve for DC3 rat granulosa cells. Cells were irradiated in the presence (solid line) or absence (dashed line) of PGE_2 at the indicated doses of X-irradiation as described in Methods. Each curve represents the average from three separate experiments, and the standard error of the means are provided. The survival curve parameters are provided in Table 1.

Table 1. DC3 Cell Radiation Survival Curve Parameters

Treatment	$D_o \pm$ S.E.M.	$D_q \pm$ S.E.M.	$n \pm$ S.E.M.
Control	1.65 ± 0.03	7.30 ± 0.46	100 ± 21
PGE_2	1.60 ± 0.0	7.26 ± 0.18	107 ± 7

Values calculated from DC3 radiation survival curves as shown in Figure 1. D_o and D_q are provided in units of Gy. The means were determined from three separate survival curves. None of the values are significantly different (α=0.05) between control cells and PGE_2-treated cells based on t-test comparisons.

with ibuprofen did not modify the radiosensitivity.

Studies for specific binding of PGE_2 by these two cell lines were conducted to determine if the lack of protection of these cell lines was associated with a lack of receptors for PGE_2 (Table 2). The results indicate that neither cell line possesses specific binding sites for radiolableled PGE_2. Binding by sheep corpora luteal cells was used as a positive control since they are known to possess specific binding sites (12). The $HSDM_1C_1$ cells were grown under three different conditions: control, dexamethsone-treated, and ibuprofen-treated, to determine if inhibition of prostaglandin synthesis might lead to up-regulation of PGE_2 receptors. Although cell cultures were continuously maintained on these treatments for three weeks prior to testing, no significant increase in the specific binding of PGE_2 by the cells was detected (Table 2).

The lack of PGE_2-induced radioprotection or PGE_2 receptors on the DC3 cells was perplexing since this cell line was derived from granulosa cells, which are highly responsive to PGE_2 (13). Therefore, the ability of PGE_2 to stimulate an increase in the cAMP concentration of the two cell lines was examined. There was a large time dependent increase in the cAMP concentration of the DC3 cells treated with PGE_2 (Table 3) and a minimal response by the $HSDM_1C_1$ cells.

Millar and Jinks reported that pretreatment of the $HSDM_1C_1$ cell line with flurbiprofen, a cyclooxygenase inhibitor, did not modify radiosensitivity (9). The ineffectiveness of flurbiprofen treatment to alter radiosensitivity might be attributed to a functioning lipoxygenase pathway through which other radioprotective eicosanoids might be synthesized. Therefore, the ability of these cells to synthesize LTC_4 was examined (Figure 2). $HSDM_1C_1$ cells were found to produce LTC_4 in amounts that were enhanced by treatment with the calcium ionophore A23187, or with ibuprofen.

Table 2. Lack of Specific Binding Sites for PGE_2

Cell Type:	PGE_2 Bound (DPM ± S.E.M., n=3):
Corpora Luteal Cells	703 ± 80
Corpora Luteal Cells + cold	305 ± 30
$HSDM_1C_1$	89 ± 10
$HSDM_1C_1$ + cold	111 ± 12
$HSDM_1C_1$ Dexamethasone	148 ± 83
$HSDM_1C_1$ Dex + cold	93 ± 5
$HSDM_1C_1$ Ibuprofen	94 ± 18
$HSDM_1C_1$ Ib + cold	114 ± 7
DC3 cells	1645 ± 350
DC3 cells + cold	1742 ± 115

"cold" indicates the addition of a 100X excess of unlabeled PGE_2 to the assay mixture. Each of the assays presented in the table utilized 50,000 cells each, with the exception of the DC3 assay which contained 1,000,000 cells. When assayed using 50,000 cells, the DC3 cell line showed a lack of specific PGE_2 binding similar to that of the $HSDM_1C_1$ cells. Both cell lines were tested using 1,000,000 cells per assay tube, but there was no magnification of specific binding. Therefore, the results of only the DC3 cells are presented to illustrate this point.

Table 3. Cellular Concentration of cAMP in Response to PGE_2

Cell Type	Control	30 Minutes	90 Minutes	180 Minutes
$HSDM_1C_1$	18 ± 3	24 ± 1	42 ± 9	110 ± 21
EtOH		17 ± 0.5	23 ± 6	66 ± 19
DC3	19 ± 1	462 ± 117	1083 ± 71	1438 ± 241
EtOH		21 ± 4	23 ± 0.1	30 ± 1

The first row of each cell type indicates the data for addition of PGE_2 in ethanol (EtOH), while the EtOH refers to the control effects of addition of EtOH alone. The final concentration of the PGE_2 in the culture medium was 28 μM. Each assay was performed in duplicate; the mean ± S.E.M. (n=3) are provided.

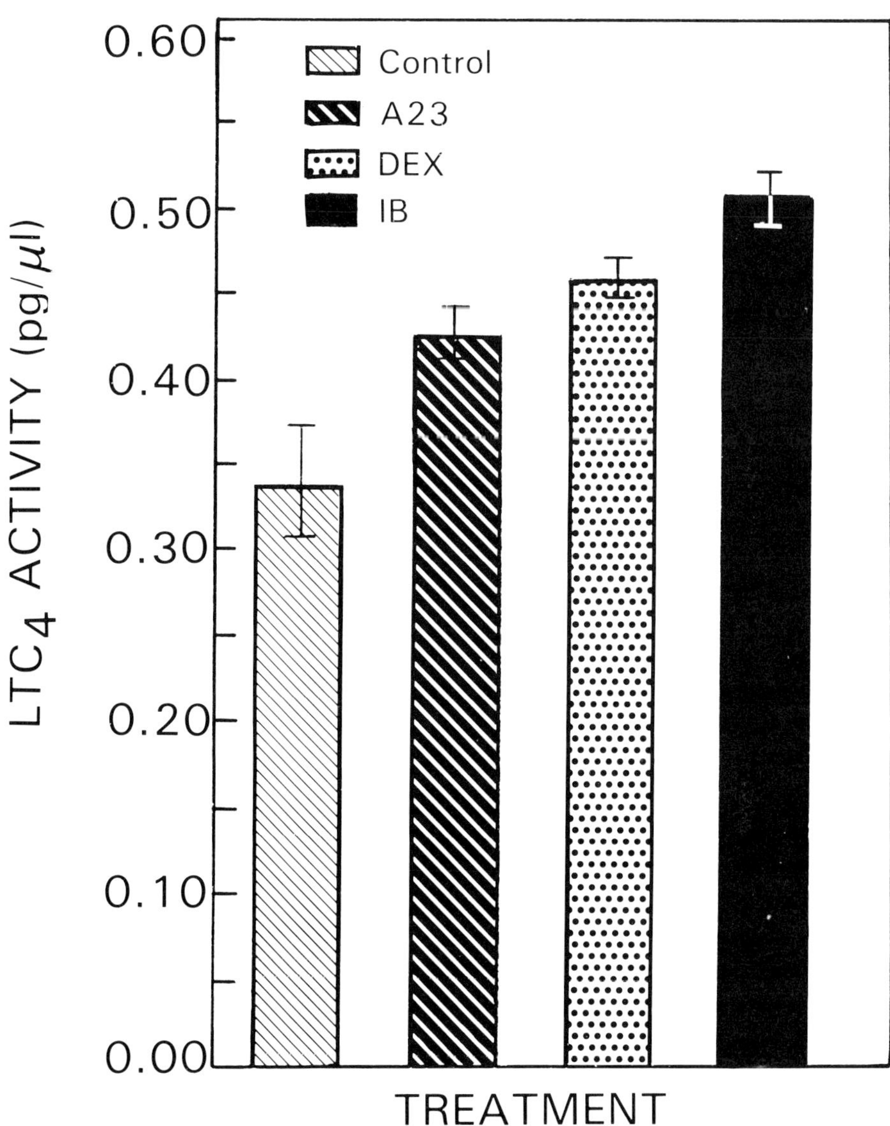

Figure 2. Production of LTC_4 by $HSDM_1C_1$ Cells. $HSDM_1C_1$ cells were plated in 24-well tissue culture plates at 10,000 cells per well. Twenty-four hours later, the medium was replaced, and the wells divided into 4 groups of 5 wells each: 1) untreated, 2) treated with 1 μM A23187, 3) 1.0 μM dexamethasone, and 4) 1.0 μM ibuprofen. Three hours later, the medium was removed from each well and assayed in duplicate for LTC_4 concentration by radioimmunoassy.

The $HSDM_1C_1$ cell line continuously produces PGE_2 in the basal state, and synthesis was further stimulated by ionizing radiation, as shown in Figures 3 and 4. The degree of stimulation was dependent on the time of sampling postirradiation and on the radiation dose (Figure 3). On day 3 postirradiation, maximum PGE_2 production was produced by 7 Gy (Figure 4). PGE_2 synthesis at this time following irradiation was 2.3 times higher than that of unirradiated cells. Interestingly, radiation doses above 7 Gy were less effective, but produced a response plateau that was still twice that of unirradiated cells. The dose response curves for the DC3 and the $HSDM_1C_1$ cells were similar, and it is apparent from Figure 1 that 7 Gy approximates the point on the survival curve at which the linear decrease in survival with increasing radiation dose begins. Therefore, it is possible that PGE_2 synthesis is still increasing proportionately for doses above 7 Gy, but is masked by the increased cell death. The cells are releasing more prostaglandins; however, there are fewer surviving cells at the higher radiation doses to participate in prostaglandin production. Therefore, prostaglandin production would continue to increase in a radiation-dose dependent manner when corrected for cell numbers but show a decrease when calculated based on media volume. This is supported by data in Figure 3 which shows that cells receiving 10 Gy produced 58% more PGE_2 on the third day postirradiation than cells that received 5 Gy irradiation, while Figure 1 shows that on day 7 after irradiation, 9 times more cells survived 5 Gy than did 10 Gy.

DISCUSSION

Pretreatment with PGE_2 did not modify the radiosensitivity of either the DC3 or the $HSDM_1C_1$ cell lines. Neither cell line appear to possess specific binding sites for PGE_2. One possibility for the lack of radioprotection in the $HSDM_1C_1$ cell line is that the cells were unable to respond because they lacked specific PGE_2 receptors. The lack of PGE_2 specific binding by the $HSDM_1C_1$ cells was further confirmed by the inability of PGE_2 treatment to elevate cellular concentrations of cAMP. However, the possibility remains that a non-receptor mediated mechanism is responsible for prostaglandin-induced radioprotection which was absent in this cell line. The data obtained for the DC3 cells regarding specific prostaglandin binding is unusual in that prostaglandin treatment increased the cAMP concentrations, yet no specific binding of prostaglandin could be detected. The increase in cAMP concentration was induced by a large concentration of PGE_2 (approximately I000X higher than the binding affinity, Kd for prostaglandin interaction with ovine luteal cells (10)) . Therefore, this response may be due either to cross-reactivity with a different prostaglandin receptor species, to a receptor possessing a very short dissociation time which makes its detection difficult, or by a receptor-independent mechanism.

Millar and Jinks reported that pretreatment of the $HSDM_1C_1$ cell line with flurbiprofen failed to modify cellular radiosensitivity (9). If the protection is receptor mediated and this cell line lacks specific receptors, then one would not expect the prostaglandin production or its inhibition to contribute to its radiation survival response curve. However, another possibility is that inhibition of the cyclooxygenase enzyme increased the amount of arachidonic acid shunted through the lipoxygenase pathway. Products of the lipoxygenase pathway have been shown to be radioprotective *in vitro* (1) and *in vivo* (2,14). By

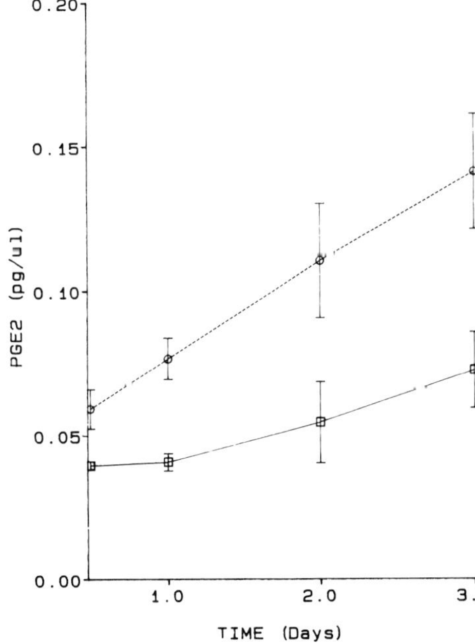

Figures 3 and 4. Time and Dose Dependence of PGE_2. Production by $HSDM_1C_1$ Cells Following Irradiation. $HSDM_1C_1$ cells were plated in 24-well tissue culture plates at 10,000 cells per well (n=5 wells/day and/or radiation dose). Twenty-four hours later, two types of experiments were conducted. In the first set of experiments cells received 5 (solid line) or 10 Gy (dashed line) of X-irradiation and the PGE_2 release into the medium was determined over time (Figure 3). In the second set of experiments, the effect of increasing radiation dose on PGE_2 release was determined on day 3 postirradiation (Figure 4). The experiments were replicated and the data combined for each figure. Standard error bars for the pooled data are provided.

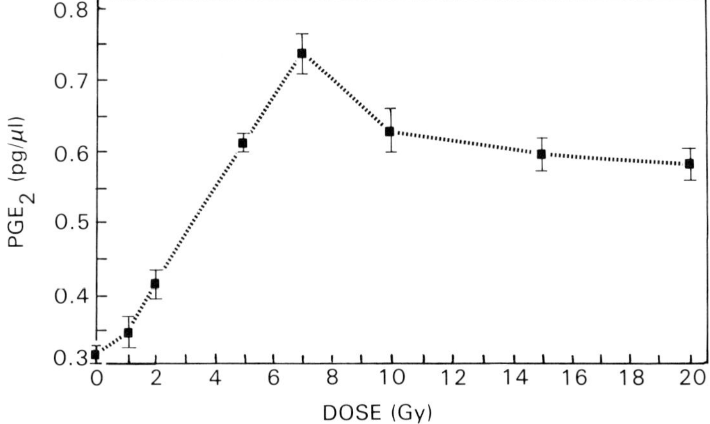

inhibiting one radioprotective metabolic pathway, another pathway may be favored. Figure 2 shows that $HSDM_1C_1$ cells produced LTC_4, and that production was increased following treatment with ibuprofen, an inhibitor of prostaglandin synthesis. Curiously, dexamethasone, an inhibitor of arachidonic acid release also stimulated LTC_4 production. It is not known at this time whether the production of LTC_4 by these cells modifies radiosensitivity. One additional factor that must be considered is the influence of increased production of prostaglandins, as occurred in the $HSDM_1C_1$ cells, on tumor growth and resistance. Presumably, the $HSDM_1C_1$ cells do not have receptors with which to respond to the increased prostaglandin synthesis. However, it is reasonable to assume that elevations in eicosanoid concentrations influence other host physiological responses in addition to those of the immune system and inflammation. For example, one of the physiological responses of host animals to transplanted $HSDM_1C_1$ tumors is an increased resorption of bone resulting from the elevation of PGE_2.

The DC3 cell line has a large D_g, 7.3 Gy, and a large *n* number of 100 (Table 1). The D_q is the dose of radiation at which a straight line drawn from the linear portion of the survival curve would intersect back to 100% survival; while the *n* number is the Y-intercept of this same line. Both values reflect enhanced radiation survival attributable to either an enhanced repair capability, or to intrinsic/extrensic protective mechanisms. The DC3 cell line is a transformed rat granulosa cell line that produces estrogens and other steroids (11,13). Estrogen has been shown to be radioprotective (15,16). Thc basis for the large radioresistance observed in the DC3 cells is not known, but it is interesting to speculate that the estrogen production provides feed-back protection. In light of the large degree of intrinsic resistance in the DC3 cell line, a prostaglandin-induced protection may not have been evident because the cells were "maximally" protected by another mechanism. This would explain why there was no increased radio-resistance in the presence of PGE_2 treatment which did elevate cAMP levels. Increased cellular concentrations of cAMP have been shown to be radioprotective (17).

In summary, the most likely explanation for the inability of PGE_2 pretreatment to modify the radiosensitivity of $HSDM_1C_1$ and DC3 cell lines is the lack of specific PGE_2 receptors.

ACKNOWLEDGEMENT

The authors would like to thank the Armed Forces Radiobiology Research Institute, Defense Nuclear Agency, for the use of the facilities. This work was supported by the Uniformed Services University for the Health Sciences, under USUHS Protocol GM8522. The views presented in this article are those of the authors. No endorsement by the Defense Nuclear Agency or the Department of Defense has been given or should be inferred.

LITERATURE CITED

1. T.L. Walden, Jr., E.V. Holahan, and G.N. Catravas. Development of a model system to study leukotriene-induced modification of radiosensitivity in mammalian cells. Prog Lipid Research 1986, 25:587-590.
2. T.L. Walden, Jr., M.L. Patchen, and T.J MacVittie. Leukotriene-induced radioprotection of hematopoietic stem cells in mice. Radiat Res 1988; 113: 388-395 .

3. W.R. Hanson, K.A Houseman, A.K. Nelson, and P.W. Collins. Radiation protection of the murine intestine by misoprostol, a prostaglandin E_1 analogue, given alone or with WR-2721, is stereospecific. Prostaglandins Leukotrienes and Essential Fatty Acids 1988; 32:101-105.
4. T.L. Walden, Jr., and J.F. Kalinich. Radioprotection by leukotrienes: Is there a receptor mechanism? Pharmacol Ther 1988; 39:379-384.
5. Allalunis-Turner, M.J., T.L. Walden, and C. Sawich. Induction of marrow hypoxia by radioprotective agents. Radiat Res 1989; 118:581-586.
6. T.A. Fitz, D.F. Contois, Y.X. Liu, D.S. Watt, and T.L. Walden, Jr. Interaction of leukotriene C_4 and chinese hamster lung fibroblasts (V79A03 cells). 1. Characterization of binding. Prostaglandins 1990; 40:417-429.
7. Y.X. Liu, D.F. Contois, D.S. Watts, T.L. Walden, Jr., and T.A. Fitz. Interaction of leukotriene C_4 and chinese hamster lung fibroblasts (V79A03 cells). 2. Subcellular distribution of binding and unlikely role of glutathione-S-transferase. Prostaglandins 1990-40:431-443.
8. Y. Furuta, N. Hunter, T. Barkley, Jr., E. Hall, and M. Lucas. Increase in radioresponse of murine tumors by treatment with indomethacin. Cancer Res 1988; 48:3008-3013.
9. B.C. Millar, and S. Jinks. Do prostaglandins affect cellular radiosensitivity in vitro? Int J Radiat Biol 1984; 46:367-373.
10. A.K. Balapure, C.E. Rexroad, K. Kawada, D.S. Watt, and T.A. Fitz. Structural requirements for prostaglandin analog interaction with ovine corpus luteum prostaglandin $F_{2\alpha}$ receptor. Biochem Pharmacol 1989; 38:2375-2381.
11. T.A. Fitz, R.M. Wah, W.A. Schmidt, and C.A. Winkel. Physiologic characterization of transformed and cloned rat granulosa cells. Biol Reprod 1989;40:250.
12. T.A. Fitz, P.B. Hoyer, and G.D. Niswender. Interactions of prostaglandins with subpopulations of ovine luteal cells. I. Stimulatory effects of prostaglandins E_1, E_2, and I_2. Prostaglandins 1984;28:119.
13. A.J.W. Hsueh, E.Y. Adashi, P.B.C. Jones, and T.H. Wells, Jr. Hormonal regulation of the differentiation of cultured ovarian granulosa cells. Endocr Rev 1984; 5:76-127.
14. T.L. Walden. Radioprotection of mouse hematopoietic stem cells by leukotriene A4 and lipoxin B4. J Radiat Res 1988; 29:255-260.
15. J. Furth, and O.B. Furth. Neoplastic diseases produced in mice by general irradiation with x-rays; incidence and types of neoplasms. Am J Cancer 1936; 28:54-65.
16. S. Katsh, and A. Edelmann. The influence of gonadectomy, sex, and strain upon the survival times of x-irradiated mice. In: Effects of Ionizing Radiation on the Reproductive System, W.D. Carlson and F.X. Gassner, eds., Pergamon Press, New York, 1964, pp 427-431.
17. D. Hess, K.N. Prasad. Modification of radiosensitivity of mammalian cells by cyclic nucleotides. Life Sciences 1981; 29:1-4.

RADIATION-INDUCED DECREASE IN RAT ABDOMINAL AORTIC REACTIVITY TO U46619: AMELIORATION WITH INDOMETHACIN AND WR2721

M.J. SCHNEIDKRAUT, M.E. WARFIELD, C.M. CUNARD, P.W. RAMWELL, and P.A. KOT

Department of Physiology and Biophysics, Georgetown University School of Medicine, 3900 Reservoir Road NW, Washington, DC 20007

INTRODUCTION

Exposure to ionizing radiation has demonstrated that vascular tissue is very radiosensitive (1-3). Besides structural changes, ionizing radiation exposure alters vascular permeability (2,3) and tone (1). Studies have shown that vascular responsiveness to exogenous vasoconstrictors are altered following irradiation (4-8). One possible explanation for this increased permeability and altered vascular reactivity is the release of vasoactive inflammatory mediators. Studies from this and other laboratories have shown that ionizing radiation exposure increases the release of thromboxane A2 (TXA2) (9-12).

The present study reviews previous investigations by this laboratory which evaluated the effect of increased endogenous TXA2 release on abdominal aortic vascular reactivity to the TXA2 mimic, 11a, 9a epoxymethano prostaglandin F2a (U46619). Data are also presented that show the effects of the radioprotectant, S-2 (3-aminopropylamino) ethyl phosphotheoic acid (WR2721), on the radiation-induced alteration in vascular reactivity. Finally, potential mechanisms for the altered aortic reactivity to this TXA2 mimic are presented.

MATERIALS AND METHODS

Irradiation.

Male Sprague-Dawley rats (200-250 g) were used in all studies. Rats were anesthetized (30 mg/kg sodium pentobarbital, i.p.) and exposed to 20 Gray (Gy) whole body irradiation in a ventro-dorsal orientation to a 7.4×10^{13} becquerel ^{137}Cs radiation source (Best Industries small animal irradiator, Arlington, VA). The rate of exposure was calibrated at 0.87 Gy/min. Sham irradiated animals were anesthetized but not irradiated (9).

Preparation of vascular rings.

Rats were re-anesthetized 2, 24, or 48 hrs after 20 Gy whole body irradiation and the animals anticoagulated with heparin (1000 USP units/kg, i.v.). A section of abdominal aorta caudal to the diaphragm and cephalad to the renal arteries was loosely ligated. The rat was then exsanguinated and the vessel segment removed. The vascular tissue was washed in cold Krebs-Ringer bicarbonate (118.2 mM NaCl, 4.7 mM KCl, 1.9 mM MgS04, 1.9 mM CaC12, 1.2 mM NaH2P04, 25 mM NaHC03, and 5.6 mM glucose; KRB) and adherent connective tissue removed (7).

Measurement of vascular reactivity.

Vascular segments were divided into 2-3 mm wide abdominal aortic rings with one ring isolated per animal. The aortic ring was suspended in a 5 ml water-jacketed (37°) tissue chamber by hooks fashioned from 26 gauge needles. One hook was attached to the glass tissue chamber and the other to an isometric tension transducer (Model UC2, Gould Instrument Co., Cleveland, OH). The tissue chamber was filled with 5 ml KRB and aerated with 95% air 5% C02. A preload tension of 1-1.5 g was applied to the tissue and the rings were allowed to equilibrate for one hour. Every 15 min during the equilibration period, the KRB was exchanged and the preload tension readjusted. Following equilibration, the developed isometric tension, induced by the addition of cumulative concentrations of U46619 (10^{-9} - 10^{-6} M, Upjohn Co., Kalamazoo, MI) or KCl (4.4 - 154 mM Sigma Chemical Co., St. Louis, MO) was recorded and compared to the response of aortic rings from sham irradiated controls (7).

Aortic Shielding.

Rats were anesthetized and randomly assigned to one of three experimental groups: 1) sham irradiated, 2) abdominal shielded - irradiated, or 3) unshielded - irradiated. Forty-eight hours later, the rats were re-anesthetized and the abdominal aortic vascular reactivity to U46619 assessed. The efficiency of the shield was previously measured at 92% using lithium iodide crystals (10).

Cyclooxygenase inhibition.

Rats were anesthetized 45 min before irradiation or sham irradiation and injected with either indomethacin (5 mg/kg, i.v.) or an equivalent volume of vehicle (154 mM NaCl plus 5.9 mM Na2C03). Four and 24 hrs after irradiation, the animals were re-injected with indomethacin (20 mg/kg, i.p.) or vehicle. Forty-eight hrs after irradiation, the rats were re-anesthetized, the abdominal aorta was removed, and the vascular response to U46619 assessed.

Radioprotectant pretreatment.

Rats were anesthetized and injected with WR2721 (200 mg/kg, i.p.) or an equivalent volume of vehicle (distilled water), 20 min before irradiation or sham irradiation. Forty-eight hrs later, the rats were re-anesthetized and the abdominal aortic responsiveness to U46619 determined (8).

Statistical analysis.

The correlation of dose versus developed isometric tension for U46619 and KCl was assessed using a Pearson product-moment correlation (r). The slope was then calculated from a semi-logrithmic plot of each dose-response curve. Comparison of the maximum contraction and slope of irradiated vessels challenged with KCl was made using an unpaired Student's t-test. Similarly, the effect of WR2721 on radiation-induced alterations in vascular reactivity to U46619 was evaluated by the unpaired Student's t-test. The effect of time following irradiation and the effect of aortic shielding on vascular responsiveness to U46619 was assessed by a multiple range Analysis of Variance plus a Dunnett's test. The effect of cyclooxygenase inhibition on the radiation-induced decrease in vascular reactivity was determined by an Analysis of Variance plus a Newman-Keuls' test. For all studies, the confidence interval was set at 95%.

RESULTS AND DISCUSSION

Aortic responsiveness to U46619 four and 24 hrs after 20 Gy whole body irradiation was unchanged from control. By 48 hrs post exposure, the slope of the U46619 dose-response curve was decreased 58.1% ($p<.05$) and the maximum contractile response was depressed 61.8% ($p<.05$) (Table 1).

Table 1. Effect of whole body gamma irradiation on vascular responses of rat aortic rings to U46619.

	Slope	Maximum Contraction (grams)
Sham irradiated	0.43 ±0.04	1.31 ±0.09
Irradiated (4 hrs)	0.33 ±0.07	1.12 ±0.22
Irradiated (24 hrs)	0.28 ±0.11	0.82 ±0.25
Irradiated (48 hrs)	0.18* ±0.08	0.50* ±0.20

Data are expressed as mean ± standard error for 6 - 35 animals per group. *$p<.05$ compared to sham irradiated control. Reproduced from Radiation Res. 117:459-468, 1989.

This indicates that a radiation-induced decrease in vascular reactivity occurs and that this altered vascular response requires more than 24 hrs in order to be observed. Furthermore, though a lethal dose of radiation was used, the altered vascular response was seen at least 24 hrs before any mortality occurred. These data agree with an earlier in vivo study in which local irradiation of rabbit ear arterioles resulted in a loss of vasomotion and vasodilation (1).

In order to determine if the radiation-induced decrease in vascular reactivity was a generalized phenonmenon, aortic rings from irradiated rats were challenged with the non-receptor mediated vasoconstrictor, KCl. This allowed an evaluation of vascular smooth muscle integrity independent of receptor injury. Irradiated aortic rings had a maximum contractile response to KCl that was not different than control (1.04 ± 0.15 versus 1.00 ± 0.16 g). The slopes of the dose-response curves were also not significantly different. Thus, the decreased aortic response to U46619 was not due to vascular smooth muscle injury (7).

Previous studies indicate that whole body irradiation will increase the in vivo synthesis of TXA2 (9-12). Other studies suggest that elevated cyclooxygenase product levels can down-regulate eicosanoid receptors (13-15). In order to test if the increased TXA2 levels were affecting the vascular response to

U46619, rats were treated with indomethacin before and for 48 hrs after whole body irradiation. Indomethacin treatment of sham irradiated rats did not alter the vascular response to U46619. Similarly, vehicle treatment of irradiated animals did not blunt the radiation-induced decrease in vascular reactivity. Indomethacin treatment before and after irradiation, blunted the radiation-induced decrease in aortic responsiveness to U46619 (Table 2). However, the improvement in vascular reactivity with indomethacin treatment was only modest, as the aortic response was also not significantly different from the vehicle treated - irradiated group (Table 2). Therefore, while increased TXA2 levels may play some role in the depressed vascular response to U46619, it is not the only mechanism involved.

Table 2. Effect of cyclooxygenase inhibition on the radiation-induced alteration in rat abdominal aortic response to U46619.

	Slope	Maximum Contraction (grams)
Vehicle - Sham	0.27 ±0.04	1.22 ±0.17
Indomethacin - Sham	0.26 ±0.02	1.26 ±0.13
Vehicle - Irradiated	0.21 ±0.03	0.78[a,b] ±0.11
Indomethacin - Irradiated	0.25 ±0.02	0.99 ±0.17

Data are expressed as mean ± standard error for 7-10 animals per group. [a]$p<.05$ compared to vehicle injected - sham irradiated group. [b]$p<.05$ compared to indomethacin treated - sham irradiated group. Reproduced from Radiation Res. 117:459-468, 1989.

Another possible mechanism for the decreased vascular reactivity to U46619 is a radiation-induced inactivation of the TXA2/PGH2 receptor. Previous studies have shown that increasing doses of radiation, dose-dependently decreased ^{3}H iloprost binding to PGI2 receptors in vitro (16). In order to test this possibility, the abdominal aorta was shielded during whole body irradiation. Shielding of the abdominal aorta blunted the radiation-induced decrease in vascular reactivity probably by direct protection of the TXA2/PGH2 receptors as well as by blunting the in vivo release of TXA2 (10) (Table 3). Thus, the partial improvement in vascular reactivity with shielding may, in part, be due to a prevention of receptor inactivation by ionizing radiation.

Finally, administration of WR2721 to rats before irradiation prevented the radiation-induced decrease in vascular reactivity to U46619 (Table 4). One can speculate that the mechanism(s) involved in

Table 3. Effect of aortic shielding on rat abdominal aortic ring vascular reactivity after whole body irradiation.

	Slope	Maximum Contraction (grams)
Sham irradiated	0.53 ±0.04	1.68 ±0.13
Shielded - Irradiated	0.44 ±0.07	1.38 ±0.21
Unshielded- Irradiated	0.36 ±0.05	1.13* ±0.14

Data are expressed as mean ± standard error for 6 - 10 animals per group. *p<.05 compared to sham irradiated control. Reproduced from Radiation Res. 117:459-468, 1989

Table 4. Effect of WR2721 on the radiation-induced alteration in vascular reactivity to U46619.

	Slope	Maximum Contraction (grams)
Vehicle - Sham	0.67 ±0.12	1.89 ±0.22
WR2721 - Irradiated	0.66 ±0.09	1.88 ±0.11

Data are expressed as mean ± standard error for six animals per group. Reproduced from Radiation Res in press.

this response is/are either direct protection of the receptor from inactivation, attenuation of receptor down-regulation by preventing the radiation-induced increase in TXA2 (12), or a combination of these actions. Further studies are needed to clarify the mechanism(s) involved in both the radiation-induced decrease in vascular reactivity as well as its attenuation by WR2721.

REFERENCES

1. Narayan, K. and Cliff, W.J. Am. J. Pathol. 106:47-62, 1982.
2. Evans, M.L., Graham, M.M., Mahler, P.A. and Rasey, J.S. Int. J. Radiat. Biol. Phys. 13:563-567, 1987.
3. Law, M.P. Adv. Radiat. Biol. 9:37-73, 1981.
4. Loyd, J.E., Bolds, J.M., Sheller, J.R., Duke, S.S., Gillette, A.W., Malcolm, A.W., Meyrick, B.O. and Brigham, K.L. J. Appl. Physiol. 62:208-218, 1987.

5. Loyd, J.E., Bolds, J.M., Wickersham, N., Malcolm, A.W. and Brigham, K.L. Am. Rev. Respir. Dis. 138:1227-1233, 1988.
6. Perkett, E.A., Brigham, K.L. and Meyrick, B. J. Appl. Physiol. 61:1875-1881, 1986.
7. Warfield, M.E., Schneidkraut, M.J., Cunard, C.M., Ramwell, P.W. and Kot, P.A. Radiat. Res. 117:459-468, 1989.
8. Warfield, M.E., Schneidkraut, M.J., Ramwell, P.W. and Kot, P.A. Radiat. Res. in press.
9. Schneidkraut, M.J., Kot, P.A., Ramwell, P.W. and Rose, J.C. J. Appl. Physiol. 57:833-838, 1984.
10. Schneidkraut, M.J., Kot, P.A., Ramwell, P.W. and Rose, J.C. J. Appl. Physiol. 61:1264-1269, 1986.
11. Schneidkraut, M.J., Ramwell, P.W. and Kot, P.A. In: Prostaglandins, Leukotrienes, and Cancer: Eicosanoids and Radiation (Eds. K.V. Honn, L.J. Marnett and P. Polgar), Kluwer Publishers, Boston, MA, 1988, pp 25-37.
12. Donlon, M., Steel, L., Helgeson, E.A., Wolfe, W.W. and Catravas, G.N. Int. J. Radiat. Biol. 47:205-212, 1985.
13. Hatmi, M., del Maschio, A., Lefort, J., de Gaetano, G., Vargaftig, B. and Cerletti, C. J. Pharmacol. Exp. Therap. 241:623-627, 1987.
14. Modesti, P.A., Fortini, A., Poggesi. L., Boddi, M., Abbati, R. and Gensini, G.F. Thromb. Res. 48:663-669, 1987.
15. Rice, M.G., McRae, J.R., Storm, D.R. and Robertson, R.P. Am. J. Physiol. 241:E291-E297, 1981.
16. Leigh, P.J., Cramp, W.A. and MacDermot, J. J. Biol. Chem. 259:12431-12436, 1984.

ANTIOXIDANTS AND PREVENTION OF THE HEPATOCELLULAR DAMAGE INDUCED BY GLUTATHIONE-DEPLETING AGENTS

A.F. CASINI, E. MAELLARO, B. DEL BELLO and M. COMPORTI

Istituto di Patologia Generale, Universita di Siena, Siena, Italy

INTRODUCTION

Previous studies from our laboratory (1-3) have shown that the intoxication of mice with three prototypical glutathione (GSH) depleting agents (bromobenzene, diethylmaleate and allyl alcohol) is followed by the development of lipid peroxidation and liver necrosis after the hepatic GSH depletion has reached critical values. The treatment of the intoxicated animals with the antioxidants Trolox C or desferrioxamine, completely prevents both lipid peroxidation and liver necrosis, while not changing at all the extent of the covalent binding of bromobenzene metabolites to liver protein. In subsequent studies, the relationships among the various antioxidant systems (namely, vit. E, GSH and ascorbic acid) of the liver cell have been investigated under conditions of severe GSH depletion, like those induced by the GSH depleting agents mentioned above. Such an abrupt loss of the GSH antioxidant system could reasonably affect the other antioxidant systems. According to some authors (4,5), in fact, GSH is directly involved in the enzymatic system ("tocopheroxy radical reductase") that reduces the oxidized form of tocopherol; on the other hand, according to others (6,7) the tocopherol regenerating system consists of ascorbic acid that is converted in the reaction to semidehydroascorbic acid radical and then to dehydroascorbic acid. Even in the latter case GSH may be involved in the reduction of the oxidized form of ascorbic acid (dehydroascorbic acid) (8,9). Alternatively, GSH depletion could affect the other antioxidant systems, by decreasing the disposition of hydrogen peroxide through GSH peroxidase. Vit. E may be consumed as a result of an increased formation of lipid peroxides in cell membranes, while ascorbate may be involved by direct interactions with oxy-radicals, especially with hydroxyl radicals.

MATERIALS AND METHODS

Male NMRI albino mice (20-30 g) were used. The animals were maintained on different diets. Some of the animals were maintained on a complete pellet diet (Altromin-Rieper), hereafter referred to as the standard laboratory diet. The remaining animals were subdivided into three groups: one group was maintained, since weanling, on a vit. E-deficient diet (10); the other two groups were maintained on the same diet (basal diet) supplemented with 30 or 65 mg of vit. E/Kg, respectively. These different dietary regimens resulted, after 40 days, in the following hepatic levels of α-tocopherol: 4-5, 90-130 and 230-300 pmol/mg protein, obtained with the vit. E deficient diet (basal diet), the basal diet supplemented with 30 mg of vit. E/Kg and the basal diet supplemented with 65 mg of vit. E/Kg, respectively. The amounts of

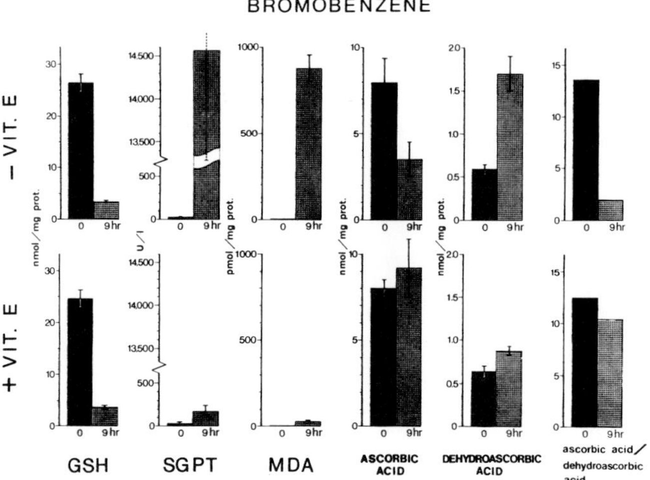

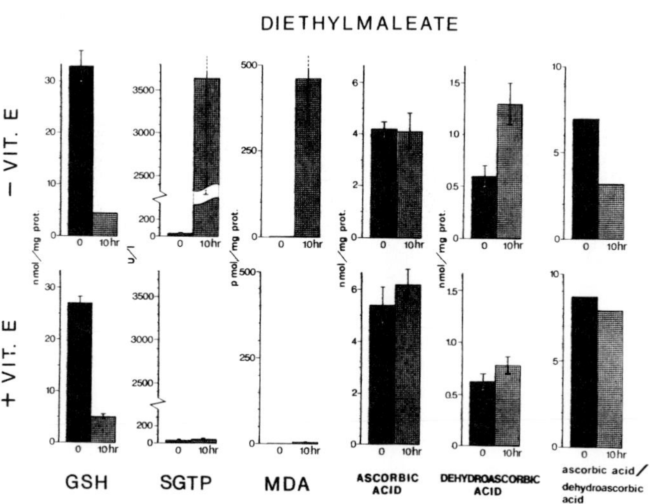

Figure 1. Hepatic glutathione (GSH) depletion, liver necrosis (SGPT), lipid peroxidation [hepatic content of malonic dialdehde (MDA)], and variation of ascorbic to dehydroascorbic acid ratio after bromobenzene or diethylmaleate intoxication in mice maintained on either a vit. E deficit diet (upper part) or the same diet supplemented with 65 mg of vit. E/Kg (lower part). Bromobenzene and diethylmaleate were given p.o. at the doses of 13 and 12 mmol/Kg body wt, respectively.

Table 1. Time-course of hepatic glutathione (GSH) depletion, liver necrosis (SGPT), lipid peroxidation (hepatic content of malonic dialdehyde, MDA) and change in hepatic α-tocopherol (vit. E), ascorbic acid and dehydroascorbic acid content after bromobenzene intoxication of mice maintained on the standard laboratory diet

Time after intoxication	0 time	3 hr	9 hr	12 hr	15 hr	18 hr
GSH (nmol/mg protein)	24.3 ± 1.7 (20)	3.7 ± 0.2 (7)	2.1 ± 0.1 (6)	2.2 ± 0.2 (15)	2.4 ± 0.3 (14)	1.9 ± 0.3 (28)
SGPT (U/l)	46 ± 5 (20)	48 ± 30 (3)	35 ± 6 (6)	63 ± 15 (12)	2578 ± 1389 (14)	4669 ± 1545 (28)
MDA (pmol/mg protein)	--	0 (3)	0 (6)	3 ± 2 (15)	189 ± 85 (14)	1097 ± 406 (11)
Vit. E (pmol/mg protein)	122 ± 6 (20)	149 ± 35 (7)	108 ± 2 (6)	86 ± 22*[a] (11)	67 ± 16*[c] (14)	45 ± 16*[c] (11)
Ascorbic acid (nmol/mg protein)	7.9 ± 0.4 (20)	11.7 ± 0.2*[c] (7)	N.D.	8.5 ± 0.7 (11)	6.6 ± 1.2 (14)	4.0 ± 0.8*[c] (16)
Dehydroascorbic acid (nmol/mg protein)	0.37 ± 0.07 (19)	1.02 ± 0.21*[b] (3)	N.D.	1.55 ± 0.24*[c] (10)	1.32 ± 0.16*[c] (14)	0.59 ± 0.38 (5)
Ascorbic acid / Dehydroascorbic acid	21.4	11.5	N.D.	5.5	5.0	6.8

For the standard laboratory diet, see Materials and Methods. Bromobenzene was given by gastric intubation at the dose of 13 mmol/Kg body wt. Results are given as means ± SE. The number of animals is reported in brackets.

*Significantly different from the 0 time value: $^{a}P < 0.05$, $^{b}P < 0.005$, $^{c}P < 0.001$.

N.D. = not determined.

vit. E added to the diet (30 or 65 mg/Kg) were selected to achieve hepatic α-tocopherol concentrations either equal to or double of that obtained with the standard laboratory diet. The intoxications were performed as reported in the Figure1. Hepatic GSH (1), liver necrosis (SGPT) (1), lipid peroxidation (hepatic content of malonic dialdehyde, MDA) (2), α-tocopherol (11), ascorbic and dehydroascorbic acid (11) were determined as previously reported.

RESULTS AND DISCUSSION

In all the intoxications vit. E was markedly decreased whenever extensive lipid peroxidation developed and, in the case of bromobenzene (Table 1), even before its onset. The ascorbic/dehydroascorbic acid ratio showed the increase of the oxidized over the reduced form in all the intoxications suggesting that this redox cycling of vit. C reflects an oxidative stress as a consequence of GSH depletion. In the case of bromobenzene (Table 1) such a change in the redox state of vit. C preceded and signaled the appearance of lipid peroxidation, whereas in the other intoxications such a change appeared to be the consequence of uncontrolled lipid peroxidation. Differences in the exent of oxidative stress induced by the three toxins can be invoked to explain this diversity.

Experiments carried out with vit. E-deficient or supplemented diets.

In mice maintained on the vit. E-deficient diet (Figure 1) all the intoxications caused the development of lipid peroxidation and liver necrosis much earlier and in a much more severe way as compared to the animals fed on the standard laboratory diet (see Table 1 for bromobenzene). Again the ascorbic/dehydroascorbic acid ratio was dramatically decreased.

In mice maintained on the same diet supplemented with 30 mg of vit. E/Kg the effects of the three intoxications (not shown) were quite similar to those obtained with the standard laboratory diet. By contrast only minor effects of the intoxications were seen in animals fed on the same diet supplemented with 65 mg of vit. E/Kg, in spite of a comparable hepatic GSH depletion (Figure 1). It must be recalled that the latter diet yielded an hepatic tocopherol concentration approximately double that obtained with the standard laboratory diet. It seems therefore that vit. E is a key factor in the expression of the hepatotoxicity of GSH-depleting agents.

ACKNOWLEDGEMENTS

This research was supported by a grant from CNR (Italy), Group of Gastroenterology. Additional fund was derived from the Association for International Cancer Research (Great Britain).

REFERENCES

1. Casini, A.F., Pompella, A. and Comporti, M. Am. J. Pathol 118: 225-237, 1985.
2. Casini, A.F., Maellaro, E., Pompella, A., Ferrali, M. and Comporti, M. Biochem. Pharmacol. 36: 3689-3695, 1987.
3. Pompella, A., Romani, A., Fulceri, R., Benedetti, A. and Comporti, M. Biochim. Biophys. Acta 961: 293-298, 1988.

4. Reddy, C.C., Scholz, R.W., Thomas, C.E. and Massaro, E.J. Ann. N. Y. Acad. Sci. 393: 193-195, 1982.
5. McCay, P.B., Lai, E.K., Powell, S.R. and Breuggemann, G. Fed. Proc. 45: 451, 1986.
6. Packer, J.E., Slater, T.F. and Willson, R.L. Nature (London) 278: 737-738, 1979.
7. Niki, E., Saito, T., Kawakami, A. and Kamiya, Y. J. Biol. Chem. 259: 4177-4182, 1984.
8. Hughes, R.E. Nature (London) 203: 1068-1069, 1964.
9. Bigley, R., Riddle, M., Layman, D. and Stankova, L. Biochim. Biophys. Acta 659: 15-22, 1981.
10. Bacharach, A.L. and Allchorne, J. In: The Biological Standard of the Vitamins (Ed. K.H. Coward), Bailliere, London, 1947, pp. 147-149.
11. Casini, A.F., Maellaro, E., Del Bello, B. and Comporti, M. In: Free Radicals in the Pathogenesis of Liver Injury (Eds. G. Poli, K.H. Cheeseman, M.U. Dianzani and T.F. Slater), Pergamon Press, Oxford, 1989, pp. 55-62.

THE EFFECTS OF OXYGEN RADICAL - MEDIATED PULMONARY ENDOTHELIAL DAMAGE ON CANCER METASTASIS

S.G. SHAUGHNESSY, D. WARNER, M.R. BUCHANAN, R. LAFRENIE and F.W. ORR

Department of Pathology and Oncology Research Group, McMaster University, Hamilton, Ont. Canada

SUMMARY

Cancer cells frequently disseminate via the bloodstream where the endothelium acts as a barrier between the circulating tumor cells and the extravascular tissue. Free radicals generated by environmental factors or host cells can cause endothelial cell injury and we have postulated that such injury could promote the metastasis of intravascular tumor cells. In mice and rats endothelial damage was induced by intravenous cobra venom factor which activates circulating leukocytes. Endothelial cell damage was demonstrated by morphology and by altered vasopermeability. When ^{125}IUdr-labelled cancer cells were injected intravenously, during periods of maximal endothelial cell injury there was a 3 fold increase in retention of these cells in the lung, 24 hours later. After 14 days there was a 3-20 fold increase in the number of metastatic tumors in CoF-treated animals. In both rats and mice, tumor cell localization was reduced 70-80% by pretreatment of the animals with catalase. In mice, endothelial injury induced by bleomycin (120 mg/kg) or by exposure to 90% oxygen for 2-4 days also significantly increased the metastasis of circulating cancer cells. Studies *in vitro* have demonstrated that rat Walker 256 cancer cells or host cells, when activated with the chemotactic peptide N-fMLP, generate oxygen-derived free radicals and can damage cultured endothelium. When fMLP-activated W256 cells were incubated with ^{3}H-2-deoxyglucose-labelled endothelial cell monolayers, there was a 27% increase in the specific release of isotope within 90 minutes. Damage correlated with tumor cell-induced chemiluminescence and was inhibited by catalase. We conclude that free radical-mediated damage to the microvasculature facilitates the metastasis of circulating cancer cells.

Vessel Wall Injury And Tumor Cell Extravasation.

Metastasis is a multi-step process involving intravasation of cells from a primary tumor, their circulation in the bloodstream, exit of these cells into extravascular tissue and finally, their growth into secondary tumors. Extravasation requires that the tumor cell pass through the capillary wall. Studies *in vitro* and *in vivo* have outlined a sequence of events by which tumor cells may cross both the endothelium and the underlying basement membrane. Following tumor cell adhesion to the endothelium, the latter cells appear to retract, thereby exposing the underlying basement membrane to which the tumor cells adhere preferentially (1). The endothelium then covers over the tumor cell (1,2). Subsequent penetration of the basement membrane may be aided by the secretion of proteolytic enzymes. Both Cathepsin B (3) and a secreted collagenase (4) have been implicated in capillary wall damage by tumor cells. The proliferation of arrested tumor cells within capillary lumens, eventually leading to vessel wall damage, has also been implicated in the process of tumor cell extravasation, (5).

Such studies have suggested that endothelial cells can act as a barrier to the exit of circulating cancer cells from the microvasculature. Since cancer cells preferentially attach to basement membranes in preference to the endothelium, we have postulated that endothelial damage facilitates metastasis by promoting the attachment of circulating tumor cells to the underlying basement membrane. Three models were chosen to test this hypothesis directly. Lung damage was induced with agents which were clinically relevant, caused a reproducible sequence of injury, and were not immunosuppresive. In all these systems, endothelial cell damage is induced by mechanisms involving the generation of oxygen-derived free radicals.

Effects of Neutrophil-Mediated Pulmonary Endothelial Injury.

Activated neutrophils can damage endothelial cells in vitro by the generation of free radicals (6,7). To test the possibility that neutrophil-mediated pulmonary endothelial cell injury promotes the metastasis of circulating cancer cells, neutrophils were activated by the intravenous injection of cobra venom factor. In both rats (8) and mice (9) this lead to complement activation and neutropenia with sequestration of neutrophils in the lung. Damage to the endothelium was confirmed by morphology and increased vasopermeability. In CoF-treated rats, increased vasopermeability was measured by leakage of ^{125}I-albumin from the circulation into lung tissue. This was detected within 5 minutes after CoF injection and increased to maximum values within 30 minutes. In mice, there was a 60-fold increase in the amount of intravascular Evans blue that was retained in the lungs after cobra venom treatment. Aggregates of neutrophils and tumor cells were observed within pulmonary capillaries 2 hours after injecting cancer cells I.V. in both CoF-treated rats and mice. Twenty-four hours after intravenous injection, there were more tumor cells in the lungs of CoF-treated animals than in controls. In CoF-treated rats, there was a 2 to 3-fold increase in the retention of radiolabelled Walker 256 carcinosarcoma cells (8). In mice, the simultaneous injection of CoF and radiolabelled fibrosarcoma cells resulted in a 3-4 fold increase in the retention of tumor cells (9). In rats and mice, pretreatment of animals with antineutrophil antiserum reduced tumor cell localization by 55 to 96% respectively. In addition, animals pretreated with catalase demonstrated a 70-85% reduction in tumor cell localization following the simultaneous injection of tumor cells and CoF. Pretreatment of animals with superoxide dismutase had no effect on tumor cell localization.

There was a direct correlation between the localization of cancer cells at 24 hours and the formation of metastasis at 14 days. In CoF-treated rats, morphometric examination and histologic sections of lung demonstrated a 5-fold increase in the percentage of lung involved with tumor (8). In CoF-treated mice there was a 3-20 fold increase in the number of metastatic pleural tumor nodules and a 410 fold increase in the area of lung involved with metastatic tumor (9). In this model, endothelial damage and its effect on metastasis were dependent upon the C5 - component of serum complement and on circulating neutrophils.

Table 1. Effects of leukocyte activation in the presence of catalase and antineutrophil antiserum

	24 Hour Cancer Cell Retention (% of negative control)		
	CoF	Catalase	Antineutrophil Antiserum
Sprague-Dawley Rats	243 ± 40	115 ± 8*	145 ± 5*
C57BL/6J Mice	392 ± 23	185 ± 46*	107 ± 14*
C5-sufficient Mice	470 ± 250	129 ± 46*	104 ± 14*
C5-deficient Mice	69 ± 8	——	——

* $P < 0.05$

The Effects Of Bleomycin And Hyperosia.

Bleomycin, a glycopeptide-derived antibiotic, is used as a chemotherapeutic agent in many treatment protocols. The drug binds to DNA in the form of an iron-bleomycin complex which can react with molecular oxygen to produce reactive oxygen species, including superoxide anion and hydroxyl radical. This leads to DNA fragmentation by the oxygenation of deoxyribose and the generation of free bases as well as the peroxidation of cell membrane lipids (10,11,12). When C57BL/6 mice were given a single I.V. injection of bleomycin (120 mg/kg), an increase in total protein as well as intravenously injected ^{125}I-albumin was observed in bronchoalveolar lavage fluids five days later (Table 2). Electron microscopy of the pulmonary capillaries, demonstrated edema of the endothelial cells as well as areas of denuded basement membrane (13,14). When radiolabelled fibrosarcoma cells were injected during this period, the percent cells retained in the bleomycin-injured lungs after 24 hours increased dramatically compared to controls. The bleomycin-treated animals also developed a greater number of metastases than did controls 14 days later.

Table 2. Effects of bleomycin and oxygen

	% Of Negative Control	
Lung injury/metastasis	Bleomycin	High Dose Oxygen
Total BAL protein	475 ± 200	1063 ± 250
^{125}I-albumin in BAL	130 ± 9	——
% cells in lungs at 24hrs	885 ± 270	3357 ± 379
Tumors at 14 days	307 ± 20	348 ± 6

Exposure to high concentrations of oxygen can also lead to vessel wall injury in pulmonary capillaries. Potential mediators of this injury are oxygen radicals, elastases or proteases, and metabolites of arachidonic acid (15). Periods of maximum injury are also associated with the adherence of neutrophils to damaged endothelium. C57BL/6 mice were exposed to an atmosphere of 90% oxygen for a period of 2-4 days (16). As with bleomycin-induced injury, tumor cell retention was significantly increased 24 hrs later, when radiolabelled fibrosarcoma cells were injected intravenously during periods of injury. After 2 weeks, more metastases were found in animals exposed to 90% oxygen.

Generation Of Free Radicals by Cancer Cells.

Walker 256 carcinosarcoma cells have been studied extensively as a experimental model for cancer metastasis in the rat. These cells are similar to leukocytes in that they carry specific receptors for the peptide, N-formyl-Met-Leu-Phe (17) and phorbol esters (18). Leukocytes and W256 cells respond to these ligands by chemotaxis, increased adhesiveness and cell swelling (17,19,20). In addition leukocytes respond by secreting proteolytic enzymes (21) and by generating oxygen-derived free radicals. Since the later response by leukocytes can cause endothelial cell injury (6,7), we postulated that W256 cells would similarily produce oxygen-derived free radicals upon fMLP addition and that this response could damage endothelial cell monolayers in vitro.

As an assay for free radical production by W256 cells we employed chemiluminescence amplified in the presence of luminol as well as the reduction of acetylated ferricytochrome c. (22). In both cases the response was linear with increasing fMLP concentrations. Low levels of background chemiluminescence were also observed in the absence of fMLP. The chemiluminescence response of W256 cells was inhibited by 50% upon the addition of either superoxide dismutase (1 mg/mL) or catalase (1000 units/mL). In addition, mannitol (5 mM), a known scavenger of hydroxyl radicals inhibited W256-promoted chemiluminescence by 66%. Under anerobic conditions, the chemiluminescence response of fMLP-activated W256 cells was greatly diminished. This inhibition was reversible when the cells were subsequently aerated (22).

The release of ^{3}H-2-deoxyglucose from cultured endothelial cell monolayers was used as an index of endothelial cell damage (23). When fMLP-activated W256 cells were incubated with prelabeled endothelial cell monolayers, there was a 27% increase in the specific release of isotope after a 90 minute incubation. A significant increase in ^{3}H-2-deoxyglucose was also observed in the absence of fMLP. Catalase (1000 units/ml) inhibited tumor cell induced release of isotope by 84% while superoxide dismutase at a concentration of 1 mg/ml, had no effect (23). Contact between the cancer cell and endothelial target was also required since the supernatant of activated tumor cells failed to promote the release of ^{3}H-2-deoxyglucose from endothelial cell monolayers. In addition, the preincubation of W256 cells with 1 uM cytochalasin B prior to their incubation with labelled endothelium resulted in an inhibition of isotope release. This was in contrast to the threefold increase in chemiluminescence observed when W256 cells were pretreated with cytochalasin B. Scanning electron micrographs of tumor cells adherent

Table 3. Effects of oxygen radical scavengers and inhibitors

Scavenger/Inhibitor	% Of Positive Control	
	Chemiluminescence	^{3}H-2-deoxyglucose Release
Catalase (1000 units/ml)	49 ± 8	17 ± 21
Superoxide Dismutase (1mg/ml)	50 ± 4	96 ± 12
Mannitol (5mM)	66 ± 4	—
Cytochalasin B, (1uM)	303 ± 13	55 ± 35

to washed endothelial cell monolayers demonstrated 60-80% fewer adherent W256 cells when the tumor cells were pretreated with cytochalasin B.

SUMMARY AND HYPOTHESIS

Using three different models of lung injury we have demonstrated that damage to the pulmonary endothelium significantly increases the localization and metastasis of intravenously injected tumor cells. In all of these models, injury to the endothelium involved the generation of oxygen-derived free radicals. We have also demonstrated that activated cancer cells can damage endothelial cells *in vitro* by the generation of oxygen-derived free radicals. In addition, preliminary experiments in our laboratory have indicated that activated cancer cells can damage basement membrane by a mechanism which involves both the secretion of a protease and the generation of oxygen-derived free radicals. Free radicals might activate a latent protease which is secreted by the cancer cell or alternatively inactivate a serum protease inhibitor. Both possibilities are currently being examined. We postulate that free radicals generated by host cells, cancer cells, or environmental agents may mediate microvascular injury and significantly promote cancer metastasis.

Supported by grants from the National Cancer Institute of Canada.

REFERENCES

1. Kramer, R.H., Gonzalez, R. and Nicolson, G.L. Inter. J. Cancer. 26: 639-645, 1980.
2. Crissman, J.D., Hatfield, J.S., Menter, D.G., Sloane, B. and Honn, K.V. Cancer Research. 48: 4065-4072, 1988.
3. Sloane, B.F., Dunn, J.R. and Honn, K.V. Science. 212: 1151-1153, 1981.
4. Nakajima, M., Welch, D.R., Belloni, P.N. and Nicolson G.L. Cancer Research, 47: 4869-4876, 1987.

5. Crissman, J.D., Hatfield, J., Schaldenbrand, M., Sloane, B.F. and Honn, K.V. Lab. Invest. 53, (No. 4): 470-478, 1985.
6. Andreoli, S.P., Mallett, C.P. and Bergstein J.M. J. Lab Clin. Med. 108 (No. 3): 190-198, 1986.
7. Andreoli, S.P., Baehner, R.L. and Bergstein, J.M. J. Lab Clin. Med. 106 (No. 3): 253-261, 1985.
8. Orr, F.W. and Warner, D.J.A. Invasion and Metastasis. 7: 183-196, 1987.
9. Orr, W.F. and Warner, D.J.A. Submitted for publication.
10. Hecht, S.M. Fed. Proc. 45: 2784-2791, 1986.
11. Kanofsky, J.R. J. Biol. Chem. 261: 13546-13550, 1986.
12. Adamson I.Y.R. and Bowden D.H. Amer J. Pathol, 77: 185-198, 1974.
13. Adamson, I., Orr, F.W. and Young, L. J.of Path. 150: 279-287, 1986.
14. Orr, F.W., Adamson, I. and Young, L. Cancer Res. 46: 891-897, 1986.
15. Davis, W.B., Rennard, S.J., Bitterman, P.B. and Crystal R. New Eng. J. Med. 309: 878-883, 1983.
16. Adamson, I., Young, L. and Orr, F.W. Lab. Invest. 57, (No. 3): 71-77, 1987.
17. Rayner, D.C., Orr, W.F. and Shiu, R.P.C. Cancer Research, 45: 2288-2293, 1985.
18. Clarke, P.R.H. and Varani, J. Cancer Research, 44: 4967-4971, 1984.
19. Varani, J. and Fantone, J.C. Cancer Research, 42: 190-197, 1982.
20. Wass, J.A., Varani, J. and Ward P.A. Cancer Letters, 9: 313-318, 1980.
21. Smith, R.J., Wierenga, W. and Iden S.S. Inflammation. 4 (No. 1): 73-88, 1980.
22. Leroyer, V., Werner, L., Shaughnessy, S., Goddard, G. and Orr, F.W. Cancer Research, 47: 4771-4775, 1987.
23. Shaughnessy, S.G., Buchanan, M.R., Turple, S., Richardson, M.and Orr, F.W. American J. of Path. 134 (No.4): 787-796, 1989.

RADIATION ENHANCED TUMOR CELL RECEPTOR EXPRESSION AND METASTASIS

J.M. ONODA and M.P. PIECHOCKI

Department of Radiation Oncology, Wayne State University, Detroit, MI 48202

INTRODUCTION

In previous studies we demonstrated a correlation between expression of the $\alpha_{IIb}\beta_3$ integrin receptor complex and metastatic potential (1,2). Increased expression of the $\alpha_{IIb}\beta_3$ receptor complex results in: 1) increased B16 (amelanotic melanoma) tumor cell adhesion to biological substrata (i.e., endothelial cell monolayers and individual components of the basal lamina such as fibronectin); 2) increased tumor cell induced platelet aggregation; and 3) increased expertimentally induced metastasis. In addition, we have identified a metabolite of the arachidonic acid cascade (i.e., 12-HETE) and an exogenous stimulator of arachidonic acid metabolism (i.e., TPA) which regulate the expression of the $\alpha_{IIb}\beta_3$ receptor (3). Our subsequent studies, using specific inhibitors of the lipoxygenase and cyclooxygenase pathways have revealed a network of biochemical events responsible for the expression of the $\alpha_{IIb}\beta_3$ complex and its causal role in regulating tumor cell adhesion, platelet aggregation and tumor cell arrest (4,5).

METHODS

Culture of B16 cells.

B16 melanoma cells were obtained from DCT Tumor Repository, Div. of Cancer Treatment, NCI, N.I.H. and cultured in Eagle's minimal essential medium (MEM) with 5% fetal calf serum. Cells were passaged every four days by harvesting with 0.25 mM Disodium ethylenediamine tetraacetate (EDTA) and subculturing at a ratio of 1:4. B16 cells (70% confluent) were exposed to 0, 25, 50 or 150 cGy of radiation [a Cesium source of radiation that delivered 100.4 cGy/minute or X-ray source (Picker unit, 280 Kev) that delivered 275 cGy/min.].

Radiation stimulates B16 cell adhesion (to fibronectin coated wells).

Three counts of constant unit area = 240 um^2 were made for each sample, 4-6 samples per radiation dose. For adhesion assays, semi-confluent monolayers of B16 cells were harvested, pelleted (4 min; 300 x g) and resuspended in MEM. Aliquots (1.0 ml) of the cell suspension were added to 2 ml vials. Immediately following irradiation, samples were incubated for 15 minutes at 37°C in humidified room air + 5% CO_2. Following incubation, 100 ul of the cell suspension (= 25,000 cells) was added to each well of a 96-well fibronectin coated (5 ug/well; 11) adhesion plate containing 100 ul MEM. Samples were incubated for 30 minutes at 37°C, rinsed and fixed with 4% formaldehyde. The adherent cells were visually counted on a Nikon diaphot inverted phase contrast microscope.

Identification of B16 cell $\alpha_{IIb}\beta_3$ receptors by immuno-fluorescence.

B16 cells were grown on glass coverslips until semi-confluent, exposed to 50 cGy and incubated for 15 min. at 37 ^{o}C. Following incubation, media was removed and samples fixed with 2% ice cold paraformaldehyde (10 min). Samples were washed (5X) with Phosphate Buffered Saline supplemented with 2mM $CaCl_2$ and 2mM $MgCl_2$ (PBS+Mg/Ca). After removing the last wash, 75 ul (50ug protein/ml) of the primary monoclonal antibody 10E5 (generously provided by Dr. Barry Coller, Stonybrook) was added to each cover slip. Monoclonal antibody 10E5 was originally raised against the human platelet GpIIb/IIIa complex (6). It's specificity for human $\alpha_{IIb}\beta_3$ and its cross reactivity with murine platelet $\alpha_{IIb}\beta_3$ and murine tumor cell $\alpha_{IIb}\beta_3$ were previously described (3,6). Following 30 min incubation (37°C, humidified room air + 5% CO_2), 1 ml of bovine serum albumin (BSA) (10 mg/ml in PBS+Mg/Ca + 1% Na Azide) was added to block non-specific binding of the secondary antibody and incubated for an additional 30 min. Primary antibody and BSA were removed and samples rinsed (3X, PBS) before addition of the secondary antibody (fluorescein isothiocyanate conjugated IgG Fraction Goat anti mouse, Cappel, West Chester, PA) (75 ul/cover slip, incubated for 30 min., 37°C, 5% CO_2). After labeling, samples were rinsed (5X, PBS+Mg/Ca) and mounted in glycerol. Fluorescence micrographs were taken with a Leitz Orthoplan Microscope using Kodak T-MAX 400 Panchromatic film.

B16 cell 12-HETE biosynthesis.

B16 cells were grown to 95% confluency in T-150 flasks and harvested using 2mM EDTA and 0.5% trypsin. Cells were washed and concentrated at 3 x 10^6 cells/ml in platelet wash (phenol red-free MEM). One ml samples of cell suspension were placed in 13 ml prosil-coated borosilicate tubes, irradiated with 250 cGy and incubated for various time points (5, 15 and 30 min-data not shown) at 37°C. Following incubation, proteins were precipitated by the addition of ice-cold acetone and centrifugation (2000 x g, 5 min., 4°C). Supernatants were evaporated under nitrogen, rehydrated in .001 N HCl and lipids extracted by octadecyl (C18) reverse phase chromatography (7). The amount of 12-HETE/sample was determined by radioimmunoassay following the manufacture's protocol (Advanced Magnetics Inc., Cambridge, MA). The experiment was repeated four times with comparable results.

Adhesion of B16 cells pretreated with NDGA.

B16 cells were treated with 50uM of the lipoxygenase inhibitor, NDGA (Nordihydroguatrietic acid) or solvent (polyethylene glycol) for 15 min. (37°C) prior to irradiation. The protocol (described above) for the adhesion assay was used.

Experimental metastasis of irradiated B16 cells.

Cells were exposed to 0, 25, 50 or 150 cGy of radiation. Following incubation (15 min., 37°C, 5% CO_2) 5.5 x 10^4 cells were injected into the lateral tail vein of unanesthetized C57BL/6J male mice, Jackson Laboratories, Bar Harbor, ME (8-9 wk old). [Note: Animal care was in accordance with institutional guidelines]. In all experiments, mice were randomly chosen from stock cages for each treatment group. All groups were injected within 20 - 30 min. post cell preparation. Mice from each group were injected in rotation so that the mean interval between irradiation and injection for each experimental group was approximately the same (i.e., 15 - 25 min. post-irradiation). All animals were maintained for 25 days after which time they were anesthetized with sodium pentobarbital (40-90 mg/kg, i.p.) and sacrificed by cervical dislocation. Lungs were removed, fixed and visible tumor colonies enumerated as previously described (8).

Statistics.

Normally distributed data were analyzed by ANOVA one-way analysis of variance using the WYSE system. Groups found to have significant F values were further analyzed by the Mann-Whitney-U Test and groups with $p<0.05$ were considered significantly different.

RESULTS

In the studies presented here, we examined low dose radiation effects on tumor metastatic potential from three perspectives. First, we found that low dose radiation (50 cGy) enhanced surface expression of $\alpha_{IIb}\beta_3$ receptors. These observations were obtained using flow cytometric analysis and fluorescence microscopy. Second, we determined radiation effects on tumor cell metastatic phenotype as quantitated by changes in tumor cell behavior favorable for metastasis - i.e., we determined that radiation stimulates expression of the $\alpha_{IIb}\beta_3$ receptor complex, thus promoting tumor cell adhesion to fibronectin in vitro and the formation of experimental metastasis in vivo. Third, we determined that low dose radiation stimulates tumor cell 12-HETE synthesis and that the LOX inhibitor, NDGA, inhibits this phenomenon.

Influence of low level radiation on tumor cell proliferation-implications for the retention of mitotic competence.

We examined the effects of various doses of radiation (i.e., 50, 100, 250 and 800 cGy) on B16 tumor cell viability using trypan blue exclusion. We determined that these levels had no significant effect on short term viability (data not shown) in that all groups of cell, even those exposed to 800 cGy gamma radiation, excluded dye if the cells were tested within 4-8 hrs post irradiation. However, when we assessed radiation effects on the mitotic competence of exposed B16 cells, we found that exposure to doses of 250 cGy (or greater) resulted in significant inhibition of tumor cell proliferation in vitro. Irradiated (50 cGy gamma radiation) of semi-confluent cultures of B16 cells (in log phase growth) had no antiproliferative effects (data not presented). Therefore, we used 50 cGy as our primary radiation dose in the studies presented below, in that we were assured that radiation induced tumor cell effects obtained would not be a result of lack of mitotic competance of irradiated cells.

Radiation effects on B16 cell adhesion.

We exposed tumor cells to non-lethal/sub-lethal gamma radiation (50 - 250 cGy). We found that all levels of radiation tested stimulated tumor cell adhesion to fibronectin; 50 cGy resulted in the highest level (i.e., percent of added cells adhering/well) of tumor cell adhesion (Figure 1). We enumerated a three-fold increase in B16 cell adhesion compared to the sham irradiated control cell adhesion. In gen-

Figure 1. Adhesion of B16 cells to fibronectin coated wells. Exposure to 0, 50, 100 or 250 cGy, in a dose-dependent fashion, significantly ($p < 0.001$) enhanced B16 cell adhesion. The difference between the 50 and 100 cGy groups was not significant. There was a significant ($p < 0.01$) difference between the 50 and 250 cGy groups. Bars represent the percent increase of adhering cells compared to sham-irradiated control cells. Bar height = mean + SEM. Inserts indicate Median: range. Triplicate counts of constant unit area = 240 um^2 were made for each sample, 4-6 samples per condition.

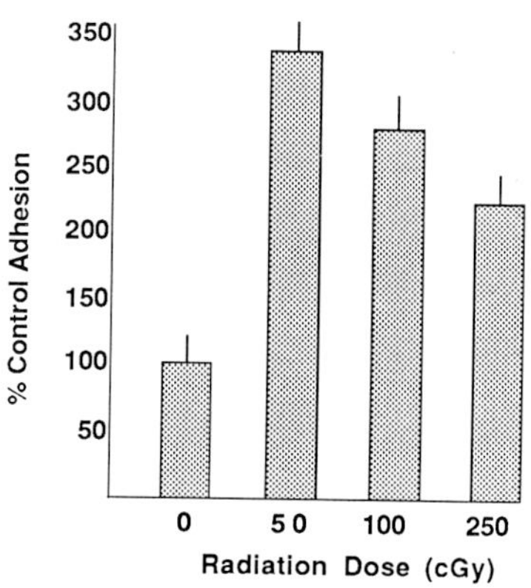

eral, the irradiated cells demonstrated an enhanced ability to adhere to fibronectin (relative to the control). However, increases in exposure above 50 cGy resulted in a gradual dose-dependent decrease in tumor cell adhesion (Figure 1), which was only marginally ($p < 0.2$) significant at 250 cGy.

Calcium dependent mechanism of radiation induced tumor cell adhesion to fibronectin - implications for the integrity of the $\alpha_{IIb}\beta_3$ integrin receptor complex.

The integrity of the IIb/IIIa integrin receptor complex and the adhesion of tumor cells to substrate is dependent on the presence of exogenous calcium (9). In order to determine the role of calcium in the radiation-induced adhesion of tumor cells, we exposed B16 cells in calcium-free or calcium supplemented media (2mM CaCl) to 50 cGy radiation (data not shown). In the absence of calcium, tumor cells exposed to 50 cGy demonstrated a 175% increase in adhesion (relative to the calcium free, sham-irradiated control), whereas tumor cells radiated in the presence of 2mM Ca++ demonstrated a 400% increase in the number of cells adherent to fibronectin (relative to the calcium supplemented sham-irradiated control). This data demonstrates the vital role of calcium in mediating the process responsible for the radiation-induced increase in tumor cell adhesion to fibronectin and are consistent with the calcium requirement for maintenance of the $\alpha_{IIb}\beta_3$ complex.

Evidence for radiation enhanced $\alpha_{IIb}\beta_3$ integrin receptor expression.

We first used flow cytometry to analyze B16 cells stained for the $\alpha_{IIb}\beta_3$ receptor using a double antibody labeling system. Data was analyzed under two key parameters: 1) an increase in the mean fluorescent intensity of populations of cells (i.e., irradiated and sham-irradiated) and 2) an increase in the percent of cells in the population that were fluorescent. These parameters are interpreted as a general increase in the number of receptor sites and an increase in the number of individuals cells with receptors on their surface, respectively. We demonstrate that 50 cGy causes a significant increase in the mean fluorescent intensity of irradiated cells compared to sham-irradiated control cells and 95% of the tumor cells exposed to 50 cGy fluoresce positively with the $\alpha_{IIb}\beta_3$ antibody label as opposed to the 22% of control cells (data not shown). Photomicrographs taken of antibody labeled cells qualitatively demonstrate a similar staining pattern. Control cells exhibit a low level of flourescence (Figure 2a) while tumor cells exposed to 50 cGy of radiation exhibit a high level of fluorescence indicative of $\alpha_{IIb}\beta_3$ receptor expression (Figure 2b). These data indicate that 50 cGy increases the number of $\alpha_{IIb}\beta_3$ receptor sites expressed on the surface of individual B16 cells and also has the ability to increase the number of cells in the population that are expressing the $\alpha_{IIb}\beta_3$ receptor to encompass 95% of the entire population. Analysis of the cells treated with 50 cGy demonstrated the occurrence of two distinct subpopulations of tumor cells that were fluorescent (data not shown). Although both subpopulations of cells were positively expressing $\alpha_{IIb}\beta_3$, the amount of fluorescence (mean fluorescent intensity) expressed by these subpopulations was different - one population is characterized by the expression of more surface receptor sites.

LOX inhibition studies.

Pretreatment of tumor cells with NDGA, a lipoxygenase inhibitor (10,11) prior to the administration of 50 cGy results in a significant inhibition of radiation-induced adhesion to fibronectin (Figure 3). Cells exposed to 50 cGy alone were the positive control and demonstrated a 250% increase in adhesion over the sham-irradiated control cells. Treatment of cells with 50 uM NDGA before radiation caused a significant decrease in the number of adhering cells compared to the untreated controls. NDGA itself, was not responsible for the inhibited adhesion; we found no significant differences between adhesion of the sham-irradiated cells and the sham-irradiated cells treated with NDGA. Although the inhibition was only incomplete, this could have been due to the fact that NDGA was not present during the actual incubation period after irradiation. These data demonstrate that inhibition of 12-HETE synthesis prior to radiation exposure significantly inhibits the radiation-induced increase of tumor cell adhesion and suggest that radiation enhanced tumor cell adhesion is dependent on a lipoxygenase pathway metabolite (i.e. 12-HETE).

12-HETE studies.

B16 tumor cells were examined for enhanced 12-HETE biosynthesis following stimulation with 50 or 800 cGy gamma radiation. Following a 15 minute post-irradiation incubation period, the samples were terminated and assayed for 12-HETE by radioimmunoassay. Radiation significantly enhanced the biosynthesis of 12-HETE (Figure 4). Although the level of 12-HETE was significantly higher in the sample exposed to 800 cGy as opposed to the sample exposed to 50 cGy, 800 cGy is lethal to B16 tumor cells. Thus, it is important to distinguish between levels of radiation which enhance 12-HETE biosynthesis sufficient to stimulate $\alpha_{IIb}\beta_3$ receptor expression and tumor cell adhesion and levels which may induce those rapid and short-term responses, but are lethal to the cell - i.e., the cells exposed to 800 cGy are not a potential source of metastatic disease.

Radiation stimulates metastasis.

We exposed B16 cell suspensions to 50-150 cGy gamma radiation. We used a tumor cell concentration and time course for injection which we previously determined would result in assurance of formation of experimental metastasis in 100% of host animals. We observed that radiation of B16 cells

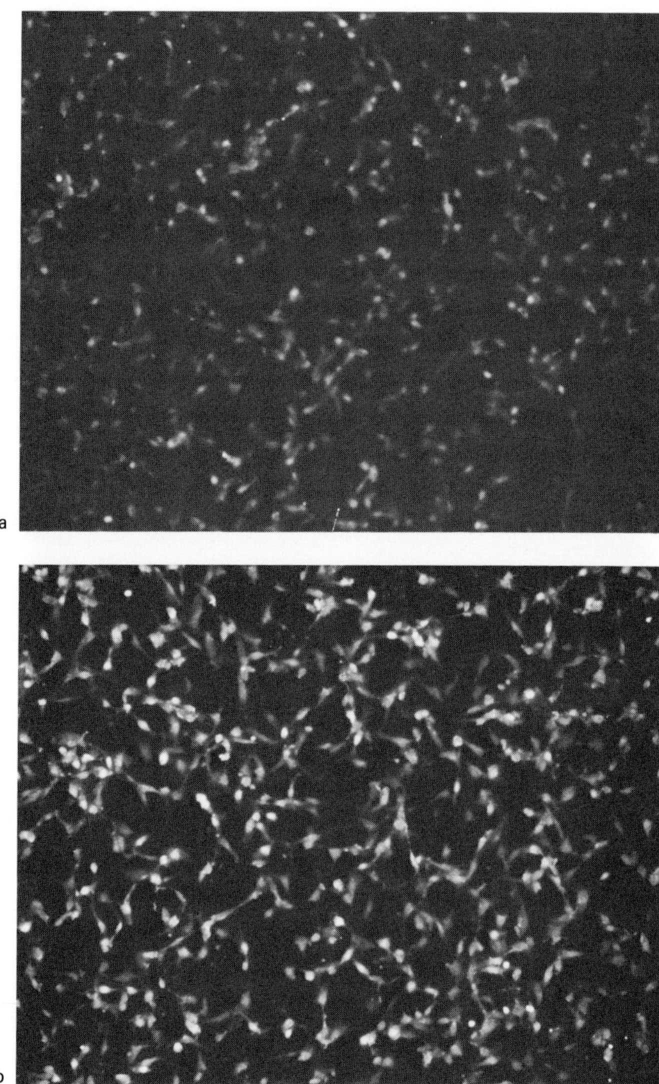

Figure 2 (a + b). Radiation stimulates B16 cell $\alpha_{IIb}\beta_3$ receptor expression. Fluorescent micrographs demonstrate that few cells (< 10%) in the control (sham-irradiated) population expressed IIb/IIIa receptors and exhibit a relatively low level of fluorescence, whereas the > 95% of the irradiated cells expressed IIb/IIIa receptors and a high level of fluorescent intensity. Tumor cells grown on coverslips, stained with monoclonal antibody to IIb/IIIa and labeled with fluorescein conjugated secondary antibody. Photos were taken under (100X) magnification.

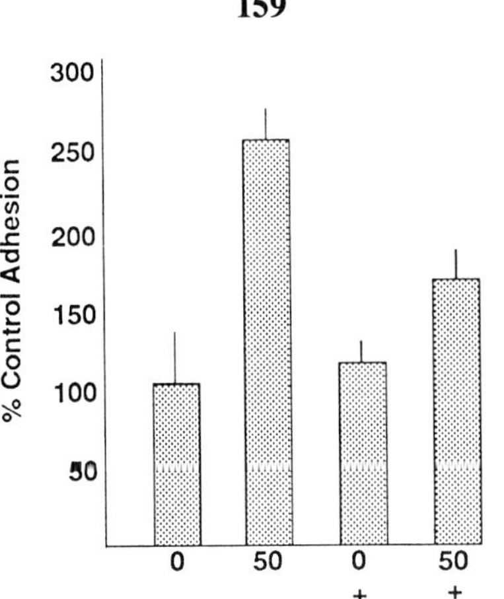

Figure 3. Adhesion of cultured B16a cells to fibronectin coated wells after exposure to 50 cGy in the presence or absence of 50uM NDGA. Pretreatment with NDGA significantly ($p < 0.01$) inhibited radiation enhanced tumor cell adhesion without effecting basal (i.e., un-stimulated) B16 cell adhesion. Experimental protocol similar to that described in Figure1.

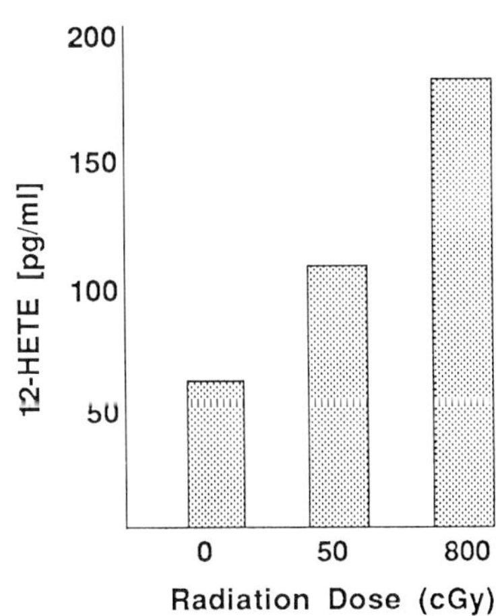

Figure 4. Radiation stimulates B16 cell 12-HETE biosynthesis. Exposure of B16 cells to 50 or 800 cGy resulted in significantly ($p < 0.001$) elevated 12-HETE levels in irradiated cells. Data is reported as pg 12-HETE/ml. Studies were run in triplicate.

(prior to their intravenous injection into syngeneic C57BL/6J host mice) significantly enhanced experimental metastasis. The data presented in Figure 5 is representative of those studies. In all groups of mice injected with irradiated B16 cells, we enumerated a significant increase (> 300% of control) in the number of pulmonary tumor colonies formed by the injected cells (compared to sham-irradiated controls). The group irradiated with 50 cGy had the highest mean number of pulmonary tumor colonies.

Figure 5. Radiation enhances experimental metastasis. B16 cells were exposed to 50 cGy, incubated for 15 min. at 37°C, and then injected intravenously via lateral tail vein (55,000 in 0.1 ml/mouse) into syngeneic C57BL/6J mice. All groups were terminated 25 days post tumor cell injection. Lungs were removed and preserved in Bouin's fixative for 24 hours prior to enumeration of macroscopic lung colonies. There was a significant ($p< 0.01$) increase in the number of pulmonary tumor colonies in the group injected with irradiated cells. Mean for the control group was 12.4 + 2.1 metastases. Bars represent median + SEM for each group, n=10.

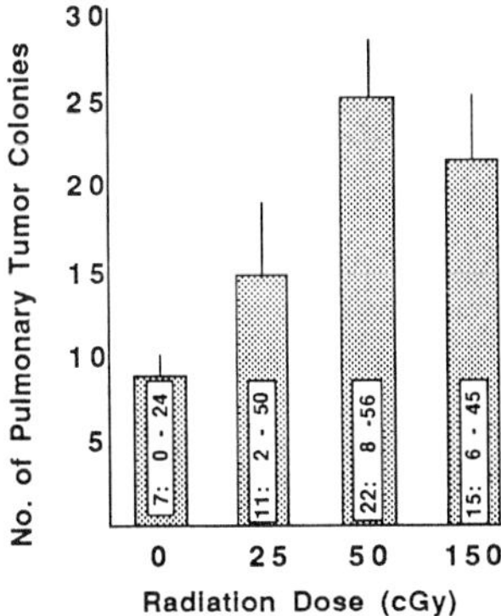

DISCUSSION

Studies assessing the effects of radiation on tumors or the host microvasculature ("tumor bed effect") have generally used high dose radiation (20-60 Gy; 12,13) and typically examined the lethal effects of radiation or the effects of irradiation at 48 hrs to > 200 days post treatment (14). Our preliminary studies indicate that enhanced expression of the IIb/IIIa integrin receptor complex on the surface of tumor cells can be observed within 15 minutes post irradiation (50 cGy), demonstrating a level of tumor cell response to irradiation which has not been critically examined. We believe that our studies provide important insight into the basic metabolism of tumor cells and open a new area of radiobiology, especially those factors which mediate the causal relationship between radiation and tumor metastatic potential. Recent reports (15-17) have demonstrated that conventional cytotoxic chemotherapy may have paradoxical effects - i.e., chemotherapy may damage the vascular endothelium resulting in enhanced metastatic disease. Our findings suggest that radiation therapy may also have paradoxical effects - i.e., radiotherapy may enhance the metastatic potential of surviving tumor cells.

REFERENCES

1. Grossi, I.M., Hatfield, J.S., Fitzgerald, L.H., Newcombe, M., Taylor, J.D., and Honn, K.V. FASEB J. 2:2385-2395, 1988.
2. Honn, K.V., Grossi, I.M., Chopra, H., Steinert, B.W., Onoda, J.M., Nelson, K.K., and Taylor, J.D. In: Advances in Prostaglandin, Thromboxane, and Leukotriene Research. B. Samuelsson, P.Y.-K. Wong, and F.F. Sun, eds., pp.439-443, 1989.
3. Grossi, I.M., Fitzgerald, L.A., Umbarger, L.A., Nelson, K.K., Diglio, C.L., Taylor, J.D. and Honn, K.V. Cancer Res., 49:1029-1037, 1989.
4. Chopra, H., Hatfield, J.S., Chang, Y.S., Grossi, I.M., Fitzgerald, L.A., O'Gara, C.Y., Marnett, L.J., Diglio, C.A., Taylor, J.D., and Honn, K.V. Cancer Res., 48: 3787-3800, 1988.
5. Honn, K.V., Grossi, I.M., Chopra, H., Steinert, B.W., Onoda, J.M., Nelson, K.K., and Taylor, J.D. In: Eicosanoids, Lipid Peroxidation and Cancer. Nigam, S., McBrien, D.L.H. and Slater, T.G., (eds.). Springer Verlag, Berlin, pp. 29-41, 1988.
6. Coller, B.S., Peerschke, E.I., Scudder, L.E., and Sullivan, C.A. J. Clin. Invest., 72: 325-338, 1983.
7. Menter, D.G., Steinert, B.W., Sloane, B.F., Taylor, J.D., and Honn, K.V. Cancer Res. 47: 2425-2432, 1987.
8. Onoda, J.M., Nelson, K.K., Grossi, I.M., Umbarger, L.A., Taylor, J.D., and Honn, K.V. Proc. Soc. Exp. Biol. Med., 187: 250-255, 1988.
9. Plow, E.F., Ginsberg, M.H. and Maruerie, G.A. In: Phillips, D.R. and Shuman, A. (eds.), Biochemistry of Platelets, pp. 160-225. Orlando, Fl: Academic Press, Inc., 1986.
10. Wess, J.A. and Archer, D.J. Int. J. Immunopharmac., 6: 1, 27-34, 1984.
11. Salari, H. Braquet, P. and Borgeat, P. Prostaglandins Leukotrienes and Medicine 13: 53-60, 1984.
12. Milas, L., Hisao, I., Hunter, N., Jones, S., and Peters, L.J. Cancer Research, 46:723-727, 1986.
13. Camplejohn, R.S. and Penhaligon, M. British J. of Radiology, 58, 443-451, 1985.
14. Milas, L., Hunter, N. and Peters, L.J. J. Radiation Oncology Biol. Phys., 13: 379-383, 1987.
15. McMillan, T.J. and Hart, I.R. Cancer Metastasis Rev., 6: 503-520, 1987.
16. Geldof, A.A., and Rao, B.R. Anticancer Research, 8: 1335-1340, 1988.
17. Poupon, M-F., Pauwels, C., Jasmin C., Antoine, E., Lascaux, V., and Rosa, B. Cancer Treatment Reports, 68: 749-758, 1984.

LEUKOTRIENE PRODUCTION BY GAMMA IRRADIATED MACROPHAGE CELLS

E. W. HUPP[1], A. HAJIBEIGI[1], and J. E. HARDCASTLE[2]

Department of Biology[1] and Department of Chemistry[2], Texas Woman's University, Denton, Texas 76204

INTRODUCTION

Irradiation of tissues and cells can liberate arachidonic acid from the phospholipids, which can then be metabolized to prostaglandins (1,2). Also, whole body gamma irradiation of animals causes significant increases in the levels of the prostaglandins and other cyclooxygenase metabolites (3,4). The release of arachidonic acid may be caused by radiation induced activation of phospholipase A_2 (2,5). Subsequent metabolism of arachidonic acid may be initiated by a radiation induced free radical mechanism and lipid peroxidation (2,5).

In parenchymal lung tissue from guinea pigs that had received whole body doses of Co-60 gamma radiation the concentrations of PGE, $PGF_{2\alpha}$ and TxB_2 increased with increase in radiation dose (3). Total body gamma irradiation of rhesus monkeys caused increased levels of PGE_2 and PGI_2 in the gastric juice (4). In both of these studies cited the increase in cyclooxygenase metabolite levels occurred in the first 2-3 hours after irradiation, and then the levels returned to normal by the second day (3,4).

X-irradiation of white pig skin causes a rapid release of arachidonic acid, followed by its metabolism into PGE_2 (2). The biosynthesis of PGE_2 increased with increase in radiation dose up to 1000 Rads, but at doses higher than 1000 Rads PGE_2 synthesis decreased. Co-60 gamma irradiation of pulmonary endothelial cells caused dose dependent arachidonic acid release and PGI_2 biosynthesis by these cells (5). The increased PGI_2 synthesis may be due to radiation induced stimulation of the cyclooxygenase activity.

Resident peritoneal cells obtained from Co-60 gamma irradiated mice synthesized larger amount of PGE_2 and LTC_4 than did unstimulated (resting) cells (6). It was suggested that arachidonic acid release, and the cyclooxygenase and lipoxygenase activities were increased by the radiation treatment.

Though there have been a number of reports concerning radiation induced stimulation of cyclooxygenase activity, we found only one report (Steel et al, 1988) of the effect of radiation on lipoxygenase activity. This report concerns studies we have been conducting for the past 3 years on lipoxygenase metabolism in gamma irradiated macrophage cell cultures.

MATERIALS AND METHODS

Macrophage cells were obtained from the peritoneal cavity of rats and were cultured in plastic flasks containing 3ml of Delbecco's modified eagle medium (DMEM, GIBCO, Grand Island, NY) supplemented with 10% fetal bovine serum (FBS, GIBCO). The cultures, each flask containing 6 X 10^6 cells, were incubated under 5% CO_2 and 95% moisturized air at 37°C. After 24 hours, nonadherent cells were removed and fresh DMEM-FBS containing 0.5 μCi/ml ^{14}C-arachidonic acid (58 μCi/mmole, Research Products International Corp., Mount Prospect, IL) was added to each culture. The cultures were incubated an additional 12 hours to complete the labelling process, then the excess radioactivity was washed away, and fresh DMEM-FBS was added to the cell cultures.

Individual ^{14}C-arachidonic acid labeled cultures were irradiated with single doses of 2 Gy, 4 Gy, 8 Gy, 16 Gy, and 32 Gy using a U.S. Nuclear Corporation GR-9 Cobalt-60 gamma irradiator. The calcium ionophore A23187 (Sigma Chemical Co., St. Louis, MO) was added to other cultures to give an ionophore concentration of 10^{-5}M per culture. These treated cultures, along with untreated control cultures, were incubated for one hour before the arachidonic acid metabolites were extracted. Cell viability in all cultures was determined by the Trypan Blue staining technique.

An alcohol-ether technique was used to extract the leukotrienes from the cell cultures. The medium was removed from the culture flask and mixed with 2-propanol and formic acid in the ratio of 1.0:0.5:0.03, respectively. After 5 minutes of mixing, the solution was transferred into a separatory funnel and 1.5 volumes of diethylether were added. The mixture was swirled for 5 minutes, and two liquid phases formed. The upper organic layer was removed and the lower aqueous phase was extracted again with ether. The ether fractions were combined, and evaporated to dryness under a stream of nitrogen. The residue was dissolved in 200 μl of methanol. All glassware used in the extraction procedure was siliconized.

High performance liquid chromatography (HPLC) and radiochemical assay were used to separate, detect and quantify the arachidonic acid metabolites produced by the macrophage cells. A Waters Associates (Milford, MA) Model 6000A pumping system with a U6K injector was used with a Partisil 5 ODS-3 (Whatman Chemical Separation Inc., Clifton, NJ) C-18 (4.6 X 250 mm) reverse phase column. The mobile phase solvent was acetonitrile:water:acetic acid (75:25:0.02, V/V/V) adjusted to pH 4.5. The mobile phase flow rate was 1 ml/min. The radioactive compounds in the HPLC eluent were detected using an in-line Radioactive Flow Detector Model CT (Radiomatic Instrument and Chemical Co. Inc., Tampa, FL).

RESULTS AND DISCUSSION

Gamma radiation did not affect cell viability significantly based on the results of Trypan Blue staining. The cells absorbed about 60% of the administered ^{14}C-arachidonic acid and after treatment released about 50% of the absorbed radioactivity. Five significant peaks were observed in the radiochromatogram from the HPLC analysis (Table 1). The most abundant ^{14}C-material was determined to be unmetabolized arachidonic acid. Another ^{14}C-substance present in large amounts has not been identified, but is thought to be a 1,2-diacylglycerol (DAG, peak 5, Table 1).

The major lipoxygenase product detected in gamma irradiated macrophage cells was leukotriene

C_4 (LTC_4). This identification was made by coelution with standard ^3H-LTC_4 and mass spectrometry. There appeared to be a general increase in LTC_4 synthesis with increase in radiation dose, though this was not significant at the 0.05 level of confidence. However, the LTC_4 production by gamma irradiated cells was significantly higher than that produced by control cells. The Ca-ionophore treated cells produced about twice as much LTC_4 as did the irradiated cells. Two other lipoxygenase metabolites were produced by the irradiated cell cultures. Though these two compounds have not been positively identified, peak 2 (Table I) coeluted with leukotriene B_4 (LTB_4) isomers, and peak 3 (Table I) coeluted with hydroxyeicosatetraenoic acid (HETE) isomers.

Table 1
Amounts of Arachidonic Acid Metabolites Produced from Irradiated, Ca-ionophore Stimulated and Unstimulated Macrophage Cultures.

Treatment	Peak 1 Mean SEM pmole (LTC_4)	Peak 2 Mean SEM pmole	Peak 3 Mean SEM pmole	Peak 4 Mean SEM pmole (AA)	Peak 5 Mean SEM
Control (5,6)*	8.33± 2.40^b	--	22.04± 11.2^d	157.92± 66.5^d	68.8± 33.5^b
2 Gy (2,2)*	16.9± 4.65^a	--	24.1± 18.4^d	433.2± 100.92^d	238.5± 169.6^a
4 Gy (3,3)*	14.2± 4.29^a	--	22.1± 1.60^d	267.0+ 58.1^d	155.0± 24.3^a
8 Gy (4,6)*	35.9± 6.56^a	16.1± 2.02^d	--	390.7± 75.2^d	126.2± 7.16^a
16 Gy (5,6)*	22.6± 4.16^a	13.0± 4.75^d	48.8± 0.23^d	231.7± 43.0^d	120.3± 21.9^a
32 Gy (5,7)*	48.6± 11.4^a	24.7± 23.6^d	34.1± 5.82^d	334.3± 64.2d	97.9± 11.6^a
Ca-ionophore (5,6)*	86.6± 14.2^c	25.9± 8.13^d	--	377.1± 53.9^d	40.3± 9.43^b

a = significantly different from b in the same column at the 0.05 level.

c = significantly different from a and b in the same column at 0.05 level.

d = not significantly different from each other in the same column.

* = first number in the parentheses indicates total experiments per treatment, and second numberis equal to the number of HPLC runs.

The total lipoxygenase metabolite level increased from about 6% of the total radioactivity in the 2 Gy extracts to about 20% in the 32 Gy extracts. Also, the LTC_4 increased from about 2% of the total radioactivity in the 2 Gy samples to about 9% in the 32 Gy samples. This data suggests radiation induced stimulation of lipoxygenase activity in general, and more specifically stimulation of the activity of LTC_4 synthetase (glutathione-S-transferase).

The amount of the post arachidonic acid compound (peak 5, Table 1), suspected to be DAG, decreased with increase in radiation dose to the cells. This data suggests that diacylglycerol lipase activity was stimulated by the gamma radiation.

Because macrophage cells suffer little damage by gamma radiation, they are good systems to study the effect of gamma radiation on arachidonic acid metabolism and associated inflammatory processes.

LITERATURE CITED

1. Allen, J. B., Sagerman, R. H., Stuart, M. J. Lancet 2:1193-1196, 1981.
2. Ziboh, V. A., Mallia, C., Morhart, E., Taylor, J. R. Proc. Soc. Exp. Biol. Med. 169:386-391, 1982.
3. Steel, L. K., Catravas, G. N. Int. J. Radiat. Biol. 42:517-520, 1982.
4. Dubois, A., Dorval, E. D., Steel, L., Fiala, N. P., Conklin, J. J. Radiation Research, 110:289-293, 1987.
5. Friedman, M., Saunders, D. S., Madden, M. C., Chaney, E. L., Kwock, L. Radiation Research 106:171-181, 1986.
6. Steel, L. K., Hughes, H. N., Walden, T. L., Jr. Int. J. Radiat. Biol. 53: 943-964, 1988.

LIPID PEROXIDATION IN LATE RADIATION INJURY OF THE RAT SPINAL CORD

K.J. LEVIN, M.D., P.H. GUTIN, M.D., M.W. MCDERMOTT, M.D., G.Y. ROSS, B.A., N. HOOPER, PH.D., M.T. SMITH, PH.D., J. R. CASHMAN, PH.D., P.M. CHAN, PH.D., R.L. DAVIS, M.D. and T.L. PHILLIPS, M.D.

Departments of Radiation Oncology, Neurological Surgery, Pharmaceutical Chemistry, Neurology, and Pathology, University of California, San Francisco, and School of Public Health, University of California, Berkeley

INTRODUCTION

Radiation therapy is a highly effective treatment for malignant gliomas and there is good evidence that increasing radiation dose results in increased survival (1,2). However, damage to the surrounding normal tissue limits the total dose of radiation which can be delivered (3). Because CNS tumors rarely metastasize, local control in these devastating conditions can translate into cure. It was thought that interstitial brachytherapy might alleviate the problem of therapeutic ratio, yet it has become quite clear that radiation necrosis is the limiting factor for this technique as well (4).

Progressive demyelination and white matter necrosis (WMN) are the sentinel histopathologic abnormalities seen in late radiation injury of the central nervous system (CNS), often occurring at sites remote from the focal high dose region (5,6). Theories as to the pathogenesis of CNS radiation injury have focused on damage to the oligodendroglial support cells and damage to the vasculature in the white matter (7,8). It has also been proposed that edema formation resulting from radiation induced changes in CNS vascular permeability may play an etiologic role (9,10). Less attention has been directed to the biochemical events which may be involved in the syndrome of late delayed radiation injury.

Given the striking propensity of injury for the white matter (5,8), the experimental evidence that radiation produces oxygen derived free radicals which initiate peroxidation reactions in fatty acids (11), and the relatively long latent period associated with CNS radiation injury, the hypothesis that lipid peroxidation chain reactions in the lipid rich myelin of the CNS white matter is responsible for the development of the progressive demyelination and WMN seen in delayed radiation injury was explored via assays for indices of lipid peroxidation. Further, the role of lipid soluble antioxidants as CNS radioprotectors was evaluated.

MATERIALS AND METHODS

Animal Model.

A standardized model of CNS radiation injury was developed with paralysis as the end point. Female F344 rats of 70-80 days were irradiated to the cervical-thoracic spinal cord (C_2-T_1) in single doses of 15-25 Gy, using 250 kVp x-rays at a dose rate of 4.24 Gy/minute. A dorsal port of 5x15 mm was placed to coincide with C_2-T_1, and treatment was done under nembutal anesthesia, 30 mg/kg, intraperitoneally (ip). Dose response curves were constructed by probit analysis and the latent period and ED50 for WMN was determined in 195 rats after 7 months of observation.

Histopathologic analysis of the irradiated segment of spinal cords from paralyzed animals was performed and demyelination and necrosis randomly distributed throughout, but mainly restricted to the white matter, was documented.

Assays for Lipid Peroxidation.

In order to test the hypothesis that lipid peroxidation is responsible for the white matter damage, assays were performed to look for the accumulation of byproducts of the peroxidation pathway, hydroxyeicosatetraenoic acids (HETEs) and malondialdehyde (MDA). Phospholipids and free fatty acids were extracted from spinal cord tissue and assayed for HETEs by reverse phase high performance liquid chromatograhpy (RPHPLC). Assays for MDA, the aldehyde breakdown product of lipid hydroperoxides, were performed via the standard TBA assay described by Smith et al. (12). Assays were also performed for the consumption of endogenous antioxidants in irradiated rat spinal cords. Vitamin C and vitamin E levels were determined via high performance liquid chromatography (HPLC) with electrochemical detection as described by Kutnick (13) and Lang (14), respectively.

Radioprotection by Antioxidants.

To further investigate the role of lipid peroxidation in CNS radiation injury, rats were placed on diets supplemented with vitamin E (diet A--1,000 mg vitamin E/kg chow) deficient in vitamin E (diet C--7.5 mg vitamin E/kg chow) and on a normal diet (diet B--50 mg vitamin E/kg chow) for 16 weeks and statistically significant differences in spinal cord vitamin E levels were documented (717 ± 35, 501 ± 19 and 197 ± 57) as seen in Figure. 1. The rats were then irradiated and the dose response curve and ED_{50} were determined.

The 21-aminosteroid U74006F, a potent and effective inhibitor of CNS tissue lipid peroxidation (15), was also tested in this context. Rats received the drug 10 mg/kg ip 30 minutes before and 2 and 24 hours after irradiation and, once again, dose response curves were constructed and the ED50 was compared with control animals.

RESULTS

Animal Model.

As seen in Figure 2, the latent period between irradiation and paralysis was found to vary indirectly with dose. That is, the higher the dose, the shorter the time to paralysis. The ED_{50} in the untreated animals was 19.6 Gy (Figure 3, 95% confidence interval 19.3-19.9 Gy). A sharp dose response curve was obtained with 0-100% paralysis noted over a dose interval of less than 3.5 Gy.

Assays.

Biochemical assays for MDA and HETEs done at intervals ranging from I hour to 148 days post irradiation at doses ranging from 10-30 Gy revealed no significant differences from control (unirradiated)

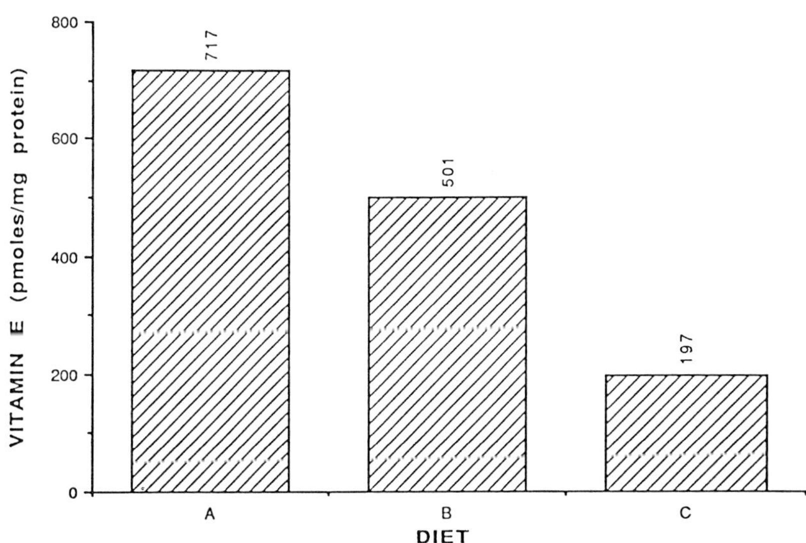

Figure 1. Spinal cord vitamin E levels from rats on supplemented (A), normal (B) and deficient (C) vitamin E diets after 16 weeks.

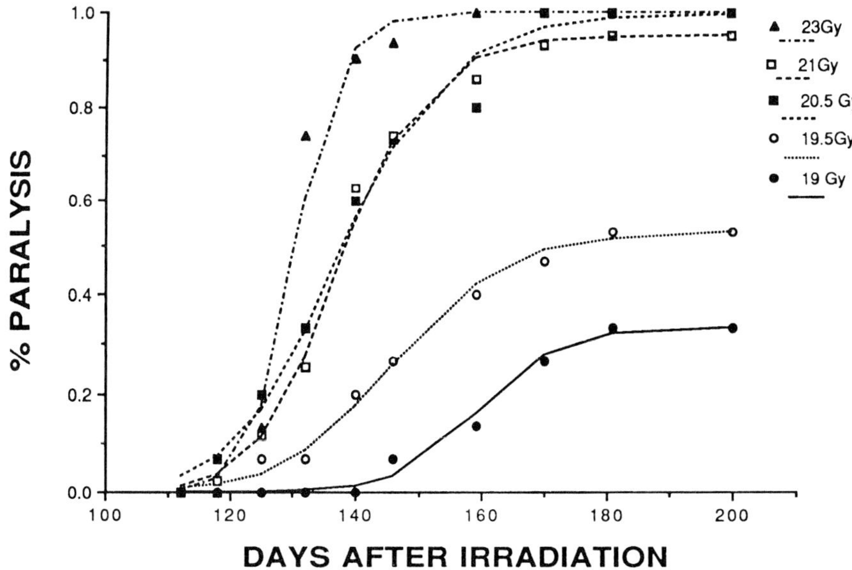

Figure 2. Time to development of paralysis after single fraction irradiation of the rat cervical-thoracic spinal cord (C_2 -T_1).

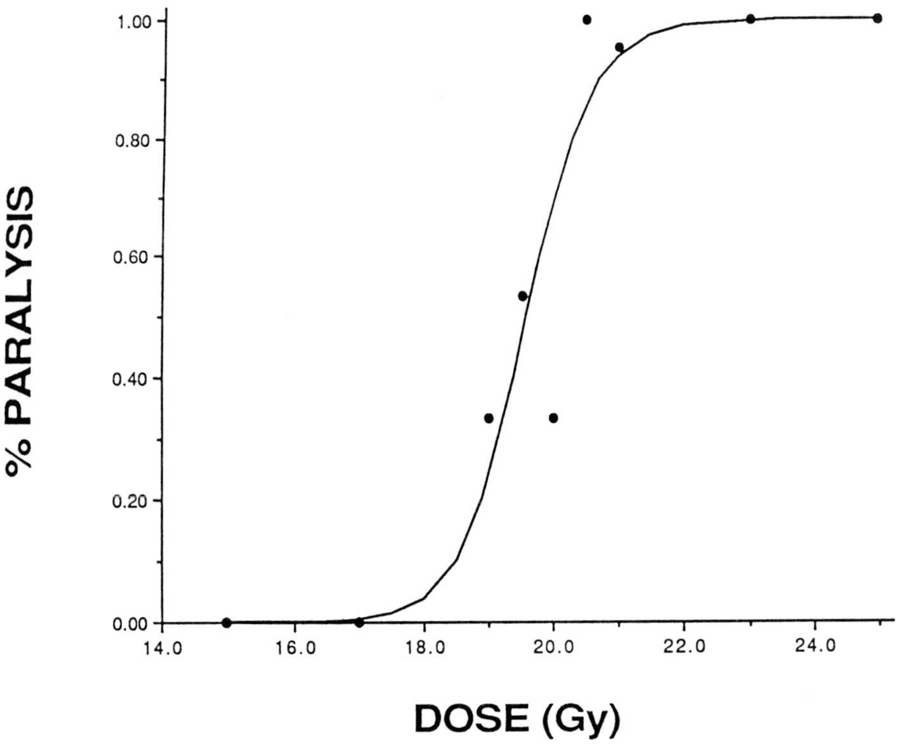

Figure 3. Percentage of paralyzed rats at 7 months after single fraction irradiation of the cervical-thoracic spinal cord (C_2 -T_1).

animals at these same time points. Similarly, assays for vitamins E and C, antioxidants which would be expected to be consumed in the process of lipid peroxidation, also revealed no significant differences from control animals over a wide range of time intervals and doses.

Vitamin E diets.

Dose response curves constructed from animals supplemented with vitamin E (diet A), made deficient in vitamin E (diet C) and on a regular diet (diet B) were found to virtually overlap, and the ED_{50}s were nearly identical at 20.4, 20.7 and 20.6 Gy, respectively, indicating that no radioprotection was offered by the vitamin E supplementation and no hypersensitivity resulted in those rats made deficient (Figure 4).

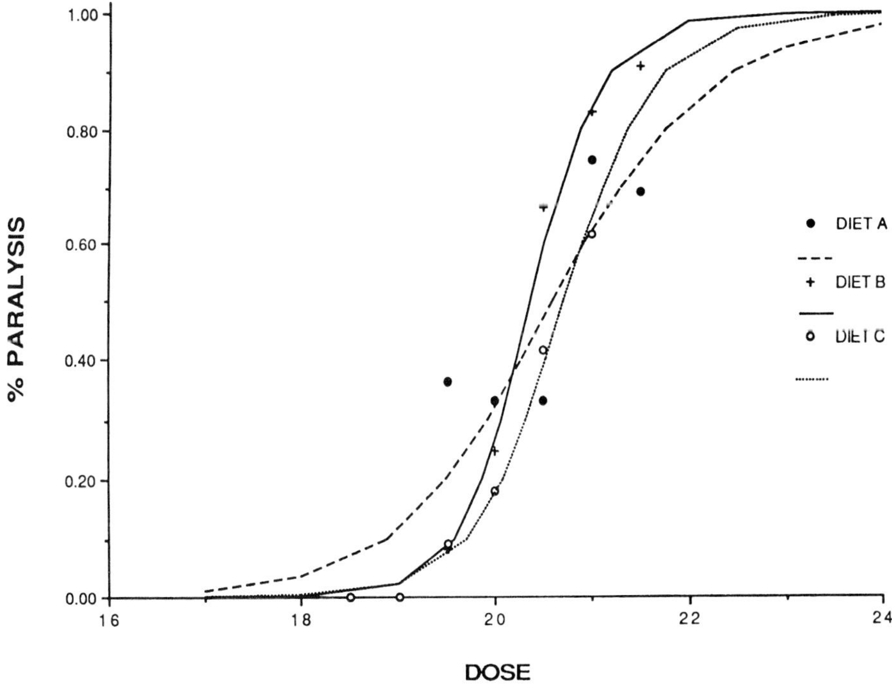

Figure 4. Percentage of paralyzed rats at 7 months on supplemented (diet A), normal (diet B) and deficient (diet C) vitamin E diets.

U74006F.

A slight rightward shift in the dose response curve was achieved in those rats treated around the time of irradiation with the 21-aminosteroid U74006F as compared with control animals (Figure 5) and the ED_{50} was found to be 20.2 Gy (95% confidence interval 19.7-20.7). This difference was, however, not statistically significant, and the confidence intervals for the two curves overlap.

DISCUSSION

In sum, a role for lipid peroxidation in the development of the progressive demyelination and WMN seen in late radiation injury has not been supported by the results of biochemical assays or by the manipulation of tissue antioxidant levels.

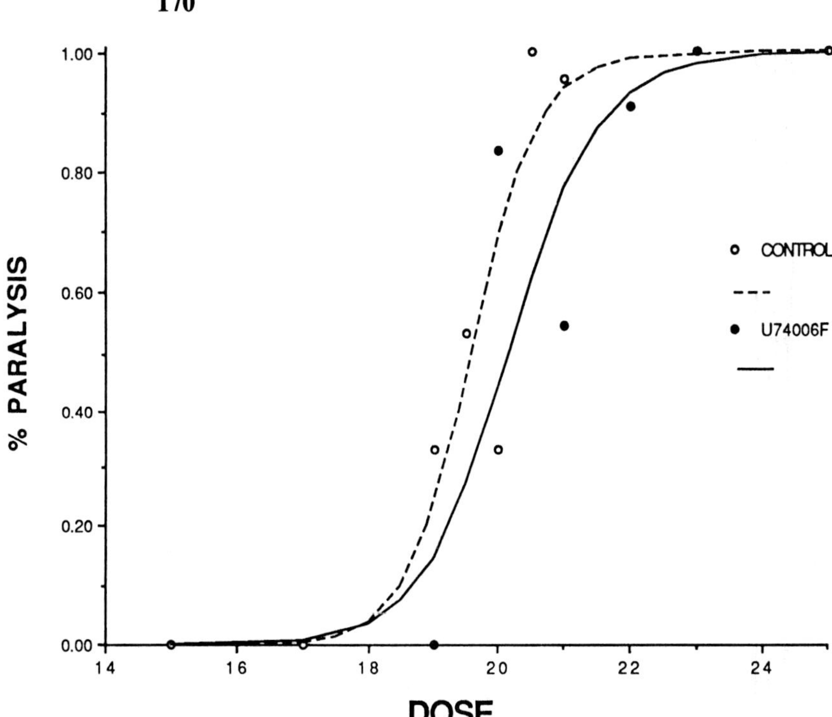

Figure 5. Percentage of paralyzed rats at 7 months after single fraction irradiation of the cervical-thoracic spinal cord (C_2 - T_1) without (---) and with (——) the 21-AS U74006F, 10 mg/kg, given 30 min before and 2 and 24 hours after irradiation.

Because concerns have developed regarding some variability in a few of the control values and the moderate doses chosen in some of the irradiated animals in which assays for MDA, HETEs, vitamin E and vitamin C were performed, assays are being repeated at specific time points using rats irradiated at 23 Gy, a dose known to result in 100% paralysis, to strengthen the data and confirm that biochemical evidence does not exist to support the hypothesis that lipid peroxidation is ongoing in the irradiated CNS. The lack of change in radiation responsiveness from the elevation and suppression of spinal cord vitamin E content, as well as from the acute administration of U74006F, both potent free radical scavengers, provides further evidence that lipid peroxidation may not be important in radiation-induced white matter injury. It also renders less likely the possibility that the accumulation of the byproducts of peroxidation and the consumption of endogenous antioxidants were events too transient or too subtle to be detected by our tissue assays.

Although a radioprotective role for U74006F was not demonstrated in this study, the drug's promising results in several experimental models of CNS injury and its lack of glucocorticoid side effects

(16), which patients with CNS radiation injury (and brain tumors) find so devastating, makes it warrant further study with larger numbers of animals and perhaps with a more prolonged course of administration to define its role in this setting.

Given that our work to date has not supported a role for lipid peroxidation in late delayed CNS radiation injury, and that the "target cell" model, implicating primary damage to glial cells or blood vessels, has been unsuccessful in elucidating a definite cause or suggesting a route of protection or treatment, our most recent work has focused on the contribution of vasogenic edema to the process. Characterization of the time course in the development of blood-brain barrier breakdown after CNS radiation and the role of polyamines, which we have found to be elevated in irradiated rat spinal cords (Gutin, P.H., unpublished data), is under investigation.

This work was supported by American Cancer Society Grant No. PDT 340.

REFERENCES

1. Gutin, P.H., Phillips, T.L., Wara, W.M., et al. J Neurosurg 60:61-68, 1984.
2. Walker, M.D., Strike, T.A., Sheline, G.E. Int J Radiat Oncol Biol Phys 5:1725-1731, 1979.
3. Sheline, G.E. Cancer 39:873-881, 1979.
4. Leibel S.A., Gutin, P.H., Wara, W.M. et al. Int J Radiat Oncol Biol Phys, 17:1129-1139, 1989.
5. Burger, P.C., Mahaley, Jr., M.S., Dudka, L., et al. Cancer 44:1256-1272, 1979.
6. Davis, R.L., Barger, G.R., Gutin, P.H., et al. Acta Neurchir Supp 33:301- 305, 1984.
7. van der Kogel, A.J. Brit J Cancer 53, Supp VII: 207-217, 1986.
8. Myers, R., Rogers, M.A., Hornsey, S. Br J Cancer 53, Supp VII 221-223, 1986.
9. Myers, R., Rogers, M.A., Hornsey, S. Radiotherapy and Oncology (in press).
10. Delattre, J.Y., Rosenblum, M.K., Thaler, H.T., et al. Brain 111:319-1339, 1988.
11. Raleigh, J.A., Kremers, W., Gabouny, B. Int J Radiat Biol 31:203, 1977.
12. Smith, M.T., Thor, H., Hartzell, P., et al. Biochem Pharcol 31:19, 1982.
13. Kutnick, M.A., Hawkes, W.C., Schaus, E.E., et al. Analytical Biochem 166:424-430, 1987.
14. Lane, J.K., Gohil, K., Packer, L. Analytical Biochem 157:106-116, 1986.
15. Braughler, J.M., Pregenzer, J.F., Chase, R.L., et al. J Biol Chem 262:10438-10440, 1987.
16. Hall, E.D., Braughler, J.M. Free Radical Biol Med 6:303-313, 1989.

THE TRANSFER RNAs OF THE IRRADIATED MOUSE SPLEEN CONTAIN QUEUINE

W. R. FARKAS, L. SZABO and T. L. WALDEN, JR.+

The University of Tennessee College of Veterinary Medicine, Knoxville, TN 37901 and +The Armed Forces Radiation Biology Research Institute Bethesda, Maryland

ABSTRACT

The post transcriptional modification of tRNA whereby a guanine residue in the first position of the anticodon of certain tRNAs is excised and replaced by queuine occurs to a lesser extent in rapidly dividing cells than in quiescent cells. In this report we show that in the sub-lethally irradiated mouse even though the spleen increased seven fold in weight during the post-irradiation period of recovery there was only a slight increase in the (q-) tRNA. In dogs the bone marrow $tRNA^{His}$ is completely (q-) however, the spleen tRNA is virtually 100% (q+). These results suggest that the presence of queuine has special importance in the metabolism of the spleen.

INTRODUCTION

The original transcripts of the tRNAs for asn, asp, his and tyr contain a guanine residue in the first position of the anticodon. This guanine is enzymatically excised and replaced by the 7-deazapurine known as queuine (1,2). The precusor tRNA is known as (q-) tRNA and the mature tRNA that contains queuine (q+) tRNA. In most cells the (q-) and (q+) isoacceptors are both present and as a general rule the ratio of (q-) to (q+) tRNA is greater in cells that are growing rapidly. This is true for tumor cells, regenerating rat liver (3,4) and fetal tissue (5). The ratio of (q-) tRNA to (q+) tRNA varies during the life cycle of Drosophila. After hatching from the egg the larvae undergo a period of very rapid growth. Afterwards, the larvae pupate and form adults. There is little growth and virtually no cell division during the adult stage. During the larval stage the (q-) tRNA predominates and just before pupation is virtually 100% of the tRNA is (q-). When the adult emerges from the pupal state (q+) tRNA represents about 10% of the queuosine family of tRNAs (6). The (q+) tRNA increases as the adult ages (7,8) and is about 50% in the two week old adult.

One of the most dramatic examples of rapid growth is the enlargement of the spleen in the sub-lethally irradiated mouse and we felt it to be of interest to determine the levels of the queuine-containing tRNA in this rapidly growing tissue. We also compared two hematopoietic tissues from the same organism with respect to their queuine content. We found that in the dog there was very little (q+) tRNA in the bone marrow, but the spleen tRNA was predomanently (q+), indicating that queuine is especially important to the spleen.

MATERIALS AND METHODS

The mice were males of the CD2F1 strain, 15 weeks old. The mice were irradiated with 800 rads from a Cobalt-60 source (100 rads per min). The mice were killed on the indicated days and the spleens weighed and kept frozen at -80° until they were extracted with phenol.

Comparison of queuine-containing tRNAs in canine bone marrow and spleen.

A dog was killed by exsanguination after receiving a lethal dose of sodium pentobarbital. The long bones were split and the marrow scooped out. The marrow was weighed, washed with ice cold phosphate-buffered saline and the tRNAs obtained by extraction with phenol as previously described for liver tRNA (1). The tRNAs from canine spleen were also extracted as previously described for liver tRNAs (1). In order to determine whether or not the tRNAs were (q+) or (q-), the spleen or marrow tRNA were charged with a radioactive amino acid of the queuosine family e.g. ^{3}H histidine and cochromatographed on RPC-5 with mouse liver tRNA charged with the same amino acid labeled with ^{14}C (9).

Queuine-Deficient Germ-free Mice.

Mice of the CD-1 strain were maintained as previously described in gnotobiotic isolators and fed a chemically defined diet that did not contain queuine (10,11). Germ-free mice fed and maintained in this manner became deficient in queuine and their tRNAs were 100% (q-). As a control the chemically-defined diet was supplemented with queuine at a concentration of 0.15 mg/liter.

Enzyme Assays.

The guanine queuine tRNA transglycosylase was assayed as described by (Howes and Farkas) (12). Superoxide Dismutase (SOD) activity was determined by the epinepherine-adenochrome method of Misra and Fridovich (13) as modified by Matkovics et al (14). The total SOD was determined in the presence and absence of cyanide. The activity in the presence of cyanide was taken as the amount of Mn-SOD. The value in the presence of cyanide was subtracted from the total SOD in order to determine the level of Cu, Zn-SOD. Catalase was determined by measuring the decrease in ultraviolet absorbance of hydrogen peroxide as described by Beers and Sizer (15). Glutathione peroxidase was determined by combining the methods of Chiu et al and Sedlak and Lindsay (16,17). In this assay the amount of reduced glutathione remaining is determined with Elman reagent after the reaction of cumenehydroperoxide with reduced glutathione. Thiobarbituric acid-reactive material which is indicative of lipid peroxidation (18) was determined by the method of Placer et al (19).

Aminoacylation of Spleen tRNA.

The tRNAs were charged with their cognate amino acid (1) and the ratio of (q+) to (q-) tRNA determined as previously described (10) using the reversed phase-5 chromatographic system described by Pearson et al (20).

RESULTS

Ratio of (Q+) to (Q-) tRNA in the Irradiated Mouse Spleen.

The mice were irradiated and on the indicated days after irradiation, groups of mice (5 to 10) were killed, the spleens washed with isotonic saline and immediately frozen at -80° until they were used. The spleens were weighed and the average spleen weight for each time point is indicated in Table I. The tRNAs were then extracted from the pooled spleens and charged with ^{3}H histidine. The ^{3}H-labeled tRNA was mixed with ^{14}C histidyl tRNA from normal unirradiated mouse liver. Since mouse liver is virtually 100% (q+) and the elution profiles of (q+) and (q-) tRNA are well known (1, 10) the liver tRNA served as a marker for identification of the peaks corresponding to (q+) and (q-) tRNA. The ratio of (q+) to (q-) $tRNA^{His}$ was determined from the area under the peaks. The data summarized in Table I shows that while the spleen weight increased seven fold there was only a slight decrease in the ratio of (Q +) to (Q-) tRNA.

Table I
Comparison of Spleen Weight and Ratio of (q-) to (q+) $tRNA^{His}$
After Whole Body Radiation

Days Post Irradiation	Spleen Weight mg	%(q-) $tRNA^{His}$
7	31	0
9	26	---
14	56	28
16	177	18
18	149	13
20	158	20
22	132	17
24	118	22

Comparison of (q+) and (q-) $tRNA^{His}$ levels in canine spleen and bone marrow.

The surprisingly high levels of (q+) tRNA in irradiated mouse spleens that had increased seven fold in mass suggested that having (q+) tRNA may be especially important for the spleen. Since both bone marrow and spleen have similar functions (in that they are both hematopoietic organs) a comparison of queuine content of canine spleen and bone marrow might add credence to this hypothesis. The results summarized in Table II shows that canine bone marrow had absolutely no (q+) $tRNA^{His}$, whereas the spleen was 48% (q+) in $tRNA^{His}$ Table II. For another member of the queuine family $tRNA^{Asp}$ the spleen was 100% (q+) and bone marrow was only 60% (q+) $tRNA^{Asp}$.

Levels of Some Enzymes involved in Oxidative Metabolism in (q+) and (q-) Germ-free Mice.

Since the spleen is a hematopoietic organ we felt it to be of interest to study the effect of queuine on some enzymes involved in oxidative metabolism. We previously showed that the Mn, SOD was about two fold higher in a murine cell line (LM cells) if queuine was added to the cell culture media (21). We compared the levels of the same oxidative enzymes in mice that were deficient in queuine and in

Table II
Comparison of Queuine Content of the tRNA from Canine Spleen and Bone Marrow

	% (q+) tRNA
Spleen tRNA ^{His}	48
Marrow tRNA ^{His}	0
Spleen tRNA ^{Asp}	100
Marrow tRNA^{Asp}	60

queuine-containing mice. Since queuine is not synthesized by mice and must be obtained either from the diet or the gut flora (10) we fed a queuine-deficient chemically-defined diet to germ-free mice. The data in Figure 1 compares the superoxide dismutase levels of mice fed a chemically-defined diet that either contained queuine or was devoid of queuine. Data obtained from conventional mice and germ-free mice fed a normal ingredient diet of commercial mouse chow is also included. Conventional mice are CD-1 mice with a normal intestinal flora fed a diet of commercial mouse chow. The data indicated that the Mn, SOD was higher in mice on the (q+) diet in liver but not kidney. The Cu, Zn SOD was also elevated in livers of the (q+) mice as was the total SOD of lung. Unfortunately there wasn't enough material to assay for Mn, SOD in lung. It is also of interest that the mice fed the CD diet irrespective of whether or not it contained queuine had higher levels of SOD than mice fed normal ingredient diets regardless of whether or not the mice were germ-free.

We also examined the levels of the two microsomal cytochromes, P-450 and B_5 and as seen in Figure 2, queuine did not have a significant effect on the levels of these two cytochromes.

Effect of Dietary Queuine on Malondialdehyde-Reactive Material in Different Tissues.

The data in Figure 3 indicates that there are small but significant increases in the amount of malondialdehyde-reactive material in germ-free mice that were fed queuine containing chemically-defined diets over the (q-) diet. The increased malondialdehyde was observed in liver and kidney but not in lung. It is of interest that there was so much more oxidized lipid in the liver and kidney of conventional over that of germ-free mice. This may be due to the high percentage of metabolism that is dedicated to control microbial growth in the body.

Effect of Dietary Queuine on Levels of Catalase and Glutathione Peroxidase.

The data in Figure 4 show that whereas there was no appreciable differences in the level of catalase there was a significant increase in glutathione peroxidase in liver and kidney but not lung in mice that were fed queuine.

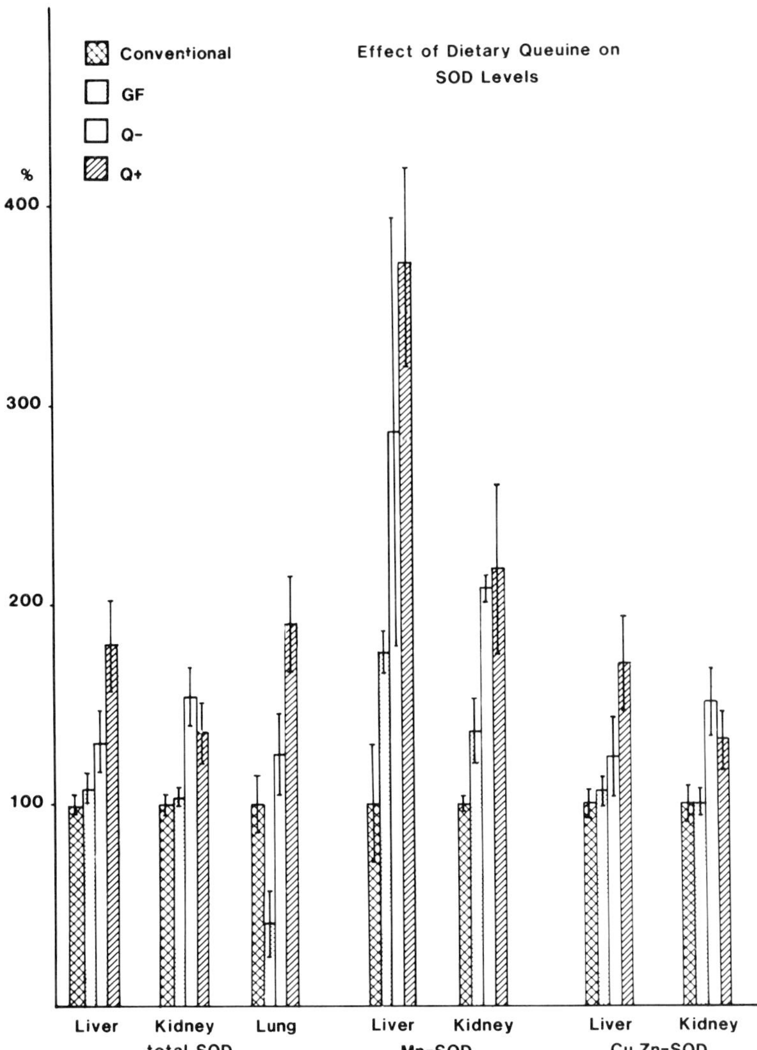

Figure 1. Effect of Dietary Queuine on Superoxide Dismutase Levels in Different Tissues. The four groups of mice were as follows. Conventional mice are not germ-free and are maintained on a normal ingredient diet of commercial mouse chow. Germ-free or GF mice are maintained in a gnotobiotic isolator and fed an autoclaved normal ingredient diet. The (q-) mice are germ-free mice fed a chemically-defined liquid diet. The (q+) mice were identical to the (q-) mice except that queuine was added to the diet at a concentration of 0.15 mg per liter. The germ-free mouse colonies were checked for sterility at least every other week.

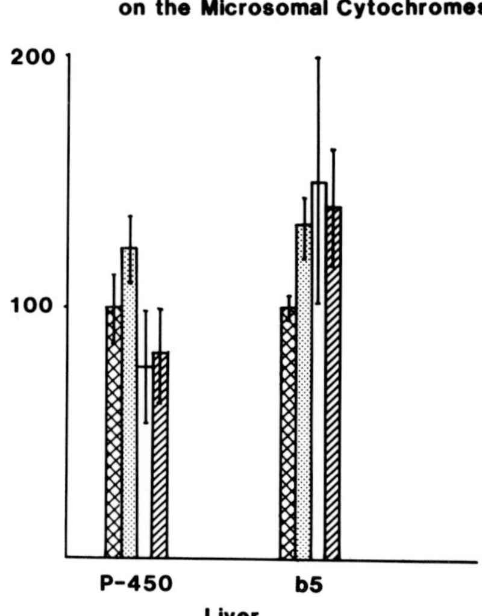

Figure 2. Effect of Dietary Queuine on Levels of Cytochrome P-450 and Cytochrome B_5. The designations are the same as in Figure 1.

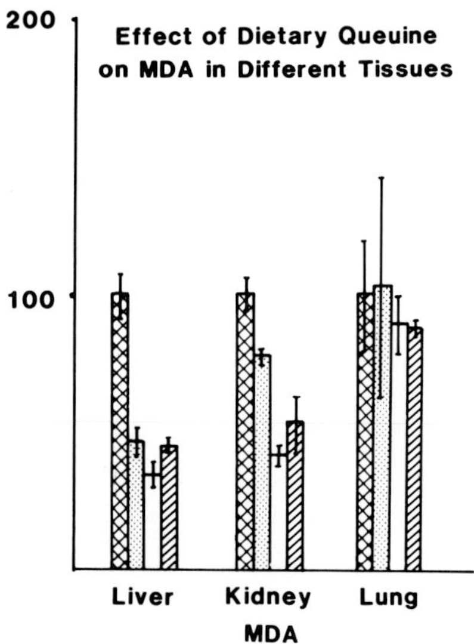

Figure 3. Effect of Dietary Queuine on Malondialdehyde in Different Tissues. The symbols are the same as in Figure 1.

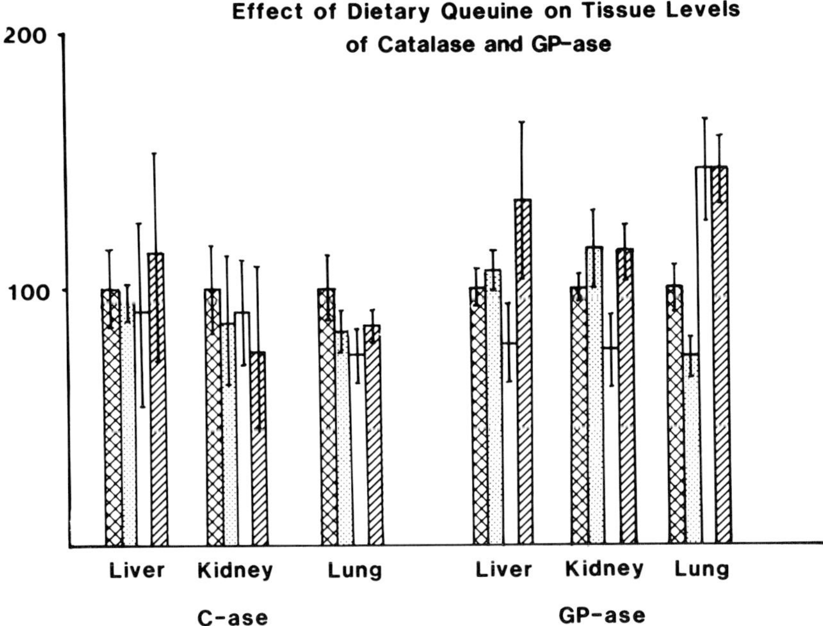

Figure 4. Effect of Dietary Queuine on Levels of Catalase and Glutathione Peroxidase in different tissues. The symbols are the same as in Figure 1.

Inhibition of Queuine Insertion by Carbon Dioxide.

In an experiment (not shown) bicarbonate was used to neutralize a compound that was being tested as an inhibitor of the enzyme that inserts queuine into tRNA. The results of this study was that bicarbonate but not the compound being tested inhibited the enzyme.

The effect of the bicarbonate was not due to a change in pH since the buffering capacity of the TES used in our standard assay at pH 7.4 was not exceeded. We determined if anions similar to bicarbonate also were inhibitors. The results shown in Table III show that neither acetate, formate, chloride or urea were inhibitors at the same concentration at which bicarbonate inhibited. These results were obtained with enzyme purified to the S-200 stage (12). When we repeated these studies with an enzyme fraction that had been purified to a greater degree (DE-32 stage) bicarbonate was no longer observed to be an inhibitor. Carbonic anhydrase catalyzes the equilibration of bicarbonate and carbon dioxide. Since the source of our enzyme was rabbit erythrocytes which are a rich source of carbonic anhydrase we added carbonic anhydrase to the reaction mix. The results shown in Table IV show that in the presence of carbonic anhydrase, bicarbonate inhibited the more purified enzyme as well as the S-200 fraction indicating that the true inhibitor is probably CO_2 and not bicarbonate.

Table III
Inhibition of Guanine, Queuine
tRNA Transglycosglase by Bicarbonate and Similar Compounds

Compound	Percent Inhibition
Bicarbonate	95.0
Acetate	3.8
Formate	18.3
Chloride	14.0
Urea	18.5

Inhibitors were all present at 10 mM. The counter ion for the anions was NH_4^+

Table IV
CO_2 is a More Potent Inhibitor than HCO_3^-

	Percent Inhibition
Control	---
Carbonic Anhydrase	5
Bicarbonate	28
Carbonic Anhydrase plus Bicarbonate	48

DISCUSSION

One of the most cogent explanations of the fact that queuine is more important to spleen than for other organs is that the tRNA from canine spleen was largely (q+) whereas in the other primary hematopoietic organ, bone marrow it was largely (q-). One could argue that this is due to the absence of the queuine insertion enzyme in bone marrow or to the inability of queuine to be transported across the plasma membrane of bone marrow cells. However, this doesn't seem to be the case since $tRNA^{Asp}$ in bone marrow was 60% (Q+). When the supply of queuine is limited $tRNA^{Asp}$ is modified before $tRNA^{His}$ (11).

We found that there was no effect of dietary queuine on the microsomal cytochromes (Figure 2) but the following interesting observation is worthy of mention. If one compares the amount of cytochrome P-450 found in the livers of the mice fed a normal ingredient diet of commercial mouse chow and the chemically-defined liquid diet there is significantly more P-450 in the mice fed the natural diet. The reason for this is that the P-450 enzymes, the role of which is to oxidize xenobiotics are inducible and their elevation indicates the extent to which ordinary food is contaminated with xenobiotics. It is also noteworthy that the level of P-450 was greater in the conventional mice than in the germ-free mice indicating that the gut flora plays a role in preventing the intestinal absorption of xenobiotics.

The malondialdehyde was significantly higher in the liver and kidney of (q+) mice than (q-) mice indicating greater degrees of oxidative activity in the presence of queuine. However, in lung there was no difference in MDA between (q+) and (q-) mice. A possible explanation of this observation may be that the constant exposure to oxygen in the lung masks any effect that queuine might have on oxidative metabolism. In support of this explanation, the levels of superoxide dismutase and glutathione peroxidase were not elevated in the presence of queuine in lung, as they were in liver and kidney.

The inhibition of queuine insertion by CO_2 is noteworthy since it has been established that there is an inverse relationship between the percentage of tRNA that is (q+) and the rate of cell growth (3,4). Since the rate of CO_2 production from mitochondrial oxidation would be elevated in rapidly growing cells this may explain the inverse relationship between rate of cell growth and the percentage of tRNA that contains queuine.

ACKNOWLEDGEMENTS

This research was supported by Grant No 89A30 from The American Institute for Cancer Research. ESO4079 from The National Institutes of Health and a grant from the Lupus Foundation of America. The authors would like to thank the Armed Forces Radiobiology Research Institute, Defense Nuclear Agency, for the use of the facilities.

REFERENCES

1. Katze, J.R. and Farkas, W.R. A Factor in Serum and Amniotic Fluid is the Substrate for the tRNA Modifying Enzyme Guanine Transferase. Proc. Nat. Acad. Sci. (USA) 76:3271-3275, (1979).
2. Okada, N.S., Okada, N., Ohgi, T., Goto, T. and Nishimura, S. Transfer Ribonucleic Acid Guanine Transglycosylase Isolated from Rat Liver. Biochemistry. 19, 395-400, 1980.
3. Okada, N., Okada, N.S., Sato, S., Itoh Y., Oda, K. and Nishimura, S. Detection of Unique tRNA Species in Tumor Tissue by E. coli Guanine Insertion Enzyme. Proc. Nat. Acad. Sci. (USA) 75:4247-4251,1978.
4. Jackson, C.D., Irving, C.C. and Sells, B.H. Changes in Rat Liver Transfer RNA Following Growth Hormone Adminstration and Regenerating Liver. Biochim. Biophys. Acta. 217:64-71, (1970).
5. Landin, R.M., Boisnard, M. and Petrissant, G. Correlation between the presence of $tRNA^{His}$ and the Erythropoietic Function in Fetal Sheep Liver. Nucl. Acid Res. 7:1635-1648, 1979.
6. White, B.N., Tener, G.M., Holden, J. and Suzuki, D.T. Activity of a Transfer RNA Modifying Enzyme during the Development of Drosophila and its Relationship to the Su(s) Locus. J. Mol. Biol. 74:635-641,1973.
7. Hosbach, H.A. and Kubli, E. Transfer RNA in Aging Drosophila: II Isoacceptor Patterns. Mech. of Ageing and Development. 10:141-149, 1979.
8. Owenby, R.K., Stuhlberg, M.P. and Jacobson, K.B. Alternation of the Q Family of Transfer RNAs in Adult Drosophila Melanogaster as a Function of Age, Nutrition and Genotype. Mech. of Ageing and Development. 11:91-103, 1979.
9. DuBrul, E.F. and Farkas, W.R. Partial Purification and Properties of the Reticulocyte Guanylating Enzyme. Biochim. Biophys. Acta. 442:379-390, 1976.
10. Farkas, W.R. Effect of Diet on The Queuine Family of tRNA of Germ-free Mice. J. Biol. Chem. 255:6832-6835, 1980.
11. Reyniers, J.P., Pleasants, J.R., Wostman, B.S., Katze, J.R. and Farkas, W.R. Administration of

Exogenous Queuine is Essential for the Biosynthesis of the Queuosine-containing Transfer RNAs in the Mouse. J. Biol. Chem. 256:11591-11594, 1981.

12. Howes, N. and Farkas, W.R. Studies on Guanylation of tRNA with a Homogeneous Enzyme from Rabbit Erythrocytes. J. Biol. Chem. 253:9082-9087, 1978.
13. Misra, H.P. and Fridovich, I. The Role of Superoxide Anion in Autoxidation of Epinephecine and a Simple Assay for Superoxide Dismutase. J. Biol. Chem. 247:3170-3175, 1972.
14. Matkovics, B., Novak, R., Hanh, H.D., Szabo, L., Varga, S.I. and Zalesna, G. A Comparative Study of Some More Important Experimental Animal Peroxide Metabolism Enzymes. Comp. Biochem. Physiol. 56B: 31-34,1977.
15. Beers, R.G. and Sizer, I.W. A Spectrophotometric Method for Measuring the Breakdown of Hydrogen Peroxide by Catalase. J. Biol. Chem. 195:133-140, 1952.
16. Chiu, D.T.Y., Stuts, F.H. and Tappel, A.L. Purification and Properties of Rat Lung Soluble Glutathione Peroxidase. Biochim. Biophys. Acta. 445:558-566,1976.
17. Sedlack, J. and Lindsay, R.H. Estimation of Total Protein-Bound and Nonprotein Sulfhydyl Groups in Tissue with Ellman's Reagent. Analyt. Biochem. 25:192-205, 1 968.
18. Patton, S. and Kurtz, G.W. α-Thiobarbituric Acid as a Reagent for Detecting Milk Fat Oxidation. J.Dairy Sci. 34:669-674,1951.
19. Placer, Z.A., Cushman, L.L. and Johnson, B.C. Estimation of Product of Lipid Peroxidation (Malonyl Dialdehyde) in Biochemical Systems. Anal. Biochem. 16:359-364, 1966.
20. Pearson, R.L., Weis, J.F. and Kelmers, A.D. Improved Separation of Transfer RNAs on Polychlorotrifluoroethylene-supported Reversed-Phase Chromatography Columns. Biochim. Biophys. Acta. 228:770-774, 1971.
21. Szabo, L., Nishimura, S. and Farkas, W.R. Possible Involvement of Queuine in Oxidative Metabolism. Biofactors, 1:241-244, 1988.

BEHAVIORAL TOXICITY OF RADIOPROTECTIVE BIOACTIVE LIPIDS

M. R. LANDAUER[1], H. D. DAVIS[1], and T. L. WALDEN, JR.[2]

Departments of Behavioral Sciences[1], and Radiation Biochemistry[2], Armed Forces Radiobiology Research Institute, Bethesda, MD 20814-5145

INTRODUCTION

The ideal radioprotective agent for use in radiotherapy and civil defense should provide effective protection with minimal behavioral disruption. The bioactive lipids are among the compounds that have demonstrated radioprotective efficacy in cellular assays or animal survival studies. Members of this group that have been determined to be radioprotective include prostaglandins, leukotrienes, and platelet-activating factor (PAF). While protective agents have been identified in both the cyclooxygenase and lipoxygenase pathways, as well as for the phospholipid derived PAF, not all bioactive lipids provide radioprotection (1). The most promising radioprotective compounds include the synthetic methylated derivative of the naturally occurring prostaglandin E_2, 16,16-dimethyl prostaglandin E_2 ($DiPGE_2$), leukotriene C_4 (LTC_4), and PAF. In our laboratory, they are maximally effective for enhancing animal survival when administered 5-10 minutes before irradiation, and provide dose reduction factors (DRF) ranging from 1.45 to 1.9 (2-4). The radioprotective mechanisms of the bioactive lipids have not been clearly elucidated, but they are believed to act through different receptor systems. Mechanisms ranging from alterations of biological mediators, such as cyclic AMP, to hypoxia and cardiovascular effects have been postulated (5,6).

Because of the important biological roles and the significant radioprotection afforded by $DiPGE_2$ (2, 7-11), LTC_4 (3, 12, 13), and PAF (4), we investigated the behavioral toxicity of these compounds. In addition, we evaluated the behavioral effects of mice exposed to the sulfhydryl radioprotector S-2 (3-aminopropylamino)ethylphosphorothioic acid (WR-2721) (14) alone and in combination with $DiPGE_2$, because previous research established that combining these agents increases the degree of radioprotection (15, 16). An ideal combination of agents should provide enhanced radioprotection without an increase in behavioral side effects. Behavioral toxicity was evaluated using a test for spontaneous locomotor activity, a paradigm recommended by the World Health Organization (17). The locomotor activity test has been determined to be a sensitive measure for assessing the behavioral toxicity of radioprotectors (18-21).

MATERIALS AND METHODS

Subjects.

Male CD2F1 male mice, 10 to 12 weeks old were obtained from Charles River Breeding Laboratory

(Raleigh, NC). They were quarantined on arrival, and representative animals were screened for evidence of disease. Mice were housed in groups of 8-10 in Micro-Isolator cages on hardwood chip contact bedding in an AAALAC accredited facility. Rooms were maintained at 21° +/- 1°C with 50% relative humidity on a 12-12 hr light-dark cycle. Commercial rodent chow (Wayne Rodent Blox) and acidified water (pH, 2.5) were freely available. All mice were euthanized by inhalation of carbon dioxide at the end of the experiment.

Drugs.

A range of doses of $DiPGE_2$, LTC_4 and PAF were administered to mice. Each mouse was tested only once. Compounds were dissolved in 4% ethanol in saline, and administered to mice subcutaneously (SC) in the nape of the neck in a volume of 100 μ1. Behavioral evaluation began immediately following drug administration. In the WR-2721 and $DiPGE_2$ combination study, all mice received two injections. The first injection was either WR-2721 (200 mg/kg) or the saline vehicle administered intraperitoneally (IP). The second injection, administered 5 min after the first, was either a SC dose of $DiPGE_2$ (0.4 mg/kg) or the vehicle, 4% ethanol in saline. Mice were placed in the test apparatus immediately after receiving the second injection.

Locomotor activity measurement.

A computerized Digiscan Animal Activity Monitor (Omnitech Electronics, Columbus, OH) was used to quantitate locomotor behavior. The apparatus used an array of infrared photodetectors spaced 2.5 cm apart to determine locomotor activity expressed as the total distance traveled. Immediately following injection of the compound(s) animals were placed into the activity monitor where ambulation was recorded every 5 min for 1 hr to ascertain the behavioral onset of the drug. Thereafter, activity was recorded at 1-hr intervals until all groups returned to control levels. All testing took place during the dark portion of the light-dark cycle.

One-way analysis of variance was used to determine significance levels for the effects of each compound on locomotor activity. Post hoc comparisons were made using Dunnett's test.

RESULTS AND DISCUSSION

Each of the three major compounds tested, $DiPGE_2$, LTC_4, and PAF, produced dose-dependent decrements in locomotor behavior (Figure 1). At the higher doses tested, the behavioral decrement induced by each compound was rapid in onset, occurring within 5-10 minutes postadministration. Locomotor activity returned to control levels by 3 hr postadministration at the highest doses evaluated.

Each of the three compounds tested has been shown to be radioprotective for animal survival when administered prior to cobalt-60 irradiation. $DiPGE_2$ at 0.4 mg/kg yields a DRF of 1.45 (16); LTC_4 at 0.4 mg/kg, a DRF of 1.9 (13); and PAF at 0.3 mg/kg, a DRF of 1.7 (4).

WR-2721 and $DiPGE_2$ alone and in combination induced almost complete cessation of locomotor activity (Figure 2). WR-2721 produced significant locomotor deficits within 15 min that lasted for 3 hr. Administration of 0.4 mg/kg $DiPGE_2$ resulted in significant decrements within 5 min of injection which

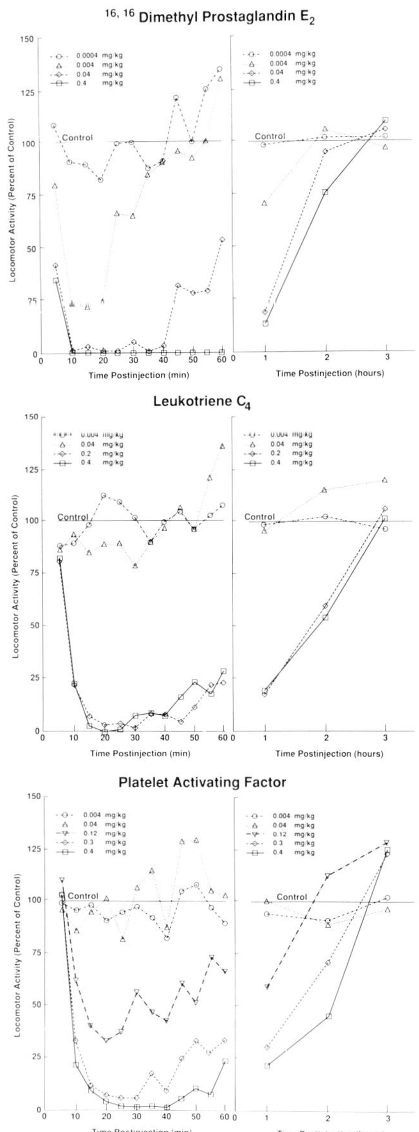

Figure 1. Onset (left) and duration (right) of locomotor deficit following administration of $DiPGE_2$, LTC_4 or PAF. Drugs were administered SC prior to testing as described in text. Data are expressed as a percent of the vehicle control group. (N = 9-13/dose).

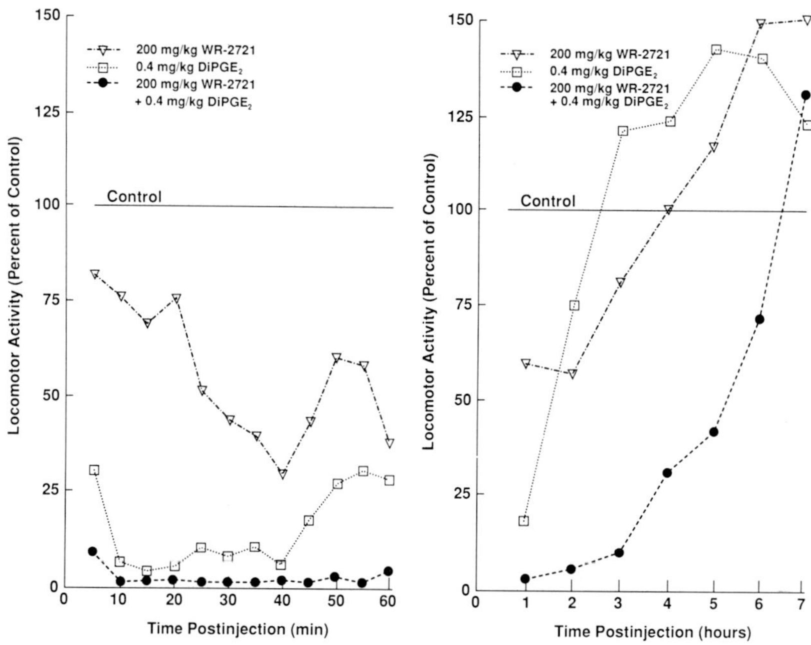

Figure 2. Effects of WR-2721 and $DiPGE_2$, alone or in combination, on onset (left) and duration (right) of behavioral decrement. WR-2721 (IP) $DiPGE_2$ (SC) or the combination was administered prior to assessment of locomotor behavior as described in text. Data are expressed as a percent of the vehicle control group (N = 8-12/group).

persisted for 2 hr. The combination of WR-2721 and $DiPGE_2$ resulted in deficits within 5 min of injection that remained below control levels for 6 hr following drug administration.

The combination of WR-2721 and $DiPGE_2$ administered to CD2F1 mice before cobalt-60 irradiation has been determined to provide a greater DRF than either compound alone (16). Pretreatment with WR-2721 provided a DRF of 1.90, while pretreatment with $DiPGE_2$ increased survival with a DRF of 1.45, and the combination yielded a DRF of 2.15. Although the combination of WR-2721 and $DiPGE_2$ enhanced radiation survival, it also produced the most severe and longest acting behavioral decrements. Therefore, increases in radioprotection also produced concomitant increases in behavioral toxicity.

The results of the research summarized in this report confirm related findings on the effects of bioactive lipids on behavior. Exogenously administered prostaglandins, including those of the E series, have been demonstrated to produce sedative or tranquilizing effects in a variety of species (22). In addition, intracerebroventricular administration of LTC_4 has been reported to decrease locomotor activity in the rat (23).

Bioactive lipids produce a variety of physiological responses. For example, $DiPGE_2$ induces diarrhea and sedative effects (18); LTC_4 produces increases in hematocrit and mean arterial blood pressure, which may be followed by prolonged hypotension (24, 25); and PAF results in profound hypotensive action, reflecting peripheral vasodilation and decreased cardiac output (26). In addition, the radioprotective phosphorothioate WR-2721 has produced hypotension, nausea, vomiting, and mild somnolence during clinical trials (27). The mechanism(s) by which these compounds exert their effects on locomotor activity, however, remain unknown.

It is not possible from these experiments to determine whether the adverse behavioral effects produced by the radioprotective compounds evaluated are mediated by a peripheral or central mechanism. Prostaglandins are capable of crossing the blood-brain barrier (28), while LTC_4 (29) and WR-2721 cannot (30). PAF can influence blood-brain barrier permeability, but does not appear to penetrate it (31). In addition, many bioactive lipids are synthesized by brain tissue (31, 32). The decrease in locomotor activity reported for these bioactive lipids may, therefore, be the result of intermediate messengers produced by the bioactive lipids administered or in response to their physiological action.

In general, the onset of behavioral decrement was highly correlated with the optimal pre-radiation administration time of the agent. The duration of the performance decrement, however, lasted considerably longer than the radioprotective effect, suggesting different mechanisms of action. Although bioactive lipids remain viable radioprotective and therapeutic agents, pharmacological concentrations of many of these compounds are behaviorally toxic, which may limit their usefulness.

ACKNOWLEDGMENTS

We wish to thank Dr. Douglas Morton of The Upjohn Company for supplying the prostaglandin used in this investigation and the Experimental Therapeutics Division, Walter Reed Army Institute of Research, Washington, DC for the WR-2721. LTC_4 and PAF were obtained from Biomol Research Laboratories (King of Prussia, PA). We are grateful to M.E. Cranford, N.K. Farzaneh, and M.E. Faccioli for their outstanding assistance in the conduct of this research. We also thank G. Ruggiero and J.F. Weiss for their helpful comments on this manuscript. This research was supported by the Armed Forces Radiobiology Research Institute, Defense Nuclear Agency, under work units 00159 and 00162. The views presented in this paper are those of the authors; no endorsement by the Defense Nuclear Agency has been given or should be inferred. Research was conducted according to the principles enunciated in the "Guide for the Care and Use of Laboratory Animals" prepared by the Institute of Laboratory Animal Resources, National Research Council.

REFERENCES

1. Walden, T.L., Jr. J. Radiat. Res., 29: 255-260, 1988.
2. Walden, T.L., Jr., Patchen, M. and Snyder, S.L., Radiat. Res., 109: 440-448, 1987.
3. Walden, T.L., Jr. Ann. NY Acad. Sci. 524: 431-433, 1988.
4. Hughes, H.N., Walden, T.L., Jr. and Steel, L.K. Abstracts of the 37th Annual Meeting of the

Radiation Research Society, p. 186, 1989.
5. Halushka, P.V., Mais, D.E., Mayeux, P.R. and Morinelli, T.A., Ann. Rev. Pharmacol. Toxicol., 10: 213-239, 1989.
6. Weiss, J.F., Kumar, K.S., Walden, T.L., Jr., Neta, R., Landauer, M.R. and Clark, E.P. Int. J. Radiat. Biol., 57:709-722, 1990
7. Hanson, W.R. and Thomas, C. Radiat. Res. 96: 393-398, 1983.
8. Hanson, W.R. and Ainsworth, E.J. Radiat. Res. 103: 196-203, 1985.
9. Hanson, W.R. In: Prostaglandin and Lipid Metabolism in Radiation Injury, (Eds. T.L. Walden, Jr. and H.N. Hughes), Plenum Press, New York, 1987, pp. 233-243.
10. Steel, L.K. and Catravas, G.N. In: Eicosanoids and Radiation, (Ed. P. Polgar), Kluwer Academic Publishers, Boston, 1988, pp. 79-87.
11. Steel, L.K., Walden, T.L., Jr., Hughes, H.N., and Jackson, W.E., III. Radiat. Res. 115: 605-608, 1988.
12. Walden, T.L, Jr., Patchen, M.L. and MacVittie, T.J. Radiat. Res. 113: 388-395, 1988.
13. Walden, T.L., Jr. Abstracts of the 37th Annual Meeting of the Radiation Research Society, p. 185, 1989.
14. Davidson, D.E., Grenan, M.M. and Sweeney, T.R. In: Radiation Sensitizers: Their Use in the Clinical Management of Cancer, (Ed. L.W. Brady), Masson, New York, 1980, pp. 309-320.
15. Hanson, W.R. Radiat. Res., 111: 361-373, 1987.
16. Landauer, M.R., Walden, T.L., Jr. and Davis, H.D. In: Frontiers in Radiation Biology, (Ed. E. Riklis), VCH Publishers, Weinheim, West Germany, in press.
17. World Health Organization, Environmental Health Criteria, Principles and Methods for the Assessment of Neurotoxicity Associated with Exposure to Chemicals. World Health Organization, Geneva, 1986.
18. Landauer, M.R., Walden, T.L., Jr., Davis, H.D. and Dominitz, J.A. In: Prostaglandin and Lipid Metabolism in Radiation Injury, (Eds. T.L. Walden, Jr. and H.N. Hughes), Plenum Press, New York, 1987, pp. 245-251.
19. Landauer, M.R., Davis, H.D., Dominitz, J.A. and Weiss, J.F. Pharmacol. Biochem. Behav. 27: 573-576. 1987.
20. Landauer, M.R., Davis, H.D., Dominitz, J.A. and Weiss, J.F. Pharmacol. Ther., 39: 97-100, 1988.
21. Landauer, M.R., Davis, H.D., Dominitz, J.A. and Weiss, J.F. Toxicology 49: 315-323, 1988.
22. Chiu, E.K.Y. and Richardson, J.S. Gen. Pharmacol. 16: 163-175, 1985.
23. Brus, R., Krzeminski, T., Juraszczyk, Z., Kurcok, A., Felinska, W. and Kozik, W. Biomed. Biochim. Acta 45: 1153-1158, 1986.
24. Landauer, M.R., Walden, T.L. Jr., Davis, H.D., Cranford, M.E. and Farzaneh, N.K. Abstracts of the 37th Annual Meeting of the Radiation Research Society, p. 185, 1989.
25. Moncada, S., Flower, R.J. and Vane, J.R. In: The Pharmacological Basis of Therapeutics, (Eds. A. Goodman Gilman, L.S. Goodman, T.W. Rall and F. Murad), Macmillan: New York, 1985, pp. 660-673.
26. Myers, A., Tores Durate, A. P. and Ramwell, P. Adv. Prostaglandin Thromboxane Leukotriene Res. 17: 833-837, 1987.
27. Kligerman, M.M., Turrisi, A.T., Urtasun, R.C., Norfleet, A.L., Phillips, T.L., Barkley, T. and Rubin, T. Int. J. Radiat. Oncol. Biol. Phys. 14: 1119-1122, 1988.
28. Bito, L.Z., Davson, H., and Hollingsworth, J.R. J. Physiol. 253: 273-285, 1976.
29. Spector, R. and Goetzl, E.J. Biochem. Pharmacol. 35: 2849-2853, 1986.
30. Utley, J.F., Marlowe, C. and Wadell, J.W. Radiat. Res. 68: 284-291, 1976.
31. Kumar, R., Harvey, S.A.K., Kester, M., Hanahan, D.J. and Olson, M.S. Biochim. Biophys. Acta 963: 375-383, 1988.
32. Murphy, S. and Pearce, B. Prostaglandins Leukotrienes Essential Fatty Acids 31: 165-170, 1988.

PROSTAGLANDINS, RADIATION, AND THERMOREGULATION

S. B. KANDASAMY and W. A. HUNT

Behavioral Sciences Department, Armed Forces Radiobiology Research Institute, Bethesda, MD 20814-5145

Changes in body temperature can be observed after radiation exposure (1), an effect that depends on the species being used. For example, radiation induces hyperthermia in cats, rabbits (2), and humans (3); a biphasic response in monkeys (a fall followed by a rise (4)); a dual effect in rats (low and high doses produce hyperthermia and hypothermia, respectively (5)); and hypothermia in guinea pigs (6). However, the mechanisms underlying hyperthermia and hypothermia due to radiation are unknown.

Normal thermoregulation apparently is controlled by a variety of putative mediators. Prostaglandins (PGs) of the E series induce hyperthermia, while D series induce hypothermia (7,8,9). In addition, a variety of endogenous peptides capable of producing opiate-like effects have been isolated from brain tissue and have been implicated in thermoregulation (10).

Exposure to ionizing radiation has been reported to increase blood levels of histamine in humans undergoing radiation therapy and in dogs following irradiation (11,12). Histamine has been implicated in radiation-induced hypotension (13), reductions in cerebral blood flow (14), and performance decrements (15). Histamine is present in the hypothalamus (16,17), and is localized in nerve terminals (18). Administration of histidine systemically or histamine centrally evokes hypothermia due to both H1 and H2 receptor activation, and it has been implicated in thermoregulation (19). It has been suggested that histamine may be a central neurotransmitter involved in many physiological functions, including thermoregulation, and could underlie radiation-induced hypothermia.

In this report, we review the work being done in our laboratory (5,6,20,21,22). Experiments were undertaken to determine (1) the effect of variable doses of ionizing radiation on body temperature in the rat (2) the effect of radiation on the brain or peripheral sites, and (3) the mechanisms that may underlie radiation-induced changes in body temperature, by comparing the effects of radiation to those of drugs with known actions and by determining if antagonists to these drugs could block the effects of radiation.

Exposure of rats to 1 Gy to 15 Gy γ radiation (60 Co) induced hyperthermia, whereas 20 Gy to 150 Gy induced hypothermia (Figure 1). The onset of these effects was rapid, and peaked within 15 min. Hyperthermia or hypothermia induced by 10 Gy or 50 Gy dose of γ radiation occurred only after whole-body or head-only exposure, not when the head was shielded, indicating that radiation-induced hyperthermia or hypothermia appear to be centrally mediated (Figure 2). Because whole-body exposure

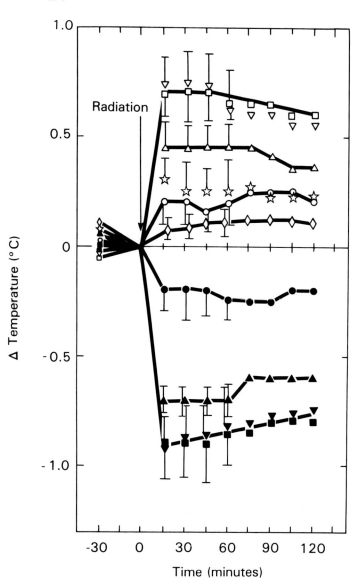

Figure 1. Changes in rectal temperature of rats exposed to variable doses of ionizing radiation: Sham radiation (◇), 1 Gy (○), 3 Gy (☆), 5 Gy (△), 10 Gy (□), 15 Gy (▽), 20 Gy (●), 50 Gy (▲), 100 Gy (▼), 150 Gy (■). Each point represents the mean ± SE of five observations, except (◇) and (□) which represent 15 observations. Zero on the ordinate represents body temperature at the time of irradiation.

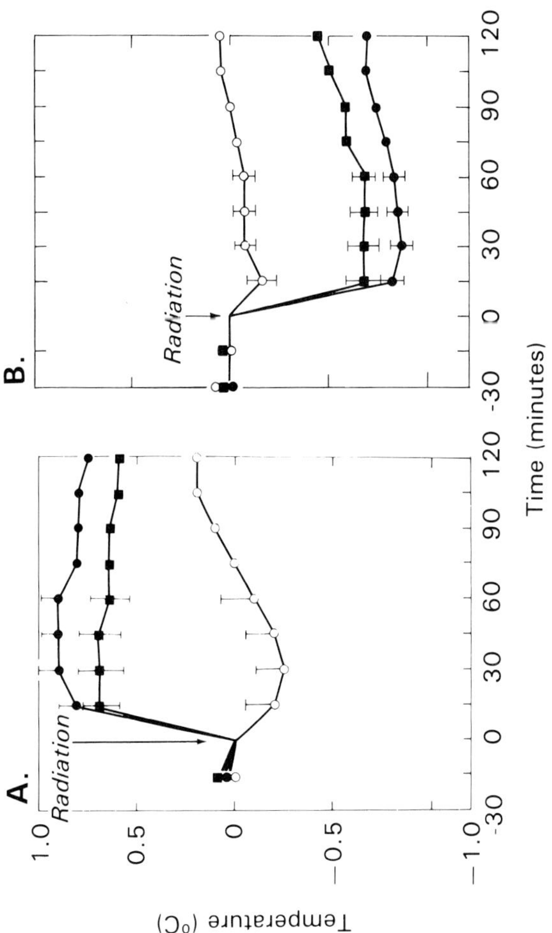

Figure 2. Effect of 10 Gy (A) or 50 Gy (B) ionizing radiation on body only (○), whole body (■), and head only (●). Each point represents the mean ± SE of six observations. Zero on the ordinate represents the temperature at the time of irradiation

resulted in the same effect as head-only exposure, subsequent studies used whole-body exposure to ionizing radiation.

Ionizing radiation induces PG synthesis (23). The observations that PGE2 and PGD2 are hyper- and hypothermic, respectively, and various anti-inflammatory agents blocked their synthesis in tissue (24) have implicated PGs in thermoregulation (8,9). Pretreatment with indomethacin, a cyclooxygenase inhibitor, attenuated radiation-induced hyper- and hypothermia (Figure 3), suggesting that these temperature responses are mediated by PGs. Similar to the effects of low and high doses of radiation, PGE2 and PGD2 produced dose-dependent hyper and hypothermia, respectively.

The effect of SC-19220, a PGE2 antagonist, was investigated on PGE2, PGD2, and radiation-induced temperature responses. The SC19220 significantly attenuated PGE2 and radiation-induced hyperthermia, but had no effect on PGD2 and radiation-induced hypothermia (Figures 4 and 5), suggesting that radiation-induced hyperthermia is mediated by PGE2.

Ionizing radiation alters β-endorphin-like immunoreactivity in the brain (25). β-endorphin induces hyperthermia (10). If radiation induces the release of β-endorphin, naloxone and similar antagonists should lower temperature. Naloxone attenuated only the hyperthermia, induced by 1-Gy and 3-Gy doses of radiation, and had no antagonistic effect on higher doses (5 Gy to 15 Gy). Because indomethacin attenuated the hyperthermia induced by all the lower doses (1 Gy to 15 Gy) studied, there may be an interrelationship between the opioid peptides and PGs. Opioids have been reported to increase the synthesis of PGs in the central nervous system (26). If radiation exposure resulted in the release of central β-endorphin, the resulting synthesis and release of PGs would be blocked by indomethacin treatment.

Taken together, these findings suggest that radiation-induced hyperthermia is mediated through the synthesis and release of PGs in the brain, and, to a lesser extent, to the release of endogenous opioid peptides.

Histamine is stored in mast cells throughout the body, including the brain; they are particularly numerous in the hypothalamus (27). Arachidonic acid is converted by the cyclooxygenase pathway, primarily to PGD2 in mast cells in humans and rats (28,29). In addition, mast cells release PGD2 and histamine after activation by various stimuli (30). The mast cell stabilizer, disodium cromoglycate, attenuated radiation-induced and PGD2-induced hypothermia (Table I), suggesting a role of central histamine in this response. The release of histamine acting on both H1 and H2 receptors may be involved in radiation-induced hypothermia, because mepyramine, an H1-receptor antagonist, and cimetidine, an H2-antagonist, not only blocked radiation-induced hypothermia but also PGD2-induced hypothermia (Table 1). Serotonin is not involved in radiation-induced hypothermia (5,6).

In summary, these results suggest that radiation-induced hyperthermia is mediated by PGE2, and histamine is involved in radiation-induced hypothermia. The attenuation of PGD2-hypothermia by disodium cromoglycate and antihistamines suggests that PGD2 acts by way of histaminergic systems.

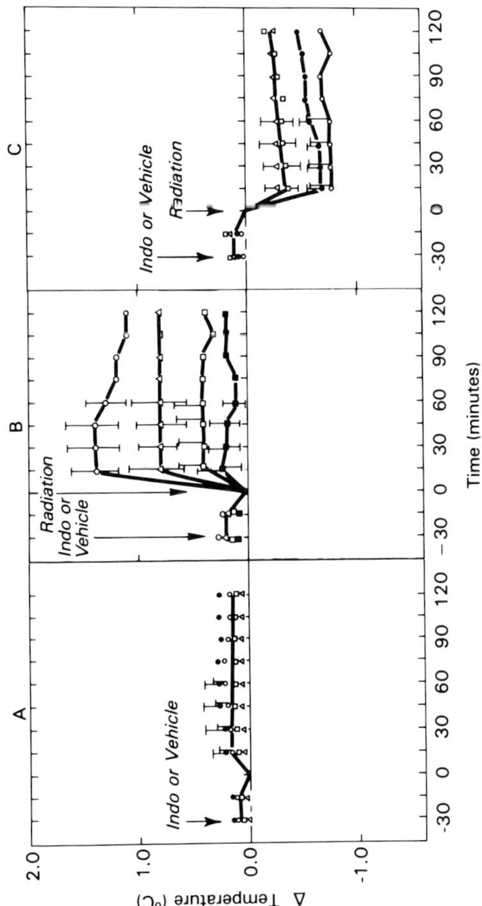

Figure 3. Effect of indomethacin, ip, (Indo) on hyperthermia and hypothermia induced by 10 Gy and 50 Gy of radiation, respectively. (A) Nonirradiated controls given indomethacin, 1 mg/kg (Δ), 3 mg/kg (○), 5 mg/kg (●), or vehicle (□); (B) 10 Gy of radiation alone (○) and in the presence of indomethacin, 1 mg/kg (Δ), 3 mg/kg (□), or 5 mg/kg (■); (C) 50 Gy of radiation alone (○) and in the presence of indomethacin, 1 mg/kg (●), 3 mg/kg (□), or 5 mg/kg (Δ). Each point represents the mean ± SE of observations on five animals. Zero on the ordinate represents the temperature at the time of the second injection.

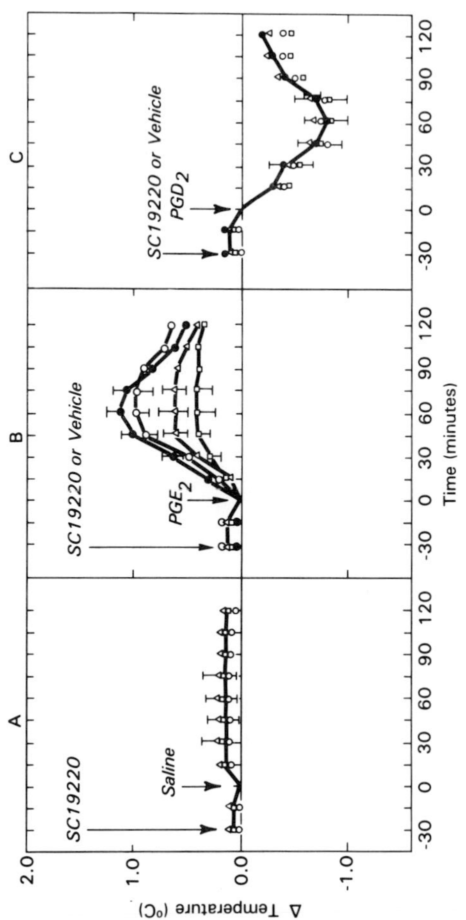

Figure 4. Effect of SC-19220, icv, on PGE2-induced and PGD2-induced hyperthermia and hypothermia, respectively. (A) Nonirradiated controls given SC-19220, 100 ng (○), 300 ng (Δ), or 500 ng (□); (B) 10 ng of PGE2 alone (●) and in the presence of SC-19220, 100 ng (○), 300 ng (Δ), or 500 ng (□); (C) 30 ng of PGD2 alone (●) and in the presence of SC-19220, 100 ng (○), 300 ng (Δ), or 500 ng (□). Each point represents the mean ± SE of observations on five animals. Zero on the ordinate represents the temperature at the time of the second injection.

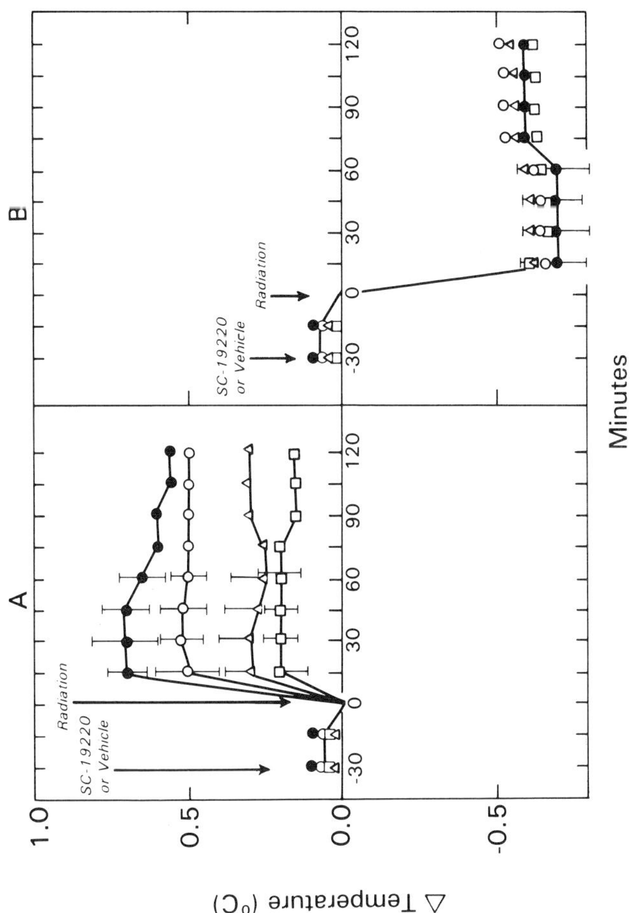

Figure 5. Effect of SC-19220, icv, on hyperthermia and hypothermia induced by ionizing radiation. (A) 10 Gy of radiation alone (●) and in the presence of SC-19220, 100 ng (○), 300 ng (Δ), or 500 ng (□); (B) 50 Gy of radiation alone (●) and in the presence of SC-19220, 100 ng (○), 300 ng (Δ), or 500 ng (□). Each point represents the mean ± SE of observation on five animals. Zero on the ordinate represents the temperature at the time of the second injection.

Table 1
Effect of disodium cromoglycate (DSCG), mepyramine, or cimetidine on radiation-induced or PGD2-induced hypothermia

	Hypothermia	
Pretreatment	Radiation-induced	PGD2-induced
DSCG	Antagonism	Antagonism
Mepyramine	Antagonism	Antagonism
Cimetidine	Antagonism	Antagonism

REFERENCES

1. Kimeldorf, D.J. and Hunt, E.L. In: Ionizing Radiation: Neural Function and Behavior (Eds. D.J. Kimeldorf and E.L. Hunt), New York, 1965, pp. 109-130.
2. Veninga, T.S. Radiat. Res. 48: 358-367, 1971.
3. Fanger, H. and Lushbaugh, C.C. Arch. Pathol. 83: 446-460, 1967.
4. McFarland, W.L. and Willis, J.A. Cerebral temperature changes in the monkey (Macaca mulatta) after 2500 rads ionizing radiation. Armed Forces Radiobiology Res. Inst. Scientific Report, SR 74-77, 1974.
5. Kandasamy, S.B., Hunt, W.A. and Mickley, G.A. Radiat. Res. 114: 42-53, 1988.
6. Kandasamy, S.B. and Hunt, W.A. Life Sci. 42: 555-563, 1988.
7. Feldberg, W. and Milton, S. In: Inflammation (Eds. J.R. Vane and S.H. Ferreira), Springer-Verlag, New York, 1978, pp. 617-656.
8. Milton, A.S. and Wendlandt, S.J. Physiol. 218: 325-336, 1971.
9. Clark, W.G. and Lipton, J.M. Neurosci. Biobehav. Rev. 9: 479-552, 1985.
10. Clark, W.G. and Lipton, J.M. Neurosci. Biobehav. Rev. 18: 299-371, 1985.
11. Lasser, E.C. and Stenstrom, K.W. Am. J. Roentgenol. 72: 985-988, 1954.
12. Cockerham, L.G., Doyle, T.F., Donlon, M.A. and Helgeson, E.A. Aviat. Space Environ. Med. 55: 1041-1045, 1984.
13. Alter, W.A., Hawkins, R.N., Catravas, G.N., Doyle, T.F. and Takenaga, J.K. Radiat. Res. 94: 654, 1983.
14. Cockerham, L.G., Cerveny, T.J. and Hampton, D.J. Aviat. Space Environ. Med. 57: 578-582, 1986.
15. Doyle, T.F., Turns, J.E. and Strike, T.A. Aerospace Med. 42: 400-403, 1971.
16. Adam, H.M. and Hye, H.K.A. Br. J. Pharmacol. 28: 137-152, 1966.
17. Lipinski, J.F., Schaumburg, H. and Baldessarini, R.J. Brain Res. 52: 403-408, 1973.
18. Snyder, S.H. and Taylor, K.M. In: Perspectives in Neuropharmacology (Ed. S.H. Snyder), New York, 1972, pp. 43-73.
19. Lomax, P. and Green, M.D. In: Temperature: Regulation, Drug Effects, and Therapeutic Implications (Eds. P. Lomax and E. Schonbaum), New York, 1979, pp. 289-304.
20. Kandasamy, S.B., Kumar, K.S., Hunt, W.A. and Weiss, J.F. Radiat. Res. 114: 240-247, 1988.
21. Kandasamy, S.B. and Hunt, W.A. In: Thermoregulation: Research and Clinical Applications (Eds. Lomax and Schonbaum), Karger, Basel, 1989, pp. 116-119.
22. Kandasamy, S.B. and Hunt, W.A. Radiat. Res. 1990, 121:84-90.
23. Pausescu, E., Chirvasie, R., Teodosiu, T. and Paun, C. Radiat. Res. 65: 163-171, 1976.
24. Vane, J.R. Nature 231: 232-235, 1971.
25. Mickley, G.A., Stevens, K.E., Moore, G.H., Deere, W., White, G.A., Gibbs, G.L. and Mueller, G.P. Pharmacol. Biochem. Behav. 19: 979-983, 1983.
26. Collier, H.O.J., McDonald-Gibson, W.J. and Sneed, S.A. Br. J. Pharmacol. 52: 116P, 1974.
27. Edvinsson, L., Cervos-Navarrp, J., Larrson, L., Owman, C.H. and Ronnberg, A.L. Neurol. 27: 878-883, 1977.

28. Abdel-Halim, M.S., Hamberg, M., Sjoquist, B. and Anggard, E. Prostaglandins 14: 633-643, 1977.
29. Forestermann, U., Heldt, R., Knappen, F. and Hertting, G. Brain Res. 240: 303-310, 1982.
30. Kawabe, H., Hayashi, H. and Hayaishi, O. Biochem. Biophys. Res. Commun. 143: 467-474, 1987.

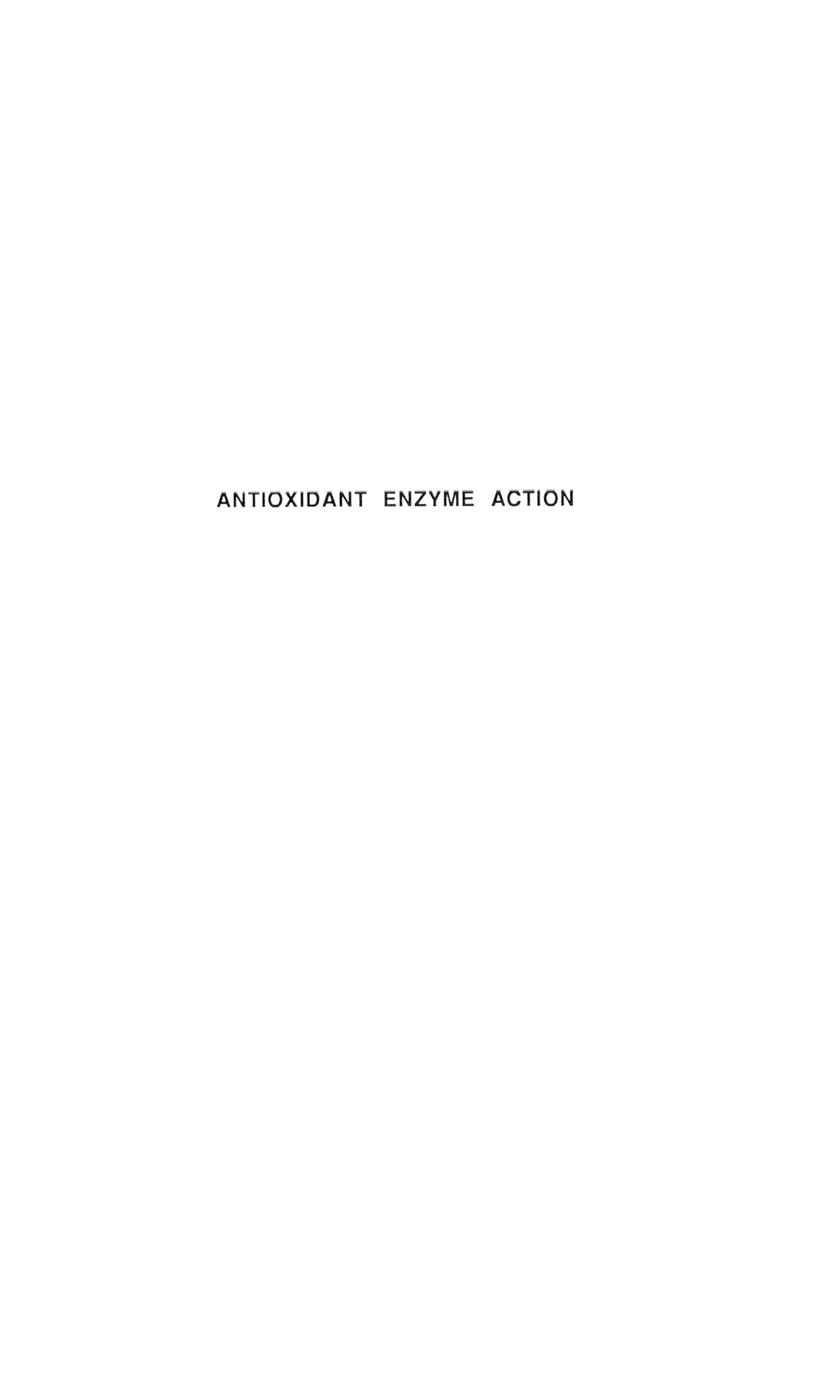

ANTIOXIDANT ENZYME ACTION

PHENOLS AND POLYPHENOLS AS ANTIOXIDANTS AND ANTICANCER AGENTS

H. L. ELFORD and B. VAN'T RIET

Molecules for Health, Inc., 3313 Gloucester Road, Richmond, Virginia 23227

INTRODUCTION

In order to replicate, a mammalian cell must replicate its genetic material which involves the synthesis of DNA. The reductive conversion of ribonucleotides to deoxynucleotides, catalyzed by the enzyme ribonucleotide reductase, is a rate limiting step in the DNA biosynthetic pathway (1). The endogenous pools of deoxynucleotides are not sufficient to support de novo DNA synthesis. Therefore, this key step in DNA synthesis represents a prime target for the development of an anticancer compound. Mammalian ribonucleotide reductase consists of two non-identical protein subunits. The larger subunit acts as a regulatory subunit since it contains the allosteric effectors (nucleotides) binding domains. The small subunits contain a pair of ferric ions and are able to generate a tyrosyl free radical which play a vital role in the reductive reaction (2). The reducing equivalents is supplied by either of two small molecular weight sulfhydryl proteins thioredoxin or glutaredoxin (1).

Importance of Polyphenolic Structure.

In our search for a chemotherapeutic agent superior to hydroxyurea to inhibit ribonucleotide reductase, we discovered polyhydroxybenzoic acid derivatives to be effective inhibitors of the enzyme and to have considerable antitumor activity in several mouse tumor models (3). This discovery came from studies to enhance the effectiveness of hydroxyurea by attaching various groups to the hydroxamic acid portion of the molecule, the structural moiety responsible for the inhibition of the enzyme. Through various structure manipulations it was found that the attachment of a vicinal polyhydroxyphenyl group to the hydroxamic acid structure resulted in 50-100 fold increase in enzyme inhibition as well as enhanced antitumor activity (4). The realization that the vicinal polyhydroxyphenyl molecular structure possessed its own inhibitory activity on mammalian ribonucleotide reductase and as a consequence had anticancer activity came from testing of other polyhydroxyphenyl compounds lacking the hydroxamic acid group. For example, methyl 3,4,5-trihydroxybenzoate inhibited the enzyme and had a ID_{50} of 30 uM, almost 20 fold better than hydroxyurea (500 uM) and had comparable antitumor activity in the L1210 leukemia model at a much lower dose (5).

The polyhydroxyphenyl compounds primarily inhibit ribonucleotide reductase and exhibit antitumor activity because of their free radical scavenging activity. They effectively destroy the tyrosyl free radical enzyme intermediate generated during the reductive reaction. The polyhydroxyphenyl hydroxamic acids, esters and amides are very good free radical scavengers (5). The ability of the hydroxybenzohydroxamic acid compounds to inhibit ribonucleotide reductase activity parallel with the compound's ability to scavenge the stable organic free radical diphenylpicrylhydrazyl (5). On the other hand, there was no appreciable difference between the various hydroxybenzohydroxamic acid's ability to complex Fe^{+3} Therefore, we continue to believe the primary mechanism of action of the polyhydroxy phenyl compounds is free radical scavenging as we proposed in the original description of these compounds (4).

The best of the first generation polyhydroxyphenyl compounds which we have synthesized and tested for enzyme inhibition and antitumor activity is 3,4-dihydroxybenzohydroxamic acid (Didox). Although this compound is not the most potent enzyme inhibitor, it exhibits the best antitumor activity in several mouse tumor models, as conducted by the National Cancer Institute (6). Didox is currently in clinical trial in England.

There have been a number of reports in the literature that polyhydroxyphenyl compounds are cytotoxic to tumor cells and exhibit antitumor activity. Among them are the reports that pyrocatechol, dihydroxy phenylalanine (DOPA) (7), and other DOPA-like compounds inhibit cell growth and produced anticancer activity in animal tumor models and have been tested in humans (8-11). In addition, naturally occurring phenolic substances isolated from mushrooms, which include γ-L-glutaminyl-4-hydroxybenzene and its glutaminyl 3,4-dihydroxy metabolite exhibit antitumor activity (12). Our laboratory was able to show that the DOPA-like compounds and 3,4-dihydroxybenzylamine could inhibit ribonucleotide reductase and were active in the L1210 tumor model (3). However, only 3,4-dihydroxybenzylamine had enzyme inhibitory activity comparable to Didox, but was not as effective antitumor agent in the L1210 leukemia model (5).

Combination Chemotherapy.

Based on the free radical scavenging property of the polyhydroxyphenyl compounds and the thesis that toxicity but not the antitumor activity of the anthracyclines (adriamycin) is due to the generation of a toxic free radical intermediate (13). Didox was tested to determine whether it could reduce adriamycin toxicity and therefore increase therapeutic effectiveness. Eugene Herman, of the FDA, found that Didox reduced toxicity in both an acute and chronic model of anthracycline toxicity in non-tumor bearing animals (14).

Encouraged by these results, Didox was tested in combination with adriamycin in the murine L1210 leukemia model. The combination chemotherapy of Didox with less than the optimal dose of adriamycin resulted in a marked enhancement of the antitumor activity of each drug administered alone and was superior to the maximum tolerated dose of adriamycin used singly (Table 1). In addition, there was less toxicity in the dually treated animals, as noted by improved exterior appearance and decreased weight loss, than in animals treated only with a comparable dose of adriamycin. Since adriamycin treatment in humans is limited to a total cumulative dose, the ability to achieve an equivalent or better therapeutic result with a significantlly reduced dose of adriamycin would permit a much longer treatment period.

Table 1. Potentiation by Didox of Sub-Optimal Dosage of Adriamycin

Treatment	Life Span (Mean)	ILS* (%)	Cures+(%)
Control	10.9	-	0
Adriamycin (6 mg/kg)[1]	14.5	33	0
Adriamycin (17 mg/kg)[2]	28.5	161	0
Didox (275 mg/kg)[A]	12.8	17	0
Didox (430 mg/kg)[B]	13.0	19	0
Adriamycin[1] + Didox[A]	28.3	159	25
Adriamycin[2] + Didox[A]	31.3	187	0
Adriamycin[1] + Didox[B]	28.3	159	25
Adriamycin[2] + Didox[B]	39.0	258	25

Adriamycin given i.p. only on day 2
Didox given on day 2, 4, and 5
* Percent increase in life span of drug-treated tumor mice compared to untreated animals
Four animals per group
\+ Survivors of 60 days and no evidence of tumor
Survivors calculated as having 60-day life span

A second important anticancer drug that Didox is particularly synergistic with is cyclophosphamide (cytoxan). Levels of cytoxan reduced to one-fourth of the optimum dose when combined with Didox produced striking synergy. A modest increase in life span (ILS) at the reduced dose of cytoxan is converted to high number of cures in the L1210 leukemia model (Table 2). This marked synergistic effect was also observed in a drug combination study of BCNU and Didox. The synergistic effect of Didox with adriamycin or cytoxan or BCNU was also observed in the Lewis lung tumor, a solid tumor model.

Table 2. Synergism of Didox and Cytoxan in the Treatment of L1210 Leukemia

Treatment	Life Span	ILS (%)	Cures* (%)
Control	8.2	-	0
Cytoxan (68 mg/kg)	10.5	28	0
Didox (494 mg/kg)	9.2	12	0
Cytoxan and Didox	60.0+	669+	100%

Cytoxan given i.p. only on day 2
Didox given i.p. only on day 2
Four animals per treatment group
* Survivors at day 60 and no evidence of tumor
\+ Survivors calculated as having life span of 60 days

The rationale for the synergy of Didox with these DNA interacting agents is attributed to Didox's ability to inhibit DNA excision-repair synthesis. Evidence for this thesis is provided by the studies of Snyder, involving several ribonucleotide reductase inhibitors in which Didox was among the most effective inhibitor of repair following u.v. radiation (15).

Radiosenitization.

Theoretically, an effective ribonucleotide reductase inhibitor would also be a radiation sensitizer through its inhibition of DNA repair as well as effect on the cell cycle. In support of this premise is the demonstration by Piver and others (16, 17) that hydroxyurea potentiated radiation therapy for cancer of the cervix. Therefore, Didox's potential to act as a radiosensitizer was tested by Russell and Brown at Stanford University (18). Exponentially growing Chinese hamster ovary cells incubated with the drug and irradiated with single fractions of x-rays resulted in an x-ray dose modification factor of 2.1 (1.8-2.4). There was a more modest enhancement of the x-radiation in regrowth delay experiments involving RIF-1 murine tumor model. There was a delay in tumor regrowth of approximately 6 days (25 days) or 30% over that seen with x-radiation alone (19 days).

Inhibition of Carcinogensis.

It should be mentioned that phenols and polyhydroxyphenyl compounds have been shown to inhibit carcinogensis in carcinogen feeding experiments in rats (19), as well as inhibit phorbol ester induction of ornithine decarbonylase activity and tumors in mouse epidermis (20).

REFERENCES

1. Reichard, P. Ann. Rev. Biochem. 57:349-374, 1988.
2. Graslund, A., Ehrenberg, A. and Thelander, L. J. Biol. Chem. 257:5711-5719, 1982.
3. Elford, H.L. and Van't Riet, B. Pharmac. Ther. 29:239-254, 1985.
4. Elford, H.L., Wampler, G.L. and Van't Riet, B. Cancer Res. 39:844-851, 1979.
5. Elford, H.L., Van't Riet, B., Wampler, G.L., Lin, A.L. and Elford, R.M. Adv. Enz. Reg. 19:151-168, 1981.
6. Elford, H.L. and Van't Riet, B. In: International Encyclopedia of Pharmacology and Therapeutics (Eds. J.G. Cory and A.H. Cory), Pergamon Press, Elmsford, N.Y., 1989, pp. 217-233.
7. Yamafuji, K. and Murakami, H. Enzymologia 35:139-153, 1968.
8. Angeletti, P.U. and Levi-Montalcini, R. Cancer Res. 30:2863-2869, 1970.
9. Chelmicka-Szorc, E. and Arnason, B.G.W. Cancer Res. 36:2382-2384, 1976.
10. Wick, M.M. Cancer Treat. Rep. 63:991-997, 1979.
11. Driscoll, J.S. J. Pharm. Sci. 68:1519-1521, 1979.
12. Vogel, F.S., Kemper, L.A.K., Boekelheide, K., Graham, D.G. and Jeffs, P.W. Cancer Res. 39:1490-1493, 1979.
13. Gianni, L., Corden, B.J. and Myers, C.E. In: Review in Biochemical Toxicology (Eds. Hodgson, et al.), Elsevier, N.Y., 1983, pp. 1-82.
14. Elford, H.L., Van't Riet, B., Wampler, G.L., Searle, A. and Willson, R.L. Proc. Am. Ass. Cancer Res. 24:326, 1983.
15. Snyder, R.D. Cell Biol. Toxicol. 1:49-57, 1984.
16. Piver, M.S., Khalil, M. and Emrich, L.J. J. Surg. Oncol. 42:120-125, 1989.
17. Stehman, F.B., Bundy, B.N., Keys, H., Currie, J.L., Mortel, R. and Creasman, W.T. Am. J. Obstet. Gynecol. 159:87-94, 1988.
18. Russell, K.J., Elford, H.L. and Brown, J.M. Submitted for publication.
19. Wattenberg, L.W. Cancer Res. 45:1-8, 1985.
20. Kozumbo, W., Seed, J.L. and Kensler, T.W. Cancer Res. 43:2555-2559, 1983.

INITIATION OF THE CYCLOOXYGENASE REACTION VIA PEROXIDASE ENZYME INTERMEDIATES

R. J. KULMACZ

Dept. of Biological Chemistry, Univ. of Illinois at Chicago, Chicago, IL 60612

Prostaglandin H synthase has two distinct catalytic activities: the cyclooxygenase activity generates a hydroperoxide PGG_2, from arachidonic acid; the peroxidase activity reduces hydroperoxides to the corresponding alcohols like PGH_2. The synthase is thus capable of both producing and destroying hydroperoxides. The metabolic progeny of PGH_2 (prostaglandins, prostacyclins, thromboxanes) are known to affect many aspects of tumor growth and metastasis (reviewed in Ref. 1).

The cyclooxygenase reaction kinetics are complex, with an early accelerative phase reflecting an auto-catalytic feedback from the product hydroperoxide, PGG_2 (2), and a later decelerative phase, reflecting irreversible self-inactivation. A free radical mechanism has been proposed (3) for the propagation of the cyolooxygenase reaction. The overall cyclooxygenase reaction can thus be described (see scheme below) by: a) hydroperoxide-dependent initiation in which the synthase is converted to a cyclooxygenase-active form; b) multiple propagation cycles dependent on fatty acid and oxygen in which PGG_2 is generated; and c) termination reactions involving either quenching of the active cyclooxygenase by antioxidants (written as AH) or self-destructive side reactions.

Initiation: E - - - - - - - >E·

Propagation: E · + RH - - - - - - - > ER·
ER · + $2O_2$ - - - - - - - >ERO_2OO ·
ERO_2OO - - - - - - - >E· + RO_2OOH

Termination E· + AH - - - - - - - > E + A·
E· - - - - - - - > $E_{inactive}$

The mechanism of the hydroperoxide-dependent initiation of the cyclooxygenase is of particular interest because it is the basis for the autocatalytic aspect of the cyclooxygenase. This feedback provides powerful and rapid generation of prostaglandins, and introduces the potential for a local amplification of the hydroperoxide level that may be used for short range intra- or extra-cellular signalling to other fatty acid oxygenases. Although the peroxidase activity of the synthase would appear to inhibit initiation of the cyclooxygenase by destroying the required hydroperoxide, evidence is accumulating that the peroxidase activity is actually an integral part of the initiation process of the cyclooxygenase.

Cyanide is a ligand for the heme prosthetic group of the synthase, with a dissociation constant of 0.19 mM (4). Cyanide has also been found to inhibit the peroxidase activity of the synthase in a non-competitive fashion with a K_i value of 0.23 mM and to interfere with initiation of the cyclooxygenase (K_i value of 0.2 mM; Ref. 4). Thus, liganding of cyanide to the synthase heme is associated with inhibition of both peroxidase activity and cyclooxygenase initiation.

Replacement of heme by mangano protoporphyrin IX in the synthase results in rather selective inhibition of the peroxidase activity (Ref. 5 and Table 1). The mangano analog of the synthase was found to require a considerably higher level of PGG_2 for effective initiation of the cyolooxygenase than did the native synthase (Table 1). On the other hand, the selective inhibition of cyclooxygenase propagation by formation of a stoichiometric indomethacin-synthase complex (6) actually decreased the level of PGG_2 needed for effective initiation (Table 1). Thus, a decreased peroxidase activity was associated with impaired initiation of the cyclooxygenase.

Table 1: Initiation in Mn Proto IX-synthase and indomethacin-synthase

	Cycloox. Initation Kp (nM PGG_2)	Peroxidase Activity (% Control)	Cycloox. Activity (% Control)
Native synthase	20	100	100
Mn Proto IX - synthase	100	<5	23
Indomethacin-synthase	10	120	4

Note: Cyclooxygenase initiation was assayed by competition with glutathione peroxidase (7). Enzymatic activities were assayed as described previously (8).

An examination of the effectiveness of a serles of hydroperoxides for reaction as peroxidase substrates indicated that the lipid hydroperoxides PGG_2 and 15-HPETE reacted rapidly, ethyl hydroperoxide reacted about 10-fold more slowly, and hydrogen peroxide about 100-fold more slowly. This ranking exactly paralleled that of the hydroperoxides effectiveness as cyclooxygenase initiators (Table 2), suggesting that the first step in the peroxidase cycle may be a crucial step in the initiation of the cyclooxygenase reaction.

Table 2
Effectiveness of hydroperoxides as peroxidase substrates and cyclooxygenase initiators.

	Cycloox. Initation Kp (μM)	Peroxidase k_1 (10^7 M^{-1} s^{-1})
Hydrogen peroxide	45	0.01
Ethyl hydroperoxide	7	0.4
15-HPETE	0.03	5
PGG2	0.02	2

Note: Cyclooxygenase initation assayed and peroxidase rate constants estimated as previously described (9,10).

Results from limited proteolytic digestions provide additional evidence consistent with a mechanistic linkage between the two activities in the synthase: there was a coordinate loss of both activities upon proteolytic cleavage in arg 253 region by trypsin, chymotrypsin or proteinase K, and coordinate protection of both activities by heme or nonsteroidal anti-inflammatory agents (11-13). The fixed ratio between the two activities observed in batches of synthase with wide variation in specific activity (12) also supports a mechanistic linkage between the two activities.

The ability of the peroxidase activity in aspirin-treated synthase to inhibit the cyclooxygenase activity of native synthase (14) points to an intramolecular, rather than intermolecular, initiation of the cyclooxygenase by the peroxidase. Reaction of the synthase with hydroperoxide leads to very rapid formation of a free radical species (Figure 1) that may be a tyrosine radical (15). This radical species may represent the key intermediate that propagates the cyclooxygenase reaction by abstracting the hydrogen atom from substrate fatty acid.

PGH synthase might thus be considered a heme-dependent peroxidase that has evolved the ability to use an oxidized peroxidase cycle intermediate for activation of a polyunsaturated fatty acid, and propagation of the cyclooxygenase reaction. The cyclooxygenase reaction can go through about 1500 cycles before a self-inactivating side reaction intervenes. This large number of cyclooxygenase cycles, each producing PGG_2, for each initiating event, each consuming PGG_2, can explain the inability of the endogenous peroxidase to suppress the cyclooxygenase by itself, and furnishes the biochemical basis for a powerful local amplification of hydroperoxide levels.

Supported by PHS grant GM30509.

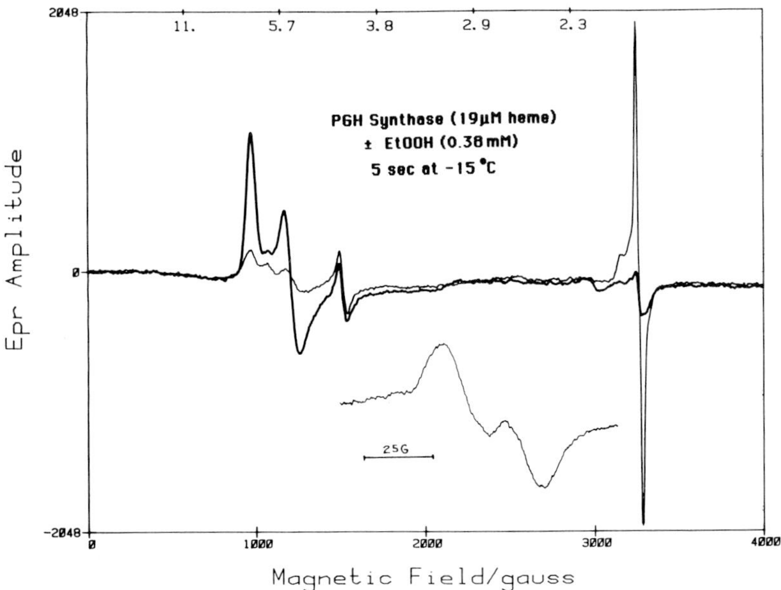

Figure 1. Electron paramagnetic spectra of synthase holoenzyme before (heavy line) and after (light line) reaction with ethyl hydroperoxide. The frequency was 9.29 MHz, the modulation amplitude 20G, the power 4 mW and the temperature 10K. The inset presents a detailed scan of the g=2 region at 0.1 mW of the reacted sample.

REFERENCES

1. Arachidonic Acid Metabolism and Tumor Promotion (S.M. Fischer and T.J. Slagal eds.) Martinus Nijhoff Publishing, Boston, 1985.
2. Hemler, M.E., Cook, H.W.J and Lands, W.E.M. (1979) Arch. Biochem. Biophys. 193: 340-345.
3. Hamberg, M. and Samuelsson, B. (1967) J. Biol. Chem. 242: 5336-5343.
4. Kulmacz, R.J. and Lands, W.E.M (1985) Prostaglandins 29, 175-190.
5. Ogino, N., Ohki, S., Yamamoto, S., and Hayaishi, O. (1978) J. Biol. Chem. 253: 5061-5068.
6. Kulmacz, R.J. and Lands, W.E.M. (1985) J Biol. Chem. 260: 12572-12578.
7. Kulmacz, R.J. and Lands, W.E.M. (1983) Prostaglandins 25: 531-540.
8. Kulmacz, R.J and Lands, W.E.M (1987) in Prostaglandins and Related Substances (Benedetto, C., McDonald-Gibson, R.G., Nigam, S., and Slater T F., eds.) pp 209-227, IRL Press, Washington DC.
9. Marshall, P.J. and Kulmacz, R.J. (1988) Arch. Biochem. Biophys. 266, 162-170.
10. Kulmacz, R.J. (1986) Arch. Biochem. Biophys. 249: 273-285.
11. Kulmacz, R J (1989) J. Biol. Chem 264: 14136-14144.
12. Kulmacz, R.J. (1989) Prostaglandins 38: 277-288.
13. Chen, Y.-N., Bienkowski, M.J., and Marnett, L.J. (1987) J. Biol. Chem. 262: 16892-16899.
14. Kulmacz, R.J., Miller, J.F., Jr., and Lands, W.E.M. (1985) Biochem, Biophys. Res. Commun. 130: 918-923.
15. Karthein, R., Dietz, R., Nastainczyk, W., and Ruf, H.H. (1988) Eur. J. Biochem. 171: 313-320.

KINETIC BASIS FOR THE IMPAIRED OXYGENATION OF EICOSAPENTAENOATE BY PROSTAGLANDIN ENDOPEROXIDE SYNTHASE

R.B. PENDLETON and W.E.M. LANDS

Department of Biological Chemistry, University of Illinois at Chicago, Chicago, Illinois 60612

Prostaglandin endoperoxide synthase (PES) oxygenates certain 20-carbon polyunsaturated fatty acids as the first committed step in the biosynthesis of prostaglandins. Both steroidal and non-steroidal anti-inflammatory agents inhibit prostaglandin biosynthesis, and therefore, it has been postulated that prostaglandin overproduction may be a pathophysiologic mechanism common to a number of chronic inflammatory and thromboembolic diseases. Epidemiologic studies have shown that many eicosanoid-related diseases are prevalent in populations that consume large amounts of n-6 polyunsaturated fatty acids (n-6 PUFA), but less frequent in populations that consume large amounts of n-3 PUFA. As neither n-3 nor n-6 PUFA can be synthesized de novo in human tissues, the common substrate acids for prostaglandin biosynthesis must be derived from the diet. The n-3 PUFA, 5,8,11,14,17-eicosapentaenoic acid (20:5n-3), is a less effective substrate for PES than the n-6 PUFA, 5,8,11,14-eicosatetraenoic acid (20:4n-6 or arachidonate). Therefore, it has also been postulated that the overproduction of prostaglandins may be inhibited by dietary n-3 polyunsaturated fatty acids [1].

PES has two distinct catalytic activities: (1) a cyclooxygenase activity that inserts two molecules of oxygen into 20:4n-6 to form the endoperoxy-hydroperoxide PGG_2, or into 20:5n-3 to form PGG_3 and (2) a peroxidase activity that reduces the 15-hydroperoxide of PGG_2 or PGG_3 to form PGH_2 or PGH_3, respectively. In addition to fatty acid and oxygen substrates, the PES cyclooxygenase activity requires the continuous presence of hydroperoxide activator, and the cyclooxygenase reaction mechanism is thought to require a meta-stable, radical-enzyme intermediate (E^*) [2]. Apparently one important function of the peroxidase activity is to generate this enzyme intermediate [3].

Figure 1 shows a proposed kinetic model of PES that integrates much of the knowledge about the cyclooxygenase and peroxidase activities. Ground state enzyme (E) reacts with hydroperoxide (ROOH, usually PGG) at the k_1 step to form EOH, an oxidized enzyme species analogous to compound I of other heme dependent peroxidases. EOH can be reduced by a single molecule of peroxidase co-substrate (AH_2) to EO, analogous to compound II, or can inactivate via k_{D6} to dead enzyme (EDD). The EOH intermediate is believed to contain a tyrosine free-radical [2] and can be converted to the active cyclooxygenase intermediate (E^*) via step k_4, or can be reduced back to ground state via step k_{3P}. E^* may have three possible fates: it can be reduced to ground state via k_{10P}; it can react with oxygen and

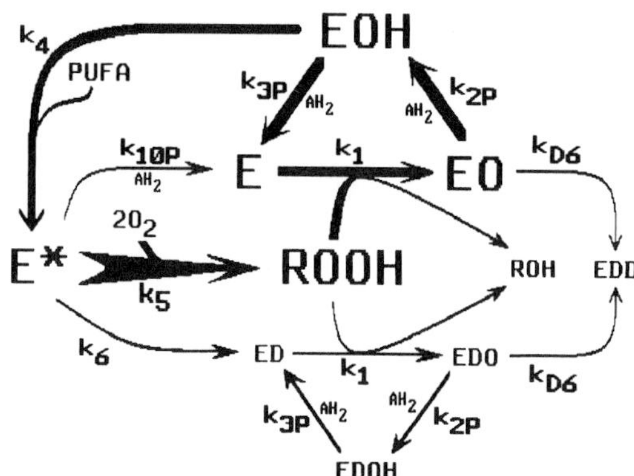

Figure 1 Kinetic model of PES oxygenation of polyunsaturated fatty acids (PUFA). Bold arrows trace the steps in peroxide (ROOH) stimulated autocatalysis. The large central arrow (k_5) represents evolution of the first reaction product, PGG. AH_2 is peroxidase cosubstrate (e.g. phenol).

fatty acid to produce hundreds or thousands of molecules of PGG (represented as step k_5); or it can inactivate via k_6 to a species that lacks cyclooxygenase activity, but retains peroxidase activity (ED) [4].

Cyclooxygenase inactivation (k_6) is distinct from the peroxidase inactivation (k_{D6}) and can account for the observation that after 120 seconds of reaction with arachidonate, about 95% of the cyclooxygenase activity is inactive, whereas about 70% of the peroxidase activity remains intact. The ED species can only react as a peroxidase (ED to EDO to EDOH to ED), and has the same kinetic rate constants as the primary peroxidase cycle (E to EO to EOH to E).

To study the validity and utility of the proposed model, the kinetic rate equations generated from Figure 1 were numerically integrated using the flux-tolerance method [5]. A computer program (OXYSIM) was written to allow for systematic study of the predicted effect of varying each kinetic rate constant [6]. Initially, the magnitudes of each of the eight kinetic constants were estimated from experimental data or taken from published results, and the effects of independently varying each constant on the oxygen consumption curve was determined. Figure 2 shows the effects of variations in the cyclooxygenase inactivation constant k_6. By carefully varying each kinetic constant, a fit was then obtained with experimentally determined time course of oxygen consumption. Figure 3 shows the surprisingly accurate prediction of the model for oxygenation of 20:4n-6, using the values for each constant given in the legend.

The oxygenation of fatty acids by PES is enzyme limited, and only 20 to 25% as much prostaglandin is produced using the substrate 20:5n-3 compared with 20:4n-6 [7]. As a first step to understanding the impaired oxygenation of 20:5n-3, PGG_2 and PGG_3 were synthesized and tested for their ability to stimulate PES in the presence of cyanide ion, a reversible hydroperoxide antagonist. Both cyclic-endoperoxy-hydroperoxides were found to be equally effective as activators of PES and

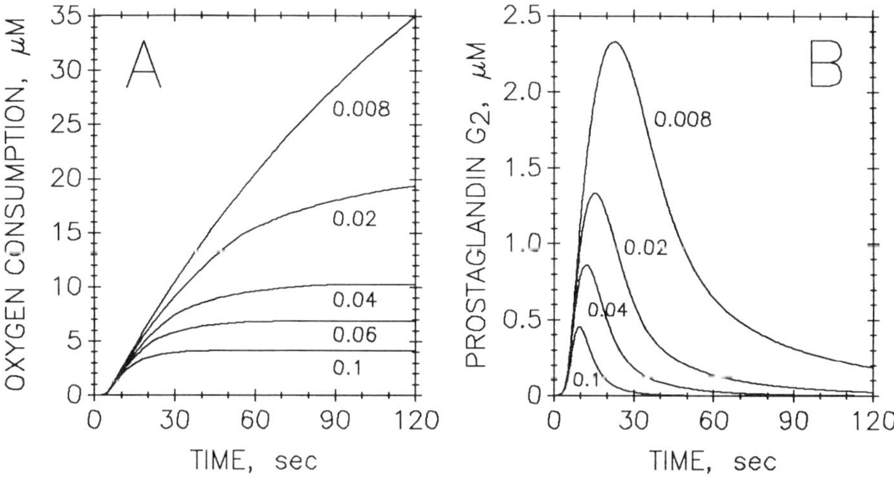

Figure 2. Simulated PES reaction kinetics: systematic variation of the rate of cyclooxygenase inactivation (k_6) on oxygen consumption (A) and PGG_2 reaction levels (B). Kinetic parameters for OXYSIM: EO=$8.5X10^{-9}$; ROOHO=$2.5X10^{-9}$; AH_2=$1X10^{-3}$; k_1=$72X10^6$; k_{2P}=$1.3X10^6$; k_{3P}=$13X10^6$; k_4=1300; k_5=26.5; k_{D6}= $12X10^{-3}$; k_{10P}=20; with BITE=0.2 [5].

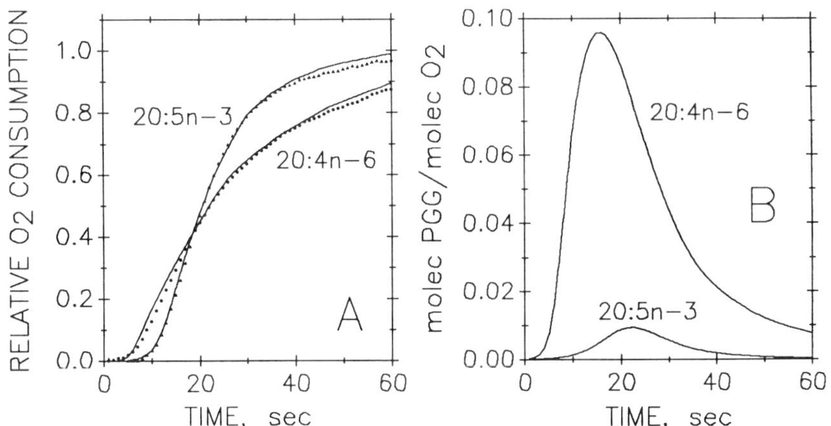

Figure 3. PES reaction kinetics: comparison of experimental (symbols) and simulated (lines) oxygen consumption (A) and PGG reaction levels (B). The impaired production of PGG_3 may account for the observed sensitivity of the 20:5n-3 reaction to suppression by glutathione peroxidase [6]. Kinetic parameters of the 20:4n-6 reaction were given in Figure 2, with k_6=0.031. For 20:5n-3: k_5=5.8 and k_6=0.068. The experimental and simulation methods are fully described in reference 5. Relative oxygen consumption equals oxygen consumption divided by total oxygen consumed at 120 seconds.

therefore the kinetics for recruitment of E* (E to EO to EOH to E* i.e., steps k_1, k_{2P}, k_{3P}, k_4, and k_{D6}) was likely to be similar or identical for both acids. To test this hypothesis, the peroxidase rate constant, k_1, was experimentally determined, and was found to be nearly identical for reaction of PES with PGG_2, PGG_3, and 15-HPETE (18 ± 4 M^{-1} sec^{-1}). Since this constant characteristics the rate of reaction between hydroperoxide and PES, it was considered to be the most sensitive to structural properties of the hydroperoxide activator. The curve fitting process was then repeated for oxygenation of 20:5n-3, however, only k_5, k_6, and k_{10P} were varied. Surprisingly, we found that only a 4.6-fold decrease in k_5 and a 2.2-fold increase in k_6 was necessary to simulate the 20:5n-3 reaction (Figure 3).

The results of these kinetic modeling studies indicate that the relatively low reactivity of PES with 20:5n-3 may result from an impaired interaction of the n-3 acid with the enzyme radical intermediate, E*, that activates the oxygenation reaction. Eicosapentaenoate differs from arachidonate only by the presence of one additional double bond at the 17 (n-3) position. Even though this part of the molecule is not modified during the oxygenation reaction, it appears that the additional structural rigidity in the alkyl chain imposed by this bond prevents optimal orientation of the acid in the enzyme's active site and results in a decreased rate of oxygen insertion (decreased k_5), and an increased rate of cyclooxygenase inactivation (increased k_6). These data may provide a detailed mechanistic rationale for the proposed health benefits of dietary n-3 polyunsaturated acids.

ACKNOWLEDGEMENT

This work was supported in part by a grant from the USPHS (HL-34422), an MSTP Fellowship (RBP), and a Pfizer Biomedical Research Award (WEML).

REFERENCES

1. W.E.M. Lands. 1986. Fish and Human Health. Academic Press, Orlando, FL.
2. Stubbe, J.A. 1989. Protein Radical Involvement in Biological Catalysis? Annu. Rev. Biochem., 58, 257-285.
3. Kulmacz, R.J., Miller, J.F. Jr., and Lands, W.E.M. 1985. Prostaglandin H Synthase: An Example of Enzymic Symbiosis. Biochem. Biophys. Res. Commun., 130, 918-923.
4. Kulmacz, R.J. 1987. Prostaglandin G_2 Levels During Reaction of Prostaglandin H Synthase with Arachidonic Acid. Prostaglandins, 34, 225-240.
5 Barshop, B.A., Wrenn, R.F., and Frieden, C. 1983. Analysis of Numerical Methods for Computer Simulation of Kinetic Processes: Development of KINSIM - A Flexible, Portable System. Anal. Biochem., 130, 134-145.
6 Pendleton, R.B. 1989. Hydroperoxide Stimulation of Prostaglandin Endoperoxide Synthase. Doctoral Thesis, University of Illinois, Urbana-Champaign.
7. Lands, W.E.M. and Pendleton, R.B. 1989. n-3 Fatty Acids and Hydroperoxide Activation of Fatty Acid Oxygenases. In: Oxygen Radicals in Biology and Medicine (Simic, Ward, and Taylor, eds.). Plenum Pub. Corp., pp 675-681.

BIOCHEMISTRY OF OXIDANT INJURY

I.U. SCHRAUFSTATTER, J.H. JACKSON, O. QUEHENBERGER, and C.G. COCHRANE

Department of Immunology, Research Institute of Scripps Clinic, La Jolla, CA 92037

INTRODUCTION

Neutrophils attracted to an area of inflammation are stimulated to produce O_2-, the degradation products of which (H_2O_2, ·OH, HOCl, etc.) are potent bactericidal as well as cytotoxic agents. In order to determine the pathways of oxidative injury, target cells were exposed to various oxidizing agents. This report will only be concerned with the effect of H_2O_2. In order to simplify the determination of kinetics a single bolus of reagent H_2O_2 was used.

DNA DAMAGE CAUSED BY H_2O_2

It has been known for a long time that ·OH causes the formation of DNA strand breaks in isolated DNA (1). It is also well established that H_2O_2 can diffuse into cells where it can form ·OH in a Fenton-type reaction as soon as it encounters transition metal. Hence it is not surprising that H_2O_2 in concentrations between 20-120 uM causes DNA strand breaks - determined by alkaline unwinding - in various target cells (2,3). These DNA strand breaks are prevented by extracellular catalase as well as by cell-permeable iron chelators (2,3). Iron chelators which do not penetrate cells (DETAPAC, short term incubation with desferal) did not prevent DNA strand break formation in whole cells, nor did ·OH scavengers prevent DNA strand break formation in intact cells, in contrast to their protective effect in isolated DNA. Presumably, a DNA-transition metal-H_2O_2 complex forms ·OH in a site-directed reaction (4). Table 1 (from Ref. 2), summarizes the effect of various scavengers on H_2O_2 induced DNA strand break formation in P388D1 cells. Cellular H_2O_2 degrading pathways - primarily catalase attenuated the effect of H_2O_2 on DNA strand break formation. An inverse correlation was found between H_2O_2 degrading capacity of various cell types and their susceptibility to DNA strand breaks (2). From these results it appears that a small fraction of H_2O_2 reaches the nucleus without being degraded on the way there, and leads to site-directed ·OH formation in the presence of transition metal.

To prove that ·OH was involved in H_2O_2 induced DNA damage, DNA base hydroxylations were determined. Formation of 8-hydroxydeoxyguanosine could be detected in whole cells exposed to H_2O_2 or other oxidants (2,5). Formation of various other base hydroxylations was shown by GC-mass spectroscopy in isolated calf thymus DNA exposed to phorbol myristate acetate stimulated neutrophils or H_2O_2 + Fe^{2+}/EGTA (6). DNA base hydroxylations were identical in quality as well as relative quantity to those previously published for $\overline{X}$-irradiation (7). The products detected were 8-hydroxyguanine, 2,6-

Table 1
Influence of Oxidant Scavengers on the Formation of H2O2-induced DNA Strand Breaks in P388D1 Cells

Scavenged species	Scavenger	Concentration	% Inhibition of DNA strand breaks
O_2^-	SOD	1 mg/ml	0
	TIRON	10 mM	0
	CuDIPS	20 μM	-9
H_2O_2	Catalase	5,000 U	100
·OH	DMTU	800 mM	0
	DMSO	1 M	36
	DMSO	0.1 M	3
	Ethanol	0.33 M	-10
	Na-benzoate	0.1 M	8
	Mannitol	0.5 M	0
	Salicylate	2 mM	5
	DMPO	0.1 M	25
Fe chelator	DFO (15 min incubation)	100 μM	1
	DFO (overnight incubation)	100 μM	86
	DFT	100 μM	90
	DTPA	100 μM	-5
	Phenanthroline	100 μM	74
Lipid Peroxides	Vitamin E (overnight preincubation)	20 μM	4

diamino-4-hydroxy-5-formamidopyrimidine, 8-hydroxyadenine, 4,6-diamino-5-formamidopyrimidine, thymine glycol, and cytosine glycol. It thus appears that neutrophils or macrophages attracted into an area of inflammation cause radiomimetic DNA damage. This may explain the increased incidence of malignancies in areas of chronic inflammation associated e.g. with ulcerative colitis, tuberculosis, osteomyelitis and schistosomiasis. Experimentally, it has been shown that stimulated neutrophils or xanthine oxidase/hypoxanthine can induce transformed foci in C3HIOT1/2 cells (8) which induce tumors in nude mice (9).

EFFECT OF H_2O_2 ON CELLULAR METABOLISM

Formation of DNA strand breaks activates poly-ADP-ribose polymerase (10,11), a nuclear enzyme which catabolizes NAD into nicotinamide and ADP-ribose, and then forms poly-ADP-ribose polymers which are attached to various nuclear proteins, e.g. histones and the polymerase itself. Kinetically, increased poly-ADP-ribose polymer formation went parallel with DNA strand break formation, and decreased as soon as DNA strand breaks were repaired. Since the turnover of ADP-ribose polymer is very high - in the order of 1 min - a major consequence of activation of poly-ADP-ribose polymerase is depletion of cellular NAD (12,13). P388DI cells exposed to 100 uM H_2O_2 lost 72% of their NAD within 10 min. Under various conditions of NAD depletion due to this pathway, consequent loss of ATP has been observed (12,14), although the mechanisms involved are not clear. Correlations between NAD and ATP depletion are, however, striking: When 7 different cell types were compared, the threshold for ATP depletion in all cells was about 60% NAD depletion. The more sensitive a particular cell was to DNA strand breaks and NAD depletion, the more sensitive it was to loss of ATP.

Addition of inhibitors of poly-ADP-ribose-polymerase (2.5 mM 3-aminobenzamide, 5 mM nicotinamide) prevented the fall of ATP with low concentrations of H_2O_2 (50-150 uM) (15). With higher concentrations of H_2O_2, the situation becomes more complicated, since H_2O_2 can directly inhibit glycolytic ATP synthesis due to inactivation of glyceraldehyde-3-phosphate dehydrogenase (16) as well as mitochondrial respiration with the ATPase (16) as its primary target. Inactivation of glyceraldehyde-3-phosphate dehydrogenase is both direct - due to disulfide formation at its active site (cys 149 - cys 153) and indirect - due to the low NAD/NADH ratio following NAD depletion. The NAD independent pathways cannot, however, account for ATP depletion at concentrations of H_2O_2 lower than 150 uM.

Since NAD synthesis from nicotinamide is ATP dependent, it appeared that ATP depletion was at least partially due to highly increased NAD synthesis. To determine this possibility, P388DI cells exposed to 150 uM H_2O_2 were pulsed with ^{3}H-adenine for 5 min intervals, and nucleotides were separated by HPLC. Between 5 and 10 min both ATP depletion and NAD synthesis were maximal. Assuming 1 mole of ATP used per mole of NAD formed NAD synthesis could account for at least 50% of the ATP lost.

With higher concentrations of H_2O_2 various other cellular pathways are disturbed, leading e.g. to an increase in free intracellular Ca^{2+} (17), and finally causing cell lysis (18). The effects of H_2O_2 on target cells are summarized in Figure 1.

DNA strand break formation (19), activation of poly-ADP-ribose polymerase (12) as well as ATP depletion (20) have all been observed in target cells exposed to stimulated neutrophils, and were largely inhibitable by catalase, indicating that the concentrations of H_2O_2 formed in these experiments were within the range produced by activated phagocytes.

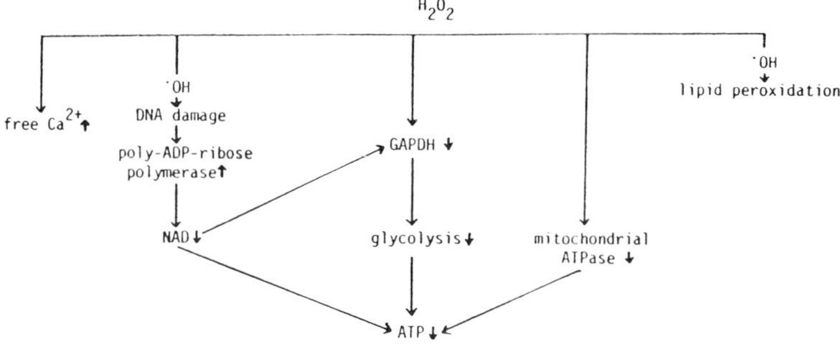

Figure 1.

EFFECT OF H_2O_2 ON ACTIVATION OF CA^{2+}-DEPENDENT ENDONUCLEASE

It has been suggested that DNA strand break formation in cells exposed to oxidants is Ca^{2+} dependent (21,22). It is, however, unlikely that increased free Ca^{2+} is involved in the DNA strand break formation described above. 1) Strand breaks occurred with concentrations of H_2O_2 (e.g.50 uM) and at time-points (30 sec) at which no increase in intracellular Ca^{2+} could be detected. 2) EGTA did not prevent DNA strand break formation, and 3) inhibitors of poly-ADP-ribose polymerase prevented the rise in intracellular free Ca^{2+}, but not the formation of DNA strand breaks (15). DNA degradation can, however, also be due to Ca^{2+}-dependent endonuclease activation (23), and if concentrations of H_2O_2 are used that will cause an increase in intracellular free Ca^{2+} (250 uM H_2O_2 in bovine endothelial cells), endonuclease activation can indeed be observed. Activation of this endonuclease leads to degradation of DNA into nucleosomal-size fragments. These fragments are observed within 3 hours after the addition of H_2O_2, and are inhibitable by EGTA, the calmodulin inhibitor calmidazolium as well as by 100 uM $ZnSO_4$, an inhibitor of the endonuclease 3-aminobenzamide - which does not prevent the formation of DNA strand breaks - also protects from endonuclease activation. Fe-chelators (e.g. phenanthroline) which protect from the initial strand break formation, similarly prevent activation of endonuclease. It hence appears, that severe DNA damage due to •OH formation, initiates a cascade of events leading to increase of free cellular Ca^{2+} and causing activation of Ca^{2+} dependent endonuclease.

CONCLUSION

The data presented indicate that H_2O_2 induced toxicity to target cells is largely a consequence of the initial formation of DNA damage. In this respect, H_2O_2 produced during the respiratory burst of activated phagocytes, an obligatory defense mechanism to fight microbial infection, mimicks the deleterious effect of ionizing radiation.

REFERENCES

1. In: Effects of ionizing radiation on DNA, Ed. Huttermann, J., Kohnlein, W., Teoule, R., Bertinchamp, A.J., Springer Verlag, Berlin, 1978.
2. Schraufstatter, I., Hyslop, P.A., Jackson, J.H., and Cochrane C.G. J. Clin. Invest. 82:1040-1050, 1988.
3. Filho, A.C.M., and Meneghini, R. Biochim. Biophys. Acta 847:82-89, 1985.
4. Yamamoto, K., Kawanishi, S. J. Biol. Chem. 264:15435-15440, 1989.
5. Floyd, R.A., Watson, J.J., Harris, J., West, M. and Wong, P.K. Biochem. Biophys. Res. Commun. 137:841-846
6. Jackson, J.H., Gajewski, E., Schraufstatter, I.U., Hyslop, P.A., Fuciarelli, A.F., Dizdaroglu, M., and Cochrane, C.G. J. Clin. Invest. 84:1644-1649, 1989.
7. Dizdaroglu, M., and Bergtold, D.S. Anal. Biochem. 156:182-188, 1986.
8. Cerutti, P.A. Science 227:375-381, 1985.
9. Weitzman, S.A., Weitberg, A.B., Clark, E.P., and Stossel T.P. Science. 227:1231-1233, 1985.
10. Benjamin, R.C., Gill, D.M., J. Biol. Chem. 255:10502-10508, 1980.
11. Smulson, M.E., Sugimura, T. Methods Enzymol. 106:438-440, 1984.
12. Schraufstatter, I.U., Hinshaw, D.B., Hyslop, P.A., Spragg, R.G., and Cochrane, C.G., J. Clin. Invest. 77:1312-1320, 1986.
13. Wielckens, K.E., Schmidt, A., George, E., Bredehorst, R., and Hilz, H. J. Biol. Chem. 258:4098-4104, 1983.

14. Sims, J.L., Berger, S.L., and Berger, N.A. Biochemistry 258:5188-5194, 1983.
15. Schraufstatter, I.U., Hyslop. P.A., Hinshaw, D.B., Spragg, R.G., Sklar, L.A., and Cochrane, C.G. Proc. Natl. Acad. Sci. 83:4908-4912, 1986.
16. Hyslop, P.A., Hinshaw, D.B., Halsey, W.A., Schraufstatter, I.U., Sauerheber, R.D., Spragg, R.G., Jackson, J.H., and Cochrane, C.G. J. Biol. Chem. 263:1665-1675, 1988.
17. Hyslop, P.A., Hinshaw, D.B., Schraufstatter, I.U., Sklar, L.A., Spragg, R.G., and Cochrane, C.G. J. Cell. Physiol. 129:356-366, 1986.
18. Schraufstatter, I.U., Hinshaw, D.B., Hyslop, P.A., Spragg, R.G., and Cochrane, C.G. J. Clin. Invest. 76:1131-1139, 1985.
19. Birnboim, H.C. Science. 215:1247-1249, 1982.
20. Spragg, R.G., Hinshaw, D.B., Hyslop, P.A., Schraufstatter, I.U., and Cochrane, C.G. J. Clin. Invest. 76:1471-1476, 1985.
21. Jones, D.B., McConkey, D.J., Nicotera, P., and Orrenius, S. J. Biol. Chem. 264:6398-6403, 1989.
22. Ochi, T., and Cerutti, P.A. Proc. Natl. Acad. Sci. 84:990-994, 1987.
23. Smith, C.A., Williams, G.T., Kingston, R., Jenkinson, E.J., and Owen, J.J.T. Nature 337:181-184, 1989.

EFFECTS OF DIETARY FISH OIL AND CORN OIL ON PROTEIN KINASE C DISTRIBUTION IN THE COLON

R. NELSON and O. HOLIAN

Department of Surgery, University of Illinois College of Medicine at Chicago, P.O. Box 6998, Chicago, Illinois 60680 USA

INTRODUCTION

The role of dietary fat in colorectal cancer causation has been problematic. Though cross cultural epidemiologic studies have shown a high correlation between quantity of fat consumption and national cancer rates, within population epidemiologic studies have been far less consistent. Only 7 case control studies have shown a positive correlation between fat consumption and colorectal cancer risk, 10 have not. None of the 4 prospective cohort studies, the strongest epidemiologic tool, have shown a positive correlation. Amongst the strongest epidemiologic evidence for fat as a risk factor is the study of Japanese migrants to Hawaii, where cancer risk in the migrant population has been shown to be associated with increased fat consumption, when compared to low risk Japanese still residing in the same region in Japan. Yet a cohort of that population of Japanese migrants residing in Hawaii followed prospectively has increased their colorectal cancer risk well beyond resident whites, while still consuming almost 25% less fat. For some anatomic sites, the risk of cancer was inversely proportional to fat intake. (1)

Because of these inconsistencies, the specific nature of fat consumed has been examined, principally experimentally. Most fat sources have been found to effect risk in a similar manner (2,3), though fish oil has not (4,5,6,7). Though epidemiologic evidence is sparse (8), all available evidence, epidemiologic and experimental, suggests that diets high in fish oil are associated with diminished colorectal cancer risk. There is good biochemical rationale to suppose that fish oil, rich in omega-3 fatty acid, would be less likely to induce or promote cancer than other unsaturated fats such as corn oil, which is rich in omega-6 fatty acid (6). However the specific mechanism by which different dietary fat sources can create physiologic changes that increase or decrease cancer risk has not been described.

We have chosen to investigate the effect of dietary fish oil and corn oil on the activity and subcellular distribution of Protein Kinase C (PKC). This enzyme is a likely mediator of the dietary tumor promoters (of which fat is one) because it plays a key role in intracellular signal transduction, is a mediator of cellular proliferative rate and is the only known receptor of an important class of tumor promoters, the phorbol esters. Its activity and localization are also effected by known physiologic tumor promoters in the colon, the bile acids (9). The effect of these dietary fat sources on PKC was investigated in the rat colon in the absence of colon specific carcinogen (1,2 dimethylhydrazine (DMH)), in rats that had been pretreated with DMH and in rats that had DMH treatment subsequent to the addition of these fats to their diets.

MATERIALS AND METHODS

21 male 5 week old Sprague-Dawley rats were randomly divided into 7 groups, 3 rats each, as follows:

1 - Rat Chow alone (Purina powdered chow Cat. #5012).
2 - Rat Chow + Corn oil, 17% by weight; total fat calories 40%.
3 - Rat Chow + Fish oil, 17% by weight.
4 - DMH, 5 weekly injections 20 mg base/kg body weight, intraperitoneally, followed by Corn oil diet as above.
5 - DMH as above followed by Fish oil as above.
6 - Corn oil as above for 3 weeks, followed by DMH as above, while the Corn oil diet was maintained to the end of the study.
7 - Fish oil as above followed by DMH as above.

All rats were sacrificed by carbon dioxide asphyxiation at the 13th week of the study, their colons removed, cleaned of feces and pericolic fat and flash frozen in liquid nitrogen. The activity of PKC in the soluble and particulate fractions of the colon was measured as described previously (10), by transfer of 32P from 32P-gamma ATP histones and expressed as picomoles/mg cellular protein (Lowry)/ minute. All colons were separated and duplicate assays performed. Results of soluble, particulate and total PKC activity, as well as the soluble/particulate PKC activity ratio (S/P PKC) were compared between groups by ANOVA, and when significant differences were found, by paired t-tests.

RESULTS

Results of PKC assays are presented in the Table below.

		PKC in pmoles/mg protein/min					
GROUP	N	SUPERNATANT		PARTICULATE		TOTAL	
1	5	32.46	+/- 9.8	110.32	+/- 34.2	142.78	+/- 35.3
2	4	43.55	9.8	192.55	16.3	236.1	13.1
3	6	51.23	23.5	220.22	39.6	271.45	46.9
4	4	40.76	13.4	196.4	43.2	237.18	53.2
5	4	61.65	36	164.2	53.2	225.85	88.5
6	4	40.96	23.3	200.68	97.5	241.65	120.2
7	3	34.47	20.4	110.43	53.6	144.9	72.8
ANOVA,	**p=**	**0.52**		**0.019**		**0.052**	

	S/P PXC Ratio	
1	0.316	+/- 0.11
2	0.229	0.07
3	0.238	0.1
4	0.208	0.04
5	0.357	0.09
6	0.199	0.03
7	0.305	0.06

ANOVA, p= 0.076

N represents the number of assays, optimally 3 rats per group and 2 assays per rat, however several rats died before sacrifice, and two outlier assay results were not tabulated. Values for PKC activity are means +/- standard deviations for the groups. Looking at the results of the ANOVA and the subsequent paired t-tests, there were no differences between groups in soluble PKC activity. In the absence of DMH treatment, corn oil (CO) and fish oil (FO) equivalently increased particulate and total PKC activity, which can best be seen in the diminished S/P PKC ratio (Groups 2 & 3). When rats were pretreated with DMH, CO similarly increased particulate PKC and lowered the S/P PKC ratio (Group 4), though FO did so less and maintained a high S/P PKC ratio (Group 5) as is seen in a low fat (6% by weight) rat chow diet (Group 1). In rats given the test diets prior to DMH treatment, CO once again augmented particulate and total PKC activity, while decreasing the S/P PKC ratio (Group 6). However FO rats had no augmentation of particulate PKC activity when compared to low fat controls and the S/P PKC ratio remained high (Group 7) as in low fat controls (Group 1).

DISCUSSION

Several studies in experimental animals have demonstrated that FO (or its constituent omega-3 fatty acid) diminishes colorectal cancer induction when compared to CO (or its constituent omega-6 fatty acid). Reddy showed diminished tumor incidence and yield in FO fed rats compared to CO fed rats, though in his initial study, the standard deviations were greater than the means and the FO group weighed significantly less than the CO group (4). This is a particular problem, as weight gain in experimental studies is a major determinant of risk independent of other factors (11). In a subsequent study by Reddy, varying ratios of FO and CO were compared for colorectal tumor induction, with equivalent weight gain in all groups, presumably through the avoidance of essential fatty acid deficiency, and FO was found again to be protective (5). Nelson found that FO resulted in significant decrease in tumor yield when compared to CO in rats fed crude rat chow diets that avoided nutritional deficiencies and which resulted in equal group weight at sacrifice (6). Minoura compared supplementation with eicosapentaenoic acid (EPA) versus linoleic acid in a similar rat colorectal carcinogenesis study and found again that there was significant protection with EPA.

Epidemiologic support for the protective effect of FO paradoxically came after the initiation of these studies from the Melbourne colorectal cancer case/control study. In that study, there were 715 cases of cancer, 727 community controls and 159 hospital controls. The relative risk of getting colorectal cancer, when comparing fish consumption between cases and controls was 0.58 (8).

The evidence that PKC is a mediator of tumor promotion is strong. Changes in the subcellular localization of the enzyme have been associated with increased mucosal proliferation in the colon and increased reactive oxygen formation, both vital elements of promotion. Phorbol esters can directly induce this translocation and bile acids, known physiologic colon tumor promoters, can do so indirectly (9). PKC was therefore an obvious choice when seeking an enzymatic mechanism for the action of dietary modulators of tumor promotion. What we have shown in this study is that in the absence of carcinogen, FO and CO have no difference in their effect on PKC activity; they both augment translocation and total activity. FO given before or after DMH treatment can however be clearly distinguished from CO in its effect on particulate and total PKC activity as well as the ratio of soluble to particulate PKC activity, in the direction of that seen in a low fat diet. Based on these data we feel that:

1. Epidemiologic inconsistencies relating fat consumption to colorectal cancer risk may have arisen from the failure to delineate dietary fat sources; not just saturated versus unsaturated, but also the specific nature of the unsaturated fat source.

2. The mechanism by which FO diminishes colorectal cancer risk compared with CO may be mediated through the effect of dietary fats on PKC activity.

3. Further studies investigating the effect of eicosanoids on tumor induction should include the very important signal transducers, especially PKC, in vitro and in human populations.

ACKNOWLEDGMENT

We are grateful to Cathy Ruiz and Ed Robins for valuable technical assistance This work was supported by the Washington Square Health Foundation.

REFERENCES

1. Stemmerman G. In Colorectal Cancer: From Pathology to Prevention? (Ed.s Seitz HK, Simanowski UA and Wright NA). Springer Verlag. Berlin. 1989. pp. 3-23.
2. Rogers AE and Nauss KM. Dig. Dis. & Sci. 30. 87s-102s. 1985.
3. Reddy BS and Maruyama H. JNCI. 77. 815-822. 1986.
4. Reddy BS and Maruyama H. Can. Res. 46. 3367-70. 1986.
5. Reddy BS and Sugie S. Can. Res. 48. 6642-47. 1988.
6. Nelson RL, Tanure JC, Andrianopoulos G, Souza G and Lands WEM. Nutr. & Cancer. 11. 215-220. 1988.
7. Minoura T, Takata T, Sakaguchi M, Takada H, Yamamura M, Hioki K and Yamamoto M. Can. Res. 48. 4790-94. 1988.
8. Kune S., Kune GA and Watson LF. Nutr. & Cancer. 9. 21-42. 1987.
9. Craven PA, Pfanstiel J and DeRubertis FR. J. Clin. Invest. 79. 532-541. 1987.
10. Hirota K, Hirota H, Aguilera G and Catt KJ. J. Biol. Chem. 260. 3243-3246. 1985.
11. Albanes D. Nutr. & Cancer. 9. 199-217. 1987.

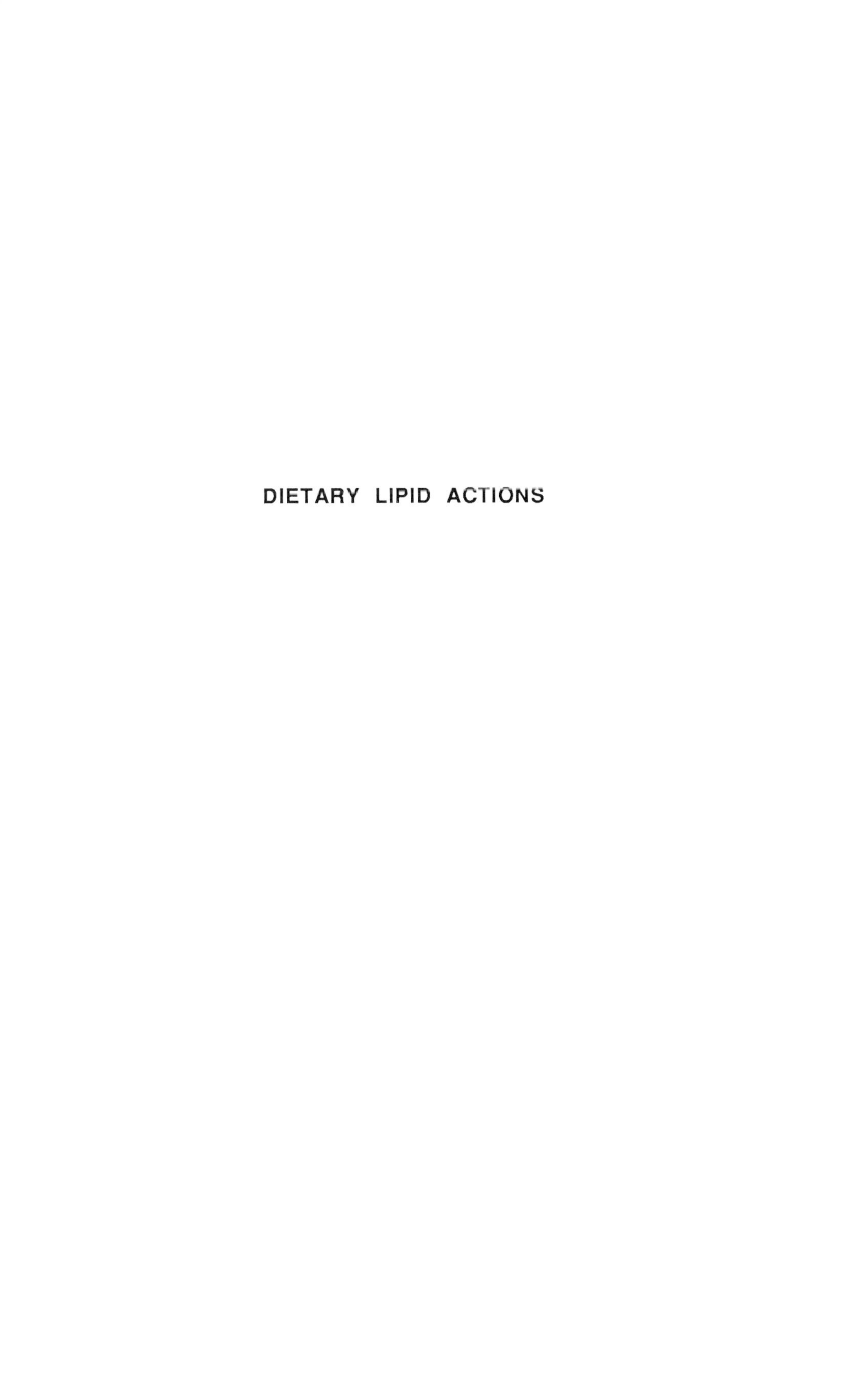

DIETARY LIPID ACTIONS

DIETARY FAT AND MAMMARY GLAND DEVELOPMENTAL GROWTH IN THE IMMATURE FEMALE MOUSE

C. W. WELSCH

Department of Pharmacology and Toxicology, Michigan State University, East Lansing, MI 48824

ABSTRACT

The purpose of this study was to determine whether or not the type of dietary fat can affect mammary gland growth processes in the immature female Balb/c mouse. Groups of immature mice were fed one of the following semi-synthetic diets containing different types of fat, i.e., 5 vegetable oil diets (5% corn oil, 20% corn oil, 20% olive oil, 20% linseed oil, 19% coconut oil-1% corn oil), 2 animal fat diets (20% lard, 19% beef tallow-1% corn oil) and 1 fish oil diet (19% Menhaden oil-1% corn oil). In addition, fishcorn oil diets (20%) containing 3 different levels of corn oil (15%, 10%, 4.5%) and fish oil (5%, 10%, 15.5%) were also examined in these studies. Immature mice were fed these diets from 21 to 45 days of age, ovariectomized at 35 days of age, injected daily with 17β-estradiol (1 μg) and progesterone (1 mg) on day 42-44 and sacrificed on day 45. Mammary ductal expansive growth through the mammary fat pad (mm, nipple to farthest end bud) was determined on the inguinal (no. 4) mammary glands. In mice fed the fish oil diets (19% Menhaden oil-1% corn oil, 15.5% Menhaden oil-4.5% corn oil, 10% Menhaden oil-10% corn oil), significantly ($P<0.05$) reduced ductal expansive growth of the mammary gland was observed when compared to mice fed the 19-20% vegetable oil or animal fat diets. No significant difference in mammary gland growth was observed among the groups of mice fed the 19-20% vegetable oil or animal fat diets. In addition, significantly ($P<0.05$) reduced mammary gland ductal expansive growth was observed in mice fed the 5% corn oil diet compared to mice fed the 20% corn oil diet. Mean body weight gains among the dietary groups of mice were not significantly influenced by diet. Thus, among the fat diets examined in this study, only the animals fed the low fat diet (5% corn oil) or the fish oil diets (19% Menhaden oil-1% corn oil, 15.5% Menhaden oil-4.5% corn oil, 10% Menhaden oil-10% corn oil) had impaired (reduced) mammae development. The results of our study clearly demonstrate that developmental growth of the mammary gland in immature female mice can be significantly affected (impaired) by diet, but by only rather extreme dietary intervention, i.e., by reducing fat content by 75% (20% to 5%) or by feeding very high levels of certain fish oils (Menhaden) that are extremely rich in n-3 polyunsaturated fatty acids such as EPA and/or DHA.

INTRODUCTION

It has been reported by numerous laboratories that the amount and type of dietary fat can significantly influence the development and/or growth of mammary tumors in rodents (1). In this communication, we have extended these studies to determine whether or not the amount and type of dietary fat can affect normal mammary gland growth processes in the immature female Balb/c mouse. For these studies we have chosen to examine four vegetable oils (corn oil, olive oil, coconut oil and linseed oil), two animal fats (beef tallow and lard) and one fish oil (Menhaden oil). Each of these fats has marked differences in their fatty acid composition and often differ sharply in their ability to influence neoplastic mammary gland growth processes.

MATERIALS AND METHODS

A total of 158 nulliparous female Balb/c mice were used in these studies. The mice were obtained from Charles River Breeding Laboratories, Inc., Wilmington, MA. They were housed in a temperature-controlled (25.5±0.5°C) and light-controlled (14 h/day) room.

The diets used in these studies are purified semi-synthetic diets prepared in our laboratory every 2 weeks (fish diets weekly), stored in plastic bags containing nitrogen gas, and kept frozen prior to feeding. The composition of the diets are as previously described (2). All the diets are isocaloric, i.e., the proportions of protein, minerals, vitamins and fiber were adjusted to keep their ratio constant with respect to calories. All mice were fed ad libitum daily; non-consumed diet was discarded daily.

The diets and experimental design of this study are provided in Tables 1 and 2. At 45 days of age, all mice were sacrificed and their inguinal (no. 4) mammary glands were excised, fixed in glacial acetic acid:100% ethanol (1:3, v/v) and stained with alum carmine for whole-mount evaluation. Developmental growth of the mammary ducts were assessed in coded whole-mount preparations by measuring the linear distance (mm) of duct expansion through the mammary fat pad, from the nipple to the most distant mammary end bud. Distance of duct expansion (penetration) through the mammary fat pad was determined by a computer-assisted image analysis system (R & M Biometrics Corp., Nashville, TN). Multigroup mean comparisons were analyzed by one-way analysis of variance in concert with the Newman-Keuls multiple comparison test. Student's t-test was used when comparing paired group means.

RESULTS

There was no significant difference among the groups of mice fed the vegetable oil and/or animal fat diets in mean nipple to end bud distance (range, 8.99 to 10.59 mm) (Table 1) . Ductal expansive growth in mice fed the fish oil diet, however, was significantly ($P<0.05$) reduced (mean, 6.18 mm) when compared to ductal growth in animals fed the vegetable oil or animal fat diets (Table 1). In mice fed the low fat diet (corn oil, 5%), ductal growth was less (mean, 8.94 mm) than that of mice fed the high fat diet (corn oil, 20%) (mean, 10.59 mm) but this difference just missed the 5% level of statistical probability ($P<0.07$) (Table 1).

The effect of different ratios of dietary corn oil and fish oil on expansive growth of the ductal system in immature mice are shown in Table 2. Corn oil/fish oil dietary ratios of 10%/10% or 4.5%/15.5%,

Table 1
Influence of Dietary Fat on Mammary Gland Development in Immature Female Balb/c Mice

Treatment[a]	No. of mice	Mean body weight (termination)	Mean Mammary gland development growth-nipple to end buddistance (mm)
Corn oil (5%)	20	19.1 ± 0.4	8.94 ± 0.45[b]
Corn oil (20%)	20	20.1 ± 0.4	10.59 ± 0.43[b]
Olive oil (20%)	20	19.8 ± 0.8	9.51 ± 0.79[b]
Linseed oil (20%)	20	19.8 ± 0.7	9.31 ± 0.58[b]
Coconut oil (19%) + Corn oil (1%)	20	20.2 ± 0.5	9.18 ± 0.59[b]
Lard (20%)	20	19.9 ± 0.6	8.99 ± 0.61[b]
Beef tallow (19%) + Corn oil (1%)	18	20.0 ± 0.3	10.32 ± 0.63[b]
Menhaden oil (19%) + Corn oil (1%)	20	18.0 ± 0.4	6.18 ± 0.60[c]

[a]Female Balb/c mice were fed the diets from 21 to 45 days of age. At 35 days, all mice were ovariectomized. From 42-44 days of age, all mice were injected s.c. daily with 17β-estradiol (1 μg) and progesterone (1 mg). The mice were sacrificed at 45 days of age, both inguinal mammary glands (no. 4) were excised and examined for developmental growth. Data are expressed as means ± standard error.

[b/c], $P<0.05$

respectively, significantly ($P<0.05$) decreased nipple to end bud distance (mean, 10.73 mm, 10.93 mm, respectively) when compared to mice fed a 20% corn oil diet (mean, 12.79 mm). Mice fed the 5% corn oil diet had significantly ($P<0.05$) reduced nipple to end bud distances (mean, 10.91 mm) when compared to mice fed the 20% corn oil diet (mean, 12.79 mm).

DISCUSSION

In this study, high levels of corn oil, olive oil, coconut oil, linseed oil, lard, beef tallow and fish oil were fed to groups of immature female Balb/c mice. Only the mice fed the fish oil diets showed altered (impaired) mammary gland development. Importantly, no significant difference in mammae development was observed in groups of mice fed the other fat (oil) diets; ductal expansive growth among these groups of mice were indistinguishable.

Table 2
Interaction Between Dietary Corn Oil and Menhaden Oil on Mammary Gland Development in Immature Female Balb/c Mice

Treatment[a]	No. of mice	Mean body weight (termination)	Mean mammary gland developmental growth nipple to end bud distance (mm)
Corn oil (5%)	10	17.9 ± 0.4	10.91 ± 0.78[b]
Corn oil (20%)	10	17.8 ± 0.5	12.79 ± 0.47[c]
Corn oil (15%)/ Menhaden oil (5%)	10	18.3 ± 0.4	12.12 ± 0.62
Corn oil (10%)/ Menhaden oil (10%)	9	18.2 ± 0.6	10.73 ± 0.61[b]
Corn oil (4.5%)/ Menhaden oil (15.5%)	9	18.1 ± 0.6	10.93 ± 0.65[b]
Corn oil (19.75%)/ Menhaden oil (10.25%)	10	18.3 ± 0.5	11.30 ± 0.58

[a]Female Balb/c mice were fed the diets from 21 to 45 days of age. At 35 days of age, all mice were ovartiectomized. From 42-44 days of age, all mice were injected s.c. daily with 17β-estradiol (1 μg) and progesterone (1 mg). The mice were sacrificed at 45 days of age, both inguinal mammary glands (no. 4) were excised and examined for developmental growth. Data are expressed as means ± standard error.

[b/c], $P<0.05$

The first laboratory to study and report the effect of dietary fat on normal mammary gland developmental processes was that of Abraham and colleagues (3). They reported that female Balb/c mice fed a high level of corn oil had considerably more mammary gland ductal epithelial growth than did mice fed a comparable level of hydrogenated cottonseed oil. The hydrogenated cottonseed oil is deficient in essential fatty acids; essential fatty acid deficiency in mice results in impaired mammary gland development (4,5), a phenomenon that can be reversed by the sole administration of linoleic acid (4). To circumvent this problem, we added a small amount of corn oil, which is rich in linoleic acid, to each of our high fat diets (coconut oil, beef tallow and Menhaden oil) that contain marginal levels of this essential nutrient. It is our experience that mice fed beef tallow or fish oil diets (20%), as their sole source of dietary fat, have significantly reduced body weight gains. In the present study, body weight gains were comparable among all dietary groups. Thus, the significant inhibitory effect of dietary fish oil on mammary gland development in immature mice was observed in animals with a normal rate of body weight gain. In our studies we also observed a suppression of mammary gland ductal growth in mice fed a low fat diet (5% corn oil) compared to mice fed a high fat diet (20% corn oil). This observation is consistent with a previous report from our laboratory (6) and by others (7).

The mechanism by which dietary fish oil suppresses mammary gland developmental processes is uncertain. The results of our study clearly demonstrate that the rate of ductal proliferation (expansive growth through the mammary fat pad) is significantly reduced in mice fed a diet rich in fish oil when compared to mice fed, e.g., a diet rich in corn oil. Thus, our data clearly support the concept that changes in dietary fat composition act by influencing mammae ductal cell proliferation. It is germane to point out that Abraham and colleagues could not demonstrate any significant difference in DNA synthesis or cell cycle kinetics (8-10) of mouse mammary tumors as a function of the type of dietary fat (e.g., corn oil vs. hydrogenated cottonseed oil or fish oil); diet was shown only to affect the rate of tumor cell loss (9, 10). Thus, according to the concept proposed by Abraham and associates, increased mammary tumor size, as a function of type of dietary fat, is a reflection primarily of cell loss, not proliferative processes. In our study, utilizing the normal mammary gland, dietary fish oil clearly suppressed mammae proliferative processes.

Altered mammae proliferative processes, as a function of the fat content of the diet, can be explained by a number of mechanisms. Potential mechanisms include the generation of lipid peroxy radicals and/or oxygen radicals (11) alteration in membrane fluidity (12), changes in intercellular communication (13), alterations in mammotrophic hormone secretion (14), enhancement of hormone and/or growth factor responsiveness (6) and alterations in eicosanoid biosynthesis (3, 5, 8, 10, 11). The concept that dietary fat may influence mammae proliferative processes via modification of eicosanoid biosynthesis is particularly attractive. Certain dietary fish oils, e.g., Menhaden oil, are especially rich in long chain n-3 fatty acids such as eicosapentaenoic acid (EPA) (20:5) and decosahexaenoic acid (DHA) (22:6). EPA and DHA modifies linoleic acid (18:2) and arachidonic acid (20:4) metabolism, thus sharply interfering with prostaglandin biosynthesis (15-17) . It is conceivable, therefore, that the inhibitory effect of dietary Menhaden oil on the developmental growth of the mouse mammary gland, as observed in our study, is manifested via an inhibition of linoleic acid utilization. Although our Menhaden oil diet was supplemented with corn oil (1%), assuring adequate RDA levels of linoleic acid, the rather large amounts of EPA and DHA in this diet could interfere with linoleic acid utilization. Indeed, in our study, suppressed normal mammae developmental growth was observed in mice fed dietary corn oil/fish oil ratios of 1: 3 (4.5% corn oil :15.5% Menhaden oil) and even 1:1 (10% corn oil; 10% Menhaden oil). Thus, if the EPA-DHA/linoleic acid utilization concept is correct, then EPA and/or DHA appear to be effective even when diets contain an abundance of linoleic acid. It is important to point out, in addition, that our observed inhibitory effect of dietary Menhaden oil on mouse mammae developmental growth cannot solely be attributed to the broad class of n-3 fatty acids, as high dietary levels of linseed oil did not, whatsoever, affect this developmental process. Linseed oil is rich (47%) in linolenic acid (18:3, n-3). Although linolenic acid can inhibit the metabolism of arachidonic acid, via cyclooxygenase, and the conversion of linoleic acid to arachidonic acid, this n-3 fatty acid does not appear to be as effective as EPA/DHA in the suppression of eicosanoid formation from arachidonic acid (12).

In summary, the results of our study provide evidence that developmental growth of the mammary gland in immature female mice can be significantly effected (impaired) by diet, but by only rather extreme dietary intervention, i.e., by reducing fat consumption by 75% (20% to 5%) or by feeding very high levels of certain fish (Menhaden) derived oils that are extremely rich in n-3 polyunsaturated fatty acids such as EPA and/or DHA. The feeding of high dietary levels of four different vegetable oils (corn oil, olive oil, coconut oil, linseed oil) and two different animal fats (lard and beef tallow) did not differentially affect developmental growth of the mammary gland.

REFERENCES

1. Welsch, C.W. Enhancement of mammary tumorigenesis by dietary fat: Review of potential mechanisms. Am. J. Clin. Nutr., 45:192-202, 1987.
2. Welsch, C.W. and O'Connor, D.H. Influence of the type of dietary fat on developmental growth of the mammary gland in immature and mature female Balb/c mice. Cancer Res. 49:5999-6007, 1989.
3. Abraham, S., Faulkin, L.J., Hillyard, L.A. and Mitchell, D.J. Effect of dietary fat on tumorigenesis in the mouse mammary gland. J. Natl. Cancer Inst., 72:1421-1429, 1984.
4. Knazek, R.A., Liu, S.C., Bodwin, J.S. and Vonderhaar, B.K. Requirement of essential fatty acids in the diet for development of the mouse mammary gland. J. Natl. Cancer Inst. 64:377-382, 1980.
5. Miyamoto, M.J., Hillyard, L.A. and Abraham, S. Influence of dietary fat on the growth of mammary ducts in Balb/c mice. J. Natl. Cancer Inst., 67:179-188, 1981.
6. Welsch, C.W., DeHoog, J.V., O'Connor, D.H. and Sheffield, L.G. Influence of dietary fat levels on development and hormone responsiveness of the mouse mammary gland. Cancer Res. 45:6147-6154, 1985.
7. Zhang, L., Bird, R.P. and Bruce, W.R. Proliferative activity of murine mammary epithelium as affected by dietary fat and calcium. Cancer Res., 47:4905-4908, 1987.
8. Hillyard, L.A. and Abraham, S. Effect of dietary polyunsaturated fatty acids on growth of mammary adenocarcinomas in mice and rats. Cancer Res., 39:4430-4437, 1979.
9. Gabor, H. and Abraham, S. Effect of dietary Menhaden oil on tumor cell loss and the accumulation of mass of a transplantable mammary adenocarcinoma in Balb/c mice. J. Natl. Cancer Inst., 76:1223-1229, 1986.
10. Gabor, H., Hillyard, L.A. and Abraham, S. Effect of dietary fat on growth kinetics of transplantable mammary adenocarcinomas in Balb/c mice. J. Natl. Cancer Inst., 74:1299-1305, 1985.
11. Bull, A.W., Nigro, N.D., Golembieski, W.A., Crissman, J.D. and Marnett, L.J. In vivo stimulation of DNA synthesis and induction of ornithine decarboxylase in rat colon by fatty acid hydroperoxides, autoxidation products of unsaturated fatty acids. Cancer Res., 44:4924-4928, 1984.
12. Berlin, E., Matusik, E.J. and Young, C. Effect of dietary fat on the fluidity of platelet membranes. Lipids, 15:604-608, 1980.
13. Aylsworth, C.F., Trosko, J.E. and Welsch, C.W. Influence of lipids on gap junction-mediated intercellular communication between Chinese hamster cells in vitro. Cancer Res., 46:4527-4533, 1986.
14. Chan, P.C. and Cohen, L.A. Effect of dietary fat, antiestrogen, and antiprolactin on the development of mammary tumors in rats. J. Natl. Cancer Inst., 52:25-30, 1974.
15. Goodnight, S.H., Harris, W.S., Connor, W.E. and Illingworth, D.R. Polyunsaturated fatty acids, hyperlipidemia and thrombosis. Arteriosclerosis, 2:87-113, 1982.
16. Culp, B.R., Titus, B.G. and Lands, W.E. Inhibitions of prostaglandin biosynthesis by eicosapentaenoic acid. Prostaglandins Med., 3:269-278, 1979.
17. Corey, R.J., Shih, C. and Cashman, J.R. Decosahexaenoic acid is a strong inhibitor of prostaglandin but not leukotriene biosynthesis. Proc. Natl. Acad. Sci. (USA), 80:3581-3584, 1983.
18. Hwang, D.H., Boudreau, M. and Chanmugam, P. Dietary linolenic acid and longer-chain fatty acids: Comparison of effects on arachidonic acid metabolism in rats. J. Nutr., 118:427-437, 1988.

MODULATION OF MAMMARY CARCINOGENESIS BY EICOSANOID SYNTHESIS INHIBITORS IN RATS FED HIGH LEVELS OF LINOLEATE

M. M. IP and C. IP

Grace Cancer Drug Center and Department of Breast Surgery, Roswell Park Cancer Center, Buffalo, NY 14263

INTRODUCTION

Diets containing relatively high amounts of polyunsaturated fat have been demonstrated to stimulate the development of a wide variety of mammary tumors in rodents (reviewed in ref. 1). Using the dimethylbenz(α)anthracene (DMBA)-induced mammary tumor model in rats, Carroll and Hopkins (2) reported that addition of as little as 3% of a linoleic acid-rich sunflower seed oil to a diet containing 17% beef tallow or coconut oil (saturated fats) was just as effective as a 20% sunflower seed oil diet in enhancing tumor development. Furthermore, rats on these diets produced twice as many tumors as those fed diets containing 20% of the saturated fats alone. These findings suggest that there may be a requirement for linoleate in mammary carcinogenesis that is not satisfied by fats such as beef tallow and coconut oil, but can be provided by adding 3% sunflower seed oil to diets containing these fats. More recently, we have shown that mammary tumorigenesis in the DMBA model was very sensitive to linoleate intake and increased proportionately in the range of 0.5% to 4% of dietary linoleate (3). Beyond this point and up to, 12% linoleate, there was no further enhancement, suggesting that the level of linoleate necessary to elicit the maximal tumorigenic response was around 4% by weight in the diet.

Several theories have been proposed to explain the stimulatory role of linoleate in mammary tumorigenesis (reviewed in ref. 4). These include effects on the endocrine system resulting in changes in the levels of mammotrophic hormones and/or tissue responsiveness to these hormones, altered intercellular communication, increased lipid peroxidation, suppression of host immune function, and reduced rate of tumor cell loss. Linoleate is the dietary precursor of arachidonic acid which can be converted to prostaglandins and thromboxanes through the cyclooxygenase pathway, and to various hydroxy and hydroxyperoxy fatty acids as well as leukotrienes through the lipoxygenase pathway. Rao and Abraham (5) first tested the eicosanoid cascade mechanism by using eicosatetraynoic acid (ETYA) to block the metabolism of arachidonic acid. They found that feeding ETYA to mice bearing a transplantable mammary tumor and maintained on a high fat diet reduced the growth of the tumor. Since then, several laboratories have reported that administration of the cyclooxygenase inhibitor indomethacin reduces the incidence, multiplicity, and/or growth of mammary tumors in rodents fed a diet containing high levels of linoleate (6-9).

The objectives of the present study were two fold. The first aim was to determine if cyclooxygenase inhibitors other than indomethacin would suppress DMBA-induced mammary carcinogenesis in rats fed a diet high in linoleate. These experiments were undertaken in an attempt to establish if the effect of indomethacin was a direct result of cyclooxygenase inhibition, or was perhaps due to some other mechanism. The second aim was to investigate the modulation of mammary tumorigenesis by drugs that can interfere with both lipoxygenase and cyclooxygenase reactions. It is essential to evaluate the significance of lipoxygenase metabolites, since diversion of arachidonic acid to this pathway as a result of cyclooxygenase blockade may lead to the production of active intermediates with anticarcinogenic potential.

Effect of cyclooxygenase inhibitors on DMBA-induced mammary carcinogenesis.

Initially, experiments were designed to follow up our observation of a specific linoleate requirement (3), in order to delineate whether the dose-dependent stimulation of mammary carcinogenesis by linoleate could be attentuated by indomethacin. Animals were treated with DMBA and then placed on 20% fat diets containing 0.5%, 4% or 12% linoleate. Half of the animals in each group received 40 mg/kg indomethacin in the diet. Results of this study, which have been published recently (10), showed that indomethacin reduced the tumor incidence, tumor number and tumor weight in the 4% and 12% linoleate groups, but not in the 0.5% linoleate group. Thus the level of linoleate in the diet seemed to influence the responsiveness to indomethacin.

In view of the above finding, two other cyclooxygenase blockers, carprofen and ibuprofen, were tested for their protective effects in rats that were fed a 20% corn oil diet (containing 12% linoleate) and treated with DMBA. Carprofen (6-chlorocarbazole-2-α-methylacetic acid) has some structural similarity to indomethacin [1-(4-chlorobenzoyl)-5-methoxy-2-methyl-1H-indole-3-acetic acid]. It is a more potent inhibitor of cyclooxygenase in vitro than ibuprofen [2-(4-isobutylphenyl) propionic acid], but is less potent than indomethacin. In this experiment, ibuprofen, at doses of 1,000 or 2,000 mg/kg in the diet, was found to have a comparable inhibitory effect on mammary carcinogenesis as indomethacin (11). Carprofen, on the other hand, was inactive in 3 separate experiments at the maximally tolerated dose of 200 mg/kg (10). The failure of carprofen to protect against tumorigenesis was independent of the linoleate effect, since negative results were obtained in rats fed either 0.5%, 4% or 12% linoleate in the diet.

Effect of indomethacin and carprofen on PGE_2 levels.

PGE_2 levels of sera collected by cardiac puncture of animals from the DMBA carcinogenesis experiments were measured as an indicator of the overall effects of diet and drug on prostaglandin synthesis (10). The rats chosen for this study were fed 20% fat diets containing 0.5%, 4% or 12% linoleate. Results of this experiment showed that linoleate alone did not significantly affect serum PGE_2 levels in non-treated rats, although a trend towards increasing PGE_2 concentration with increasing dietary linoleate was evident. As expected, both indomethacin and carprofen reduced serum PGE_2 levels, regardless of the linoleate content of the diet.

Further evaluation of the effect of both drugs on PGE_2 production was focused on the proliferating mammary gland as a target tissue. Normal mammary gland contains very few epithelial cells and may not be an appropriate model due to the limitation and sensitivity of the system. Consequently, we decided to employ the procedure of implanting the animals with silastic pellets containing estradiol and progesterone to stimulate the proliferation of the mammary epithelium. Similar to the serum data, PGE_2 content in the mammary tissue was elevated with increasing levels of dietary linoleate. Treatment with indomethacin or carprofen substantially depressed the concentration of PGE_2 in the hormonally-stimulated gland (10). At least in this tissue, we also found carprofen to be a more potent inhibitor of PGE_2 synthesis than indomethacin.

Studies were then carried out to examine the effect of these two drugs on PGE_2 content in mammary tumors. Our data showed that PGE_2 levels in the tumors varied over a wide range and no correlation was observed between PGE_2 levels and tumor size or linoleate content of the diet. Because of the large standard errors associated with the sample means, it was difficult to detect significant trends due to treatment with either indomethacin or carprofen. In our hands, tumor PGE_2 is a poor indicator for the availability of linoleate as a precursor or for the efficacy of drugs which inhibit the cyclooxygenase pathway of arachidonate metabolism.

Effect of cyclooxygenase plus lipoxygenase inhibitors on DMBA-induced mammary carcinogenesis.

Since indomethacin and carprofen block the cyclooxygenase pathway, an increase in lipoxygenase-activated products as a result of diversion of substrate flow into this arm cannot be ruled out. In the next series of experiments, we proceeded to examine the effects of two drugs which can inhibit both enzymes. Rats were fed a 20% corn oil diet containing either 100 mg/kg of timegadine [3-amino-1-(3-trifluoromethylphenyl)-2-pyrazoline hydrochloride from Leo Pharmaceuticals] or 250 mg/kg of BW-755C [N-cyclohexyl-N"-4-(2-methylquinolyl)-N'-2-thiazolylguanidine from Wellcome Research Laboratories]. In contrast to the cyclooxygenase inhibitor results, both compounds were found to stimulate DMBA-induced mammary carcinogenesis as indicated by an increase in tumor incidence and tumor number (11). In addition, timegadine also decreased tumor latency and BW-755C increased tumor weight. These experiments, taken in conjunction with the indomethacin and ibuprofen data, suggest that certain metabolite(s) in the lipoxygenase-activated pathway might normally function as an inhibitor of malignant proliferation.

DISCUSSION

The role of linoleate in regulating tumor development has not been clearly elucidated. Linoleate, via the intermediate arachidonic acid, can serve as a precursor to a host of biologically active compounds emanating from both the cyclooxygenase and lipoxygenase reactions. With the use of specific inhibitors to these enzymes, results of the current study highlight the complexity of the concept of eicosanoid modulation as a mechanism by which linoleate stimulates neoplastic progression. We have found that two related prostaglandin synthesis inhibitors, indomethacin and carprofen, have different effects on tumorigenesis, although both agents suppressed PGE_2 levels in blood and mammary gland. It is noteworthy that both inhibitors reduced PGE_2 levels in hormonally-stimulated mammary tissue, since its proliferative activity is probably a better approximation of the growth of a small clone of transformed epithelial cells than the normal quiescent gland.

The lack of an effect of carprofen in cancer chemoprevention was unexpected, since other functionally similar compounds such as indomethacin and flurbiprofen, which are competitive inhibitors of the cyclooxygenase enzyme, have been shown to protect against chemically-induced mammary tumorigenesis in rodents (7,12,13). It is possible that these drugs may produce characteristic changes in selective constituents of the eicosanoid spectrum which obviously will not be detected by measuring only one metabolite. For example, indomethacin and ibuprofen have been shown to stimulate lipoxygenase activity in addition to their inhibitory effect on cyclooxygenase (14). If carprofen does not have the same effect, then one might speculate that an increase of lipoxygenase products, rather than a decrease of cyclooxygenase products, might be protective of tumorigenesis. Results of the timegadine and BW-755C experiments are certainly consistent with this interpretation.

The degree of inhibition or stimulation in the synthesis of individual components of the eicosanoid tree will most likely be drug-specific. Subtle shifts in the balance of the overall pattern may be critical in determining whether the carcinogenic process will be arrested or accelerated. Another caveat that has to be taken into consideration in interpreting our results is that local prostaglandin synthesis by the mammary tissue may not be an important event in controlling neoplastic expression. These drugs might differentially affect the cells of the immune system and thus impact on tumor development by an indirect mechanism. It is evident that in further elaboration of the role of the linoleate-eicosanoid axis in modulation of tumorigenesis, we need to define not only the target tissue but also the complete profile of arachidonic acid metabolism in response to these inhibitors.

This work was supported by NIH grant CA 35641 and by NIH core grant CA 24538.

REFERENCES

1. Welsch, C.W. and Aylsworth, C.F. J. Natl. Cancer Inst. 70: 215-221, 1983.
2. Carroll, K.K. and Hopkins, G.J. Lipids 14: 155-158, 1979.
3. Ip, C., Carter, C.A. and Ip, M.M. Cancer Res. 45: 1997-2001, 1985.
4. Welsch, C.W. Am. J. Clin. Nutr. 45: 192-202, 1987.
5. Rao, G. and Abraham, S. J. Natl. Cancer Inst. 58: 445-447, 1977.
6. Hillyard, L.A. and Abraham, S. Cancer Res. 39: 4430-4437, 1979.
7. Carter, C.A., Milholland, R.J., Shea, W.K. and Ip, M.M. Cancer Res. 43: 3559-3562, 1983.
8. Kollmorgan, G.M., King, M.M., Kosanke,S.D. and Do, C. Cancer Res. 43: 4714-4719, 1983.
9. Hubbard, N.E., Chapkin, R.S. and Erickson, K.L. Cancer Lett. 43: 111-120, 1988.
10. Carter, C.A., Ip, M.M. and Ip, C. Carcinogenesis 10: 1369-1374, 1989.
11. Ip, M.M., Mazzer, C., Watson, D. and Carter, C.A. Proc. Am. Assoc. Cancer Res. 30: 182 (Abstr. No. 721), 1989.
12. McCormick, D.L. and Moon, R.C. Brit. J. Cancer 48: 859-861, 1983.
13. McCormick, D.L., Madigan, M.J. and Moon, R.C. Cancer Res. 45: 1803-1808, 1985.
14. Vanderhoek, J.Y. and Bailey, J.M. J. Biol. Chem. 259: 6752-6756, 1984.

ENHANCEMENT OF COLONIC CARCINOGENESIS BY DIETARY FAT: ROLE OF ESSENTIAL, OXIDIZED, POLYUNSATURATED AND SATURATED FATTY ACIDS

A. W. BULL

Oakland University, Department of Chemistry, Rochester, MI 48309

The major factor affecting the development of intestinal carcinogenesis in both animals and man appears to be environmental in origin. Clearly, the major environmental factor affecting the colon is the diet and the most important tumor enhancing component of the diet appears to be the type and level of fat (1). There have been numerous studies investigating the relationship between the risk of colon tumor formation and the fat content of the diet. A majority, but certainly not all, studies in animals have suggested that animals consuming high levels of dietary fat develop more tumors than animals consuming lower levels of fat. More recently it has been shown that the particular fatty acid content of the dietary fat is often as important as the total amount of fat (2). The present paper will examine a few selected mechanisms by which dietary fat could enhance intestinal tumorigenesis.

No discussion of the role of dietary fat in intestinal carcinogenesis would be complete without mention of the role of bile acids as possible colon tumor promoters. Tumorigenesis studies have been performed in which bile acids were either applied directly to the colonic mucosa, fed in the diet, or measured in the luminal contents under conditions found to lead to an alteration in the bile acid content (3). In most cases, there is a close positive correlation between the exposure of the colonic mucosa to bile acids and the development of colonic tumors. However, in spite of these data, there is evidence to suggest that diet related factors other than bile acids also act to influence colonic tumorigenesis. It is these other factors which will be the focus of the current paper.

The particular fatty acid composition of dietary fat has been shown to be important for tumorigenesis. For example, Reddy and Maeura have shown that dietary fats containing relatively high levels of polyunsaturated fatty acids enhance tumorigenesis more than fats containing monounsaturated or saturated fatty acids (2). Similar results were demonstrated by Sakaguchi et al. using purified ethyl esters of linoleic or stearic acid as the source of dietary fat (4). Thus, polyunsaturated fatty acids clearly lead to enhanced tumorigenesis relative to more saturated fatty acids.

The observations that the degree of fatty acid unsaturation is important for promotion of colon tumors raises a number of questions as to the mechanism for this effect. There are two obvious possibilities which have been explored experimentally. The first concerns the role of essential fatty acids and the second concerns the formation of unsaturated fatty acid oxidation products and the potential biological activity of these products. Both these possibilities will be considered in the following discussion.

In a number of experiments by different groups, the essential fatty acid requirement for optimal tumorigenesis has been investigated in the breast, pancreas, and colon. In the breast and pancreas, the EFA level for optimal tumorigenesis is well in excess of that required for proper nutrition. For example, Ip and co-workers reported that a dietary level of 4.4% EFA was optimal for development of mammary tumorigenesis in rats (5). Whereas the generally accepted nutritional requirement of EFA for laboratory rats is 0.6% of the diet.

A similar titration of the EFA requirement for colonic tumorigenesis has been reported and the results indicate some important differences between the colon and other organs (6). In the colon experiment, diets were prepared containing various mixtures of safflower oil, beef fat, or medium chain triglyceride oil (MCT). The EFA level, as % linoleate, varied from 1.28% to <0.03% as determined by extraction and gas chromatographic analysis. Colon tumors were induced by two weekly injections of azoxymethane and the animals killed six months after the start of the experiment. The results are summarized in Table 1. The incidence of large bowel tumors was dependent on the dietary linoleate content. Rats consuming diets containing less than 0.1% linoleate showed a statistically significant reduction in tumor incidence compared to rats fed diets containing 0.6% to 1.28% linoleate. In contrast to the results in the mammary gland, the tumor incidence did not increase as the EFA content of the diet was raised from 0.6% to 1.28%. It is also noteworthy that rats fed 20% beef fat (0.34% linoleate) had the highest incidence of tumors of any dietary group.

Table 1
Effect of diets containing different linoleate levels on colon tumor formation.

Dietary Linoleate[a] (%)	Tumor Incidence (%)	Tumor Multiplicity Tumors/TBA (±S.D.)[b]
1.28	72.4	2.0 ± 0.9
0.6	73.3	2.1 ± 1.4
0.11	55.2	2.3 ± 1.3
0.08	39.3	1.8 ± 1.2
<0.03	37.9	1.7 ± 0.9
0.34[c]	88.8	3.3 ± 3.3

a) unless otherwise noted, diets contained 5% total fat
b) mean no. of tumors per tumor bearing animal
c) diet contained 20% beef fat

To assess the overall EFA status of the animals, the triene/tetraene ratio in the plasma, liver, and colon was measured. Ratios of greater than 0.4 are generally indicative of an EFA deficiency. The plasma and liver triene/tetraene ratios were well in excess of 0.4 in the two groups consuming 0.08% and <0.03% linoleate. Thus it is apparent these animals were EFA deficient. On the other hand, the colonic content of 20 carbon fatty acids and consequently the triene/tetraene ratio was low relative to the other organs. Thus the colon did not indicate an EFA deficient state. In fact, the low level of eicosanoic acids suggests the tissue has a relatively low requirement for these compounds. This is consistent with the observation that colon tumorigenesis is not affected until the EFA level is much lower than the required daily amount.

The major role of EFA is generally believed to be to provide precursors for the biosynthesis of prostaglandins and other eicosanoids. If in fact the colon does have a low requirement for EFA, how does one reconcile this fact with the observation that inhibitors of prostaglandin biosynthesis also inhibit colon tumor growth? It is conceivable that the EFA requirement changes as the colonic tissue undergoes transformation from normal to malignant tissue. Investigation of this possibility could yield important clues to the carcinogenic process.

In addition to the role of EFA, there are other effects of fat which contribute to the carcinogenic process. For example, in the experiment described above, rats fed 0.34% EFA as part of a 20% fat diet had the highest tumor incidence and multiplicity of any animals in the study. Since tumorigenesis was maximal at less than the highest EFA level, non-EFA dependent fat effects must also be involved. Part of these non-EFA effects may involve oxidation products of unsaturated fatty acids, including the monounsaturates .

The initial products of the autoxidation of unsaturated fatty acids are hydroperoxy fatty acids. Subsequent reactions of the hydroperoxides yield hydroxy and keto-fatty acids. These oxidation products of unsaturated fatty acids induce ornithine decarboxylase activity and stimulate DNA synthesis when they are instilled into the colon of rats. On the other hand, the unoxidized parent fatty acids do not stimulate these markers of cell proliferation.

A structure-activity study to define the structural requirements for the stimulation of colonic mucosal cell proliferation determined that an oxygen-containing moiety adjacent to a carbon-carbon double bond was essential for the induction of mitogenesis (7). There is no difference in mitogenic potency between molecules in which the oxidized center is a hydroperoxide, alcohol, or ketone. This raises the possibility that oxidized fatty acids are metabolized to a common intermediate which initiates mitogenesis. We have suggested this ultimate mitogen might contain an enone or dienone functionality (7).

The ability of the colonic mucosa to metabolize hydroperoxy fatty acids to enone containing derivatives has recently been investigated *in vitro. A* hydroperoxide derived from linoleic acid, specifically 13-hydroperoxyoctadecadienoic acid (13-ROOH) was incubated with colonic homogenates prepared from male Sprague-Dawley rats. The products were extracted, analyzed by HPLC, and identified by UV, NMR, and GCMS. The major products produced by the colonic homogenates were 13-hydroxyoctadecadienoic acid and a series of isomers of 2,4-dienones of octadecadienoic acid.

The product profiles from these incubations were significantly less complex than those obtained from the decomposition of hydroperoxy fatty acids in a number of non-enzymatic systems (8,9). In particular, there was no detectable production of epoxy fatty acids nor their hydrolysis products. Thus, incubation of 13-ROOH with homogenates of colonic mucosa results in the production of relatively large amounts of unsaturated carbonyl compounds in preference to the formation of the myriad of other possible hydroperoxide derived products. These data lend support to the hypothesis that the mitogenic activity of oxidized fatty acids derives from the production of enone or dienone compounds.

A summary of the metabolism of 13-ROOH by colonic homogenates is shown in Scheme 1. As presented, the exposure of the colonic mucosa to 13-ROOH is followed by reduction of the hydroperoxide to an alcohol. Dehydration of the alcohol to the 2,4-dienone would account for the generation of a compound capable of reaction with cellular nucleophiles. It is also conceivable that direct dehydration of 13-ROOH occurs which provides an alternate route to generation of the dienone. Depending on the cellular constituent reacting with the dienone an alteration in cellular physiology can be envisioned.

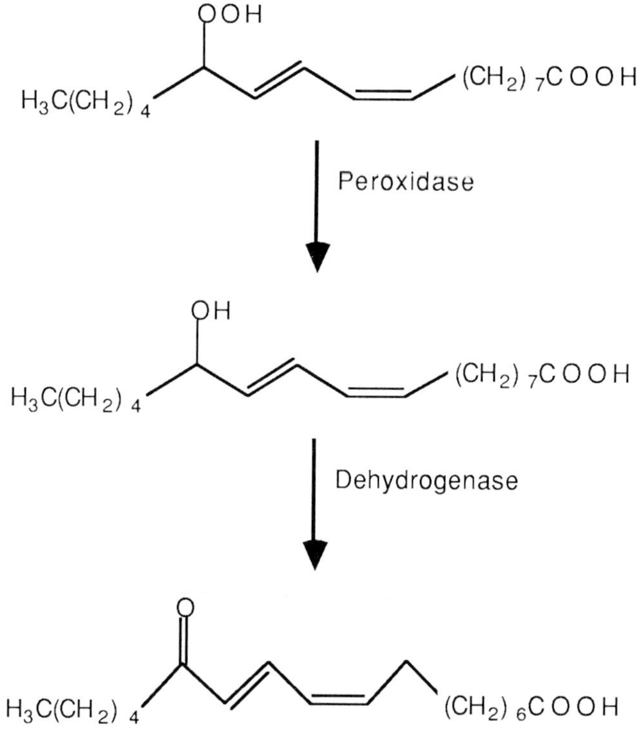

OOH

$H_3C(CH_2)_4$ $(CH_2)_7COOH$

Peroxidase

OH

$H_3C(CH_2)_4$ $(CH_2)_7COOH$

Dehydrogenase

O

$H_3C(CH_2)_4$ $(CH_2)_6COOH$

Scheme 1 f 13-ROOH by colonic hc

Scheme 1. Possible pathway for metabolism of 13-ROOH by colonic homogenates.

The topics considered above summarize a few of the major hypotheses for the mechanism by which dietary fat enhances intestinal tumorigenesis. The discussion is by no means all inclusive as a number of additional possibilities have been presented elsewhere. It is entirely possible that the enhancement of colonic tumorigenesis by dietary fat is a combination of several different biochemical events, mediated by distinct chemical entities. Whether these events occur simultaneously or in some definite temporal sequence is presently unknown as is the potential interaction between the different chemical species.

REFERENCES

1. Abraham, S. (ed.) Carcinogenesis and Dietary Fat Kluwer Academic Publishers, Norwell, MA 1989.
2. Reddy, B.S., and Maeura, Y. J. Nat'l Cancer Inst. USA 72: 745-750,1984.
3. Reddy, B.S., Weisburger, J.H., and Wynder, E.L. In: Carcinogenesis: A Comprehensive Survey, Vol. 2, (eds. Slaga, T.J., Sivak, A., and Boutwell, R.K.) Raven Press, New York, 1978, pp. 453-464.
4. Sakaguchi, M, Hiramatsu, R., Takada, H., Yamamura, M., Hioki, K., Saito, K., Yamamoto, M. Cancer Res. 44:1472-1477,1984.
5. Ip, C., Carter, C.A., and Ip, M.M. Cancer Res. 45:1997-2001,1985.
6. Bull, A.W., Bronstein, J.C., and Nigro, N.D. Lipids 24: 340-346,1989.
7. Bull, A.W., Nigro, N.D., and Marnett, L.J. Cancer Res. 48:1771-1776,1988.
8. Dix, T.A., and Marnett, L.J. J. Biol. Chem. 260: 5351-5357,1985.
9. Gardner, H.W., Weisleder, D., and Nelson, E.C. J. Org. Chem. 49:508-515, 1984.

EICOSANOID SYNTHESIS IN MAMMARY TUMORS OF RATS FED VARYING TYPES AND LEVELS OF N-3 AND/OR N-6 FATTY ACIDS

O. R. BUNCE, S. H. ABOU-EL-ELA, and A. E. WADE

Department of Pharmacology and Toxicology, University of Georgia, Athens, Georgia

INTRODUCTION

In previous studies (1,2), we have shown that the incidences of dimethylbenzanthracene (DMBA) induced mammary tumors are decreased in animals fed diets containing the n-6 fatty acid, gamma-linolenic acid (GLA) as contained in primrose oil (PO); and the n-3 fatty acids contained in menhaden oil (MO). Synthesis of eicosanoids was decreased in mammary fat pads of control rats and in mammary tumors of DMBA-treated rats by feeding high fat diets containing the n-3 fatty acids. Feeding a GLA source increased the ratio of monoenoic to dienoic eicosanoids compared to feeding either 20% corn oil (CO) or MO diets (2). In a study designed to explore mechanism(s) by which n-3 and/or n-6 polyunsaturated fatty acids (PUFAs) inhibit or promote mammary tumorigenesis, difluoromethylornithine (DFMO) and/or indomethacin were given during mammary tumor promotion in rats fed high n-3 and/or n-6 fat diets (3). This study demonstrated that diets containing high n-6 fatty acids enhance synthesis of cyclooxygenase, lipoxygenase, and ornithine decarboxylase (ODC) in mammary tumors. However, promotion of tumorigenesis by a 20% corn oil diet was not inhibited by blocking cyclooxygenase and/or ODC activities without significantly blocking 5-lipoxygenase. The combination of DFMO with a diet containing an n-3/n-6 fatty acid ratio of 1.2 profoundly inhibited (72%) tumor promotion. This study demonstrated that simultaneous inhibition of the arachidonic acid cascade (both cyclooxygenase and lipoxygenase) as well as polyamine synthesis may be necessary to achieve the greatest inhibition of tumorigenesis. The present study was designed to determine the optimal levels of n-3 fatty acids and/or GLA needed in a 20% fat diet to significantly inhibit mammary tumor promotion.

The biochemical mechanism(s) involved in tumor promotion through which n-3 and/or n-6 PUFAs inhibit or promote mammary tumorigenesis were also explored.

METHODS

Experimental design.

At 50 days of age 200 virgin female Sprague-Dawley rats were each administered 10 mg DMBA by intragastric intubation as described previously (1). Three weeks post-DMBA the animals were randomly divided into 8 groups of 25 rats each and placed on dietary regimens containing 20% fat derived from corn oil (CO), primrose oil (PO), black currant oil (BCO), borage oil (BO), or varying ratios of MO/CO as shown in Figure 1. Table 1 gives the percentages of the various fatty acids in the oils. During the period

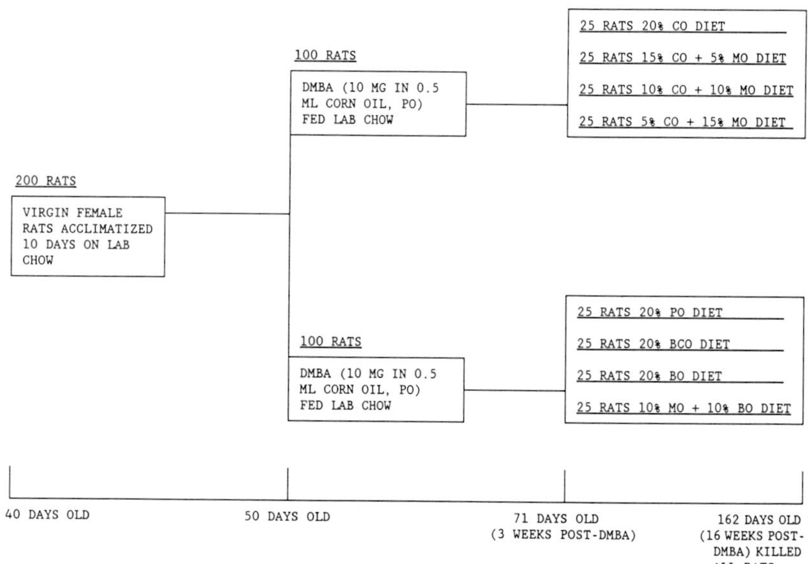

Figure 1. Schedule of Diets and Treatments

of high fat feeding, tumor latency, number and position were determined. At 16 weeks post-DMBA surviving rats were killed, and the total number of tumors, the location and the size of each tumor were noted. Mammary tumors were fixed in buffered formalin for histopathological examination according to the criteria of Van Zwieten (4). Only histologically confirmed malignant mammary tumors were used in data analyses.

Eicosanoid and ODC Analyses.

Malignant tumors were finely minced and appropriate tissue aliquots were incubated in 1 ml Krebs buffer for 1 h at 37°C according to the method described in detail by Abou-El-Ela (3). The stable metabolite of prostaglandin E, bicyclic PGE, and leukotrienes B_4 and C_4 were analyzed by radioimmunoassay (RIA) using kits purchased from Amersham Corp., Arlington Heights, IL. PGE_1 was analyzed by RIA using kits purchased from Advanced Magnetics Inc., Cambridge, MA. The PGE_1 antibody showed 23% cross-reactivity with PGE_2. Postmicrosomal cytosol fractions from tumors were prepared by differential centrifugation (3), and ODC was assayed by measuring the release of $^{14}CO_2$ from L-(1-^{14}C) ornithine hydrochloride, as described by Russell and Snyder (5).

Results and Discussion.

As shown in Table 2, incidences of mammary tumors at 16 weeks post-DMBA were 80% in rats fed the 20% CO diet, 84% in rats ingesting 20% PO, 67% in rats fed 20% BCO, 88% in rats fed 20% BO, 60% in rats fed the 15% MO + 5% CO diet, and 67% in rats fed the 10% MO + 10% CO, 83% in rats fed

Table 1
Percentage Fatty Acid Composition of Oils

Fatty Acid		Corn[a]	Primrose[b]	Borage[c]	Black Currant[c]	Menhaden[d]
14:0		–	–			8.35
16:0		11.2	6.5	10.5	8.5	15.17
16:1		–	0.2	1.1	0.4	11.62
16:2		–	–	–	–	2.37
16:3		–	–	–	–	1.96
10:4		–	–	–	–	1.73
18:0		2.1	1.5	3.5	1.75	2.67
18:1		25.0	7.5	16.5	12.5	9.5
18:2	n-6	59.9	75.0	38.0	37.5	1.81
18:3	n-6	0.5	9.0	25.0	19	–
18:3	n-3	–	–	–	16.5	1.82
18:4		–	–	–	–	3.47
20:1		–	–	3.0	–	1.32
20:4	n-6	–	–	–	–	2.3
20:5	n-3	–	–	–	–	16.03
22:1		–	–	1.5	–	–
22:5		–	–	–	–	3.92
22:6	n-3	–	–	–	–	10.83
24:1		–	–	1.5	–	–
Others		0.1	0.5	–	–	4.37

[a]Assay provided by Best Foods, Englewood Cliffs, N.J.
[b]Assay provided by Efamol Research, Inc., Nova Scotia, Canada
[c]Assay provided by Traco Labs, Inc., Champaign, Ill.
[d]Assay provided by Zapata Haynie Corp., Reedville, Va.

the 5% MO + 15% CO and 92% in rats fed the 10% MO + 10% BO diet. Tumor multiplicity was lowest in the PO-fed rats and highest in the BO-fed rats. Based on previous studies (1-3), we expected to observe greatest inhibition of tumorigenesis in animals that had been fed either diets with high level of GLA or the diet with the optimal mixture of n-3 to n-6 fatty acids (MO + CO diet). Tumor incidence was, as expected, lowest in rats fed the 15% MO + 5% CO diet. Tumor burden was lowest in the 15% MO + 5% CO and 10% MO + 10% CO-fed rats and highest in the BCO fed rats. There were no significant differences in tumor latencies. Contrary to our previous study (1), GLA containing diets showed enhancement of tumorigenesis rather than inhibition. However, in the previous study, (1) the diets were stored refrigerated rather than frozen (-20°) under nitrogen, and fresh diet was placed in the food hopper three times a week rather than daily as in the present study. On the other hand, of the diets containing GLA, only the BCO diet showed inhibition of mammary tumorigenesis. BCO is unique among vegetable oils for having both alpha-linolenic acid (ALA) and GLA. Thus, it is questionable whether GLA in BCO contributed to the inhibition of tumorigenesis. Lawson and Hughes (6) have shown that the GLA position

Table 2
Effects of 20% Fat Diet with Varying Levels of n-3 and n-6 Fatty Acids on Mammary Tumor Development at 16 Weeks After DMBA Administration

Diet[a]	Tumor Incidence	Total No. of Tumors[b]	Latency Period[c] (week)	No. of Tumors/ Tumor Bearing Rat[c]	Tumor Burden/ Tumor Bearing Rat (g)[c]
20% CO	20/25 (80%)[d,e,f]	81	10.4 ± 0.6[g]	4.0 ± 0.5[g,h,i]	2.1 ± 0.4[g,h]
20% PO	21/25 (84%)[d,f]	56	11.2 ± 0.6[g]	2.8 ± 0.33[i]	2.1 ± 0.3[g,h]
20% BCO	16/24 (67%)[d,e]	78	10.5 ± 0.7[g]	4.4 ± 0.68[g,h]	2.7 ± 0.4[g]
20% BO	21/24 (88%)[d,f]	92	10.6 ± 0.6[g]	4.6 ± 0.7[g]	2.5 ± 0.4[g,h]
15% MO + 5% CO	15/25 (60%)[e]	49	11.6 ± 0.7[g]	3.3 ± 0.53[g,h,i]	1.6 ± 0.4[h]
10% MO + 10% CO	14/21 (67%)[d,e]	40	11.8 ± 0.7[g]	3.2 ± 0.36[g,h,i]	1.5 ± 0.2[h]
5% MO + 15% CO	20/24 (83%)[d,e,f]	79	10.9 ± 0.6[g]	4.1 ± 0.4[g,h,i]	2.1 ± 0.3[g,h]
10% MO + 10% BO	23/25 (92%)[f]	65	11.7 ± 0.4[g]	2.9 ± 0.37[h,i]	1.9 ± 0.3[g,h]

a CO, corn oil; PO, primrose oil; BCO, black currant oil; BO, borage oil; MO, menhaden oil.

b Tumors were diagnosed as tubulopapillary, tubular, squamous and compact tubular carcinomas.

c Mean ± SEM (N=15-23). The values for tumor burden per tumor bearing rat are shown after square root transformation and compared among dietary groups using one-way analysis of variance.

d,e,f Tumor incidences were compared using Chi-square procedure without continuity correction. Incidences which are significantly ($p<0.007$-0.05) different are followed by different superscripts.

g,h,i Comparison among the dietary groups was made using one-way analysis of variance. Means which are significantly ($p<0.05$) different are followed by different superscripts.

in the triacylglycerol of BCO and PO is in the 3-position and in the 2-position in BO. Therefore, it is possible that variations in triacylglycerol composition may lead to differences in biological activities among the various GLA-containing oils. When the Pearson correlation coefficient was determined between dietary n-3/n-6 ratios and mammary tumor incidences in rats fed combinations of MO + CO, the value of r=0.91. These data show that inhibition of mammary tumor promotion by long chain n-3 fatty acids is best achieved by an n-3/n-6 of approximately 1.2. Interestingly, when a 10% MO diet was combined with either 10% BO or 10% CO tumor incidence was significantly changed (Table 2). However, GLA in BO appears to contribute to promotion rather than inhibition of mammary tumorigenesis. Eicosanoid analysis and ODC activity showed that feeding n-3/n-6 ratio of 1.2 (15% MO + 5% CO) significantly reduced the products of the cyclooxygenase and lipoxygenase (PGE_1, PGE, LTB_4, LTC_4) and ODC activity as shown in Table 3 and 4. It is well established (7) that n-3 fatty acids competitively inhibit the metabolism of arachi-

Table 3
Influence of Diets on Eicosanoid Synthesis in Mammary Tumors at 16 Weeks Post - DMBA

Diet[a]	PGE[b]	PGE_1[b]	LTB_4[b]	LTC_4[b]
20% CO	870 ± 20[c]	262 ± 15[e,f]	65.2 ± 4.3[c]	42.2 ± 2.7[c,d]
20% PO	260 ± 8[f]	342 ± 17[c]	38.7 ± 2.0[d]	41.0 ± 3.9[d]
20% BCO	233 ± 13[f]	348 ± 28[c]	26.5 ± 1.0[e,f]	25.8 ± 0.9[e]
20% BO	395 ± 19[e]	337 ± 15[c,d]	41.3 ± 4.0[d]	28.0 ± 1.8[e]
15% MO + 5%CO	100 ± 6g	80 ± 6[g]	18.8 ± 1.1[f]	16.0 ± 1.7[f]
10% MO + 10%CO	265 ± 15[f]	103 ± 6[g]	27.3 ± 1.4[e]	18.3 ± 1.3[f]
5% MO + 15%CO	673 ± 21[d]	224 ± 7[f]	43.7 ± 4.0[d]	42.2 ± 2.6[c,d]
10% MO + 10%BO	378 ± 18[e]	295 ± 8[d,e]	22.0 ± 2.0[e,f]	48.8 ± 2.7[c]

a CO, corn oil; PO, primrose oil; BCO, black currant oil; BO, borage oil; MO, menhaden oil.

b Mean ± SEM (n=6-15). PGE, PGE_1, LTB_4 and LTC_4 values are expressed as nanograms of eicosanoid synthesized per gram of tissue per hour.

c,d,e,f,g Comparisons among the dietary groups were made using one-way analysis of variance. Means which are significantly ($p<0.05$) different are followed by different superscripts.

Table 4. Influence of Diets on Ornithine Decarboxylase Activity in Mammary Tumors at 16 Weeks Post-DMBA

Diet[a]	Ornithine decarboxylase activity (nmol CO_2/h/mg protein)
20% CO	58.6 ± 0.68[c]
20% PO	61.6 ± 1.04[b]
20% BCO	4.1 ± 1.2[f]
20% BO	55.4 ± 1.5[d]
15% MO + 5% CO	41.0 ± 0.8[f]
10% MO + 10% CO	49.3 ± 0.8[e]
5% MO + 15% CO	58.8 ± 0.8[b,c]
10% MO + 10% BO	50.2 ± 0.6[e]

donate via the cyclooxygenase and lipoxygenase pathways; however, our data (3) suggest that n-3 fatty acids also inhibit ODC activity. In conclusion, simultaneous inhibition of the arachidonic acid cascade (both cyclooxygenase and lipoxygenase as well as polyamine synthesis appear to be necessary for inhibition of mammary tumor promotion by high n-6 fatty acids.

REFERENCES

1. Abou-El-Ela, S.H., Prasse, K.W., Carroll, R. and Bunce, O.R. Lipids 22: 1041-1044, 1987.
2. Abou-El-Ela, S.H., Prasse, K.W., Carroll, R., Wade, A.E., Dharwadkar, S. and Bunce, O.R. Lipids 23: 948-954, 1988.
3. Abou-El-Ela, S.H., Prasse, K.W., Farrell, R.L., Carroll, R.W., Wade, A.E. and Bunce, O.R. Cancer Res. 49: 1434-1440, 1989.
4. Van Zwieten, M.J. In: The Rats as Animal Model in Breast Cancer Research (Ed. Van Zwieten, M.J.), Martinus Nijhoff, Boston MA., 1984, pp. 53-134).
5. Russell, D.H. and Snyder, S.H. Proc. Natl. Acad. Sci. USA 68: 1420-1427, 1968.
6. Lawson, L.D. and Hughes, B.G. Lipids 23: 313-317, 1988.
7. Karmali, R.A. Am. J. Clin. Nutr. 45: 225-229, 1987.

IMMUNOMODULATION

LIPOXIN FORMATION DURING NEUTROPHIL-PLATELET INTERACTIONS: A ROLE FOR LEUKOTRIENE A_4 AND PLATELET 12-LIPOXYGENASE

C. N. SERHAN, S. FIORE and K.-A. SHEPPARD

Hematology Division, Department of Medicine, Brigham and Women's Hospital and Harvard Medical School, Boston, MA 02115

INTRODUCTION

The lipoxins are a series of biologically active eicosanoids which contain a conjugated tetraene structure as a characteristic feature (1). The two main compounds which carry biological activities are positional isomers: one designated lipoxin A_4 (5S,6R,15S-trihydroxy-7,9,13-trans-11-cis-eicosatetraenoic acid) and the other lipoxin B_4 (5S,14R,15S, trihydroxy-6,10,12-trans-8-cis-eicosatetraenoic acid). Multiple pathways have been documented in vitro which can lead to the formation of lipoxins (1-4). It appears that the biosynthetic pathways utilized are species-, cell type- and substrate-specific. One route, documented with results from both isotopic oxygen studies as well as the identification of alcohol trapping products, involves the transformation of 15-HETE to a 5(6)-epoxytetraene by leukocytes (1). When this intermediate (15S-hydroxy-5,6-epoxy-7,9,13-trans-11-cis-eicosatetraenoic acid) was synthesized and incubated with purified cytosolic epoxide hydrolase, it was quantitatively converted into LXA_4 (5). During the formation of lipoxins from exogenous 15-HETE by human neutrophils (an event which may occur in cell-cell interactions), an inverse relationship is observed between leukotriene and lipoxin production (6). Thus, the generation of epoxide-containing intermediates by human PMN appears to play a pivotal role in the biosynthesis of both leukotrienes and lipoxins.

Aside from its role as an intermediate in the formation of leukotrienes within its cell type of origin, it is now recognized that the epoxide LTA_4 can also be released by or escape from cells to be transformed via transcellular routes (7). In general, lipoxygenases catalyze the oxygenation of 1,4-cis-pentadiene structures of polyunsaturated fatty acids (8). Since LTA_4 also contains a 1,4-cis-pentadiene which is not within its conjugated triene structure, it was of interest to determine whether LTA_4 plays a role in the biosynthesis of lipoxins. Here, we discuss recent evidence for: (i) the conversion of LTA_4 by 15-LO to a 5(6)epoxytetraene; (ii) Ca^{2+} mobilizing actions of LTA_4 in human PMN; (iii) the lack of LTA_4 conversion to lipoxins by human PMN; and (iv) the transformation of LTA_4 to lipoxins by the 12-LO of human platelets.

RESULTS AND DISCUSSION

LTA_4 as substrate for the 15-LO.

Before examining whether LTA_4 could be converted to lipoxins by various cell types, we tested if

LTA_4 could serve as a substrate for the soybean (SB) 15-LO. The time course of this conversion is shown in Figure 1. LTA_4 was added to sodium borate buffer (1 ml, 0.1 M, pH 8.5) at 4°C, and the UV spectrum recorded (left insert). Upon addition of ~4 µg of the 15-LO, a rapid increase in absorbance at 300 nm was observed, suggesting the formation of a conjugated tetraene chromophore. The insert (right) shows the UV spectrum at 25 min of an aliquot of this material, which gave a triplet of absorption at 288, 302 and 317 nm. When this sample was treated with $NaBH_4$ and analyzed by RP-HPLC (6), the products formed coeluted with the aqueous hydrolysis products of authentic 5(6)-epoxytetraene. Neither the aqueous hydrolysis products of LTA_4 (i.e., 6-trans-LTB_4 and 12-epi-6-trans-LTB_4) nor LTA_3 were converted to tetraenes by the SB 15-LO under similar conditions. These findings indicate that LTA_4 can serve as a substrate for the 15-LO to give a 5(6)-epoxytetraene.

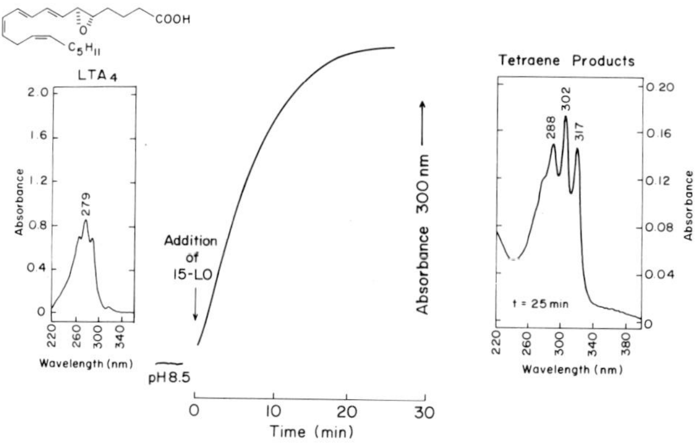

Figure 1. Transformation of LTA_4 by soybean 15-LO.

Exogenous LTA_4 and human neutrophils.

Since human PMN possess a 15-LO, it is possible that extracellular LTA_4 could be transported and converted to its 15-hydroperoxy derivative (i.e., 5(6)-epoxytetraene). To test this, PMN (30 x 10^6 cells/ml) were incubated with either LTA_4 (30 nmol) or LTA_4 with A23187 (2.5 µM). In neither case did PMN generate lipoxins from exogenous LTA_4 (n=3). Further experiments were performed with 100,000 g supernatants prepared from purified PMN, which converted LTA_4 to LTB_4. In these incubations, however, neither lipoxins nor the ω-oxidation products of LTB_4 were detected. Together, these findings suggest that extracellular LTA_4 is not converted to the 5(6)-epoxytetraene upon exposure to human PMN (10).

Transcellular metabolism of LTA_4 implies that during this event: (i) LTA_4 must first "exit" the PMN; (ii) come in contact with the plasma membrane of the "acceptor cell"; and (iii) traverse or gain access to intracellular compartments prior to its enzymatic conversion. Within this temporal framework, several cellular responses may be affected by LTA_4. To test this, Ca^{2+} mobilization was monitored as an early and sensitive signal involved in PMN activation (11). When added to fura-2-loaded PMN, LTA_4 provoked a rapid and transient increase in $[Ca^{2+}]_i$ (max within 8-10 sec), which returned to baseline within 60-90 seconds. Ca^{2+} mobilization was dose-dependent (10^{-12}-10^{-6}M) and evident at concentrations as low as 10^{-11}M. At 1 μM, LTB_4 and LTA_4 were quantitatively similar, while within the range of 10^{-10}-10^{-8}M LTB_4 proved to be more effective. Prior exposure to EGTA (3 mM) did not diminish the amplitude or extent of $[Ca^{2+}]_i$ mobilization by LTA_4. Results from trapping studies revealed that LTA_4 was intact during the initial phase of Ca^{2+} mobilization (t_o-10 sec) stimulated by LTA_4 and that neither LTB_4 nor its ω-oxidation products were detected within this interval (11). Their formation from extracellular ^3H labeled LTA_4/cold LTA_4 was observed only at intervals >30 sec of exposure to PMN. These results, along with those obtained with 5(6)- and 14(15)-epoxytetraenes, suggest that these eicosanoid epoxides possess intrinsic activities (11).

The ability of eicosanoid epoxides to mobilize $[Ca^{2+}]_i$ may serve to amplify cellular responses either within their cells of origin or by acting upon adjacent cells during transcellular metabolism (i.e. homotypic cell-cell interactions). Along these lines, we have found that phospholipid bilayers can enhance the stability of LTA_4 as well as the epoxytetraenes by protecting the epoxides from non-enzymatic hydrolysis (12). Thus, the biological half-life of these intermediates as well as the response they evoke may be increased during their association with membranes. Together, these results indicate that, although LTA_4 can be converted by the SB-15-LO to an epoxytetraene, exogenous LTA_4 is not transformed to lipoxins by human PMN. In this case, extracellular LTA_4 appears to serve as a signal to mobilize Ca^{2+} which may, in turn, amplify PMN responses.

Transformation of LTA_4 to lipoxins.

Previously, we reported that human platelets can utilize and transform PMN-derived eicosanoids (9). To determine if PMN-derived LTA_4 can be transformed to lipoxins by platelets, LTA_4 was incubated with washed platelets (10). Following extraction, products were analyzed with a gradient RP-HPLC equipped with a rapid spectral detector and chromatographic software (6). An isogram plot showed that each product carried a conjugated tetraene chromophore. Materials beneath the major peaks co-eluted with the all-transisomers of LXA_4 and LXB_4 as well as both synthetic and PMN-derived LXA_4 (10). In addition, platelets also generated the recently identified 7-cis-11-trans-LXA_4 (6) from LTA_4. The identity of the platelet-derived LXA_4 was substantiated by GC/MS analysis of its C value and prominent ions present in the mass spectrum of its trimethylsilyl derivative (10).

The conversion of LTA_4 to lipoxins was enhanced by platelet agonists, including thrombin (10). Cycloxoygenase inhibitors (indomethacin, aspirin) did not significantly alter lipoxin generation by platelets, while esculetin (an LO inhibitor (13)), completely blocked their formation. Further studies with platelet-derived 100,000 g supernatants, which displayed 12-LO activity with C20:4 and no detectable 15-LO activity, provide a role for the human platelet 12-LO and its ω-6-oxygenase activity in converting LTA_4 to lipoxins (10). These results suggest a direct action on LTA_4 by the 12-LO to generate lipoxins via a delocalized cation intermediate. A similar intermediate has been proposed in the biosynthesis of lipoxins from a common substrate (14).

CONCLUSIONS

In summary, although LTA_4 is converted to an epoxytetraene by SB 15-LO (Figure 1), results obtained with both intact human PMN and platelets as well as their respective 100,000 g supernatants revealed a differential profile of LTA_4 utilization. PMN, which contain an active 15-LO, did not transform exogenous LTA_4 to lipoxins, while platelets, as well as their 100,000 g supernatants which display 12-LO activity, transform LTA_4 to lipoxins (10). Recently, Edenius et al. (15) reported that LTA_4 is converted to lipoxins by platelets, and Garrick et al. (16) showed that LTA_4 is converted to lipoxins by mesangial cells. Our results are consistent with these observations and provide evidence for a novel biosynthesis route for the formation of lipoxins, namely the conversion of LTA_4 by the human 12-LO. In addition, we have found that costimulation of neutrophils and platelets via receptor-mediated routes can lead to the generation of lipoxins in vitro (10). Thus, in addition to interactions between the 5- and 15-LO, lipoxins can also be generated by interactions between the 5-LO and 12-LO. Since LXA_4 is found in the bronchoalveolar lavage of patients with selected pulmonary diseases (17), this new route of lipoxin formation may contribute, at least in part, to their production.

ACKNOWLEDGMENTS

The authors wish to thank Mary Halm Small for skillful preparation of this manuscript. This work was supported in part by NIH grants #AI26714 and GM38765 (CNS). CNS is a recipient of the J.V. Satterfield Arthritis Investigator Award from the National Arthritis Foundation and is a Pew Scholar in the Biomedical Sciences.

REFERENCES

1. Serhan, C.N. and Samuelsson, B. Adv. Exp. Med. Biol. 229:1-14, 1988.
2. Kuhn, H., Wiesner, R., Alder, L., Fitzsimmons, B.J., Rokach, J. and Brash, A.R. Eur. J. Biochem. 169:593-601, 1987.
3. Ueda, N., Yokoyama, C., Yamamoto, S., Fitzsimmons, B.J., Rokach, J., Oates, J.A. and Brash, A.R. Biochem. Biophys. Res. Commun. 149:1063-1069, 1987.
4. Walstra, P., Verhagen, J., Vermeer, M.A., Klerks, J.P.M., Veldink, G.A. and Vliegenthart, J.F.G. FEBS Lett. 228:167-171, 1988.
5. Puustinen, T., Webber, S.E., Nicolaou, K.C., Haeggstrom, J., Serhan, C.N. and Samuelsson, B. FEBS Lett. 207:127, 1986.
6. Serhan, C.N. Biochim. Biophys. Acta 1004:158-168, 1989.
7. Dahinden, C.A., Clancy, R.M., Gross, M., Chiller, J.M. and Hugli, T.E. Proc. Natl. Acad. Sci. USA 82:6632-6636, 1985.
8. Hamberg, M. Biochem. Biophys. Res. Commun. 117:593-600, 1983.
9. Marcus, A.J., Broekman, M.J., Safier, L.B., Ullman, H.L., Islam, N., Serhan, C.N., Korchak, H. and Weissmann, G. Biochem. Biophys. Res. Commun. 109:130-137, 1982.
10. Serhan, C.N. and Sheppard, K.A. 85:772-780, 1990.
11. Luscinskas, F.W., Nicolaou, K.C., Webber, S.E., Veale, C.A., Gimbrone, M.A., Jr. and Serhan, C.N. Biochem. Pharmacol., 39:355-365, 1990.
12. Fiore, S. and Serhan, C.N. Biochem. Biophys. Res. Commun. 159:477-481, 1989.

13. Sekiya, K., Okuda, H. and Arichi, S. Biochim. Biophys. Acta 713:68-72, 1982.
14. Corey, E.J. and Mehrotra, M.M. Tetrahedron Lett. 27:5173-5176, 1986.
15. Edenius, C., Haeggstrom, J. and Lindgren, J.A. Biochem. Biophys. Res. Commun. 157:801-807, 1988.
16. Garrick, R., Shen, S.-Y., Ogunc, S. and Wong, P.Y.-K. Biochem. Biophys. Res. Commun. 162:626-633, 1989.
17. Lee, T.H., Crea, A.E.G., Gant, V., Spur, B.W., Marron, B.E., Nicolaou, K.C., Reardon, E., Brezinski, M. and Serhan, C.N. (Submitted).

INVOLVEMENT OF ARACHIDONIC ACID METABOLITES IN THE TRANSCRIPTIONAL REGULATION OF CSF-1 GENE EXPRESSION BY TUMOR NECROSIS FACTOR

M. L. SHERMAN, B. L. WEBER, R. DATTA, and D. W. KUFE

Laboratory of Clinical Pharmacology, Dana-Farber Cancer Institute and Department of Medicine, Harvard Medical School, Boston, MA 02115

INTRODUCTION

The macrophage-specific colony stimulating factor (CSF-1) regulates the hematopoietic stem cell formation of monocyte/macrophage-containing colonies (1). CSF-1 also stimulates the production of several biologic factors including prostaglandin E, plasminogen activator, interleukin 1, granulocyte-specific colony stimulating factor, interferon, myeloid colony stimulating activity and tumor necrosis factor (TNF) (2). In contrast to the known pleiotropic effects of CSF-1, the regulation of CSF-1 gene expression has not been extensively examined. Recent studies have demonstrated that phorbol esters and the granulocyte/macrophage-specific colony stimulating factor induce CSF-1 gene expression in MIA-PaCa cells, normal human monocytes, and during monocytic differentiation of human leukemia cells (3-6). Furthermore, the CSF-1 gene has been shown to be constitutively expressed in a variety of human ovarian, breast and lung carcinoma cell lines (7).

TNF is a regulatory cytokine which has multiple effects on hematopoietic cell growth and differentiation. TNF also induces monocytic differentiation of human HL-60 promyelocytic leukemia cells (8). Recent studies have demonstrated that TNF induces secretion of CSF-1 by monocytes both in vitro and in vivo (9,10). In the present study, we examined the involvement of arachidonic acid metabolites in the transcriptional regulation of CSF-1 gene expression by TNF in HL-60 cells during monocytic differentiation.

MATERIALS AND METHODS

Cell culture.

The HL-60 promyelocytic cells were grown as previously described (11,12). Human recombinant TNF (Asahi Chemical Industry Co, New York, NY) had a specific activity of 2.3×10^6 U/mg and contained less than 10 pg endotoxin/mg protein by the Limulus lysate assay.

Preparation of RNA and Northern blot hybridization.

Total cellular RNA was isolated by the guanidine isothiocyanate-cesium chloride technique as described (11,12). Total cellular RNA (20 ug) was subjected to electrophoresis in a 1% agarose/2.2 M formaldehyde gel, transferred to nitrocellulose paper, and hybridized to one of the following ^{32}P-labeled DNA probes: 1) the 0.57-kb AccI/EcoRI fragment of a human CSF-1 cDNA purified from the pc-CSF-12 plasmid (13); and 2) the pA1 plasmid containing a 2.0-kb PstI insert of the chicken beta-actin gene (14).

Run-on transcriptional analyses.

HL-60 cells (10^8 cells per treatment) were washed with ice-cold phosphate-buffered saline, nuclei were isolated by lysis in 0.5% NP-40 buffer and ^{32}P-labeled RNA was extracted as described (11,12).

Plasmid DNAs containing various cloned inserts were digested with restriction endonucleases as follows: 1) the 2.0-kb PstI fragment of the chicken beta-actin pA1 plasmid; and, 2) the 1.6-kb SalI/EcoRI fragment of the pc-CSF-12 plasmid. The digested DNA was run in a 1% agarose gel, transferred to nitrocellulose filters by the method of Southern and hybridization was performed with 10^7 cpm of ^{32}P-labeled RNA per ml hybridization buffer for 72 h at 42°C.

RESULTS AND DISCUSSION

The effects of TNF on the expression of CSF-1 gene transcripts were first examined during induction of monocytic differentiation (12). Total cellular RNA was isolated from HL-60 cells, separated by agarose/formaldehyde gel electropheresis, transferred to nitrocellulose and hybridized with a ^{32}P-labeled CSF-1 cDNA probe. There was a 20-fold increase in the level of CSF-1 transcripts after 3 h of exposure to TNF. This increase was transient and the level of CSF-1 transcripts returned to that of control cells by 24 h. TNF had no effect on levels of actin transcripts.

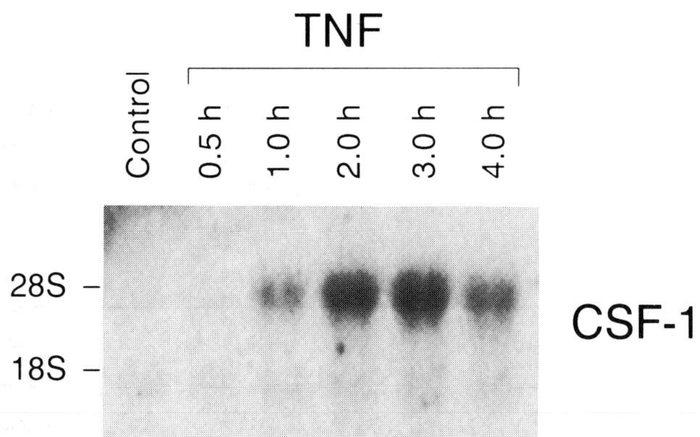

Figure 1. Effects of TNF on CSF-1 RNA levels in HL-60 cells. Northern blot analysis of RNA levels was performed in HL-60 cells after treatment with TNF (200 U/ml). Total cellular RNA (20 ug/lane) was hybridized to a 0.57 kb ^{32}P-labeled CSF-1 DNA probe. The control lane represents RNA from untreated HL-60 cells. (Reproduced in part from the Journal of Clinical Investigation 1990, vol. 85 (in press) by copyright permission of the American Society for Clinical Investigation.)

We were also interested in asking the question whether the induction of CSF-1 by TNF was at the level of transcription. Run-on transcriptional assays in isolated nuclei were performed to determine the mechanisms responsible for the regulation of CSF-1 gene expression by TNF. While a low level of CSF-1 gene transcription was detectable in untreated HL-60 cells, exposure to TNF for 1 and 2 h increased CSF-1 gene transcription by 4-fold and 6-fold, respectively (12).

We next asked the question whether arachidonic acid metabolism is also involved in CSF-1 expression. The induction of CSF-1 RNA by TNF was examined after treatment of HL-60 cells with 4-bromophenacyl bromide (BPB) and quinacrine, inhibitors of phospholipase A_2 activity and arachidonic acid production. TNF-induced increases in CSF-1 transcripts were blocked by both BPB and quinacrine in a concentration-dependent manner. For example, 1 uM BPB inhibited TNF-induced increases in CSF-1 transcripts by 57%, while 5 and 10 uM BPB completely blocked this induction. Similarly, 2 and 5 uM quinacrine inhibited the induction of CSF-1 mRNA by 38 and 64%, respectively, while 10 uM quinacrine completely inhibited the effects of TNF on CSF-1 gene expression (12).

Previous studies had shown that the cyclooxygenase metabolite PGE_2 is a potent regulator of monokine production (15). Thus, we first studied the effects of the cyclooxygenase inhibitor indomethacin on CSF-1 gene expression. Indomethacin alone had no effect on CSF-1 expression, and in combination with TNF had no detectable effect on the induction of CSF-1 RNA. However, the expression of CSF-1 RNA was blocked in a dose-dependent manner by PGE_2 treatment of TNF-induced HL-60 cells (Figure 2). PGE_2 decreased the accumulation of CSF-1 transcripts by 78% and 89% at concentrations of 1 nM and 10 nM, respectively. Furthermore, treatment of HL-60 cells with 200 U/ml TNF and 1 uM PGE_2 inhibited CSF-1 gene transcription by 89% as compared to cells treated with TNF

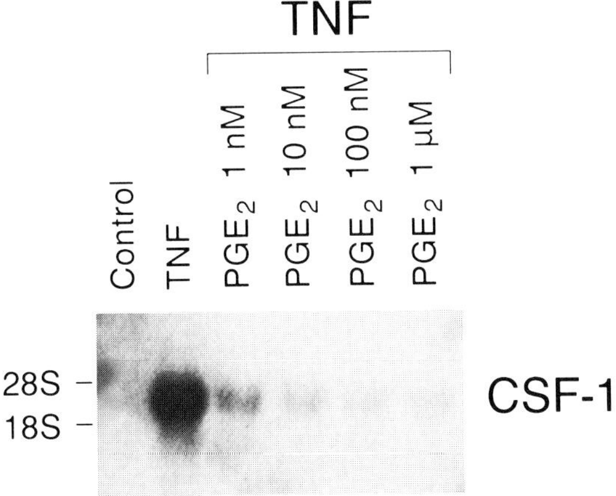

Figure 2. Effects of PGE_2 on TNF induction of CSF-1 gene expression. HL-60 cells were treated with TNF for 3 h in the presence of varying concentrations of PGE_2, and monitored for CSF-1 RNA by Northern blot analysis using a 0.57 kb ^{32}P-labeled CSF-1 DNA probe. The control lane represents RNA from untreated HL-60 cells. Reproduced in part from the Journal of Clinical Investigation, 1990, vol. 85 (in press) by copyright permission of the American Society for Clinical Investigation.

alone. Since we had previously shown that TNF treatment of HL-60 cells had no significant effect on the production of cAMP and that PGE_2 increased cAMP levels in both untreated and TNF-stimulated HL-60 cells (16), it was also of interest to determine if the effects of PGE_2 on CSF-1 transcripts could be mimicked by the addition of exogenous cAMP. Indeed, decreases in the induction of CSF-1 transcripts by TNF were observed in HL-60 cells treated with dibutyryl cAMP. Thus, both PGE_2 and cAMP were potent inhibitory signals for the induction of CSF-1 transcripts by TNF. These findings suggest that the effects of PGE_2 may be due, at least in part, to cAMP metabolism. Recent results have demonstrated that the induction of TNF mRNA is also inhibited by the cyclooxygenase metabolite PGE_2 (17). Thus, cAMP appears to represent a common inhibitory signal for induction of both the CSF-1 and TNF genes.

The stimulation of phospholipase A_2 and production of arachidonic acid by TNF is thus associated with induction of certain genes involved in monocytic differentiation. Arachidonic acid formation is the rate-limiting step in the synthesis of leukotrienes, lipoxins and prostaglandins. This cascade of secondary messengers may be involved in the regulation of genes requlred for the proliferation, differentiation and activation of monocytes.

ACKNOWLEDGMENT

Reproduced in part from the Journal of Clinical Investigation, 1990, vol. 85 (in press) by copyright permlsslon of the American Society for Clinical Investigation.

REFERENCES

1. Stanley, E.R., Guilbert, L.J., Tushinski, R.J. and Bartelmez, S.H. J. Cell. Biochem. 21:151-159, 1983.
2. Warren, M.K. and Ralph, P. J. Immunol. 137:2281-2285, 1986.
3. Ralph, P., Warren, M.K., Lee, M.T., Csejtey, J., Weaver, J.F., Broxmeyer, H.E., Williams, D.E., Stanley, E.R. and Kawasaki, E.S. Blood 68:633-639, 1986.
4. Horiguchi, J., Sariban, E. and Kufe, D. Mol. Cell. Biol. 8:3951-3954, 1988.
5. Horiguchi, J., Warren, M.K. and Kufe, D. Blood 69:1259-1261, 1987.
6. Horiguchi, J., Warren, M.K., Ralph, P. and Kufe, D. Biochem. Biophys. Res. Commun. 141:924-930, 1986.
7. Horiguchi, J., Sherman, M.L., Sampson-Johannes, A., Weber, B.L. and Kufe, D.W. Biochem. Biophys. Res. Commun. 157:395-401, 1988.
8. Trinchieri, G., Kobayashi, M., Rosen, M., Loudon, R., Murphy, M. and Perussia, B. J. Exp. Med. 164:1206-1225, 1986.
9. Oster, W., Lindermann, A., Horn, S., Mertelsmann, R. and Herrmann, F. Blood 70:1700-1703, 1987.
10. Kaushansky, K., Broudy, V.C., Harlan, J.M. and Adamson, J.W. J. Immunol. 141:341-3415, 1988.
11. Sariban, E., Luebbers, R. and Kufe, D.W. Mol. Cell. Biol. 8:340-346, 1988.
12. Sherman, M.L., Weber, B.L., Datta, R., and Kufe, D.W. J. Clin. Invest. 85:442-447, 1990.
13. Kawasaki, E.S., Ladner, M.B., Wang, A.M., Van Arsdell, J., Warren, M.K., Coyne, M.Y., Schweickart, V.L., Lee, M-T., Wilson, K.J., Boosman, A., Stanley, E.R., Ralph, P. and Mark, D.F. Science 230:291-296, 1985.
14. Cleveland, D.W., Lopata, M.A., MacDonald, R.J., Cowan, N.J., Rutter, W.J. and Kirschner, M.W. Cell 20:95-105, 1980.
15. Kunkel, S.L., Spengler, M., May, M.A., Spengler, R., Larrick, J. and Remick, D. 1988. J. Biol. Chem. 263:5380-5384, 1988.
16 Imamura K., Sherman, M.L., Spriggs, D. and Kufe, D. J. Biol. Chem. 263:10247-10253, 1988.
17. Horiguchi, J., Spriggs, D., Imamura, K., Stone, R., Luebbers, R. and Kufe, D. Mol. Cell. Biol. 9:252-258, 1989.

MODULATION OF SPLEEN AND THYMUS LYMPHOID SUBSETS BY IN VIVO ADMINISTRATION OF DI-M-PGE2 IN NORMAL AND TUMOR-BEARING MICE

A. MASTINO, C. FAVALLI, S. GRELLI*, and E. GARACI

Department of Experimental Medicine and Biochemical Sciences, II University of Rome. Via O. Raimondo. 00173, *Ist. Med. Sper. CNR; Rome. Italy

INTRODUCTION

Prostaglandin E2 (PGE2) have been implicated both in experimental tumor growth and in the modulation of immune response (reviewed in 1, 2). Regarding to their immunomodulating action, PGE2 are known to exert a suppressive activity after in vitro and in vivo treatment. However, in some conditions, they are also able to cause enhancing effects on the immune system (3,4,5). We have previously demonstrated that the in vivo administration of 16,16 dimethyl-PGE2-methyl ester (di-M-PGE2), a long-acting synthetic analog of PGE2, causes differential effects on the immune response in normal or tumor-bearing mice and that these effects could be related to the inhibition of tumor growth (reviewed in 6). Thus di-M-PGE2 has been clearly shown to inhibit in normal mice a variety of immune functions as the number of plaque forming cells from spleen, the seric hemagglutinin titers or the delayed hypersensitivity reaction to sheep erythrocytes, as well as natural klller (NK) activity or mitogen induced IL-2 production. On the other hand, PGE2 has been able to enhance the same functions in B-16 melanoma tumor-bearing mice (7,8,9).

The effects of PGE or PGE analogues on different cellular compartment and subsets of the immune system have been limitedly studied (10,11,12). Moreover, no informations regarding the effects of in vivo PGE2 administration on phenotipically identified lymphocyte subsets in the murine system, are actually available. Considering the central role of different lymphocyte subsets both in the control and in the effector phase of the immune response, we have studied the effect of in vivo administration of di-M-PGE2 on spleen cell subsets in normal and tumor-bearing mice. In order to understand if the modifications of spleen cell subsets could be related to alteration at thymus level, we have also examined the distribution of thymus subsets following in vivo administration of di-M-PGE2. In this work we report the results of a systematic study, performed by means of flow cytometry using specific antibodies.

MATERIALS AND METHODS.

Mice.

Six-week old inbred C57BL/6NCrBR mice, purchased from Charles River, (Calco, Como, Italy) were used in all experiments.

Tumors.

B-16 Melanoma, obtained originally from Dr. M.G. Zupi (Istituto Regina Elena, Rome, Italy), was mantained in vivo by serial subcutaneous (s.c.) transplantation in C57B1/6 mice. In all the experiments performed, tumors were freshly excised from tumor bearing mice, minced in Hanks' balanced salt solution (HBSS) and strained through a fine stainless-steel mesh. Cell suspensions obtained in this way were collected by centrifugation, washed twice, counted and resuspended to the desired concentration. Cellular viability, determined by trypan blue exclusion, ranged 10-20%. Mice received 2 x 10^5 viable B16 melanoma cells s.c. in the right flank.

PGE2 administration.

Mice were randomized, divided into control and experimental groups (4-9 animals each) and injected i.p. which control diluents or di-M-PGE2, respectively (500 µg/Kg once a day for 4 consecutive days). Spleen and thymus cell subsets were analyzed at various times after the last injection.

Cell preparation.

Spleen and thymus cells were obtained from normal or B-16 melanoma bearing mice, both treated or not with di-M-PGE2, by gentle teasing of spleens and thymuses in RPMI 1640 (Flow Laboratories, Irvine, Ayrshire, UK). The resultant cell suspension was filtered through a nytex mesh, washed twice with RPMI 1640, counted and resuspended in phosphate buffered salt solution (PBSS) at 2 x 10^7/ml cells. Spleens and thymuses were individually processed in non sterile conditions.

Immunofluorescence staining.

Samples were prepared by transferring 50 µl of cell suspension, collected from each animal, into 12x75 mm round-bottom polystyrene tubes (Falcon, B.D. Co., Lincoln Park, NJ) containing PBSS as unstained control, or the following antibodies: fluorescein conjugate monoclonal antibody anti-mouse Thy-1.2, fluorescein conjugate goat anti-mouse Ig, phycoerythrin conjugate anti-mouse L3T4, fluorescein conjugate anti-mouse Lyt-2 (Becton Dickinson Mountain View, Ca). Staining was performed at 4°C for 30 minutes. After treatment cells were washed twice in PBSS containing 0.02% sodium azide and used immediately.

Flow cytometry analysis.

Analysis was performed using a FACS analyzer (Becton Dickinson, FACS Systems, Mountain View, CA). Thresholds and gates were selected by using electronic volume, and side scatter, in order to exclude red blood cells. Data usually collected as "list mode" were obtained from 10,000 cells for each analysis. The following elaboration of data was performed by Consort 30 Software (Becton Dickinson) running on HP 9,000/ 217 computer (Hewlett-Packard Co., Fort Collins, CO). The proportion of cells showing background fluorescence was selected by marker setting, according to unstained control sample, allowing the computer to quantify positive cells with subsequent subtraction of background fluorescence.

RESULTS

Effect of Prostaglandins E2 on spleen cell in normal mice.

The administration of di-M-PGE2 24 hr after the last injection caused a dramatic fall of the absolute numbers, in both Thy-1.2+ positive and Ig+ positive subsets, due to an evident decrease of spleen cellularity. However T-cells seem to be more affected by di-M-PGE2 inhibition than B-cells (Table 1). Analysis of T major subsets indicated that CD8+ cells are more sensitive to di-M-PGE2 than CD4+ cells. These modifications were still persistent 4 days after the last di-M-PGE2 inoculation, but a certain ongoing recovery was shown (Table 1).

Table 1. Effect of di-M-PGE$_2$ on spleen lymphocyte subsets

	Millions of Positive cells ± S.D.				
	Control	Hours after administration			
		24		96	
Thy 1.2+	81.71 ± 6.38	35.81 ± 2.68	(43.8%)a	58.87 ± 4.40	(72.1%)
CD8+	59.88 ± 8.09	31.55 + 1.25	(52.7%)	46.28 ± 4.51	(77.3%)
CD4+	44.66 ± 4.13	20.04 ± 1.15	(44.9%)	34.83 ± 4.81	(78.0%)
IG+	21.77 ± 1.75	8.68 ± 1.07	(39.9%)	11.14 ± 1.36	(51.2%)

a) Percentage variation.

Effect of di-M-PGE2 on thymus in normal mice.

Quantitative modifications of thymocyte subsets showed a drastic reduction of CD4+CD8+ double positive cells 24 hr after the last injection of di-M-PGE2 (Table 2). Single positive CD4+ or CD8+ thymocytes were also reduced; on the other hand, the number of double negative thymocytes was increased. The results obtained 96 hr after the last injection showed slight differences in single positive or double negative subsets respect to the control mice, while the decrease of the absolute number of double positive thymocytes was still clearly evident (Table 2).

Effect of di-M-PGE2 in tumor-bearing mice.

Following the study of the effect of di-M-PGE2 on lymphoid subsets in normal mice, we have examined the effect of di-M-PGE2 administration in B-16 melanoma tumor bearing mice. We have recently seen that the growth of this experimental tumor is characterized by a progressive remarkable reduction of Thy-1.2+ positive spleen cells (unpublished results). In order to investigate a possible modulation of T-cell subsets in tumor-bearing mice, the administration of di-MPGE2 was started on day

Table 2. Effect of di-M-PGE2 on thymus lymphocyte subsets

	Millions of Positive cells ± S.D.				
	Control	Hours after administration			
		24		96	
DNa	3.62 ± 1.60	21.39 ± 2.25	(590.9%) b	9.17 ± 1.83	(253.3%)
DP	127.06 ± 9.84	15.13 ± 1.56	(11.9%)	58.15 ± 4.11	(47.8%)
CD4+	18.40 ± 5.71	9.79 ± 0.70	(53.2%)	10.95 ± 0.73	(59.5%)
CD8+	6.55 + 4.12	1.84 + 0.18	(28.1%)	2.35 ± 0.56	(35.9%)

a) DN=Double negative CD4/CD8; DP=Double positive CD4/CD8
b) Percentage variation.

18 after tumor inoculation. On day 22 after tumor inoculation (i.e. 24 hr after the last injection of di-M-PGE2) spleen cells were analyzed by flow cytometry. Results showed that di-M-PGE2 were able to partially restore the percentage of Thy-1.2+ cells in B-16 tumor-bearing mice. The analysis of T cell subsets indicated that the partial restoration of Thy-1.2+ cell was principally ~ due to the increase of CD4+ cell percentage, while no modification in CD8+ cells, respect to untreated control was observed (Table 3).

Table 3. Effect of di-M-PGE2 on spleen lymphocyte subsets in B-16 tumor-bearing mice

	Percentage of Positive cells ± S.D.				
	Control	B-16		B-16+Di-M-PGE2a	
Thy 1.2+	50.81 ± 4.12	33.80 ± 3.46	(66.5%)	45.15 ± 3.57	(88.9%)
Ig+	38.49 ± 8.09	31.19 ± 1.61	(81.0%)	34.04 ± 3.66	(88.4%)
CD4+	32.59 ± 2.67	23.04 ± 1.49	(70.7%)	28.20 ± 3.90	(86.5%)
CD8+	19.33 + 1.13	13.48 + 1.25	(69.7%)	13.31 ± 1.10	(68.9%)

a) treatment was started 18 hr after tumor inoculation and flow cytometry analysis was performed 24 hr after the last injection.

DISCUSSION

The analysis of the quantitative modifications in spleen or thymus cell subset after di-M-PGE2 administration, showed some new interesting informations about the in vivo modulatory effect of PGE2 in the immune system. The evidence that the T cell compartment seems to be more sensitive to di-M-PGE2, than the B cell one, cleary confirms the peculiar modulation of the immune response by PGE2 Thus, the immune suppressive action of PGE2 in normal mice should not be simply attributed to their non specific inhibition of cell proliferation. Drugs able to exert such inhibition, as cyclophosphamide, are known to preferentially decrease the B spleen cell and to increase the percentage of T cells (13). Moreover, considering that the CD8+ spleen cells seem to be more down regulated by di-M-PGE2 in vivo than CD4+ cells, it has to be excluded that the immunosuppressive activity of PGE2 in normal mice could be mediated by a selective differentiation or by an enrichment of the CD8+ subset. This result is in agreement with previous in vitro studies (10). The alteration of T cell compartment is detectable not only at the periphery, but also at the central level as it is suggested by the dramatic modifications in the thymocytes subsets. Similar effects were also observed in adrenalectomized mice, demostrating that they are not corticosteroid-mediated (data not shown). The transient increase of absolute number of double negative thymocytes 24 hr after the last injection, indicate that some of the immunosuppressive effects of di-M-PGE2 at periphery level are related to an intrathymic block in the differentiation of T cell. Different results were observed in B-16 tumor-bearing mice. In this case in vivo di-M-PGE2 administration caused an increase of Thy-1.2+ spleen cells percentage mainly due to the CD4+ subset enrichment. No absolute number increase T cell was really observed in treated tumor bearing mice, but the redistribution in the percentage of T cell subset could at least partially, explain some enhancing effect of di-M-PGE2 on T cell function, in B-16 melanoma tumor-bearing mice, previously shown by as.

REFERENCES

1. Goodwin, J.S. Prostaglandins and Immunity. Martinus Nijhoff, Boston, 1985.
2. Thaler-Dao, H., Crastes de Paulet A., Paoletti R. Icosanoid and Cancer. Raven Press, New York, 1984.
3. Mertin, J., Stackpoole, A., Shumway, S.J. Transplantation 18: 396-02, 1984.
4. Hacker-Shahin, B., Droge, W. Cell. Immunol. 91: 43-51, 1985.
5. Quill, H., Gaur, A., Phipps, R.P. J. Immunol. 142: 813-818, 1989.
6. Favalli, C., Mastino, A., Garaci, E. In: Prostaglandins and Cancer Research (Ed. E. Garaci, R. Paoletti, M.G. Santoro), Springer-Verlag, Berlin, 1987, pp. 245-253.
7. Favalli, C., Garaci, E., Etheredge, E., Santoro, M.G., Jaffe, B.M. J. Immunol. 125: 351-359, 1980.
8. Garaci, E., Mastino, A., Jezzi, T., Riccardi, C., Favalli, C. Cell. Immunol. 106: 43-52, 1987.
9. Jezzi, T., Mastino, A., Marini, S., Pica, F., Favalli, C., Garaci, E. Int. J. Immunophatol and Pharmacol. 2: 31-40, 1989.
10. Ceuppens, J.L., Goodwin, J.S. Cell. Immunol. 70 41-54, 1982.
11. Goodwin, J.S., and Clay, J.A. Int. J. Immunopharmac. 8: 867-873, 1986.
12. Whittum-Hudson, J., Ballow, M., Zurier, R.B. Immunopharmacol. 16: 71-78, 1988.
13. Turk, J., Parker, D. Immun. Rev. 65: 99-113, 1982.

RECEPTOR MODULATION OF LIPID METABOLISM

G PROTEIN INVOLVEMENT IN SIGNAL TRANSDUCTION

J. N. FAIN

Department of Biochemistry, University of Tennessee, Memphis, TN 38163

This chapter is concerned with the role of G proteins in the regulation of signal transduction by ligands which bind to high affinity receptor proteins on the cell surface. Some of these receptors transmit information from the exterior surface of the cell into internal signals or second messengers. Other receptors alter reactions such as ion fluxes without an intracellular messenger.

A specific example of a plasma membrane receptor that alters intracellular metabolism without the release of any intracellular messenger is the nicotillic cholinergic receptor. This receptor complex is an ion channel that is activated as the result of a conformational change in shape resulting from receptor binding (1,2). However, there is another mechanism for activation of ion channels involving a conformational change in G proteins as a result of ligands binding to receptors (3,4). This involves mechanisms similar to those by which ligand receptor omplexes are able to regulate the activity of adenylate cyclase and phospholipase C.

The effects of ligands that are mediated through activation of enzymatic processes in the plasma membrane can be divided into four general categories. The first category is the adenylate cyclase cascade where a variety of hormones either inhibit or stimulate adenylate cyclase thus altering the level of cyclic AMP which acts as a regulator of a protein kinase that phosphorylates serine or threonine residues in proteins (5,6). The second is the phosphoinositide cascade where hormones activate a phosphoinositide specific phospholipholipids that degrades phosphatiltylinositol 4,5-bisphosphate (PIP_2) resulting in the release of diacylglycerol and inositol 1,4,5-trisphosphate (IP_3) (7,8). The IP_3 releases Ca^{2+} from intracellular stores (7,9) and this results in activation of a Ca^{2+}-calmodulin protein kinase B (10) and other Ca^{2+}-dependent processes. The diacylglycerol activates another protein kinase known as protein kinase C (11) . Thus these two enzymatic cascades alter the activity of three different protein kinases and these in turn cause covalent modifications of target proteins.

The receptors involved in the adenylate cyclase and phospholipase C cascades have two major common features. All the receptors have seven transmembrane spanning hydrophobic regions (seven-helix motif) and have no known enzymatic activity. Furthermore all these receptors are present as complexes with guanine nucleotide binding (G) proteins. A conformational change induced by binding of the hormone to the receptor causes an alteration in the conformation of the G protein and this in turn is linked to activation of adenylate cyclase or phospholipase C on the inner surface of the plasma membrane.

Receptors of the third and fourth type have only one transmembrane spanning unit per receptor molecule. One group of receptors have guanylate cyclase activity and convert GTP to cyclic GMP which activates a serine-threonine protein kinase. Only one protein is involved with a hormone-binding domain in the extracellular region and catalytic activity in the intracellular domain (12). It is as yet unclear why a more complex mechanism involving three proteins is used for the generation of cyclic AMP.

The fourth group of ligand receptors also have only one transmembrane spanning region. These receptors phosphorylate proteins on tyrosine residues. It is also unclear what the link is between the tyrosine protein kinase activity of the receptor and the hormonal response.

The four receptor types mentioned above along with the ion channel receptors with no enzymatic activity and multiple transmembrane spanning regions can account for most of the known plasma membrane ligand receptors. It should also be noted that there are two additional mechanisms by which ion channels can be regulated besides having a ligand-binding subunit as part of the ion channel complex. One is via G proteins and the other is secondary to altered phosphorylation of these channels as a result of changes in intracellular second messengers (4).

The four most important intracellular messengers are cyclic AMP, cyclic GMP, inositol trisphosphate (IP_3) and diacylglycerol. The latter two are formed by cannibalization of a minor plasma membrane phospholipid and the former from common metabolic intermediates (ATP and GTP). All act as activators of protein kinases that phosphorylate target proteins on serine or threonine residues thus changing their enzymatic activity (Figure 1). The role of G proteins in formation of these messengers is

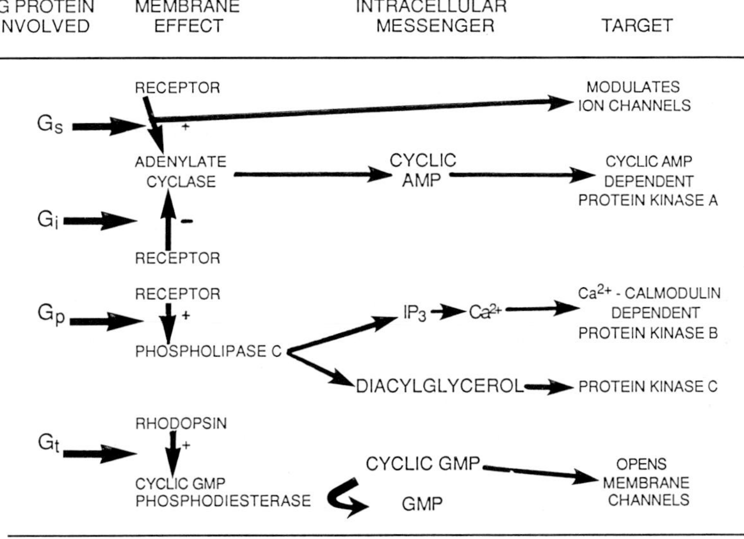

FIGURE 1. The role of G proteins in second messenger generation and regulation of ion channels.

also illustrated in Figure 1. There are other effects of G proteins on ion channels in membranes that do not involve second messengers (Figure 1) . One involves G_t and will be discussed later in this chapter. The other example shown in Figure 1 is G_s modulation of ion channels.

There has been substantial indirect evidence for some time that ligands such as β catecholamines have effects on metabolism and muscle contraction that cannot be attributed solely to cyclic AMP. Only recently it was found that in vesicles of cardiac sarcolemma or skeletal muscle T-tubules the active G_s α subunit containing bound GTP or GTPγS stimulates Ca^{2+} channels (14).

The first evidence that receptors with the seven-helix motif work through G proteins (G stands for guanine nucleotide binding) was the discovery in the laboratory of Martin Rodbell that GTP was required for activation of adenylate cyclase (13). The role of GTP was unclear for some time and especially since, while it was required for glucagon activation of adenylate cyclase activity in liver membranes, it actually decreased the binding of glucagon to liver membranes. Eventually it was discovered that hormones bind much more tightly to receptors when they are coupled to G proteins in the inactive state. In the inactive state the heterotrimeric G protein has GDP bound to the α subunit. In the presence of a ligand binding to the receptor occurs and GTP is exchanged for bound GDP on the G protein. The α subunit of the G protein with bound GTP then dissociates from the β-γ subunits and activates adenylate cyclase (14-16).

The rapid dissociation of the hormone-receptor complex from the G protein after bound GDP is exchanged for GTP appears to be a device to permit many G proteins to be formed per hormone receptor complex. This provides for an additional step of amplification in hormonal response that is missing when the hormone-receptor complex is an active enzyme as is the case for guanylate cyclase. Hormone antagonists actually bind to hormone receptors that interact with G proteins much more tightly than do agonists because the receptor-antagonist is unable to induce conformational changes that result in exchange of GDP for GTP. This is supported by the finding that catecholamine antagonist binding in not influenced by GTP. In contrast both catecholamine agonist binding and agonist displacement of antagonist binding are reduced by GTP.

If many G proteins are activated per hormone-receptor complex then how is the hormone signal terminated when the level of hormone decreases? The GTP bound α subunit once activated has no mechanism to perceive whether the level of hormone has increased or decreased. G protein activation is really a hit rather than occupancy mechanism. As long as the hormone is bound to the receptor the production of a membrane-bound messenger occurs but G proteins have a built in mechanism for inactivation. This involves hydrolysis of the bound GTP to GDP by the α subunit after a finite time. The α subunit of the G protein is in effect a GTPase enzyme with a very low turnover number since it degrades only bound GTP. The GDP that is formed does not dissociate from the α subunit but remains bound. The GDP-bound (inactive) α subunit rebinds the γ and β subunits and presumably forms a complex with the receptor which remains inactive until another molecule of hormone binds to the receptor and the bound GDP is exchanged for GTP. The G_s (the s stands for stimulatory) protein is involved in activation of adenylate cyclase. The G_i (i stands for inhibitory) proteins are involved in inhibition of adenylate cyclase .

Opiates, adenosine and α-2-adrenergic amines all lower cyclic AMP in target cells and inhibit adenylate cyclase activity of membranes from these cells (17). The binding of these agonists to their receptors is reduced by GTP and they stimulate GTPase activity of target membranes as seen with hormones that stimulate adenylate cyclase. The toxin produced by *Bordetella pertussis* covalently modifies the inhibitory G protein by attaching an ADP-ribose moiety derived from NAD (18).

In contrast the toxin produced by *Vibrio cholerae* also uses NAD to ADP-ribosylate the α subunit of the G_s but not the G_i protein. The diarrhea seen in cholera is due to the cholera toxin and is secondary to high levels of cyclic AMP in the gut. When the G_s α subunit is ADP-ribosylated by cholera toxin it remains in the active state with bound GTP. In effect after ADP-ribosylation the self-destruct mechanism for inactivation of G_s is circumvented and the message stays active because of the covalent modification involving ADP-ribosylation (18).

There is substantial indirect evidence that G proteins are involved in the regulation of phospholipase C (8). However, as yet it has not been possible to reconstitute this signal pathway in phospholipid vesicles using a known G protein, phospholipase C and the appropriate receptor. This has been achieved with the G proteins involved in both activation and inactivation of adenylate cyclase and was proof that three separate proteins are required for signal transduction with regard to cyclase activation.

Guanine nucleotides affect the binding of hormones that stimulate phospholipase C and it has been possible to see activation of GTPase activity in membranes upon addition of these ligands (8). Further indirect evidence for a G_p (p stands for phospholipase C activation) protein was the finding that in some membranes agonist activation of phospholipase C was only seen in the presence of GTPγS a non-hydrolyzable analog of GTP (19). GTP γS substitutes for GTP in the activation of adenylate cyclase by hormones. The G protein involved in regulation of phospholipase C in some cells differs from G_s and G_i in that it is apparently not a substrate for either cholera or pertussis toxins. In the brain both phospholipase C and polyphosphoinositides are much more abundant than in other cells. Muscarinic cholinergic stimulation of phospholipase C can be seen in brain membranes using exogenous phosphoinositides (19). The enzyme(s) that are activated degrade phosphatidylinositol as well as polyphosphoinositides (19).

The best understood G protein is G_t originally known as transducin (15,20,21). This protein has a heterotrimeric structure and its α subunit is ADP-ribosylated by both cholera and pertussis toxins. It binds GTP upon activation and is deactivated by hydrolysis of the bound GTP to GDP. The structure of G_t is very similar to that of the other G proteins. The capture of a single photon of light by rhodopsin results in the formation of around 500 activated G_t molecules. This process is the first stage of amplification in visual excitation (20,21).

Rhodopsin is the photosensitive protein in the discs of the rod cells of the eye and consists of opsin, a protein, and II-cis-retinal, the prosthetic group. The opsin part consists of a protein with the seven helix motif (7 transmembrane spanning regions) and shows remarkable structural similarity to hormone receptors that interact with G proteins. These proteins differ only in that light presumably interacts with the II-cis-retinal chromophore located near the center of rhodopsin in the membrane while hormones interact with specific sites on the receptor rather than with a prosthetic group (20,21).

Both light and hormonal activation result in displacement of bound GDP on G proteins. However, $G_{t\alpha}$ activates a cyclic nucleotide phosphodiesterase in rods which degrades cyclic GMP to GMP. This results in a decrease in the permeability of Na^+ channels in rods and hyperpolarization. The amplification factor per single photon is at least a million. In the visual regulatory cascade one photon of light results in 500 activated $G_{t\alpha}$ subunits and each activated $G_{t\alpha}$ subunit decreases the entry of 2,000 Na^+ ions (20,21).

The activation of cyclic GMP phosphodiesterase in the eye involves relief from an inhibitory constraint. The phosphodiesterase as isolated consists of three subunits and the active $G_{t\alpha}$ binds to one of the subunits without catalytic activity known as the inhibitory subunit. This results in dissociation of the complex and the phosphodiesterase is now catalytically active. Just as in cyclic AMP activation of protein kinase A the phosphodiesterase is active only as long as the active $G_{t\alpha}$ binds to its inhibitory subunit. After a finite time the GTP bound to $G_{t\alpha}$ is degraded to bound GDP and the inactive $G_{t\alpha}$ now dissociates from the inhibitory subunit of the phosphodiesterase (20,21).

Early models for the structure of receptors without enzymatic activity did not have them spanning the membranes. However we now know that receptors that interact with G proteins actually span the plasma membrane at least 7 times and therefore have three loops as well as a tail extending into the cytoplasmic space. Theoretically activation of G proteins should not require receptors to extend into the cytosol. It now appears that the major role of the loops and tail is actually to serve as sites for phosphorylation by protein kinases (22). Apparently a large part of the desensitization processes involved in light adaptation and so-called down regulation to hormones upon continued occupancy of receptors is mediated through increased phosphorylation of receptors on the third loop or the cytosolic tail. These sequences have many serine and threonine residues. Protein kinases A, B and C are all able to phosphorylate receptors and reduce their sensitivity to further stimulation. The product of the receptors linked to adenylate cyclase is cyclic AMP and among the substrates for protein kinase A is the receptor itself. In addition the occupancy of receptors seems to increases their sensitivity to phosphorylation by endogenous protein kinases.

The insulin and EGF receptors have both been isolated from cell membranes in recent years and sequenced (23-25). Both receptors have a single transmembrane helix per subunit and have tyrosine kinase activity. However, the link between this tyrosine kinase activity and the cellular responses is still unknown (23,26). It has been possible to construct a chimeric receptor with the extracellular insulin binding region of the insulin receptor linked to the intracellular tyrosine kinase domain of the EGF receptor and demonstrate increased tyrosine kinase activity of this chimera upon binding of insulin (25).

Another receptor with a single transmembrane spanning region is that for platelet-derived growth factor (PDGF). Studies of hormone action and tumor virology converged when it was realized that the retroviral oncogene v-sis encoded one of the subunits of the PDGF receptor with tyrosine protein kinase activity (27). The viral form of the erb-B oncogene encodes a truncated receptor for EGF in which the tyrosine kinase activity is locked in the on position even in the absence of EGF. Alterations in the structure of growth factor receptors resulting in high basal tyrosine protein kinase activity stimulates oncogenesis. We are still unclear about the mechanisms involved. Studies analyzing the proteins phosphorylated on tyrosine residues when growth factors are added or the oncogenes inserted into cells have been very frustrating.

The binding of PDGF to its receptor stimulates a number of responses within minutes besides activation of tyrosine kinase (27). One of these is increased breakdown of phosphoinositides. This response is puzzling since the known mechanisms for activation of phospholipase C involve receptors with seven transmembrane domains and G proteins. The simplest explanation is that the phospholipase C is phosphorylated on tyrosine residues by the PDGF receptor and this represents an alternative mechanism for activation of phospholipase C. Wahl *et al.* (28) reported that EGF treatment of A-431 cells (a tumor cell line expressing very high levels of EGF receptors) resulted in phosphorylation of a phospholipase C isozyme. Further studies should provide more information about this unique mechanism for activation of phospholipase C. However, activation of phospholipase C in the same cells by bradykinin which is thought to work through G proteins was not associated with increased tyrosine phosphorylation of the phospholipase C.

The recent work from the laboratory of Williams (27) has shown that phosphoinositide breakdown and many of the other early responses to PDGF are not sufficient to stimulate DNA synthesis in CHO cells. Tyrosine kinase activity appears to be necessary but insufficient for stimulation of DNA synthesis. However, the stimulation of phosphatidylinositol kinase by PDGF was lost in cells with an altered receptor that was able to stimulate phosphoinositide breakdown but not DNA synthesis. When the normal receptor is stimulated by PDGF there is a physical association of the receptor with a unique lipid kinase that phosphorylates the 3 rather than the 4 position on the inositol ring of PI resulting in formation of phosphatidylinositol 3-phosphate. This unique lipid appears to be a poor substrate for brain phospholipase C (29) and may serve as a lipid intracellular messenger. Ordinarily in cells under basal conditions the ratio of phosphatidylinositol-3-phosphate to phosphatidylinositol 4-phosphate is very low (30).

This chapter has reviewed the role of G proteins in signal transduction. Much has been learned in recent years about the mechanisms involved in the regulation of cyclic AMP, IP_3, diacylglycerol and cyclic GMP levels. We are also just beginning to unravel the complex interactions between these messengers that result in the specific and unique response of a given cell to a particular hormone. However, within the past twenty years we have come to realize the key role of G proteins in signal transduction.

We now know that the receptors involved in the regulation of adenylate cyclase and phospholipase C by hormones, eicosanoids and neurotransmitters have two major features in common. These receptors have seven transmembrane spanning hydrophobic regions (seven-helix motif) and no known enzymatic activity. Furthermore all these receptors can be isolated as complexes with guanine nucleotide binding (G) proteins. A conformational change induced by binding of the hormone to the receptor causes an alteration in the conformation of the G protein and this is linked to activation of adenylate cyclase or phospholipase C on the inner surface of the plasma membrane. In the inactive state, the heterotrimeric G proteins have GDP bound to the α subunit. In the presence of a hormone-receptor complex and GTP the exchange of bound GDP for GTP occurs. The α subunit with bound GTP then dissociates from the β-γ subunits and activates adenylate cyclase.

REFERENCES

1. Guy, H.R. and Hucho, F. Trends Neurosci. 10: 318-321, 1987.
2. Krueger, B.K. FASEB J. 3: 1906-1914, 1989.
3. Rosenthal, W., Hescheler, J., Trautwein, W. and Schultz, G. FASEB J. 2: 2784-2790, 1988.
4. Casey, PJ. and Gilman, A.G. J. Biol. Chem. 263: 2577-2580, 1988.
5. Taylor, S.S. J. Biol. Chem. 264: 8443-8446, 1989.
6. Krebs, E.G. Biochem. Soc. Trans. 13: 813-820, 1985.
7. Berridge, M.J. and Irvine, R.F. Nature 341: 197-205, 1989.
8. Fain, J.N., Wallace, M.A. and Wojcikiewicz, R.J.H. FASEB J. 2: 2569-2574, 1988.
9. Streb, H., Irvine, R.F., Berridge, M.J. and Schulz, I. Nature 306: 67-69, 1983.
10. Cheung, W.Y. The Harvey Lecture Series. Academic Press 79: 173-216, 1985.
11. Nishizuka, Y. Science 233: 305-312, 1986.
12. Garbers, D.L. J. Biol. Chem. 264: 9103-9106, 1989.
13. Rodbell, M., Birnbaumer, L., Pohl, S.L. and Krans, M.J. J. Biol. Chem. 245: 1877-1882, 1971.
14. Brown, A.M. and Birnbaumer L. Am. J. Physiol. H401-H410, 1988.
15. Gilman, A.G. Ann. Rev. Biochem. 56: 615-649, 1987.
16. Levitzki, A. Science 241: 800-806, 1988.
17. Limbird, L.E. FASEB J. 2: 2686-2695, 1988.
18. Moss, J. and Vaughan, M. Advances in Enzymology and Related Areas of Molecular Biology 61: 303-379, 1988.
19. Claro, E., Wallace, M.A., Lee, H.-M. and Fain, J.N. J. Biol. Chem., in press, 1989.
20. Stryer, L. Ann. Rev. Neurosci. 2: 87-119, 1986.
21. Stryer, L. Sci. Amer. 255: 42-50, 1987.
22. Sibley, D.R., Benovic, J.L., Caron, M.G. and Lefkowitz, R.J. Endocrine Rev. 2: 38-56, 1988.
23. Rosen, O.M. Science 237: 1452-1458, 1987.
24. Schlessinger, J. Biochemistry 27: 3119-3123, 1988.
25. Yarden, Y. and Ullrich, A. Biochemistry 27: 3113-3119, 1988.
26. Czech, M.P., Klarlund, J.K., Yagaloff, K.A., Bradford, A.P. and Lewis, R.E. J. Biol. Chem. 263, 11017-11020, 1988.
27. Williams, L.T. Science 243, 1564-1570, 1989.
28. Wahl, M.I., Nishibe, S., Suh, P.-G., Rhee, S.G. and Carpenter, G. Proc. Natl. Acad. Sci. USA 86, 1568-1572, 1989.
29. Lips, D.L., Majerus, P.W., Gorga, F.R., Young, A.T. and Benjamin, T.L. J. Biol. Chem. 264, 8759-8763, 1989.
30. Stephens, L., Hawkins, P.T. and Downes, C.P. Biochem. J. 259, 267-276, 1989.

REGULATION OF PROTEIN KINASE C

Y. A. HANNUN, MD

Departments of Medicine and Cell Biology, Duke University Medical Center, Durham, N.C. 27710

INTRODUCTION

Protein kinase C has emerged as a key element in the transduction of the effects of growth factors, hormones, and neurotransmitters (1). The enzyme was initially discovered by Nishizuka and coworkers who defined a proteolytically activated kinase from rat brain. A number of discoveries by that group led to the recognition of the significance of protein kinase C as an important regulator of tumor promotion, cell regulation, and cell differentiation. Initial characterization of the enzyme by Nishizuka and coworkers led to the identification that the proenzyme could be activated in the presence of membranes and calcium. Further studies led to the identification that the neutral lipid, diacylglycerol (DAG), caused potent activation of the enzyme and significantly reduced its calcium requirement to the low micromolar and high nanomolar range, rendering the enzyme active at physiologic concentrations of calcium in the presence of DAG. This finding led Nishizuka and coworkers to implicate protein kinase C in the pathways mediating the effects of "calcium-mobilizing" agents in what had been termed as the "phosphatidylinositol (PI) cycle" (1). In this cycle, the action of a number of extracellular agents leads to the activation of phospholipase C which results in the cleavage of inositolphospholipids yielding inositol trisphosphate and DAG. Inositol trisphosphate mobilizes intracellular calcium while DAG activates protein kinase C. Another major discovery by Nishizuka's group related to the finding that phorbol esters, potent tumor promoters, could directly activate protein kinase C with a mechanism similar to that of DAG. This finding again implicated protein kinase C in mediating the effects of phorbol esters on tumor promotion, cell differentiation, and a variety of other biological responses such as granule secretion and hormone release (1).

Further studies on protein kinase C regulation have led to more detailed examination of the *in vitro* mechanism of regulation of this enzyme by phospholipids and DAG and to the identification of a number of additional modulators of protein kinase C activity. This review will discuss the different modalities of regulation of protein kinase C *in vitro* and extend those studies to physiologic regulation of protein kinase C in cellular systems.

PROTEIN KINASE C IS A FAMILY OF ISOENZYMES

Protein kinase C has been cloned by a number of investigators from different species. The most significant result was the finding that protein kinase C exists as a family of closely related isoenzymes with at least 8 isoenzymes identified so far. The major isoenzymes a, b, and c are products of distinct genes with the b form existing in 2 isoforms that are alternatively spliced products of the same gene (2).

The linear structure of protein kinase C isoenzymes show similar organization into 4 constant regions and 5 variable regions (Figure 1). The carboxy terminus region of the enzyme shows high homology to other serine and threonine kinases and to some tyrosine kinases. The amino terminus domain has unique sequence compared to other protein kinases. The major isoenzymes of protein kinase C can be separated on hydroxyapatite chromatography, and their in vitro regulation has been studied without delineation of any significant differences amongst the 3 different isoenzymes (3). Further insight into the structure/function organization of protein kinase C has been obtained from studies based on the proteolytic cleavage of protein kinase C into a 32 kDa aminoterminus and a 50 kDa carboxyterminus. The 50 kDa carboxyterminus shows intrinsic catalytic activity that is no longer regulated by phospholipid, DAG, or calcium. The aminoterminus 32 kDa domain is able to bind phorbol esters in the presence of phospholipid and calcium suggesting that it is the lipid binding domain which imparts regulation to the intact enzyme (4). Additionally, a pseudosubstrate site at the aminoterminus of the regulatory domain has been identified which shares a consensus sequence for protein kinase C substrates but lacks a phosphorylatable serine or threonine. It has been hypothesized that this pseudosubstrate keeps the substrate site of the intact enzyme in an inaccessible form (5). The action of protein kinase C activators may then be to release the pseudosubstrate from the catalytic domain of protein kinase C rendering the enzyme capable of phosphorylating exogenous substrates.

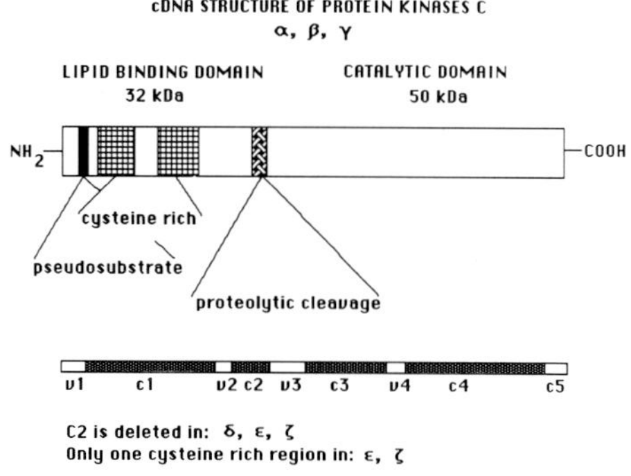

Figure 1. Linear structure of protein kinase C isoenzymes as deduced from cDNA sequencing

IN VITRO MECHANISMS OF REGULATION OF PROTEIN KINASE C

Investigation on the mechanisms of regulation of protein kinase C has led to the identification of a number of mechanisms for modulating protein kinase C activity in vitro (Table 1). These mechanisms are briefly discussed below:

Calcium/phospholipids/DAG.

Protein kinase C is primarily activated in vitro in the presence of phospholipid, calcium and DAG. The enzyme shows strong dependence on anionic phospholipids, especially phosphatidylserine (PS). No other cation has been found that could totally replace calcium as a cofactor for activation.

To investigate the in vitro mechanisms of protein kinase C activation by lipids and DAG, we devised mixed micellar methodologies that allow kinetic analysis of enzyme regulation in vitro (6). Detergent/lipid mixed micelles are homogenous structures whereby a small and defined number of lipid molecules are present in individual mixed micelles that retain the primary physical characteristics of detergent micelles such as uniform size and composition. Utilizing mixed micellar methodologies, we evaluated the stoichiometry and mechanism of protein kinase C regulation by DAG and phorbol esters. Activity of protein kinase C was found to depend on the composition of micelles, but not on the actual detergent used or the number of micelles in the reaction assay. That is, enzyme activity is sensitive to the mol ratio of PS and DAG compared to detergent, but not to the absolute concentration of lipid cofactors. Monomeric protein kinase C was found to interact with a single micelle in the presence of 4 - 6 molecules of PS, 1 or more molecules of calcium and a single molecule of DAG. These studies indicated that the enzyme is sensitive to the micro environment of a single mixed micelle and its activity is modulated by the local concentration of phospholipid and DAG (7). Mixed micellar analysis was also extended to study the structure/activity relationships of DAG activation of protein kinase C. These studies revealed that the enzyme was stereospecifically activated by the sn-1,2-diacylglycerol stereoisomer and that activation required the presence of the 2-ester moieties as well as the 1-hydroxyl group. This highly specific activation of the enzyme by DAGs strongly suggest that the enzyme directly interacts with DAG (8).

TABLE I: IN VITRO REGULATION OF PROTEIN KINASE C

Ca^{2+}/phospholipid/DAG
Autophosphorylation
Cations e.g. Pb^{2+}, Zn^{2+}
Fatty acids
Lysophospholipids
Sphingosine and lysosphingolipids
Pharmacologic inhibitors,
e.g. certain anti-tumor agents

Mixed micellar analysis was also extended to the evaluation of phorbol ester binding and activation of protein kinase C with the finding that phorbol esters activate protein kinase C with a mechanism similar to that of DAG.

The kinetic interrelationships between the lipid cofactors and calcium and the effects of lipid activators on substrate dependency of protein kinase C were also examined. These results allowed the definition of a two-step mechanism for protein kinase C activation. In the first step, soluble enzyme interacts with mixed micelles in the presence of calcium and PS. In this state, the enzyme remains inactive but is able to bind MgATP. In the following step, DAG interacts with micelle-bound enzyme and causes enzyme activation presumably by releasing the pseudosubstrate from the substrate site on the catalytic domain of the enzyme. In this form, the enzyme is able to act on exogenous substrate and induce phosphorylation (7).

Autophosphorylation.

The enzyme has been found to undergo autophosphorylation in vitro and in reconstituted systems. Unlike autophosphorylation of calcium/calmodulin dependent kinases, autophosphorylation of protein kinase C results in only modest changes in its kinetic properties, its regulation by lipids, and its association with surfaces (9).

Effects of other cations.

Cations other than calcium have been found to modulate protein kinase C activity. Lead has been found to stimulate the PS and DAG dependent activity of partially purified protein kinase C from rat brain (10). Zinc has also been found to increase the affinity of protein kinase C for phorbol esters in T lymphocytes (11).

Fatty acids.

Protein kinase C has been found to be activated by arachidonic acid as well as by other cisunsaturated fatty acids in *in vitro* systems (12). Activation of the enzyme by fatty acids occurs in the absence of PS and DAG and is only partially enhanced by calcium. Recently, it has been shown that protein kinase C isoenzymes may display partial selectivity in their response to arachidonic acid. Lipoxin A and other eicosanoids were also able to stimulate protein kinase C activity in a similar manner (13).

Lysophospholipids.

A number of lysophospholipids and especially lysophosphatidylcholine were found to have a biphasic effect on protein kinase C with stimulation at lower concentrations (up to 20 1M) and with inhibition at higher concentrations. Stimulation by lysophospholipids required the presence of PS and calcium but could occur independent of the presence of DAG (14).

Sphingosine and lysosphingolipids.

Initial screening of naturally occurring lipid molecules that could regulate protein kinase C activity led to the discovery that sphingosine and other long-chain amino bases were potent inhibitors of protein kinase C (15). The mechanism of interaction of sphingosine with protein kinase C was investigated using mixed micellar methodologies. Sphingosine was found to be a competitive inhibitor of DAG/phorbol ester but not of PS or calcium. According to the two-step model of protein kinase C activation, sphingosine was found to inhibit the second step. That is, sphingosine was found to prevent the interaction of DAG with membrane-associated protein kinase C, i.e., the PS.PKC.Ca^{2+} complex. Sphingosine appears to interact with PS through an ionic interaction between the positively charged amine on sphingosine and the negatively charged phosphate of PS. This interaction prevents the subsequent interaction of DAG with PS which is a requirement for the activation of protein kinase C by DAG.

Consistent with its lipid nature, sphingosine inhibition of protein kinase C was found to display surface dilution kinetics whereby the inhibitory effect of sphingosine could be reduced by surface dilution (i.e., by increasing the membrane or mixed micellar surface). Similar surface dilution kinetics were obtained in the analysis of inhibition of protein kinase C by sphingosine in cellular systems (16).

Structure function activity studies of protein kinase C inhibition by sphingosine resulted in the identification of a requirement for the free amine of sphingosine and of a minimum hydrophobic character to the molecule. Sphingosine analogs with less than 11 carbons were found to be inactive with activity increasing progressively with increasing carbon numbers, peaking at the C_{18} sphingosine (16). Interestingly, it was discovered that substitutions at the 1-hydroxyl position did not significantly affect the ability of sphingosine analogs to inhibit protein kinase C activity. This observation led to the identification that all members of the class of lipid molecules termed lysosphingolipids are inhibitors of protein kinase C. Lysosphingolipids may be considered to derive from parental sphingolipids by a single deacylation step, i.e., lysosphingolipids lack the amide-linked fatty acid moiety of sphingolipids. Therefore, for each sphingolipid there exists (at least _in vitro_) the corresponding lysosphingolipid which shares the same head group at the 1-position but lacks the fatty acid at the 2-position. While none of the parental sphingolipids inhibited protein kinase C activity, all lysosphingolipids did. This raised the possibility that lysosphingolipids, some of which have been already known to accumulate in the sphingolipidoses, may play a pathogenetic role in these diseases through inhibition of protein kinase C (17).

Sphingosine has been evaluated by a number of investigators for its effects in various cell systems (18). Wherever examined, sphingosine has been found to inhibit phorbol ester-induced responses, and may therefore, be considered as an anti-tumor promoter. In addition, sphingosine has been found to have effects independent of protein kinase C inhibition, such as inhibition of tissue factor activity _in vitro_. The selectivity of sphingosine has not been fully evaluated. Among different possible targets involved in signal transduction, sphingosine appears to have selectivity against protein kinase C over other kinases and lipid metabolizing enzymes. Further studies are required to evaluate the selectivity of sphingosine and to determine its appropriate use as a probe to evaluate the role of protein kinase C in various cell systems.

Pharmacologic inhibitors.

A number of pharmacologic inhibitors of protein kinase C have been described. We have been particularly interested in the study of anti-tumor agents and their effects on protein kinase C. These studies have led to the identification that aminoacridines are potent and reversible inhibitors of protein kinase C (19). Also, the iron complex of adriamycin has been found to be a very potent inhibitor of enzyme activity (20). Both aminoacridines and adriamycin share similar structural features, namely the possession of a hydrophobic character as well as a free amine. Kinetically, aminoacridines and adriamycin iron-III share similar mechanisms of action with sphingosine. They inhibit enzyme activity by interacting with phospholipid moieties and prevent activation of the enzyme by DAG. Because of its role in mediating the action of tumor promoters, protein kinase C should be seriously considered as a target for the action of anti-tumor agents.

While the list of possible modulators of protein kinase C activity is still growing, the physiologic relevance of modulation of protein kinase C by these different lipid cofactors and cations has not been evaluated. These various _in vitro_ modulators may bespeak complex networks of protein kinase C regulation that could operate over short term as well as long term intervals to fine-tune protein kinase C activity in cellular systems.

CELLULAR MECHANISMS OF REGULATION OF PROTEIN KINASE C

Physiologically, protein kinase C is primarily regulated by the operation of the PI cycle and the subsequent generation of endogenous DAG (1). Cellular activation of protein kinase C is associated with "translocation" of the enzyme from the cytosolic to the membranous fraction. This has served as a useful parameter to evaluate for endogenous activation of protein kinase C. Biochemically, this appears to involve an increased resistance of membrane-associated enzyme to chelator extraction during fractionation of cells once the enzyme is activated. Whether this is simply due to an increased affinity of the enzyme to membranes in the presence of DAG/phorbol esters or due to other conformational changes of the enzyme and/or interaction with other membrane proteins is to be evaluated.

TABLE II: CELLULAR REGUALTION OF PROTEIN KINASE C
PI turnover
Translocation
Down regulation
Complex DAG generation
Sphingolipid cycle
Transcriptional activation

Prolonged activation of protein kinase C with phorbol esters leads to down regulation of the enzyme, probably through proteolytic digestion through the action of endogenous proteases. Although this has been used as a pharmacologic tool to deplete cells of protein kinase C activity, recent evidence points to the presence of down regulation-resistant protein kinase C that could be a reflection of the differing sensitivities of different isoenzymes for proteolytic action (21) .

Our recent studies have led us to evaluate physiologic regulation of protein kinase C under different situations (Table 2). These mechanisms will be briefly discussed:

Complex DAG formation.

Activation of human platelets with thrombin results in PIP_2 hydrolysis and DAG formation. It is now known, however, that DAG could be potentially formed from phospholipids other than PIP_2 and from PI-glycan anchors as well as through the *de novo* synthesis from glycerol 3-phosphate (26 and Figure 2). Our earlier studies on the role of protein kinase C in platelet activation led us to define a necessary but insufficient role for protein kinase C in the secondary rather than the primary phase of platelet aggregation (22). This raised the question that DAG formation may persist in platelets beyond the initial phase of PIP_2 hydrolysis. We, therefore, investigated for DAG formation in c-thrombin stimulated platelets. The treatment of platelets with fully stimulating concentrations of c-thrombin resulted in a multiphasic DAG response. Under similar conditions, only an early and single peak of IP_3, calcium mobilization, and arachidonic acid-labeled DAG were detected. The successive phases of DAG production led to accumulation of DAG levels above baseline. The accumulated DAG, in turn, correlated with the extent of platelet secretion and the aggregatory response (23).

These studies suggest that the temporal regulation of DAG production is tightly controlled in stimulated platelets. Moreover, these studies have two important implications. First, DAG production may be compartmentalized in platelets with different phospholipid precursors in different subcellular fractions serving as precursors for the different phases of DAG. Second, the different phases of DAG may lead to the activation of different isoenzymes of protein kinase C. Further studies are required to investigate these possibilities.

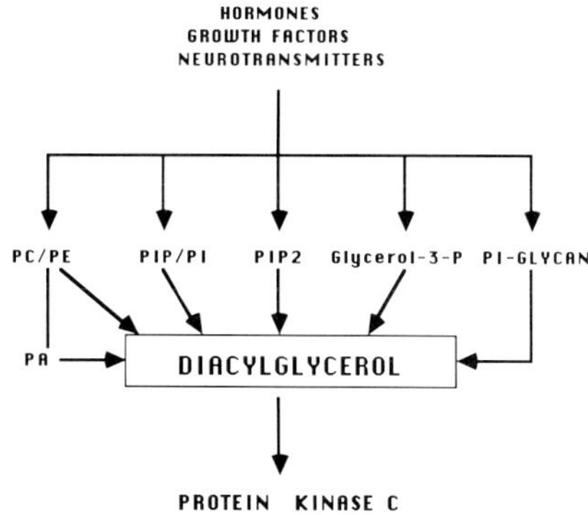

Figure 2. Potential pathways for the generation of intracellular diacylglycerol levels.

Transcriptional regulation of protein kinase C.

While the formation of DAG may serve as an appropriate signal to activate protein kinase C for short term cellular responses, a number of long-term cellular responses are suspected to involve protein kinase C activation without detectable PI turnover. In HL-60 human promyelocytic leukemia cells, both vitamin D_3 and phorbol myristate acetate (PMA) induce similar differentiation of the leukemic cells into a monocytic phenotype. Moreover, both vitamin D_3 and PMA cause phosphorylation of common cellular proteins following treatment of HL-60 cells. Finally, it has been observed that treatment of HL-60 cells with vitamin D_3 results in an increase in phorbol ester receptor number indicating possible increases in protein kinase C levels.

We investigated the mechanism and significance of protein kinase C regulation by vitamin D_3 in HL-60 cells. Vitamin D_3 treatment of HL-60 cells resulted in a dose- and time-dependent increase in phorbol ester receptor number and in protein kinase C activity. The increase in protein kinase C levels was found to be due to transcriptional regulation of the b isoenzyme of protein kinase C with a peak response of 4 to 5-fold increase in transcriptional rate of the gene for b protein kinase C occurring at 12 h following treatment with vitamin D_3. While vitamin D_3 caused no detectable changes in DAG levels in HL-60 cells, phosphorylation of protein kinase C substrates was found to parallel the increase of protein kinase C levels (24). These results suggest that protein kinase C may be activated by increasing the levels of protein kinase C which would lead then to increased substrate phosphorylation in the presence of baseline DAG levels. Transcriptional regulation of protein kinase C may be an important mechanism for long-term modulation of the protein kinase C pathway of cellular regulation. It may also be a particularly important pathway for mediating the action of hormones and cellular agonists that act independent of cell surface receptors.

Sphingomyelin turnover.

The finding that sphingosine and lysosphingolipids are inhibitors of protein kinase C in vitro raised the possibility that endogenous formation of sphingolipid breakdown products may serve to regulate protein kinase C. These considerations led us to evaluate sphingolipid metabolism in response to cellular stimulation. Treatment of HL-60 cells with vitamin D_3 resulted in early and reversible turnover of sphingomyelin (Figure 3). This turnover appeared to occur in response to the activation of a neutral sphingomyelinase by vitamin D_3. The products of sphingomyelin hydrolysis were ceramide and phosphorylcholine (25).

The physiologic significance of sphingomyelin hydrolysis and ceramide generation in the induction of HL-60 cells were investigated using bacterial sphingomyelinase. Bacterial sphingomyelinase, which causes sphingomyelin hydrolysis and ceramide formation, acted in synergy with subthreshold concentrations of vitamin D_3 to induce HL-60 cell differentiation along a monocytic/macrophage-like phenotype (25).

These studies demonstrate the existence of a regulated sphingomyelin cycle that functions in leukemia cell differentiation. The implications of these observations are two-fold. First, these studies suggest that ceramide may act as a second messenger in response to inducers of cell differentiation. Second, sphingolipid metabolism may function to yield sphingosine and other lysosphingolipids that may cause inhibition of protein kinase C, although no such products have been detected in HL-60 cells.

Figure 3. Sphingomyelin turnover and phosphorylcholine generation in HL-60 cells stimulated with vitamin D_3. HL-60 cells were prelabeled with $[^3H]$-choline and then treated with vitamin D_3 for the indicated time intervals. Sphingomyelin was extracted from the lipid fraction and analyzed on thin layer chromatography. Phosphorylcholine was extracted from the aequeous phase of a Bligh-Dyer extract of the cells and analyzed by thin layer chromatography. (Reproduced with permission for the J. Biol. Chem.)

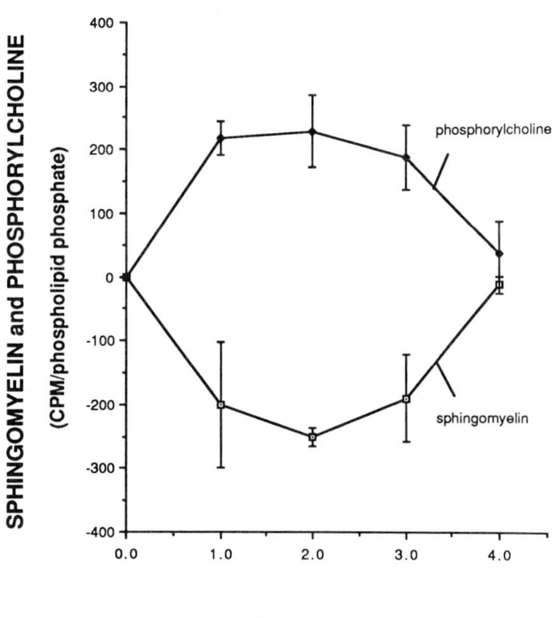

CONCLUSIONS

Protein kinase C is subject to complex regulation in vitro by a number of lipid molecules, lipid breakdown products, and cations. Other than for the endogenous formation of DAG, the physiologic significance of these in vitro regulatory mechanisms is not established.

Recent studies have resulted in the identification of complex cellular mechanisms involved in protein kinase C regulation. In addition to DAG generation from PIP_2 hydrolysis, protein kinase C appears to be activated when DAG is generated from the hydrolysis of other phospholipids and possibly from the hydrolysis of the PI-glycan protein anchor as well as de novo synthetic pathways. Long-term regulation of protein kinase C activity may also occur at the transcriptional level which may be important for such cellular responses as differentiation and long-term potentiation. Finally, the existence of a regulated sphingolipid cycle has been identified and the relation of sphingolipid metabolism to protein kinase C regulation is under investigation.

REFERENCES:

1. Nishizuka, Y. (1986) Science 233, 305-312
2. Nishizuka, Y. (1988) Nature 334, 661-665
3. Huang, K.P., Nakabayashi, H., and Huang, F.L. (1986) Proc. Natl. Acad. Sci. USA 83, 8535-8539
4. Lee, M.H., and Bell, R.M. (1986) J. Biol . Chem. 261, 14867-14870
5. House, C., and Kemp, B.E. (1987) Science 238, 1726-1728
6. Hannun, Y.A., Loomis, C.R., and Bell, R.M. (1985) J. Biol. Chem. 260, 10039-10043
7. Hannun, Y.A., and Bell, R.M. (1987) in Cell Calcium and the Control of Membrane Transport (Mandel, L.J., and Eaton, D.C., eds) pp. 230-240, Rockefeller University Press, New York
8. Ganong, B., Loomis, C.R., Hannun, Y.A., and Bell, R.M. (1986) Proc. Natl. Acad. Sci. USA 83, 1184-1188
9. Huang, K.P., Chan, K.F., Singh, T, J., Nakabayashi, H., and Huang, F.L. (1986) J. Biol. Chem. 261, 12134-12140
10. Markovac, J., and Goldstein, G.W. (1988) Nature 334, 71-73
11. Csermely, P., Szamel, M., Resch, K., and Somogyi, J. (1988) Biochem. Biophys. Res. Commun. 154, 578-583
12. Murakami, K., Chan, S.Y., and Routtenberg, A. (1986) J. Biol. Chem. 261, 15424-15429
13. Hansson, A., Serhan, C.N., Haeggstrom, J., Ingelman-Sundberg, M., and Samuelsson, B. (1986) Biochem. Biophys. Res. Commun. 134, 1215-1222
14. Oishi, K., Raynor, R.L., Charp, P.A., and Kuo, J.F. (1988) J. Biol. Chem. 263, 6865-6871
15. Hannun, Y.A., Loomis, C.R., Merrill, A.H., Jr., and Bell, R.M. (1986) J. Biol. Chem. 261, 12604-12609
16. Merrill, A.H., Jr., Nimkar, S., Menaldino, D., Hannun, Y.A., Loomis, C., Bell, R.M., Tyagi, S.R., Lambeth, J.D., Stevens, V.L., Hunter, R., and Liotta, D.C. (1989) Biochemistry 28, 3138-3145
17. Hannun, Y.A., and Bell, R.M. (1987) Science 235, 670-674
18. Hannun, Y.A., and Bell, R.M. (1989) Science 243, 500-507
19. Hannun, Y.A., and Bell, R.M. (1988) J. Biol. Chem. 263, 5124-5131
20. Hannun, Y.A., Foglesong, R.J., and Bell, R.M. (1989) J. Biol. Chem. 264, 9960-9966
21. Kariya, K., and Takai, Y. (1987) FEBS Lett . 219, 119-124
22. Hannun, Y.A., Greenberg, C.S ., and Bell, R.M. (1987) J. Biol. Chem. 262, 13620-13626
23. Werner, M., Bielawska, A., and Hannun, Y.A. (submitted)
24. Obeid, L.M., Okazake, T., Karolak, L.A., and Hannun, Y.A. (1990) J. Biol. Chem. 265:2370-2374
25. Okazaki, T., Bell, R.M., and Hannun, Y.A. J. Biol . Chem. (1989) J. Biol. Chem, 264:19076-19080
26. Bishop, W.R. and Bell, R.M. (1988) Oncogene Res. 2, 205-218

MODULATED INTERCELLULAR COMMUNICATION: CONSEQUENCE OF EXTRACELLULAR MOLECULES TRIGGERING INTRACELLULAR COMMUNICATION

J.E. TROSKO, B.V. MADHUKAR, C. HASLER, and C.C. CHANG

Department of Pediatrics/Human Development, Michigan State University, East Lansing, Michigan 48824

INTRODUCTION: Concept of Cell Communication in Homeostasis.

The objective of this brief review is to examine how eicosanoids and other bioactive lipids might affect the carcinogenic and other toxic endpoints. Tactically, this can be achieved either by a thorough analysis of all the detailed technical reports related to experiments in which eicosanoids and cancer have been studied or by an analysis of emerging concepts related to the molecular and cellular mechanisms of carcinogenesis. In this review, we have chosen to see how the eicosanoid relate to the multi-stage or initiation/promotion/progression concept of carcinogenesis (1) and the concept of intercellular communication (2). In addition, we will offer an alternative hypothesis to the prevailing concept in carcinogenesis, namely, "carcinogens as mutagens" (3). In brief, it has been generally assumed that if a chemical, such as various eicosanoids, produce oxygen-radical species, and influence cancer, they do so by damaging DNA and by causing mutations which lead to cancer. It will be our view that the critical molecular targets for the eicosanoids and their metabolites are membrane and cytosolic molecules, not the DNA.

In a multi-cellular, higher organism, such as the human being, self-regulation and orchestration of the diverse biochemical, cellular, and physiological functions is referred to as homeostasis. Reactions within cells, between different cells within a tissue and between cells of different tissues must be coordinated in a precise manner in order for growth, development and maintenance of tissue and physiological functions to be normal and adaptive.

Because the multi-cellular organism is more than a collection of independently-acting cells, the hierarchial (4) and cybernetic (5) concepts, which stress the interactions between cells, helped to explain how the organisms is "greater than the sum of the parts". In modern biological terms, this homeostatic regulation to regulate whether a cell will divide, differentiate, or if differentiated, respond to stimuli in an adaptive manner, is mediated by three basic forms of communication transmitted by ions and molecules. Extra-, intra-, and intercellular communication mechanisms have evolved with the appearance of multi-cellular organisms in an integrative manner in order to maintain homeostatic control of cell proliferation, differentiation and adaptive physiological functions of the multi-cellular organism (6) [Figure 1].

The term, extracellular communication, depicts the process by which one cell can communicate with another over extra-cellular space via molecules, such as hormones, biologically active peptides,

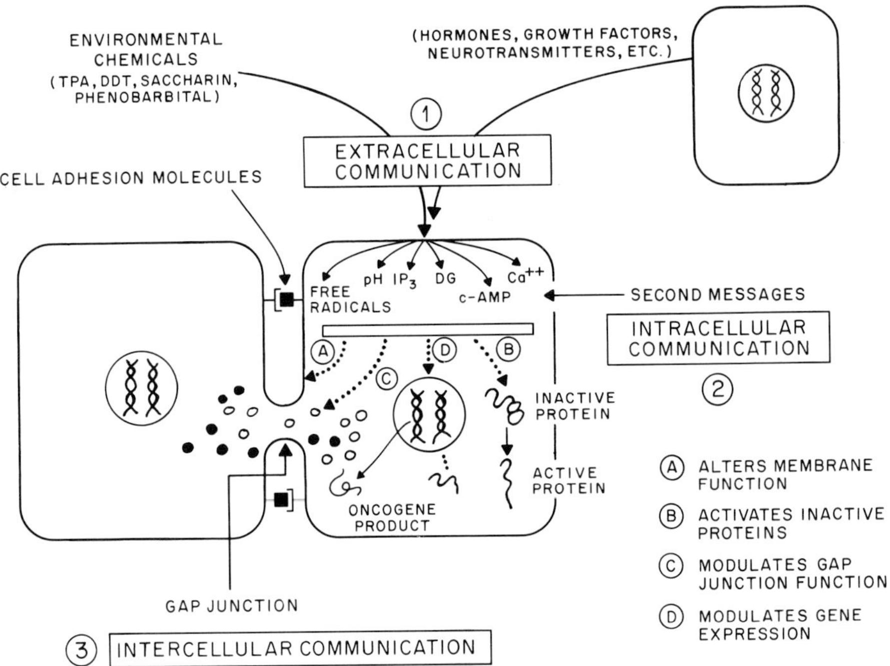

Figure 1. The heuristic schemata characterizes the postulated link between extracellular communication and intercellular communication via various intracellular transmembrane signalling mechanisms. It provides an integrating view of how the neuroendocrine-immune system ("mind or brain/body connection") and other multi system coordinations could occur. While not shown here, activation or altered expression of various oncogenes (and "anti-oncogenes") could also contribute to the regulation of gap junction function. [From Trosko et al (61) with permission from Pergamon Press, New York].

lymphokines and neurotransmitters. In the broadest sense, influences external to the cell, such as extracellular matrices or cell adhension molecules, could also be viewed as being able to communicate, information to a cell, extracellularly. After a cell receives this molecular signal, depending on whether it is receptor-dependent or independent, and or the specific molecular/biochemical consequence of that interaction, specific molecular/biochemical reactions occur. This constitutes the process of intracellular communication, whereby, in spite of thousands of different endogenous biologically active extracellular molecules that interact with cells, only a few generic "second" message systems translate the communication signals to adaptive cellular responses of cellular proliferation, differentiation or a differentiated function. Alterations in cellular pH, intracellular free calcium, cyclic AMP levels, generation of free radicals, and activation of protein kinases act as diverse "second" messages to mediate the action of a wide range of structurally diverse endogenous biologically active extracellular communicating molecules.

If all cells of the multi-cellular organism existed independently of their neighbors, the interaction of cells would involve only extra- and intracellular communication processes. In fact, a third form, intercellular communication, involves the transfer of ions and molecules below approximately 1000 daltons via a membrane-protein structure, the gap junction, between contiguous cells (7). These gap junctions are found in most cells of multi-cellular metazoans. To date, a small family of genes, coding for a series of proteins having a high degree of homology (8), have been identified. Gap junctions have been implicated in the regulation of cell proliferation, developmental processes, differentiation of cells, metabolic cooperation in nonexcitable tissues and synchronization of electronic signals in excitable tissues (9). Early embryonic development (10), synchronization of heart cells (11), secretion in pancreatic cells (12), uterine function during labor (13), as well as developmental, metabolic and functional regulation between astro-glial neuron function (14) have been linked to gap junctions.

The significance of mentioning gap junctional intercellular communication in this review is that both endogenous, and exogenous extracellular communicating molecules, can modulate (up or down regulate) intercellular communication. There is strong evidence that the modulation is mediated by several biochemical/biophysical mechanisms which involves the second-messages or intracellular communication mechanisms. This conceptual model could help delineate a scientific mechanisms to explain multi-system effects, such as those seen in neuroendocrine-immune responses (15).

Chemicals, either endogenous or exogenous, could, by triggering changes in intracellular calcium, pH, free radicals, cyclic AMP, or protein kinases, either increase or decrease gap junction function at either the transcriptional, translational or post-translational levels (epigenetic levels) (16). This latter point illustrates a major point, in that exogenous chemicals can "mimic" the effect of endogenous chemicals. Since these chemicals induce the same second message intracellular communication mechanisms, the cell is unable to distinguish the exogenous signal from the endogenous signal. The biological consequence of modulating gap junctional communication by either endogenous or exogenous extracellular communicating molecules could be either adaptive or maladaptive, therapeutic/pharmacological or toxicological (17).

Carcinogenesis: A Disease of Homeostatic Dysfunction.

If a normal cell is characterized by being homeostatically regulated, cancer cells, which do not contact inhibit or have lost growth control, and do not terminally differentiate, must be viewed as having dysfunctional homeostasis (18). The transition from a normal, contact-inhibited cell to a malignant cell is the result of an evolution of phenotypes involving multiple steps (19). The multiple nature of this carcinogenic process has been conceptualized as consisting of an initiation/promotion/progression stage (20). In addition, based on the assumption that cancer is a "disease of differentiation" (21, 22), "a stem-cell disease" (23,24) ["Oncogeny as partially blocked ontogeny" (25)], the initiation process appears to be one that irreversibly blocks a stem cell from terminally differentiating. While the mechanism of initiation is not known, mutagenesis appears to be involved, since the process is irreversible and mutagens seem to be good initiators (26). Experimental evidence seems to be consistent with the idea that initiation does block terminal differentiation (27).

Promotion, on the other hand, is, operationally, up to a point, a potentially reversible or interruptible process. It is the process by which a single initiated stem cell is clonally amplified. Promoters are, by definition, mitogens for, at least, the initiated cells. Any mitogenic stimuli (e.g., wound healing, cell death, growth stimuli due to growth factors or hormones, and chemical agents which block mitogen-suppressors), which cause the stem or progenitor cells to divide has the potential to act as a tumor promoter. If the mitogenic stimuli induces both normal and initiated cells to proliferate, the daughter cells of the normal stem cell should terminally differentiate. The initiated cell, however, would proliferate but not terminally differentiate. In effect, these non-differentiated cells would accumulate in the tissue as dysfunctional foci of cells [Figure 2]. However, not all promoters seem to be mitogenic for the normal cells of the target organ. For example, barbital sodium, which is a promoter of the kidney tubules, urinary blad-

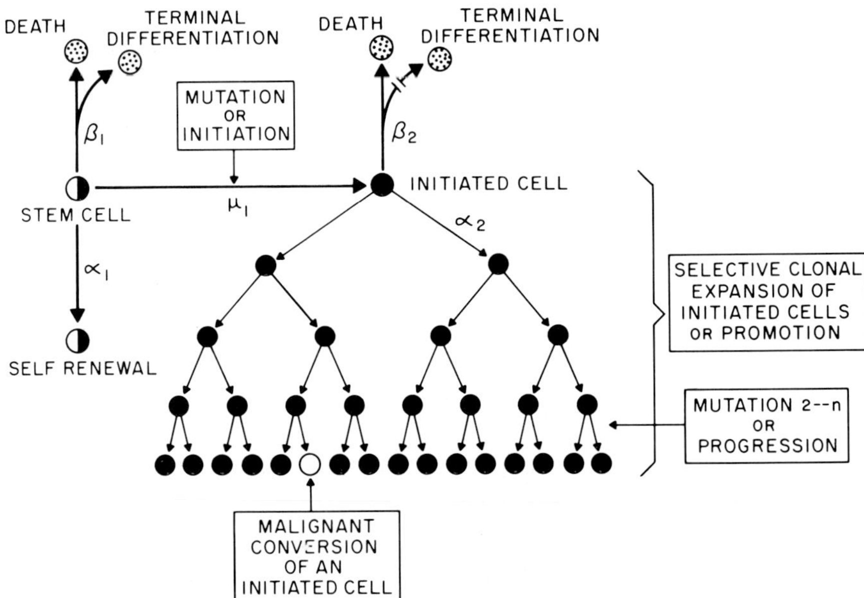

Figure 2. The initiation/promotion/progression model of carcinogenesis. β_1 = rate of terminal differentiation and death of stem cell; β_2 = rate of death, but not of terminal differentiation of the initiated cell ( ); α_1 = rate of cell division of stem cells; α_2 = rate of cell division of initiated cells; μ_1 = rate of the molecular event leading to initiation (i.e., possibly mutation); μ_2 = rate at which second event occurs within an initiated cell. (From Trosko, J.E., Chang, C.C., Madhukar, B.V., Oh, S.Y., Bombick, D., and El-Fouly, M.H., Gap Junctions, Hertzberg, E.L., Ed., Alan R. Liss, New York, 1988, 435. With permission).

der and liver of the Fischer 344 rat, does not induce persistent DNA synthesis in the bladder or hepatocytes. Enzyme altered foci in the liver, papillomas in the skin and polyps in the colon might be viewed as non-terminally differentiated cells derived from a single initiated cell (28).

Assuming that cell communication is needed for normal growth control and differentiation, and given that cancer cells do not have normal growth or do not terminally differentiate, one could predict that cancer cells ought to be dysfunctional as far as cell communication is concerned. Loewenstein and co-workers were the first to observe that many cells derived from tumors were, in fact, dysfunctional in their ability to perform gap junctional intercellular communication (29). While there have been several reports that not all cancer cells seem to have dysfunctional cell communication (30), a variety of alternative explanations for these observations have been made, including the phenomenon of "selective" communication between cells of the tumor and the surrounding normal cells (31). Furthermore, there have been reports correlating the loss of gap junctional communication with the metastatic potential of cells (32,33).

To fit these observations into the initiation/promotion/progression model, the hypothesis that chemical tumor promoters (or any physical promoting condition such as compensatory hyperplasia after wounding or tissue necrosis) allowed initiated cells to escape the suppressing effect of surrounding normal cells (34), tumor promoters have been shown to inhibit gap junctional intercellular communication in a reversible fashion (35,36). Further evidence of the role of gap junctional communication in carcinogenesis comes from the observation that anti-tumor promoting retinoids, which reduced the frequency of chemically induced transformants of CH_3-l0T1/2 cells in vitro, increased gap junctional communication in these cells (37).

Stem Cells, Oncogenes and Growth Factors in Carcinogenesis.

With the development of the oncogene concept, there is a necessity to integrate it with the multi-stage nature of carcinogenesis. Initial observations, suggesting two oncogenes were needed to "immortalize" and transform certain cells, in vitro, seemed to fit, superficially, into the initiation/promotion phases of carcinogenesis (38). However, further observations because, in other cells, only a single oncogene was needed to transform these cells (39) or that there did not seem to be a correlation between the expression of some oncogenes, such as ras, and tumorigenicity because of the existence of anti-tumor suppressor genes (40,41), seemed to render simple correlations of certain oncogenes and the initiation/promotion model as naive.

To look at the problem in a different light, it should first be noted that cellular oncogenes have been defined as DNA sequences which normally influence cell growth and differentiation. These cellular oncogenes, when overexpressed, misregulated or mutated, have been postulated to cause a cell to become cancerous (i.e., become homeostatically dysfunctional). There are oncogenes, which code for growth factors, growth factor receptors or transmembrane mitogenic signalling elements, and which code for nuclear proteins (42). Several of the oncogenes, of the former class, such as the activated H-ras, src, neu, as well as the T-antigen of the papilloma virus (43-54), have been correlated with the down regulation of gap junctions.

Growth factors have been shown to act as promoters, in vitro (55,56) and In vivo (57,58). Epidermal growth factor (EGF) and transforming growth factor-beta (TGF-β) have also been shown to down regulate gap junctional communication in several cell lines and strains in vitro (59, 60) .

Cells that are contact-inhibited should be gap junctionally coupled. These tumor promoting conditions, which allow the clonal expansion of the initiated cells, should, by logic, remove contact-inhibition, and therefore, gap junctional communication. The observations cited above seem to be consistent with that hypothesis, in that chemical promoters, which are "growth factors" for the initiated cells, oncogenes, which code for growth factors or growth factor receptors, and growth factors, themselves, all down regulate gap junctional communication. In effect, while each of these down-regulators of gap junctional communication probably works via different biochemical mechanisms, the end-result is the same, namely, the initiated cell no longer is suppressed by the surrounding normal cells (6).

One additional concept has to be accounted for in these complex carcinogenic process. Two major hypotheses exist for explaining the origin of the tumor. One is that the carcinogenic process blocks or partially blocks a stem cell from terminally differentiating ["oncogeny as partially blocked ontogeny" (25)]. The other is that retro- or dedifferentiation of the differentiated cell occurs after exposure to a carcinogen or exogenously transfected oncogene.

In the case of blood cancers the stem cell theory seems to be consistent with the facts. In solid tumors, while the clonal nature of tumors would be consistent with the stem cell theory, one could argue that a de-differentiated cell, after initiation, could also explain the clonal nature of tumors.

Recent information related to liver carcinogenesis might, however, help resolve this question. The rat liver "oval" cell has been speculated to be a stem or progenitor cell for the hepatocytes (61). Recent karyotyping of normal hepatocytes has shown most of them to be aneuploid. On the other hand, cells in the preneoplastic foci appear to be diploid (62,63). If a minimum of two genetic hits is required for neoplastic transformation (64), cells which are polyploid would not only be harder to transform because of more normal genes which must be mutated, but also, during the de-differentiation process after initiation, they would have to lose complete sets of chromosomes to become diploid. This seems highly unlikely.

Even more interesting, the oval cell, which does have gap junctional intercellular communication (65), does not communicate with the hepatocyte, which also can gap junctionally communicate with other hepatocytes (66). The oval cell expresses the 43 Kda gap junction protein while the mature hepatocyte expresses the 32 Kda protein. Most interestingly, the cells of preneoplastic lesions in the liver express the 43 Kda protein, suggesting these cells communicate amongst themselves but not with the surrounding normal cells ["selective communication" (67)]. If during further evolution, another genetic event occurs such that these selectively communicating cells lose all ability to communicate, the cell now might be considered a carcinoma.

If this hypothesis is correct, implications for cancer therapy and risk assessment become focussed, in that one objective would be to find ways to restore gap junctional communication in cancer cells (68) and the other would be to identify the cells at risk and to determine factors which promote initiated stem cells.

Eicosanoids and Carcinogenesis.

Eicosanoids, a family of oxygenated C_2O fatty acids (including prostaglandins, leukotrienes and related hydroxy-fatty acids (69), has been implicated in a number of clinical conditions, including inflammation, postischemic injury, degenerative diseases of aging including cancer (70). Diets high in polyunsaturated fatty acids have been implicated in the development and progression of cancer (71,72). For example, Linoleic acid has been shown to act as a tumor promoter in animals treated with carcinogens, as well as to increase the incidence of metastases (73). Although the exact mechanism is not yet known, some have speculated it might be linked to the metabolism of arachidonic acid.

Since cell-cell contact has been shown to be an important modulator of cell sensitivity to hyperoxia and radiation (74) and to play a role in the tumor promotion (28) and metastasis phase of carcinogenesis (32,33), a possible connection between eicosanoids and gap junctional communication seems to be a reasonable idea.

When it was shown that some protease inhibitors, which prevented the production of superoxide anion radicals from phagocytic cells, also were inhibitors of phorbol ester induced tumor promotion in mouse skin (75), one of the early hypotheses for the mechanism of action of tumor promotion was formulated (76,77). More recently, the same line of reasoning extended to liver tumor promotion, when inducers of cytochrome P-450 or of peroxisomes, both potential sources of free radicals or other active states of oxygen, were shown to be tumor promoters (78-80). Moreover, many studies have implicated dietary unsaturated fatty acids, free radical generating chemicals and several eicosanoid metabolites with the tumor promotion and metastatic stages of carcinogenesis (71-73, 79-82).

One of the mechanisms to explain the possible role of the unsaturated fatty acid and eicosanoid involvement in promotion phase of carcinogenesis was the production of free radical species which, by analogy to their production by x-rays, could damage DNA (83, 84) .

However, this hypothesis had several logical problems, not the least of which was, if promotion was the consequence of free-radical damage caused by eicosanoid metabolism, then how does one explain the fact that tumor promoters such as the phorbol esters were not mutagenic. Also, if promoters worked via free-radical induced DNA damage, "Why was the tumor promotion process a potentially reversal process?" or "Why aren't tumor promoters tumor initiators?"

When it was shown that tumor promoters, such as the phorbol esters, could inhibit gap junctional communication (a membrane target), it wasn't long before it was shown that many unsaturated fatty acids, arachidonic acids and other free-radical generating chemicals could down-regulate gap junctional communication in a variety of cell types in vitro (66,71,85-88).

Although the biochemical mechanisms which modulate gap junctional communication at the transcriptional, translational and post-translational levels are not known, it is clear that there are several distinct mechanisms [i.e., activation of protein kinase C, intracellular changes in pH, free Ca^{++} , C-AMP, and free radical damage] (89). In the case of phorbol esters, protein kinase C activation and free radical production are triggered in cells.

Since tumor promotion involves cell proliferation of, at least, the initiated cells (90) and since elevated arachidonic acid has been linked to cell proliferation during tissue repair or tumor promotion (91), the question arises whether arachidonic acid and its metabolites might be the "cause" or "consequence" of the tumor promotion process. However, while there was some evidence consistent with the hypothesis that TPA induced skin promotion involved arachidonic acid, Fischer et al (92) seemed to dissociate the TPA induced oxidant generation from the tumor promotion process.

In the liver, where cell interaction between the hepatocyte and non-parenchymal cells is necessary for normal physiological function, agents, which trigger responses in hepatocytes, apparently do so by an indirect effect. The endogenous or exogenous chemicals can induce the production and release of eicosanoids in the non-parenchymal cells, which then interact with the hepatocytes, which do not produce eicosanoids (93,94). The evidence for this is that inhibitors of cyclo-oxygenase and phospholipase A2 block the physiological responses in the liver caused by arachidonic acid and other like factors.

In the case of liver injury, one might have to distinguish cell removal (as in the case of partial hepatectomy) from cell death caused by non-genotoxic agents (carbon tetrachloride) and from selective proliferation of initiated cells caused by xenobiotic chemicals under noncytotoxic conditions (i.e., perioxisome proliferators, phenobarbital, polybrominated biphenyls). In all cases, eicosanoids are produced. However, the case of the partial hepatectomy, the surviving hepatocytes are not injured and probably give rise to the new hepatocytes. In the latter cases, evidence indicates that the "oval" or epithelial cells are the precursors to the new hepatocytes (95), since they might be more resistant to the toxic effects of the hepatotoxicants because they have restricted metabolizing capabilities (96).

While there are observations interpreted as indicating that chemical tumor promoters, free radical generating chemicals and eicosanoid might act as DNA damaging agents, a number of studies have been shown to cast doubt on that interpretation. For example, many techniques to measure free radical damage to DNA could easily produce artifacts and be misinterpreted (97-100). Also, many of these free radical producing agents are, as stated above, not complete carcinogens or tumor initiators (81,101), nor do they induce DNA damage (102-106) or mutations (28,107). In those cases where clastogenicity is induced by these free-radical generating chemicals (108), the question is whether these events are the consequence of cells dying as a result of non-DNA lesions, such as membrane damage (99). Membrane would be expected to be the target of these eicosanoid and free radical generating chemicals, as has been shown with arachidonic acid activated ion channels (109,110) and phosphorylation of plasma membrane protein (111).

Therefore, under conditions where non-cytotoxic, mitogenic stimuli trigger the loss of contact-inhibition or inhibition of gap junction function (i.e., activation of protein kinase C), the eicosanoids might not play a significant role. In cases of chemically induced cell death or mechanical injury, localized high, but not cytotoxic, levels of eicosanoids could, by blocking cell to cell communication, stimulate regenerative hypoplasia. Whereas, if the levels of eicosanoids reach cytotoxic levels, especially in vitro, or in cases of massive acute toxicity, these levels themselves might be cytotoxic.

REFERENCES

1. Pitot, H.C., Goldsworthy, T. and Moran, S. J. Supramol. Struct. Cellul. Biochem. 17:133-146, 1981.
2. Sheridan, J.D. In: Cell-to-Cell Communication, edited by DeMello, W.C. New York: Plenum Press, 1987, p. 187-222.
3. Ames, B.N., Magaw, R. and Gold, L.S. Science 236:271-280, 1987.
4. Brody, H. Perspect. Biol. Med. 17:71-92 1973.
5. Potter, V.R. Perspect. Biol. Med. 17:164-183 1974.
6. Trosko, J.E., Chang, C.C., Madhukar, B.V. and Oh, S.Y. In: Cell-Cell Communication, edited by DeMello, W.C. Boca Raton, FL: CRC Press, 1989, p. 111-131.
7. Loewenstein, W.R. Physiol. Rev. 61:829-913, 1981.
8. Saez, J.C., Spray, D.C. and Hertzberg, E.L. In Vitro Toxicol. (In Press)
9. Pitts, J.D. and Finbow, M.E. J. Cell sci. 4:239-266, 1986.
10. Lee, S., Gilula, N.B. and Warner, A.E. CELL 51:851-860, 1987.
11. Demello, W.C. Prog. Biophys. Mol. Biol. 39:147-182, 1982.
12. Meda, P., Bruzzone, R., Chanson, M., Bosco, D. and Orci, L. Proc. Natl. Acad. Sci. U.S.A. 84:4901-4904 1987.
13. Cole, W.C. and Garfield, R.E. Amer. J. Physiol. 251:411-420, 1986.
14. Massa, P.T. and Mugnaini, Neurosci 14:695-709, 1985.
15. Pert, C.B., Ruff, M.R., Weber, R.J. and Herkenham, M. J. Immunol. 135:820-826, 1985.
16. Spray, D.C., Saez, J.C., Burt, J.M., et al. In: Gap Junctions, edited by Hertzberg, E. and Johnson, R. New York: Alan R. Liss, Inc., 1988, p. 227-244.
17. Trosko, J.E. and Chang, C.C. Pharmacol. Rev. 36:137-144 1984.
18. Iverson, O.H. In: Progress in Biocybernetics, edited by Wiener, N. and Schade, J.P. Amsterdam: Elsevier Publishing Company, 1965, p. 76-110.
19. Nicolson, G.L. Cancer Research 47:1473-1487, 1987.
20. Weinstein, I.B., Gattoni-Celli, 5., Kirschmeier, P., Lambert, M., Hsiao, W., Backer, J. and Jeffrey, A. J. Cellul. Physiol. 3:127-137, 1984.
21. Markert, C. Cancer Research 28:1908-1914, 1968.
22. Pierce, G.B. Am. J. Pathol. 77:103-118, 1974.
23. Till, J.E. J. Cell. Physiol. 1:3-11, 1982.
24. Nowell, P.C. Science 194:23-28, 1976.
25. Potter, V.R. Br. J. Cancer 38:1-23, 1978.
26. Trosko, J.E. and Chang, C.C. In: Methods for Estimating Risk of Chemical Injury: Human and Non-Human Biota Ecosystems, edited by Vouk, V.B., Butler, G.C., Hoel, D.G. and Peakall, D.B. Chichester, England: John Wiley and Sons, 1985, pp. 181-200
27. Yuspa, S.H. and Morgan, D.L. Nature 293:72-74, 1981.
28. Trosko, J.E., Chang, C.C. and Medcalf, A. Cancer Invest. 1:511-526, 1983.
29. Loewenstein, W.R. Ann. New York Acad. Sci. 137:441, 1966.
30. Weinstein, R.S. and Pauli, B.U. In: Junctional Complexes of Epithelial Cells, edited by Stoker, M. Chichester, England: John Wiley and Sons, Ltd., 1987, pp. 240-260.
31. Yamasaki, H., Hollstein, M., Mesnil, M., Martel, N. and Aguelon, A.M. Cancer Research 47:5658-5664, 1987.
32. Kanno, Y. Japan. J. Physiol. 35:693-707, 1985.
33. Nicolson, G.L., Dulski, K.M. and Trosko, J.E. Proc. Natl. Acad. Sci. U.S.A. 85:473-476, 1988.
34. Yotti, L.P., Chang, C.-C. and Trosko, J.E. Science. 206:1089-1091, 1979.
35. Trosko, J.E. and Chang, C.C. In: Banbury Report 31: New Directions in the Qualitative and Quantitative Aspects of Carcinogen Risk Assessment, edited by Battey, R. Cold Spring Harbor, New York: Cold Spring Harbor Laboratory, 1988, pp. 139-170.
36. Murray, A.W. and Fitzgerald, D.J. Biochem. Biophys. Res. Commun. 91:395-401, 1979.
37. Mehta, P.P., Bertram, J.S. and Loewenstein, W.R. J. Cell Biol. 108:1053-1065, 1989.

38. Land, H., Parada, L.F. and Weinberg, R.A. Nature 304:596-602, 1983.
39. Birrer, M.J., Segal, S., DeGrave, J.S., Kaye, F., Sausville, E.A. and Minna, J.D. Molec. Cell Biol. 8:2668-2673, 1988.
40. Koi, M. and Barrett, J.C. Proc. Natl. Acad. Sci. U.S.A. 83:5992-5996,1986.
41. Geiser, A.G., Der, C.J., Marshall, C.J. and Standbridge, E.J. Proc. Natl. Acad. Sci. U.S.A. 83:5209-5213, 1986.
42. Weinberg, R.A. Science 230:770-776, 1985.
43. Vanhamme, L., Rolin, S. and Szpirer, C. Exp. Cell Res. 180:297-301, 1989.
44. Atkinson, M.M., Anderson, S.K. and Sheridan, J.D. J. Memb. Biol. 91:53-64, 1986.
45. Atkinson, M.M. and Sheridan, J. J. Cell Biol. 99:401a, 1984.
46. Azarnia, R., Reddy, S., Kimiecki, T.E., Shalloway, D. and Loewenstein, W.R. Science 239:398-400, 1988.
47. Azarnia, R. and Loewenstein, W.R. Molec. Cell. Biol. 7:946-650, 1987.
48. Azarnia, R. and Loewenstein, W.R. J. Memb. Biol. 82:191-205, 1984.
49. Azarnia, R. and Loewenstein, W.R. J. Memb. Biol. 82:213-220, 1984.
50. El-Fouly, M.H., Warren, S.T., Trosko, J.E. and Chang, C.C. Am. J. Hum. Genet. 39:A30, 1986.
51. Bignami, M., Rosa, S., Fulcone, G., Tuto, F., Katoh, F. and Yamasaki, H. Molec. Carcinogenesis 1:67-75, 1988.
52. El-Fouly, M.H., Trosko, J.E. and Chang, C.C. In Vitro Toxicol. (In Press)
53. El-Fouly, M.H., Trosko, J.E., Chang, C.C. and Warren, S.T. Molec. Carcinogenesis (In Press)
54. Chang, C.C., Trosko, J.E., Kung, H.J., Bombick, D. and Matsumura, F. Proc. Natl. Acad. Sci. U.S.A. 82:5360-5364, 1985.
55. Harrison, J. and Auersperg, N. Science 213:218-219, 1981.
56. Gansler, T. and Kopelovich, L. Cancer Letters 13:315-323, 1981.
57. Chester, J.F., Gaissert, H.A., Ross, J.S. and Malt, R.A. Cancer Research 46:2954-2957, 1986.
58. Rose, S.P., Stahn, R., Passovoy, D.S. and Herschman, H. Experientia 32:913, 1976.
59. Madhukar, B.V., Oh, S.Y., Chang, C.C., Wade, M.H. and Trosko, J.E. Carcinogenesis 10:13-20, 1989.
60 Maldonado, P.E., Rose, B. and Loewenstein, W.R. J. Memb. Biol. 106:203-210, 1988.
61. Trosko, J.E., Chang, C.C. and Madhukar, B.V. Toxicol. In Vitro 1989.(In Press)
62. Sargent, L.M., Xy, Y., Sattler, G.L., Meisner, L. and Pitot, H.C. Proc. Amer. Assoc. Cancer Res. 30:208, 1989.
63. Saeter, G., Schwarze, P.E., Nesland, J.M. and Seglen, P.O. Br. J. Cancer 59:198-205, 1989.
64. Potter, V.R. Carcinogenesis 2:3175-3179, 1981.
65. Jone, C., Trosko, J.E. and Chang, C.C. In Vitro Cell. Devel. Biol. 23:214-220, 1987.
66. Saez, J.C., Bennett, M.V.L. and Spray, D.C. Science 236:967-969, 1987.
67. Enomoto, T. and Yamasaki, H. Cancer Research 44:5200-5203, 1984.
68. Trosko, J.E. Eur. J. Cancer Clin. Oncol. 23:599-601, 1987.
69. mith, W.L. Biochem. J. 259:315-324, 1989.
70. Poot, M., Esterbauer, H., Rabinovitch, P.S. and Hoehn, H. J. Cell. Physiol. 137:421-429, 1988.
71. Aylsworth, C.F., Welsch, C.W., Kabara, J.J. and Trosko, J.E. Lipids 22:445-454, 1987.
72. Welsch, C.W. and Aylsworth, C.F. J. Natl. Canc. Inst. 70:215-221.
73. Chapkin, R.S., Hubbard, N.E., Buckman, D.K. and Erickson, K.L. Cancer Research 49:4724-4728, 1989.
74. Kavanagh, T.J., Raghu, G., Masta, S.E. and Martin, G.M. In: Oxy-Radicals in Molecular Biology and Pathology, New York: Alan R. Liss, Inc., 1988, p. 301-312.
75. Troll, W., Witz, G., Goldstein, B., Stone, D. and Sugimura, T. In: Carcinogenesis - A Comprehensive Survey, edited by Hecker, E., Fusening, N.E., Kunz, W., Marks, F. and Thielmann, H.W. New York: Raven Press, 1982, p. 593-597.
76. Cerutti, P.A. Science 227:375-381, 1985.
77. Kensler, T.W. and Taffe, B.G. Adv. Free Radical Biol. Med. 2:347-387, 1986.
78. Goldstein, B.D., Czerniecki, B. and Witz, G. Environ. Health Perspect. 81:55-57, 1989.
79. Reddy, J.K. and Lalwani, N.D. CRC Crit. Rev. Toxicol. 12:1-58, 1984.
80. Slaga, T.J., Klein-Szanto, A.J.P., Triplett, L.L., Yotti, L.P. and Trosko, J.E. Science 213:1023-1025, 1981.
81. Klein-Szanto, A.J.P. and Slaga, T.J. J. Invest. Dermatol. 79:30-34, 1982.
82. Copeland, E.S. Cancer Research 43:5631-5637, 1983.
83. Birnboim, H.C. Science 215:1247-1249, 1982.
84. Birnboim, H.C. Carcinogenesis 7:1511-1517, 1986.
85. Agarwal, R. and Daniel, E.E. Amer. J. Physiol. 250:495-505, 1986.

86. James, J.L., Friend, D.S., MacDonald, J.R. and Smuckler, E.A. Lab. Invest. 54:268, 1986.
87. Ruch, R.J. and Klaunig, J.E. Toxicol. Appl. Pharmacol. 94:427-436, 1988.
88. Trosko, J.E., Aylsworth, C., Jone, C. and Chang, C.C. In: Arachidonic Acid Metabolism and Tumor Promotion, edited by Fischer, S.M. and Slaga, T.J. Boston: Martinus Nijhoff, Publishing, 1985, p. 169-197.
89. Spray, D.C. and Bennett, M.V.L. Ann. Rev. Physiol. 47:281-303, 1985.
90. Trosko, J.E., Chang, C.C., Madhukar, B.V. and Oh, S.Y. In: Cell-Cell Communication, edited by DeMello, W.C. Boca Raton, FL: CRC Press. (In Press)
91. Saez, J.C., Spray, D.C. and Hertzberg, E.L. In Vitro Toxicol. (In Press)
92. Fischer, S.M., Baldwin, J.K., Jasheway, D.W. and Patrick, K.E. Carcinogenesis 8:521-524, 1987.
93. Altin, J.G. and Bygrave, F.L. Molec. Cell. Biochem. 83:3-14, 1988.
94. Haussinger, D. J. Hepatol. 5:259-266, 1989.
95. Evarts, R.P., Nagy, P., Nakatsukasa, H., Marsden, E. and Thorgeirsson, S.S. Cancer Research 49:1541-1547, 1989.
96. Tsao, M.S., Smith, J.D., Nelson, K.G. and Grisham, J.W. Exp. Cell Res. 154.38-52, 1984.
97. Trosko, J.E. Mutagenesis 3:363-366, 1989.
98. Bradley, M.O., Taylor, V.I., Armstrong, M.J. and Galloway, S.M. Mutation Research 189:69-79, 1987.
99. Taningher, M., Bordone, R., Russo, P., Grilli, S., Santi, L. and Parodi, S. Anticancer Res. 7:669-680, 1987.
100. Brambilla, G., Carlo, P., Finollo, R. and Ledda, A. Carcinogenesis 6:1285-1288, 1985.
101. Trosko, J.E. and Chang, C.C. In: Banbury Report 31: Carcinogen Risk Assessment: New Directions in the Qualitative and Quantitative Aspects, edited by Hart, R.W. and Hoerger, F.G. Cold Spring Harbor, NY: Cold Spring Harbor Laboratory, 1988, p. 139-170.
102. Corn, B.W., Liber, H.L. and Little, J.B. Radiat. Res. 109:100-108, 1987.
103. Gabrielson, E.W., Rosen, G.M., Grafstrom, R.C., Strauss, K.E., Miyashita, M. and Harris, C.C. Cancer Research 48:822-825, 1988.
104. Gupta, R.C., Goel, S.K., Early, K., Singh, B. and Reddy, J.K. Carcinogenesis 6:933-936, 1985.
105. Bradley, M.O. and Erickson, L.C. Biochim. Biophys. Acta 654:135-141, 1981.
106. Capranico, G., Babudri, N., Casciarri, G., et al. Chem. -Biol. Interact. 57:189-201, 1986.
107. Fujii, T., Shizaki, M., Fujiki, H. and Sugimura, T. Mutation Research 110:263-269, 1983.
108. Kinsella, A.R., Gainer, H.St. and Butler, J. Carcinogenesis 4:717-719, 1983.
109. Kim, D. and Clapham, D.E. Science 244:1174-1176, 1989.
110. Ordway, R.W., Walsh, J.V. and Singer, J.J. Science 244:1176-1178, 1989.
111. Chan, T.M., Chen, E., Tatoyan, A., Shargill, N.S., Pleta, M. and Hochstein, P. Biochem. Biophys. Res. Commun. 139:439-445, 1986.

GROWTH FACTOR REGULATION OF PROSTAGLANDIN H SYNTHASE GENE EXPRESSION

R. R. GORMAN, M. J. BIENKOWSKI and A. H. LIN

Department of Cell Biology, The Upjohn Company, Kalamazoo, MI 49001

Over the past 20 years, the prostaglandin H synthase (PGHS) (EC 1.14.99.1) has been one of the most heavily studied enzymes in lipid biochemistry (1-3). The purified enzyme is a homodimer of 70-kDa subunits that contain 3.5% carbohydrate of the high mannose type by weight (4-7). The enzyme contains an Fe^{3+} protoporphyrin IX prosthetic group and catalyzes both the bisdioxygenation of arachidonic acid to the hydroperoxyendoperoxide PGG_2 and the reduction of PGG_2 to the hydroxyendoperoxide PGH_2. The apoprotein of PGHS can be readily cleaved by trypsin to form two protein fragments: a 33-kDa fragment that contains the amino terminus and a 38-kDa fragment that includes the carboxyl terminus and the aspirin-binding site.

Despite the large amount of information that has been accumulated, little is known about the factor(s) that regulate PGHS gene expression. The cloning of the PGHS has provided the tools necessary to study the molecular basis of PGHS gene expression (8,9). In this report, we show that recombinant PDGF-BB (rPDGF) induces PGHS mRNA levels but that peak mRNA induction occurs after maximal PGE_2 synthesis is achieved. These data suggest that rPDGF-stimulated PGE_2 biosynthesis does not depend upon de novo PGHS synthesis in NIH-3T3 cells, but that rPDGF does regulate PGHS gene expresslon.

MATERIALS AND METHODS

Actinomycin D, cycloheximide, acetylsalicylic acid, indomethacin, Na_4 EDTA, phenylmethylsulfonyl fluoride, Triton X-100, sodium deoxycholate, and sodium dodecyl sulfate were purchased from Sigma. rPDGF was purchased from AMGEN Biochemicals (Thousand Oaks, CA). All PGE_2 enzyme-linked immunoassay reagents were purchased from Cayman Chemical (Ann Arbor, MI).

Cell Culture.

NIH-3T3 cells were obtained from American Type Culture Collection and were maintained in Dulbecco's modified Eagle's medium supplemented with 10% fetal calf serum. After reaching approximately 80% confluency, the medium was replaced with Dulbecco's modified Eagle's medium containing 0.5% fetal calf serum, and the cells were cultured for an additional 18 h. The serum-starved cells were then exposed to rPDGF (20 ng/ml) and incubated for the appropriate time interval. The same basic protocol was used for PGE_2 measurements, PGHS mRNA analysis, and immunoblot studies.

mRNA Measurement.

Total cellular RNA was isolated using guanidine thiocyanate solubilization and subsequent cesium chloride centrifugation (10,11,12). The RNA was linked to the membrane by UV cross-linking and hybridized to a ^{32}P-labeled prostaglandin H synthase cDNA probe labeled to 1 x 10^9 dpm/μg by random priming. The probe was a 1.6-kilobase EcoRI fragment of ovine PGH synthase cDNA corresponding to nucleotides 1-1609 and was the kind gift of Dr. David L. DeWitt (Michigan State University). The cDNA was subcloned into pUC19 and passaged in Escherichia coli DH5a, and the insert was recovered by EcoRI digestion.

Immunoblot of Prostaglandin H Synthase.

Lysates were electrophoresed on a 10% sodium dodecyl sulfate-polyacrylamide gel, electroblotted onto a nitrocellulose membrane, and hybridized to a 1:400 dilution of rabbit anti-sheep prostaglandin H synthase antibody (raised against homogeneous sheep seminal vesicle PGHS provided by Dr. L.J. Marnett Wayne State University). Immuno complexes were visualized with ^{125}I-protein A followed by autoradiography.

Measurement of Prostaglandin E_2

Prostaglandin E_2 was measured by enzyme-linked immunoassay (EIA) according to Pradelles et al. (13).

RESULTS

Exposure of serum-starved NIH-3T3 cells to 20 ng/ml rPDGF resulted in the stimulation of PGE_2 synthesis (Figure 1). PGE_2 synthesis was rapid, with a measurable increase over basal levels within 10 min, a 4-fold increase at 60 min, and maximal synthesis after 2 h (Figure 1). The addition of 10 μM exogenous arachidonate to the serum-starved cells resulted in the immediate synthesis of large amounts of PGE_2. The amount of PGE_2 formed in 30 min from 10 μM exogenous arachidonate was more than twice as large as the levels formed in 2 h in response to rPDGF (data not shown). These data suggest that there was sufficient PGHS in resting cells before the addition of rPDGF to fully account for all subsequent rPDGF-stimulated PGE_2 synthesis, and that *de novo* synthesis of enzyme should not be required. To assess our findings further, we inhibited protein synthesis with 36 μM cycloheximide and measured rPDGF- and arachidonate-stimulated PGE_2 biosynthesis. Cycloheximide pretreatment did inhibit (>90%) rPDGF-stimulated PGE_2 biosynthesis, but did not influence arachidonic acid-stimulated PGE_2 synthesis (data not shown). These data suggested that new protein synthesis was required for rPDGF-stimulated PGE_2 synthesis, but not necessarily PGHS.

In an attempt to understand these seemingly anomalous data, we measured PGHS mRNA levels by Northern analysis and enzyme levels by immunoblot in rPDGF-stimulated NIH-3T3 cells. The time course of PGHS mRNA accumulation in rPDGF-stimulated NIH-3T3 cells is shown in Figure 2. The PGHS transcript (2.9 kilobases) was readily detected in the serum-starved cells (zero time), and there was no change in PGHS mRNA levels at 30 or 60 min after the addition of rPDGF. After 2 h, when rPDGF-

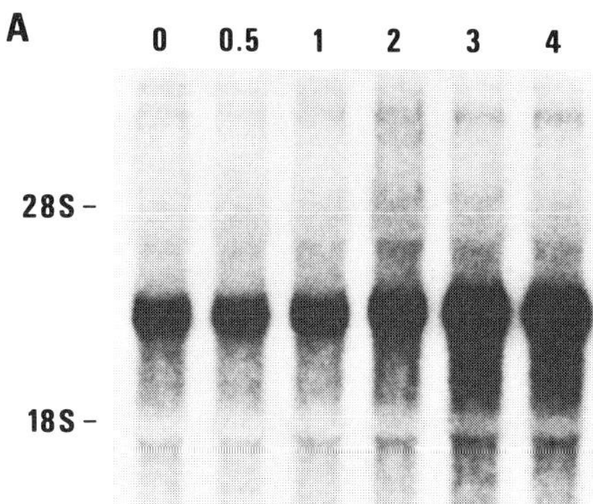

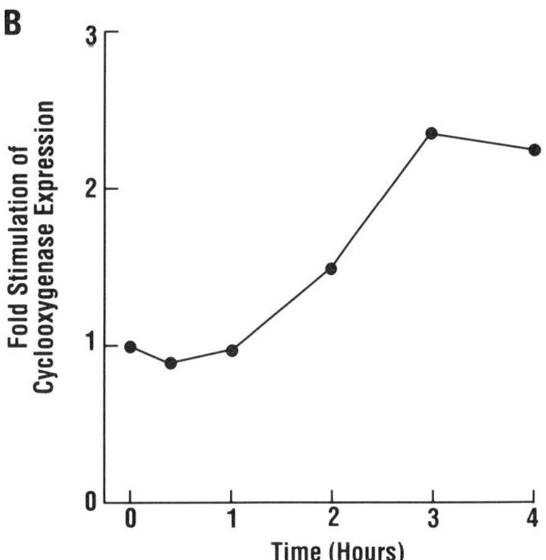

Figure 1. Time course of rPDGF-stimulated PGE_2 synthesis. NIH-3T3 cells (0.6-0.8 x 10^6/well) were cultured for 18 h in 0.5% fetal calf serum and then exposed to 20 ng/ml rPDGF. Samples were removed from the cultures at the indicated times, and the amount of PGE_2 was quantitated by EIA. Data are reported as mean $\pm$ S.E. of triplicate determinations.

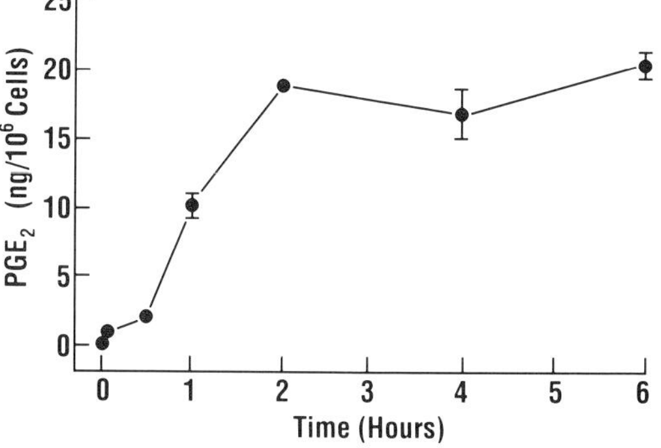

Figure 2. Northern analysis of PGHS mRNA levels in rPDGF-stimulated cells. NIH-3T3 cells (5 x 10^6/dish) were cultured as described for Figure 1 and stimulated with 20 ng/ml rPDGF. At zero time and 0.5, 1, 2, 3, and 4 h after the addition of rPDGF, RNA was isolated and purified as described under "Materials and Methods". The purified RNA was electrotransferred to Nytran and hybridized to a 1.6-kilobase EcoRI fragment of PGHS cDNA probe. mRNA levels were quantitated by densitometry, with the zero time level taken as 1.0.

stimulated PGE_2 synthesis was already maximal (Figure 1), there was 60% increase in PGHS mRNA levels. The maximal induction (250%) of PGHS mRNA levels occurred 3 h after rPDGF stimulation (Figure 2). Over the same time course where PGHS mRNA levels were increasing, we quantified PGHS protein levels.

Figure 3 shows an immunoblot of PGHS protein levels in NIH-3T3 cells during log growth (serum) and in serum-starved cells before (0 min) and from 5 min to 6 h after the addition of 20 ng/ml rPDGF. Although the experiment was repeated several times, there was no consistent difference in enzyme levels regardless of growth conditions and whether or not rPDGF was present. Notice that the proteolysis products (33 and 38 kDa) of the enzyme were also detected; and again, there were no significant differences among the treatments.

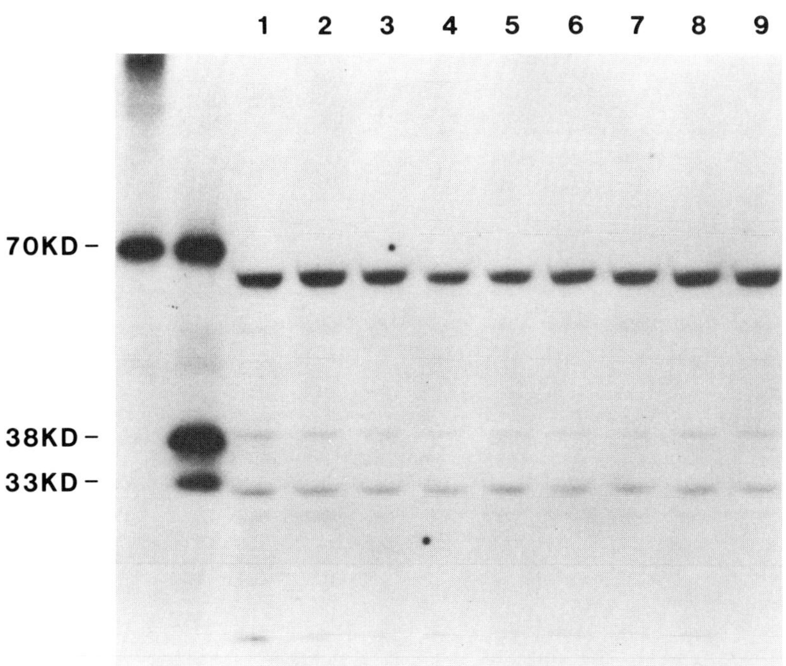

Figure 3. Immunoblot of PGHS enzyme levels in rPDGF-stimulated cells. NIH-3T3 cells (5 x 10^6/dish) were cultured either in 10% serum (designated "serum") or in 0.5% serum as described for Figure 1. At zero time, PGHS levels were quantitated in both the serum cells and the serum-deprived cells. Some of the deprived cells received 20 ng/ml rPDGF, and PGHS levels in these cells were determined by immunoblot at 5,10, and 15 min and 1, 2, 4, and 6 h. Molecular size standards were purified sheep PGHS (70 kDa) and proteolized sheep enzyme (38 and 33 kDa).

DISCUSSION

The rate-limiting step in eicosanoid biosynthesis is usually thought to be the liberation of arachidonic acid from membrane phospholipids. This concept arose form the observation that only free nonesterified arachidonic acid was a suitable substrate for the immediate synthesis of eicosanoids. However, recent papers (14,15,16) have suggested that the level of PGHS may be regulated by agents such as interleukin-1, PMA, and PDGF and that subsequent prostaglandin biosynthesis is, in some cases, dependent upon *de novo* synthesis of PGHS.

NIH-3T3 cells are an excellent model in which to study the correlation between growth factor-stimulated PGE_2 production and PGHS gene expression. Following exposure to rPDGF, NIH-3T3 cells synthesize PGE_2, with maximal synthesis by 2 h. rPDGF-stimulated PGE_2 synthesis was inhibited (>90%) by cycloheximide. Paradoxically, the addition of exogenous arachidonic acid to NIH-3T3 resulted in the immediate synthesis of levels of PGE_2 that exceeded PGE_2 synthesis in response to rPDGF. These data showed that there was more than enough active PGHS in NIH-3T3 cells to fully support all rPDGF-stimulated PGE_2 without the need for *de novo* synthesis of enzyme. Subsequent Northern analysis showed that rPDGF did induce PGHS mRNA levels, but that the induction lagged behind rPDGF-stimulated PGE_2 synthesis. Immunoblot measurements showed no detectable increase in PGHS following stimulation with rPDGF.

All of our data suggest that *de novo* PGHS synthesis is not obligatory for rPDGF-stimulated PGE_2 synthesis in NIH-3T3 cells. Since PGHS is autoinactivated by the conversion of PGG_2 to PGH_2, the delayed induction of PGHS mRNA levels following rPDGF stimulation may be a natural consequence of the cell replacing inactive enzyme resulting from rPDGF-stimulating PGE_2 synthesis. This mechanism was recently postulated in cultured human umbilical endothelial cells (16).

The fact that cycloheximide can severely inhibit rPDGF-stimulated PGE_2 synthesis has been interpreted by others to show that *de novo* PGHS is required to support PGE_2 synthesis (13). Although our data show that cycloheximide does inhibit rPDGF-stimulated PGE_2 synthesis, it has no influence on arachidonate-stimulated synthesis. Since the arachidonate-mediated PGE_2 synthesis is much larger than that elicited by rPDGF, cycloheximide cannot be acting by inhibiting the synthesis of new PGHS. We believe that cycloheximide is inhibiting the synthesis of a protein(s) that are involved in transducing the signal between the growth factor receptor and the phospholipase that releases arachidonate from membrane phospholipids. Such a protein, called phospholipase-activating protein, has been recently described (17). Alternatively, cycloheximide might be inhibiting the synthesis of a regulatory protein that is required for PGHS gene expression.

Another possibility could be that rPDGF induces the expression of a second PGHS that is coupled to the PDGF receptor and whose mRNA is not readily detected by our probe. Thus, the possibility remains that there is differential mRNA splicing or even a second gene. We are now exploring these possibilities, but believe that our data clearly divorce the majority of rPDGF-stimulated PGE_2 synthesis from PGHS gene expression and subsequent enzyme synthesis.

REFERENCES

1. Samuelsson, B. Progr. Biochem. Pharmacol. 51:109-128, 1969.
2. VanDorp, D. Ann. N.Y. Acad. Sci. 180:181-189, 1971.
3. Lands, W., Lee, R. and Smith, W. Ann. N.Y. Acad. Sci. 180:107-122,1971.
4. Miyamoto, T., Ogino, N., Yamamoto, S. and Hayashi, O. J. Biol. Chem. 251:2629-2636,1976.
5. Hemler, M., Lands, W.E.M. and Smith, W.L. J. Biol. Chem. 251:5575-5579,1976.
6. VanderOuderaa, F.J., Buytenhak, M., Nugteren, D.H. and VanDorp, D.A. Biochim. Biophys. Acta. 487:315-331,1977.
7. Matsaers, J.H.G.M., VanHalbeek, H., Kamerling, J.P. and Oliegenthart, J.F.G. Eur. J. Biochem. 147:569-574,1985.
8. DeWitt, D.L. and Smith, W.L. Proc. Natl. Acad. Sci. U.S.A. 85:1412-1416,1988.
9. Merlie, J.P., Fagan, D., Mudd, J. and Needleman, P. J. Biol. Chem. 263:3550-3553, 1988.
10. Chirgwin, J.M., Przybyla, A.E., McDonald, R.J. and Rutter, W.J. Biochemistry 18:5294-5299, 1979.
11. Glisin, V., Crkvenjakov, R. and Byus, C. Biochemistry 13:2633-2637,1974.
12. Ullrich, A., Shine, J., Chirgwin, J., Pictet, R., Tischer, E., Rutler, W.J. and Goodman, H.M. Science 196:1313-1319,1977.
13. Pradelles, P., Grassi, J. and Maclouf, J. Anal. Chem. 57:1170-1173,1985.
14. Habenicht, A.J.R., Goerig, M., Grulich, J., Rothe, D., Gronwald, R., Loth, U., Schletter, G., Kommerell, B. and Ross, R. J. Clin. Invest. 75:1381-1387.
15. Whitely, P.J. and Needleman, P. J. Clin. Invest. 74:2249-2253, 1984.
16. Wu, K.K., Hatzakis, H., Lo, S.S., Seong, D.C., Sanduja, S.K. and Tai, H.H. J. Biol. Chem. 263:19043-19047,1988.
17. Clark, M.A., Conway, T.M., Shorr, R.G.L. and Crooke, S.T. J. Biol. Chem. 262:4402-4406,1987.

ENHANCED EICOSANOID RELEASE IN RAS-TRANSFORMED CELLS

G. A. JAMIESON, Jr., K. A. FLEM, H. A. ELKOUSY, S A. HOLLIDAY, and G. D. LEIKAUF

Division of Molecular Toxicology, Department of Environmental Health, University of Cincinnati College of Medicine, Cincinnati, OH 45267

INTRODUCTION

Our laboratory is studying the spectrum of ionic and biochemical events which are activated seconds to minutes after the addition of mitogens to quiescent fibroblasts. Previous work determined serum and bradykinin to rapidly stimulate phospholipases A_2 and C in human fibroblasts (1-4). Activation of these phospholipases results in the production of a variety of lipid-derived "second messengers" (including arachidonate and its metabolites, diacylglycerol and inositol trisphosphate). These messengers stimulate a variety of cellular processes which are thought to be important components of the mitogenic response - including changes in cellular ion fluxes (2-8), activation of protein kinases (7,8), and induction of rapid transcriptional events (9,10).

After examining phospholipase activation in normal fibroblasts we proceeded to determine whether these cellular responses were altered upon oncogenic transformation. In these studies we used a normal diploid human fibroblasts and its SV40 transformed counterpart (SV40/WI-38). We determined bradykinin, while capable of activating phospholipases A_2 and C in WI-38 cells, did not stimulate these activities in the SV40 transformed cells (11). This difference was traced to a reduced level of bradykinin receptor expression in SV40/WI-38 cells (5% of parental receptor levels). These studies lead us to conclude that transformation reduces bradykinin receptor expression in human fibroblasts.

In contrast to these observations other studies have determined transformation (by ras or dbl) to increase bradykinin receptor expression in rodent fibroblasts (12-14). We had determined previously that serum stimulated enhanced arachidonate release in ras-transformed NIH/3T3 cells (15) and we hypothesized this increased arachidonate release might be due to an altered expression of a bradykinin coupled phospholipase A_2 activity in these cells. In the current study we examined the ability of bradykinin to stimulate arachidonate release in ras-transformed cells and characterized the arachidonate metabolites which were are released by cells subsequent to stimulation with bradykinin.

MATERIALS AND METHODS

Cell Culture.

NIH/3T3 cells and ras-transformed NIH/3T3 cells were grown in DMEM containing 10% bovine calf serum in a 95% air, 5% CO_2 atmosphere at 37°C. Cultures were as follows NIH/3T3 cells and K-ras (DT)

transformants (R. Bassin, NIH); H-ras transformants (V.P. Sukhatme, Univ. of Chicago). Cells were subcultured onto 60 mm dishes for experiments.

Analysis of Arachidonate Acid Release.

Cells were incubated with 0.1-0.2 uCi/ml of [^{3}H]-arachidonate (NEN) 4-6 hours (previously determined to maximally label phospholipids) in a Hepes-buffered DMEM which contained 0.1% fatty acid free BSA in an air incubator (37°C). Cells were then washed free of labeling medium and assays performed using medium containing fatty-acid free BSA throughout. Assays were initiated by addition of fresh medium containing bradykinin, Ca ionophore, serum or other factors. After 5 minutes aliquots of the medium were removed, microfuged to insure the absence of any particulate/cellular material and then an aliquot assayed for [^{3}H]-arachidonate acid and its metabolites by scintillation counting.

HPLC Analysis of Eicosanoid Metabolism.

To investigate the array of arachidonic metabolites produced we qualitatively analyzed release assay medium by radiochromatographic HPLC separation. Briefly, cells were labeled with [^{3}H]-arachidonic acid and treated with bradykinin and other agonists as described above. Before separation prostaglandin B_2 was added to each sample (to allow the estimation of recoveries), and the sample acidified (pH = 3.5) and extracted 3 times with 2 volumes of ethyl acetate. Samples were dried with purified N_2, and then quantitatively injected onto a ODS-Ultrasphere column. Gradient, reverse-phase HPLC allowed for the identification of major cyclooxygenase and lipoxygenase products. Identification of the eicosanoids produced was by co-elution of the radio-labeled products with authentic standards (monitored by UV-absorbance with a multi-wavelength detector).

ELISA Analysis of Released Eicosanoids.

An alkaline phosphatase enzyme immunoassay (Advanced Magnetics) was adapted for use with goat anti-rabbit coated 96-well plates. Briefly, cells were serum-deprived for 4 hr. prior to the initiation of release assays. The medium (phenol-red free) from a release assay was removed, acidified with formic acid and then extracted 3 times with ethyl acetate to extract the PGE_2. Samples were dried under purified N_2 resuspended in ELISA assay buffer and then incubated in the presence of PGE_2 alkaline phosphatase and rabbit anti-PGE_2 overnight. Microtiter plates were washed and then developed using a ELISA amplification kit (BRL). PGE_2 standard was obtained from Sigma Chemical Co.

RESULTS

Initially we examined whether serum stimulated the release of arachidonate-derived material from normal or ras-transformed NIH/3T3 cells. Arachidonic acid release was determined to be greatly enhanced in the ras-transformed NIH/3T3 versus that observed in the parental NIH/3T3 cells (see Figure 1). As ras-transformation had been shown to elevate bradykinin receptor expression in rodent fibroblasts (12,13) we next tested the effects of bradykinin in this system. Bradykinin stimulated the release of arachidonate-derived material from ras-transformed cells but not from NIH/3T3 cells. Bradykinin stimulated release was equivalent to that obtained with serum (see Figure 1). Bradykinin or serum

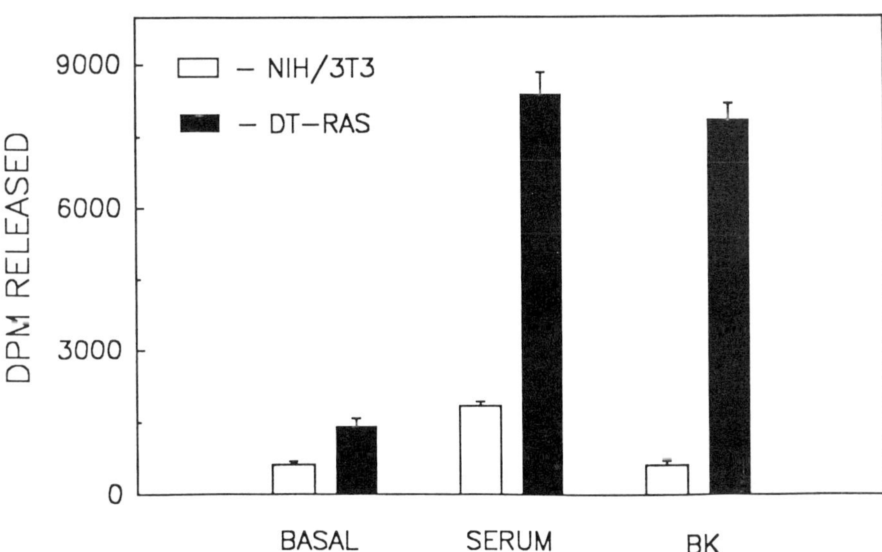

Figure 1 - Stimulation of release of arachidonate-derived material from normal and RAS-transformed NIH/3T3 cells. Confluent cultures were serum-deprived and prelabeled with [^{3}H]-arachidonic acid for 4 hours as described in METHODS. Assays were for 5 min and stimuli were 10% FBS or bradykinin (100 ng/ml).

routinely stimulated the release of 6 to 10 percent of the total [^{3}H]-label present in the monolayer during the 5 minute assay period.

As bradykinin stimulated arachidonate-release to levels equivalent to those obtained with serum we continued our analyses using a defined stimulus, (i.e. bradykinin) and the K-ras transformed NIH/3T3 cells (DT cells). Bradykinin stimulated release of arachidonate-derived material was determined to be a rapid event - maximum release was obtained within 3-5 minutes of stimulation with bradykinin.

We next characterized the nature of the arachidonate-derived material which was released into the assay medium. Assay mixtures from bradykinin-stimulated cultures were extracted with ethyl acetate and subjected to gradient, reverse-phase HPLC (16). A typical HPLC radiochromatogram is presented in Figure 2. Prostaglandin E_2 is the major eicosanoid product released. Peaks representing lesser amounts of PGD_2 and 6-keto-PGF_{1a} flank the PGE_2 peak.

To quantitate the amount of PGE_2 released from ras-transformed NIH/3T3 cells we used an ELISA assay. Depending upon the experiment 50-75 ng of PGE_2 were released from a confluent 60 mm culture dish into the assay medium within 5 minutes after the addition of bradykinin. The time course of PGE_2 release into the medium paralleled the time course observed for the release of radiolabeled product.

Having determined serum and bradykinin to stimulate the release of large quantities of PGE_2 from ras-transformed cells, but not NIH/3T3 cells, we next wished to determined which phospholipid(s) were

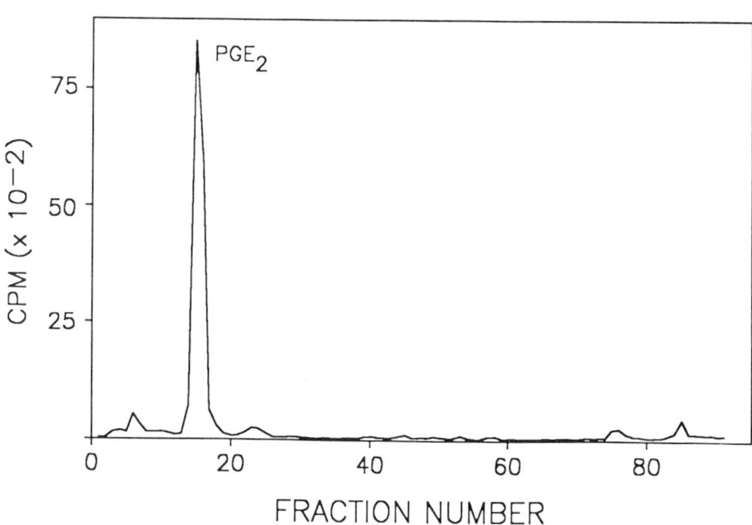

Figure 2 - HPLC Radiochromatogram of eicosanoids. Cells were prelabeled with [^{3}H] arachidonic acid for 4 hours prior to removal of radiolabeling media and stimulation with bradykinin (100 ng/ml) for 5 minutes. The assay medium was extracted with ethyl acetate and the extract, after evaporation under N_2, was analyzed by gradient HPLC as described in METHODS. The single large peak migrated at the position of the internal PGE_2 standard.

the source of the released arachidonate metabolites. Mock- and bradykinin-stimulated monolayers were extracted by the method of Bligh and Dyer (17) and phospholipids analyzed by thin layer chromatography. The levels of phosphatidylinositol and phosphatidylcholine initially decreased rapidly, consistent with the rapid release of arachidonate-derived material we observed, but then rapidly recovered to basal levels. Analyses of phosphatidylinositol metabolism failed to reveal large increases in inositol phosphate metabolism subsequent to stimulation of DT cells with bradykinin or the Ca ionophore A23187. As strong stimuli of arachidonate release did not activate inositol phosphate release we have initially concluded the arachidonate release we observe is mediated via a phospholipase A_2 activity and not the result of the sequential phospholipase C and diacylglycerol lipase activities on phosphatidylinositides.

Finally we examined the ability of bradykinin to stimulate arachidonate release from H-ras versus K-ras transformed NIH/3T3 cells. We determined that in contrast to the ability of both serum and Ca ionophore to rapidly activate the release of arachidonate-derived material from either H-ras or K-ras transformed NIH/3T3 cells that bradykinin stimulated release from only the K-ras line (DT cells; see Figure 3). Currently we are examining whether this observation reflects differential expression of bradykinin receptors in these two cell types or a K-ras specific coupling of the bradykinin receptor to phospholipase A_2.

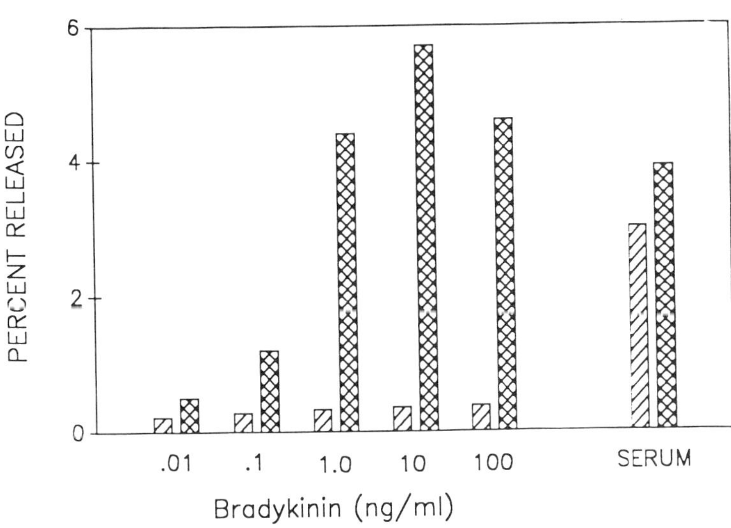

Figure 3. Bradykinin stimulated eicosanoid release in H-RAS and K-RAS transformed NIH/3T3 cells. Assays were performed as described in Figure 1 with the indicated concentrations of bradykinin and serum at 10%. Values represent the percent of the total DPM present in the cell monolayer released during the assay period. Striped - H-ras transformants; Hatched - K-ras transformants.

SUMMARY

In the current study we have examined the ability of serum, Ca ionophore and bradykinin to stimulate phospholipase A_2 in normal and ras-transformed NIH/3T3 cells. We determined serum and Ca ionophore to rapidly stimulate the release of arachidonic acid derived material from both H-ras and K-ras-transformed NIH/3T3 cells. The release of arachidonic acid metabolites is significantly elevated in ras-transformed cells over that observed in parental NIH/3T3 cells. Bradykinin stimulates the rapid release of arachidonic acid metabolites in K-ras transformed NIH/3T3 cells but not in H-ras transformed NIH/3T3 cells. This suggests either a K-ras specific coupling of the bradykinin receptor to phospholipase A_2 or differential expression of the bradykinin receptors on the cell lines used in the current study. Analysis by reverse-phase HPLC determined the major eicosanoid released in response to bradykinin, serum, or Ca ionophore to be prostaglandin E_2. Current studies are examining whether the prostanoids released in response to bradykinin stimulation are subsequently dehydrated (to PGA_2 and PGJ_2) and then accumulate intracellularly as noted by Narumiya and co-workers (see pages 439-448 of the current volume).

ACKNOWLEDGMENTS

The authors would like to thank Robin Lerchen for technical assistance and the support of NIH S07-RR05408, NIEHS ES 00159. KAF and HAE were Duke Futures Summer Interns.

LITERATURE CITED

1. Jamieson, G.A., Jr. and Villereal, M.L.: Arch. Biochem. Biophys. 252:478, 1987.
2. Muldoon, L.L., Jamieson, G.A., Jr. and Villereal, M.L.: J. Cell Physiol. 130:29, 1987.
3. Jamieson, G.A., Jr., Etscheid, B.G., Muldoon, L.L. and Villereal, M.L.: J. Cell Physiol. 134:220, 1987.
4. Vicentini, L.M., Miller, R.J. and Villereal, M.L.: J. Biol. Chem. 259:6912, 1984.
5. Mix, L.L., Dinerstein, R.J. and Villereal, M.L.: Biochem. Biophys. Res. Comm. 119:69, 1984.
6. Muldoon, L.L., Dinerstein, R.J. and Villereal, M.L.: Am. J. Physiol. 294:C140, 1985.
7. Palfrey, H.C., Nairn, A.C., Muldoon, L.L. and Villereal, M.L.: J. Biol. Chem. 262:9785, 1987.
8. Muldoon, L.L., Jamieson, G.A., Jr., Kao, A.C., Palfrey, H.C. and Villereal, M.L.: Am. J. Physiol. 253 (Cell Physiol 22):C219, 1987.
9. Joseph, L.J., Le-Beau, M.M., Jamieson, G.A., Jr., Acharya, S., Shows, T.B., Rowley, J.D., and Sukhatme, V.P.: Proc. Natl. Acad. Sci. USA 85:7164, 1988.
10. Jamieson, G.A., Jr., Mayforth, R., Villereal, M.L.: J. Cell Physiol. 139:262, 1989.
11. Etscheid, B.G., Jamieson, G.A., Jr., Toscas, K. and Villereal, M.L.: Am. J. Physiol. 259:C549-556, 1990.
12. Parries, G., Hoebel, R. and Racker, E.: Proc. Natl. Acad. Sci. (USA) 84:2648, 1987.
13. Downward, J., de-Gunzburg, J., Riehl, R. and Weinberg, R.A.: Proc. Natl. Acad. Sci. USA 85:5774, 1988.
14. Ruggiero, M., Srivastava, S.K., Fleming, T.P., Ron, D., and Eva, A.: Oncogene 4:767, 1989.
15. Jamieson, G.A., Jr., Sukhatme, V.P., McArdle, R.A. and Villereal, M.L.: J. Cell Biol. 105:108a, 1987.
16. Powell, W.S.: Methods of Enzymology 86:467, 1982.
17. Bligh, E.G., Dyer, W.J.: Canad. J. Biochem. Physiol. 37:911, 1957.

STIMULATION OF de novo SYNTHESIS OF PROSTAGLANDIN H SYNTHETASE (PHS) IN RAT TRACHEAL EPITHELIAL CELLS BY TPA INVOLVES ACTIVATION OF PROTEIN KINASE C

Z.M. DUNIEC, P. NETTESHEIM, and T.E. ELING

LMB & LPP, National Institute of Environmental Health Sciences, Research Triangle Park, NC 27709

INTRODUCTION

Elevated prostaglandin production is believed to be involved in tumor promotion. Several tumor promoters of different chemical structure, including the best known and most potent 12-0-tetradecanoylphorbol-13-acetate (TPA), stimulate arachidonic acid (AA) metabolism in a variety of cell types (1,2). TPA-stimulated prostaglandin production as well as many other pleiotropic responses of TPA are thought to result from the activation of protein kinase C (PKC), the putative receptor for TPA (3,4).

AA metabolism is tightly regulated at several enzymatic steps, the most important being: 1) release of AA from cellular phospholipids by specific phospholipases (A_2 and C, ref. 5) and 2) conversion of released AA into prostaglandins by PHS (6). The rate limiting step was thought to be release of AA from its cellular stores (7). Lately it has been suggested that resynthesis of PHS after autoinactivation which occurs during AA metabolism may be of equal importance as the rate limiting step. Recent reports postulate that de novo synthesis of PHS is stimulated by different biologically active agents (8-10) including TPA (11).

In a previous paper (12) we have shown that TPA was the only factor which stimulated PGE_2 production in the transformed rat tracheal epithelial cell line, EGV-4T, grown in serum-supplemeted medium. Various peptide growth factors were ineffective.

In the present study we have further examined the mechanism responsible for the stimulation of PGE_2 production by TPA using the cell line EGV-6aigT which can grow in serum-free medium and thus avoiding other potentially interfering substances.

METHODS

EGV-6aigT cell cultures were maintained in serum-free medium, i.e. Ham's F-12 supplemented with insulin, transferrin, EGF (all from Sigma) and other growth promoters including bovine serum albumin (ICN Immunobiologicals) and bovine pituitary extract (Clonetics Corp.).

The cultures grown to about 75% confluency were subjected to 24 hr starvation (Ham's F-12 with no supplements) prior to subsequent experimentation.

To measure the release of AA from endogenous phospholipids cells were pretreated with ^{3}H-AA (New England Nuclear) followed by treatment with different agents. Media were then analysed by RP-HPLC as described previously (13).

PHS activity was estimated by measuring the metabolism of exogenous AA. Cells pretreated with various inhibitors or vehicle were incubated for 4 hr with TPA (Chemsyn Science Lab.) followed by 30 min incubation with exogenous AA (Nu Check Prep.).

To measure PGE_2 production media were analysed by radioimmunoassay using a specific anti-PGE_2 antibody (Advanced Magnetics) as described previously (14).

To determine mRNA expression total cytoplasmic RNA was isolated (15), separated, transferred to nitrocellulose membranes (16) and identified by hybridization to a 1.6 kb PHS RNA probe (Oxford Biomedical Research), labeled with ^{32}P-CTP by in vitro transcription.

RESULTS AND DISCUSSION

It is well established that TPA increases prostaglandin production in a variety of cells (1), including the rat tracheal epithelial cell lines EGV-4T and EGV-6aigT, used in our studies. The mechanism by which TPA causes enhancement in prostaglandin production could involve 1) increased release of AA from phospholipids (by phospholipases), 2) activation of PHS, 3) stimulation of de novo synthesis of PHS or 4) all of the above.

To test the first possibility cells were incubated for 24 hr with 10 μCi of ^{3}H-AA followed by 30 min incubation with calcium ionophore A23187 (10 μM) or TPA (50 nM), and media were analysed by HPLC. Calcium ionophore A23187 stimulated the release and subsequent metabolism of AA to PGE_2, the major eicosanoid produced by these cells, while TPA had no effect. These data indicate that, in contrast to A23187, TPA does not increase PGE_2 levels via stimulation of phospholipases. However, when cells were pretreated with TPA and then incubated with 10 μM exogenous AA, which bypasses phospholipases, an increase in PGE_2 production was observed. This suggests that TPA either elevated PHS levels or increased the activity of PHS. The increase in PGE_2 synthesis was dependent on TPA concentration and required 4 hr of incubation with TPA (with 2 hr lag phase) for maximum activity. Subsequently, a slow decrease occurred and PGE_2 synthesis reached control levels after 12 to 24 hr of incubation with TPA. TPA-stimulated PGE_2 production was blocked by indomethacin (PHS inhibitor) and by dexamethasone (purported phospholipase A_2 inhibitor) in a concentration dependent manner (Table 1).

To test for de novo synthesis of the enzyme cells were treated with actinomycin D (transcriptional inhibitor) and cycloheximide (protein synthesis inhibitor). As shown in Table 1, both of these inhibitors reduced TPA enhancement of PGE_2 production suggesting that TPA stimulated de novo synthesis of PHS. Furthermore, TPA significantly enhanced recovery of PHS activity in cells in which PHS activity was irreversibly inhibited by pretreatment with aspirin (Table 1) .

Since it is well established that many, if not all, TPA responses are mediated by PKC (3,4), we determined whether PKC inhibitors such as staurosporin would block the TPA induced stimulation of PGE_2 synthesis in EGV-6aigT cells. The results showed that PKC inhibitors abolished the stimulatory effect of TPA on PGE_2 production (Table 1). Thus, taken together our findings indicate that TPA effects on PHS synthesis are mediated by PKC.

The results obtained by measurement of PGE_2 production were confirmed by Northern blot analysis of EGV-6aigT RNA. TPA treatment enhanced PHS mRNA levels while actinomycin D blocked the increase in PHS transcripts following TPA treatment. Staurosporin (PKC inhibitor) prevented TPA stimulated increase in PHS transcripts.

Table 1.
Influence of different inhibitors on PGE_2 production stimulated by TPA.

	Treatment	PGE_2 production (ng/10^5 cells) (mean + S.D.)	
A)	None	1.41 ± 0.21	(n=3)
	Indomethacin (10^{-6}M)	0.02 ± 0.02	(n=3)
	TPA (50 nM)	2.61	(n=2)
	Indomethacin + TPA	0.01 ± 0.00	(n=3)
B)	None	1.19 ± 0.05	(n=3)
	Dexamethasone (10^{-6}M)	0.72 ± 0.07	(n=3)
	TPA (50 nM)	2.44 ± 0.11	(n=3)
	Dexamethasone + TPA	1.20 ± 0.10	(n=3)
C)	None	1.78 ± 0.15	(n=11)
	Actinomycin D (10 μg/ml)	1.96 ± 0.22	(n=3)
	TPA (50 nM)	3.17 ± 0.36	(n=12)
	Actinomycin D + TPA	1.70 ± 0.04	(n=3)
D)	None	1.70	(n=2)
	Cycloheximide (10 μg/ml)	1.47 ± 0.10	(n=3)
	TPA (50 nM)	3.83 ± 0.29	(n=3)
	Cycloheximide + TPA	1.53 ± 0.12	(n=3)
E)	None	1.78 + 0.15	(n=11)
	Staurosporin (100 nM)	1.45 ± 0.09	(n=3)
	TPA (50 nM)	3.17 ± 0.36	(n=12)
	Staurosporin + TPA	1.68 ± 0.12	(n=3)
F)	None	2.98 ± 0.24	(n=6)
	Aspirin (300 μM)	1.94 ± 0.07	(n=6)
	washed twice and treated:		
	None	1.77 ± 0.32	(n=5)
	TPA (50 nM)	8.08 ± 0.71	(n=4)

Nutrient starved cells were pretreated 30 min (4 hr for dexamethasone) with listed inhibitors followed by 4 hr incubation with TPA and 30 min incubation with 10 μM of exogenous AA. Media were analysed by RIA.

In summary, our data indicate that TPA enhances PGE_2 production by stimulation of de novo synthesis of PHS and that this process involves activation of PKC.

REFERENCES

1. Levine, L. Adv. Cancer Res. 35: 49-79, 1981.
2. Levine, L. and Fujiki, H. Carcinogenesis 6: 1631-1634, 1985.
3. Nishizuka, Y. Nature 308: 693-698, 1984.
4. Ashendel, C.L. Biochim. Biophys. Acta. 822: 219-242, 1985.
5. Blackwell, G.J. and Flower, R.J. Br. Med. Bull. 39: 260-264, 1983.
6. Needleman, P., Turk, J., Jakschik, B.A., Morrison, A.R. and Lefkowith, J.B. Ann. Rev. Biochem. 55: 69-102, 1986.
7. Lapetina, E.G. Trends Pharmacol. Sci. 3: 115-118, 1982.
8. Habenicht, A.J.R., Goerig, M., Grulich, J., Rothe, D., Gronwald, R., Loth, U., Schettler, G., Kommerell, B. and Ross, R. J. Clin. Invest. 75: 1381-1387, 1985.
9. Casey, M.L., Korte, K. and MacDonald, P.C. J. Biol. Chem. 263: 7846-7854, 1988.
10. Raz, A., Wyche, A. and Needleman, P. Proc. Natl. Acad. Sci. USA 86: 1657-1661,1989.
11. Wu, K.K., Hatzakis, H., Lo, S.S., Seong, D.C., Sanduja, S.K. and Tai, H.H. J. Biol. Chem. 263: 19043-19047, 1988.
12. Duniec, Z.M., Eling, T.E., Jetten, A.M., Gray, T.E. and Nettesheim, P. Exp. Lung Res. 15: 391-408, 1989.
13. Henke, D., Danilowicz, R. and Eling, T. Biochim. Biophys. Acta. 876: 271-279, 1986.
14. Morrison, A.R., McLaughlin, L., Bloch, M. and Needleman, P. J. Biol. Chem. 259: 13579-13583, 1984.
15. Gilman, N. In: Current Protocols in Molecular Biology (Eds. F.M. Ausubel, R. Brent, R.E. Kingston, D.D. Moore, J.G. Seidman, J.A. Smith and K. Struhl), Greene Publishing Associates & Wiley-Interscience, J.Wiley & Sons, New York, Chichester, Brisbane, Toronto, Singapore, 1988, p.403-416.
16. Selden, R.F. ibid. p.491-498.

MITOGENIC EFFECTS OF EICOSANOIDS IN HUMAN AIRWAY EPITHELIAL CELLS

G. D. LEIKAUF, H.-E. CLAESSON, C. A. DOUPNIK, and R. G. GRAFSTROM

Pulmonary Cell Biology Laboratory, Departments of Environmental Health, and Physiology and Biophysics, University of Cincinnati Medical Center, Cincinnati, Ohio 45267-0182, and Departments of Toxicology and Physiological Chemistry, Karolinska Institut, Stockholm, Sweden S104-01

INTRODUCTION

Uncontrolled epithelial cell growth is a hallmark of many forms of cancer and, in the lung, the airway epithelium represents an important target site for initiation by environmental agents (1). Epithelial proliferation and hyperplasia are common sequelae of chronic irritation and inflammation, and thus have been linked to the promotion phase in multistage carcinogenesis (2). Understanding the local processes that provide a micro-environment selective for clonal explanation of pre-carcinogenic cells could therefore be useful in evaluating the complex relationships between inflammation and cancer.

Diverse environmental stimuli can initiate inflammatory responses in the lung which in turn are often accompanied by phospholipase activation and subsequent synthesis of specific eicosanoids. Marked increases in 5-lipoxygenase product formation with conversion of eicosatetraenoic acid to 5-hydroperoxyeicosatetraenoic acid, leukotriene A_4, leukotriene B_4 or leukotriene C_4 has been demonstrâted in human lung homogenates and airway preparations (3). The resulting increased leukotriene formation can have a wide range of pathophysiologic consequences, including heightened airway reactivity (4), glycoprotein secretion (5), and activation of epithelial ion transport (6,7). Recently, eicosanoids have been found to influence growth and differentiation of several non-respiratory cell types including fibroblasts (8), vascular smooth muscle (9), and epidermal cells (keratinocytes and melanocytes) (10,11). In this study we examine the effects of selected 5-lipoxygenase products on growth of human airway epithelial cells.

MATERIAL AND METHODS

Methods used in this study are similar to those described elsewhere (12). Briefly, human airway epithelial cells were grown from tracheobronchial tissue explants and transferred onto collagen/fibronectin-coated dishes by the methods described by Lechner and associates (13). Cells were grown in a MCDB-153 based medium supplemented with hydrocortisone, insulin, transferrin, phosphoethanolamine, ethanolamine, epidermal growth factor, 3,3'5-triiodo-L-thyronine, and bovine pituitary extract (12). Cell preparations produced by this method retain human karotype, express epithelial keratin, possess a specialized plasma membrane, and are capable of differentiating into a ciliated epithelium.

Colony-forming efficiency was measured with cells seeded at 250-500 cells/cm^2 for 24h, and grown without (control) or with selected concentrations of leukotriene B_4 (5S,12R-dihydroxy eicosatetraenoic acid) or its non-biologically active stereoisomer 5S,12S-dihydroxyeicosatetraenoic acid. To examine the effect of secondary prostaglandin formation, a cyclooxygenase inhibitor, 1.0 uM indomethacin, was added lh before leukotriene B_4 addition and cells were grown throughout with both compounds present in the medium. Cells were grown for 7-9 days with one medium change at 4 days. At the end of this period, cultures were fixed in phosphate-buffered saline containing 10% formaldehyde, stained with 0.25% crystal violet, and colonies (containing 16 or more cells) counted with a dissecting microscope.

Values of colony forming efficiency were averaged for determinations from duplicate or triplicate trials from each donor (n=4-6) and normalized to appropriate paired controls of either 4 ul of 50:50 ethanol:water (leukotriene vehicle) in 4 ml culture medium (final volume percent = 0.05 ethanol) or the same vehicle with 1.0 uM indomethacin. (Vehicle control = 154+19 and vehicle control + indomethacine = 161+23 colonies/60 mm dis, $\bar{x}\pm$S.E.)

RESULTS AND DISCUSSION

Colony forming efficiency of human airway epithelial cells was stimulated by leukotriene B_4, but not 5S,12S-dihydroxyeicosa-tetaenoic acid. Leukotriene B_4 increased colony forming efficiency at concentration as low as 0.01 pM with a maximal effect at 1-100 pM (see Table 1). Higher concentrations of leukotriene B_4 (10^{-7} and $3X10^{-7}$) yielded colony forming efficiencies of 154 $\pm$ 12 and 110 $\pm$ 11, respectively. In contrast, 5S,12S-dihydroxyeicosatetaenoic acid produced no change in growth in concentrations up to 10 nM. Previously, we reported that cysteinyl-leukotrienes C_4 and D_4 were also potent mitogens, while leukotriene E_4 was inactive (12). These results indicate that these compounds affect cell growth through a stereospecific mechanism likely to require a leukotriene-receptor(s), rather than by a nonspecific effect due solely to fatty acid addition, since 5S,12S-dihydroeicosatetraenoic and leukotriene E_4 share this property with the active compounds leukotriene B_4 and C_4.

Addition of indomethacin produced no significant enhancement in the leukotriene B_4 response. For example, at 0.001, 0.1 and 10 nM leukotriene B4 plus 1.0 uM indomethacin addition resulted in the following change in colony forming efficiency 162+14, 163+11, and 167+17%, respectively ($\bar{X}$+S.E., n=8). Although these values are significantly different from control (vehicle + indomethacin), none were significantly different from leukotriene B_4 alone at equivalent doses (see Table 1). Human airway epithelial cells when grown in culture express cyclooxygenase activity that can be stimulated with calcium ionophore (12). In isolated canine tracheal epithelium, we and others have observed that high levels of cysteinyl-leukotrienes can stimulate prostaglandin formation, an effect not seen with leukotriene B_4 (6-7). Similarly, indomethacin potentiated the mitogenic effects of leukotriene C_4, but not leukotriene B_4 in human airway epithelial cells. Thus, this potentiation may be due to diminished secondary prostaglandin E_2 formation which has been reported to inhibit growth of other cell types (see Axelrod this conference).

TABLE 1. MITOGENIC EFFECT OF 5-LIPOXYGENASE EICOSANOIDS ON HUMAN AIRWAY EPITHELIAL CELLS.

	Colony Forming Efficiency (Percent Control)					
	Concentration (M)					
Compound	10^{-18}	10^{-16}	10^{-14}	10^{-12}	10^{-10}	10^{-8}
LTB_4	115(15)	96(8)	149(23)*	183(27)*	190(39)*	156(12)*
5,12diHETE	99(2)	100(4)	97(5)	94(15)	105(8)	93(7)
LTC_4	110(7)	131(14)	185(33)*	220(26)*	323(36)*	249(30)*
LTD_4	102(5)	104(4)	105(8)	136(13)*	162(19)*	169(20)*
LTE_4	100(7)	107(4)	100(3)	100(5)	108(16)	100(5)

Human airway epithelial cells were grown in growth-factor supplemented MCDB-153 for 7-9 days, fixed, stained, and colonies (consisting of $\geq$16 cells) counted. Values are means with standard error in parenthesis (LTB_4 n=9, 5S,12S-diHETE n=4, LTC_4-E_4 n=6). Data for leukotriene C_4-E_4 from reference 12. *Value significantly different from control $p<0.05$.

Previously, we found that cell interactions between leukocytes and endothelial cells resulted in increased leukotriene biosynthesis by two independent mechanisms -- through endothelial cell activation of leukocyte 5-lipoxygenase, and through transfer leukocyte-derived leukotriene A_4 to endothelial cells for subsequent (and greater) metabolism into cysteinyl leukotrienes and leukotriene B_4 (14). In preliminary tests with human airway epithelial cells, exogenous leukotriene A_4 was converted principally to leukotriene B_4, suggesting that transcellular metabolism is also possible in this cell type (12,15). Further, because we found only weak 5-lipoxygenase activity and leukotriene B_4 formation after calcium ionophore stimulation of human airway epithelial cells, any enhancement of leukotriene A_4/B_4 formation at the local site of epithelial inflammation is likely the result of leukocyte infiltration, activation, and eicosanoid cometabolism. Such an outcome may thereby be significant in providing an unique pro-proliferative environment substantiating hyperplastic growth.

Lastly, we compared the effectiveness of leukotriene C_4 with that of leukotriene B_4 in preliminary tests with cells from the same donors. Leukotriene C_4 produced a greater maximal response (0.1 nM LTC_4 = 467+48 and 0.1 nM LTB_4 = 166+11%, $\bar{x}$+S.E., n=3); this was consistent with the results presented in Table 1 in which data from different donors are compared. Thus, the relative mutogenic effect of 5-lipoxygenase products for human airway epithelial cells is $LTC_4 > LTB_4 \geq LTD_4 > LTE_4$ =5S,12S-diHETE. This relationship is like that reported for human glomerular epithelial cells (16), but differs from that for human epidermal cells (10), confirming that leukotriene-mediated responses act through tissue/somatic-specific mechanisms thought to control transducer/selector/effector expression in each cell type.

In summary, leukotriene B_4 is a potent mitogen for human airway epithelial cells much like cysteinyl-leukotrienes, but unlike the cysteinyl leukotrienes, this response is independent of secondary prostaglandin formation. Thus, leukotriene B_4 formation at local sites of inflammation may alter epithelial cell growth and thereby provide a positive growth micro-environment characteristic of the tumor promotion phase of carcinogenesis.

ACKNOWLEDGEMENTS

We thank Elizabeth Summers and Joan Abbinante for valued technical assistance. This study was supported in part by the Health Effects Institute, an organization jointly funded by the United States Environmental Protection Agency (Assistance Agreement X812059) and automotive manufactures, the National Institutes of Environmental Health (ES-00159), King Gustat V 80th Birthday Foundation and Swedish Cancer Society (2891-B90-01XA). The contents of this article do not necessarily reflect the views or policies of the Health Effects Institute, Environmental Protection Agency, or automotive manufacturers.

REFERENCES

1. Harris, C . C . Cancer Res . 47 :1-10, 1987 .

2. Argyris, T.S. CRC Crit. Rev. Toxicol. 14:211-258, 1985.
3. Drazen, J.M. and Austen, K.F. Am. Rev. Respir. Dis. 136: 985-998, 1987 .
4 Leikauf, G.D., Doupnik, C.A., Leming, L.M., and Wey, H.E. J. Appl . Physiol . 66 :1838-1845, 1989.
5. Marom, Z ., Shelhamer, J.H., Bach, M.K., Morton, D.R., and Kaliner, M. Am. Rev. Respir. Dis. 126:449-451, 1982.
6. Leikauf, G.D., Ueki, I.F., Widdicombe, J.H., Nadel, J.A. Am. J. Physiol . 250: F47-F53, 1986 .
7. Eling, T., Danilowiez, R., Sivorajah, K., Henke, D., Yankaskas, J ., and Boucher, R . J . Biol . Chem . 261: 12841-12849, 1986 .
8. Baud, L., Perez, J., Denis, M., and Ardaillou, R. J. Immunol. 138: 1190-1195, 1987 .
9. Palmberg, L., Claesson, H-E., and Thyberg, J. J. Cell Sci. 88: 151-159, 1987 .
10. Kragballe, K., Desgarlais, L., and Voorhees, J. Br. J. Dermatol. 113: 43-52, 1985 .
11. Abdel-Malek, Z.A., Swope, V.B., Amornsiripanitch, N., and Nordlund, J.J. Cancer Res. 47:3141-3146, 1987.
12. Leikauf, G.D., Claesson, H-E., Doupnik, C.A., Hybbinette, S., and Grafstrom, R. G. Am. J . Physiol. 259:L255-261, 1990.
13 . Lechner, J. F. and LaVeck, M.A. J. Tissue Culture Methods 9: 43-48, 1985 .
14. Claesson, H-E. and Haeggstrom, J. Eur. J. Biochem. 173: 93-100, 1988 .
15. Bigby, T. D., Lee, D.M., Aldrich, A.J., Kattan, F., and Gruenert, D.C. FASEB J. 3:A315, 1989.
16. Baud, L., Sraer, J., Perez, J., Nivez, M-P., and Ardaillou, R. J. Clin. Invest. 76: 374-377, 1985 .

EICOSANOID MODULATION OF RECEPTOR EXPRESSION

LIPOXYGENASES, INTEGRIN RECEPTORS, AND METASTASIS

K. V. HONN, I.M. GROSSI, Y.S. CHANG, and Y. CHEN

Depts. Radiation Oncology, and Chemistry, Wayne State University, Detroit, MI 48202

Failure of tumor cells to arrest and form stable adhesions to the endothelium may be viewed as a critical barrier to the formation of a successful metastatic lesion. This suggests that agents (i.e., receptors, platelets, hemodynamic factors, eicosanoids, etc.) which regulate initial tumor cell arrest and adhesion are of significant importance in the development (or prevention) of a successful metastasis (1).

We previously reported evidence for a glycoprotein complex related to the platelet $\alpha_{IIb}\beta_3$ integrin receptor on the membrane surface of human and rodent tumor cell lines (2,3,4) (Figure 1). Recently, the authentic mRNAs of α_{IIb} and β_3 subunits were identified in mouse B16a cells (5). The platelet $\alpha_{IIb}\beta_3$ complex has a well established role as an adhesion receptor in cell-cell, and cell-matrix interactions, interacting with several adhesion proteins (i.e., fibronectin, fibrinogen, von Willebrand factor, vitronectin, etc.) (6,7). Because tumor cells metastasis is a series of events requiring tumor cell-host cell interactions, it seems reasonable that the tumor cell $\alpha_{IIb}\beta_3$ glycoprotein may serve as a receptor for tumor cell-platelet interactions (3), and mediate, in part, tumor cell adhesion to endothelial cells (8), and subendothelial matrix (4,8). Moreover, the level of mRNAs and surface expression of the $\alpha_{IIb}\beta_3$ from subpopulations of B16 amelanotic melanoma tumors correlates positively with their ability to induce aggregation of homologous platelets (r=0.90), adhere to fibronectin (r=0.97), and form lung colonies (r=0.90) in experimental metastasis assays (9).

Considerable evidence in the literature has suggested that eicosanoids (i.e., lipoxygenase and cyclooxygenase metabolites of arachidonic acid) modulate homotypic adhesion of tumor cells, as well as heterotypic adhesion of tumor cells, such as to normal cells and to various inert and biological substrata (1,10-12). We recently reported that tumor cell expression of $\alpha_{IIb}\beta_3$ and tumor cell adhesion to fibronectin and endothelial cell monolayers increased following tumor cell pretreatment with the lipoxygenase metabolite of arachidonic acid 12-hydroxyeicosatetraenoic acid (12-HETE) (4) are important during the arrest and adhesion phases of hematogenous metastasis (8). This effect was demonstrated to be specific for the 12(S)- enantiomer, as the 12(R)- enantiomer, and other monohydroxy fatty acids had no effect (Figure 2). Pretreatment of the tumor cells with the phorbol ester, TPA mimicked these results (2,9). Phorbol esters are known to enhance arachidonic acid metabolism by a number of tumor cell lines (13), and the effect of TPA may be mediated via tumor cell metabolism of arachidonic acid to the lipoxygenase metabolite 12(S)-HETE, as 12(S)-HETE is the major lipoxygenase product produced by several tumor cell lines (14-16). Further, tumor cells stimulated with TPA in the presence of lipoxygenase inhibitors (i.e., BW755c, NDGA) demonstrate an inhibition in surface

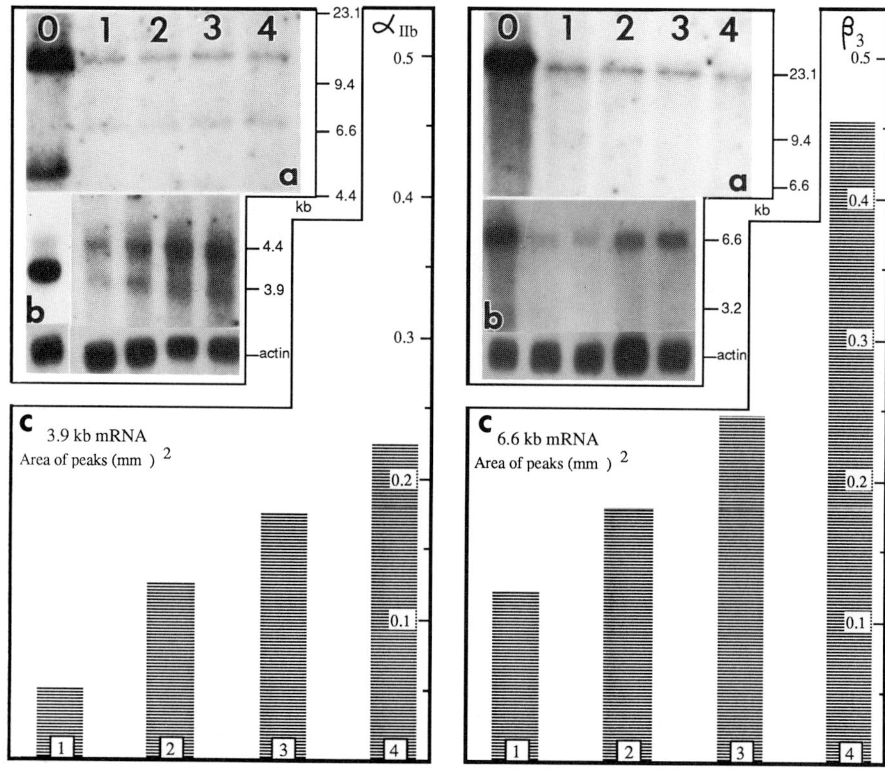

Figure 1. Northern blot analysis of mRNA from the cells of four B16a elutriated fractions. Five μg of mRNA from the B16a cells and HEL cells (possitive control) was denatured in 2.2 M formaldehyde and 50% formamide and separated in 1% formaldehyde agarose gel. The RNA's were transferred to nitrocellulose membrane, and filters were prehybridized and hybridized with α_{IIb} (a) and β3 (b) cDNA probes labeled by random primer oligo labeling system. The filters were deprobed and rehybridized with a b-actin cDNA probe for quantitation of the mRNA's. Ten μg of genomic DNA from the four B16a subpopulations and HEL cells were digested with Eco R1, separated by 0.8% agarose gel electrophoresis, and transferred to nitrocellulose membranes for Southern blot analysis of genomic DNA. The filters were prehybridized and hybridized with α_{IIb} (c) and β3 (d) cDNA probes. Hind III cut lambda DNA's were used as DNA size markers. The sizes of $\alpha_{IIb}$and β3 mRNA's and DNA size markers are in kilobases.

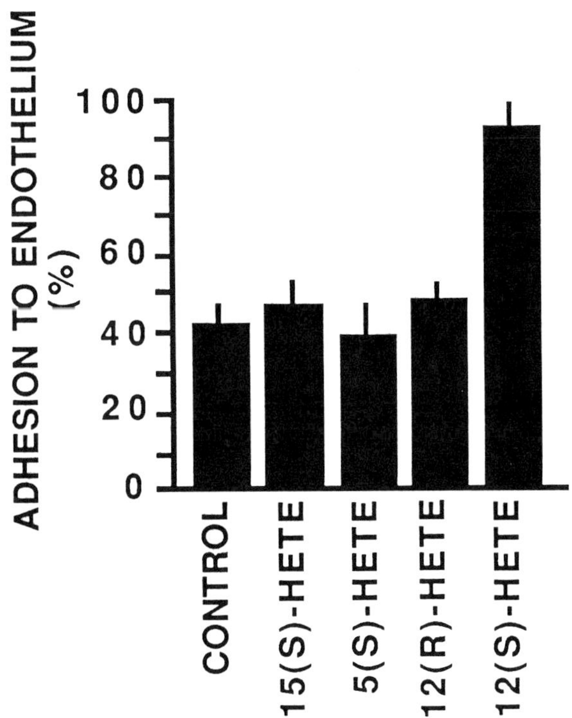

Figure 2. Adhesion of rat Walker 256 tumor cells to rat aortic endothelial cells. Only tumor cells treated with 12(S)-HETE (0.1μM) demonstrate increased adhesion to endothelial cell monolayers. 5(S)-, 15(S)-, and 12(R)-HETE had no significant effect on tumor cell adhesion (n=4; X±SD).

expression of $\alpha_{IIb}\beta_3$, and inhibition in the TPA-stimulated ability of tumor cells to adhere to relevant substrata. However, TPA stimulation of tumor cells in the presence of cyclooxygenase inhibitors (i.e., indomethacin, ASA) revealed no inhibition of receptor expression and no inhibition of TPA-stimulated tumor cell adhesion (Figure 3).

In addition to lipoxygenase metabolites of arachidonic acid, a lipoxygenase metabolite of linoleic acid is also implicated as a mediator in normal cell adhesion. A lipoxygenase metabolite produced by endothelium was reported by Buchanan and collegues (17) to decrease platelet adhesion to endothelial cell monolayers. This metabolite was later identified as 13-HODE (18). We have demonstrated previously that 13-HODE antagonizes the increased expression of $\alpha_{IIb}\beta_3$ expression of tumor cells induced by either 12-HETE or TPA, as well as 12-HETE or TPA stimulated tumor cell adhesion (8). 13-HODE is hypothesized to influence the thromboresistance of vascular endothelium (18), possibly by

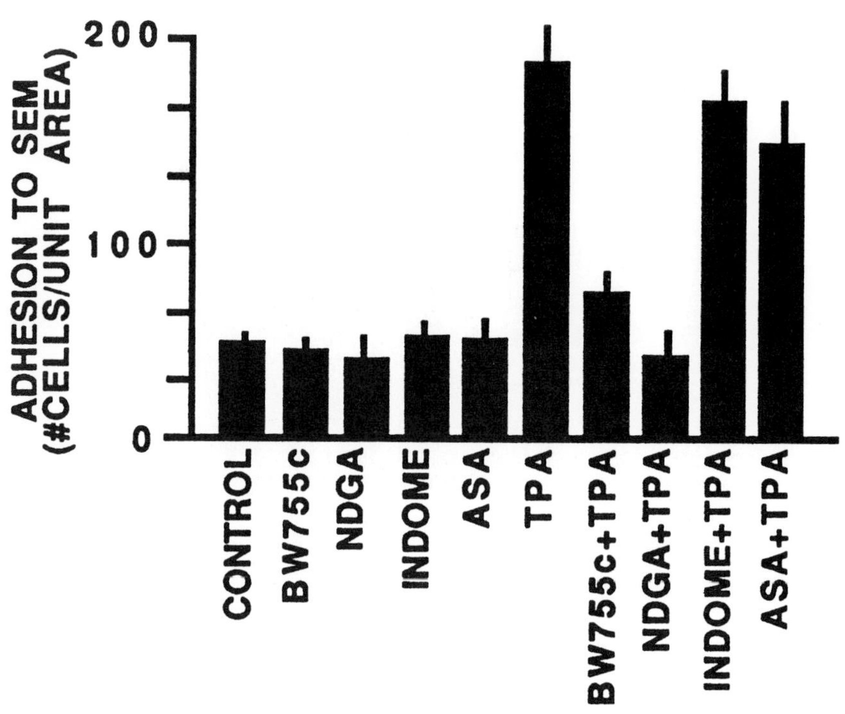

Figure 3. Adhesion of rat Walker 256 tumor cells to rat aortic endothelium subendothelial matrix (SEM). Lipoxygenase inhibitors (BW755c and NDGA) inhibit TPA stimulated tumor cell adhesion whereas cyclooxygenase inhibibors (indomethacin and ASA) have no effect TPA stimulated tumor cell adhesion. None of the inhibitors demonstrate a significant effect on basal tumor cell adhesion (n=4; X±SD).

increasing endothelial cell synthesis of prostacyclin (PGI_2), a potent antiplatelet agent (19). Numerous investigators have reported that exogenous PGI_2, an endothelial cyclooxygenase metabolite, and PGI_2 analogs inhibit lung colony formation by various tumor lines (11,20,21). Further, PGI_2 has also been demonstrated to inhibit stimulated [i.e., TPA, 12(S)-HETE] tumor cell expression of $\alpha_{IIb}\beta_3$, and tumor cell adhesion to endothelial cells, subendothelial matrix, and fibronectin (Figure 4). Prostacyclin also inhibits tumor cell-platelet interactions (22,23), and homotypic tumor cell interactions (24).

Tumor cell adhesion to endothelial cell monolayers is followed by endothelial cell retraction and tumor cell migration to the subendothelial matrix (25,26). We have previously demonstrated that tumor cell adhesion to endothelial cells and subendothelial matrix is enhanced in the presence of homologous platelets (22,27). In vivo, platelets are the predominant host cells associated with arrested tumor cells (28,29). Maximum platelet activation by the arrested tumor cell is demonstrated at a time coincident with

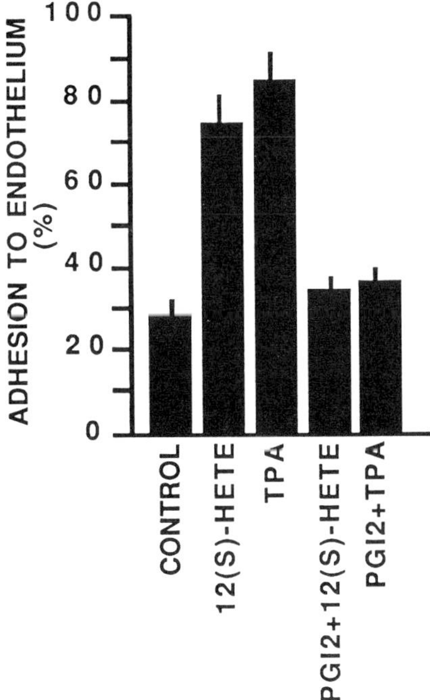

Figure 4. Inhibition of 12(S)-HETE and TPA enhanced adhesion of rat Walker 256 tumor cells to rat aortic endothelial cells by prostacyclin (PGI_2) (n=4; X±SD).

the induction of endothelial cell retraction (29). These observations suggest that the platelet or a platelet-derived agent (or agents) may enhance endothelial cell retraction during tumor cell-platelet-endothelial cell interactions. Several lines of evidence suggest that 12(S)-HETE may be a key mediator in tumor cell- or platelet enhanced tumor cell-induced endothelial cell retraction. Firstly, 12(S)-HETE has been demonstrated to be the principle lipoxygenase metabolite product of arachidonic acid in B16 amelanotic melanoma and Lewis lung carcinoma tumor lines (14-16). Secondly, exogenous 12(S)-HETE has been demonstrated to increase theexpression of tumor cell $\alpha_{IIb}\beta_3$ (8), increase the expression of the vitronectin receptor ($\alpha_v\beta_3$) on endothelial cells [a receptor which has been demonstrated by Buchanan and collegues (30) to play a role in integrin mediated tumor cell adhesion to endothelium], increase tumor cell adhesion to relevant substrata (4,8), and increase lung colonization by pretreated tumor cells (Figure 5). Thirdly, studies revealed that exogenous 12(S)-HETE induces tumor cell shape change after a reorganization of cytoskeletal microfilaments and intermediate filaments (31) (this cytoskeletal reorganization may play an important role in cell surface expression of integrins). Finally,

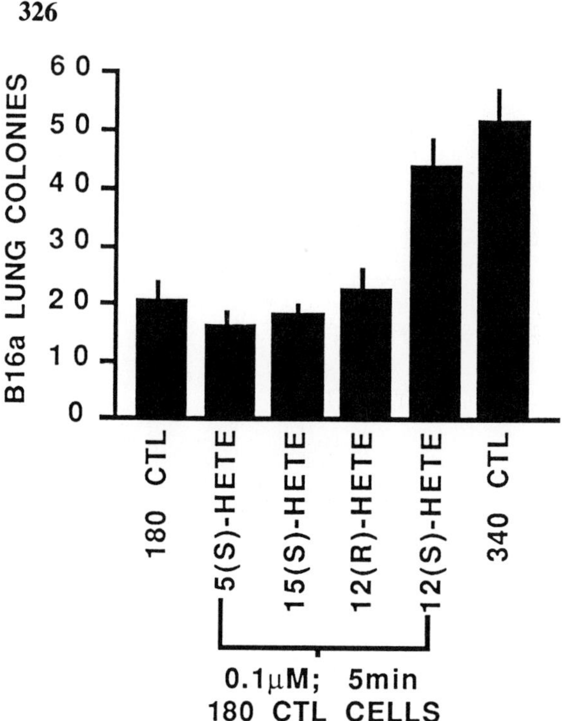

Figure 5. Enhancement of pulmonary tumor colony formation of low-metastatic subpopulations of B16 amelanotic melanoma cells (180F) to that of the high-metastatic subpopulation (340F) by treatment with 12(S)-HETE prior to tail vein injection. 5(S)-, 15(S)-, and the biologically inactive enantiomer, 12(R)-HETE had no effect on pulmonary tumor colony formation (n=12; X±SD).

12(S)-HETE may transfer from cell of original synthesis to adjacent cells [i.e, platelet to endothelial cell (32)]. 12(S)-hydroxyeicosatetraenoic acid may also act directly on endothelial cells. Exogenous 12(S)-HETE, but not 12(R)-HETE (or other monohydroxy fatty acids) has been demonstrated to induce endothelial cell retraction (Figure 6) and exposure of the subendothelial matrix, which results in increased tumor cell adhesion. In addition, the action of 12(S)-HETE on endothelial cell monolayers is nondestructive and reversible, which supports the observation that invasive tumor cells penetrate and spread under endothelial cells which later reform as confluent monolayers (26). We have recently reported that endothelial cell monolayers treated with 12(S)-HETE demonstrate a loss of cell-cell junctions and cobblestoned morphology, as well as cytoskeletal rearrangements producing contractions of filopodia into blebs, and retraction/detachment of the endothelial cells' peripheral surfaces from the subendothelial matrix (33). This retraction of endothelial cells from subendothelial matrix provides pockets into which tumor cells could invade.

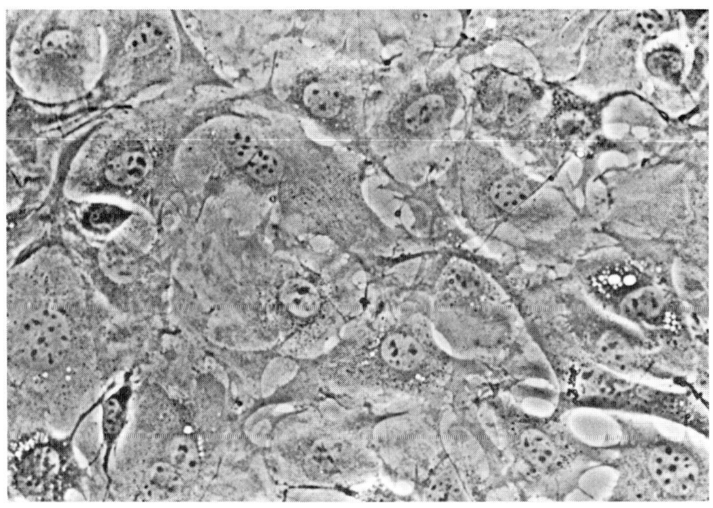

a

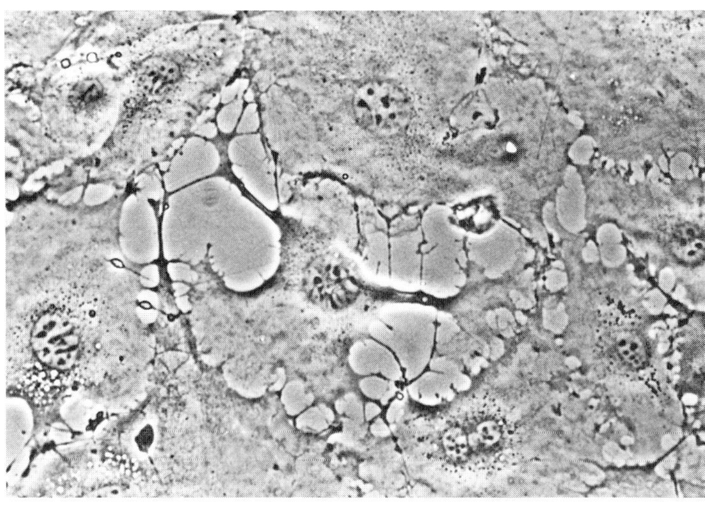

b

Figure 6. Endothelial cell retraction induced by 12(S)-HETE. Normal murine pulmonary vein microvessel endothelial cells (A) upon stimulation by 12(S)-HETE undergo a nondistructive retraction which is seen as maximal at 60 min post treatment (B; arrows).

We originally proposed (8,12) that tumor cell-platelet-endothelial cell/subendothelial matrix interactions were mediated in part by arachidonic acid metabolites synthesized by these respective cell types. We now postulate that the lipoxygenase metabolite 12(S)-HETE plays a specific and unique role in tumor cell metastasis. Platelet arachidonic acid metabolism to the cyclooxygenase metabolite thromboxane A2 and the lipoxygenase metabolite 12(S)-HETE results upon tumor cell induced platelet activation (34). 12(S)-hydroxyeicosatetraenoic acid has been demonstrated to transfer between cell types during their interaction (32). We postulate that transfer of platelet 12(S)-HETE to tumor cells and endothelial cells during the interaction of these cell types leads to the summation of three separate events which may enhance tumor cell adhesion to endothelial cells and ultimately to the subendothelial matrix. The first event is the increased expression of the tumor cell $\alpha_{IIb}\beta_3$ receptor which may facilitate tumor cell adhesion to endothelial cells. The second event is the increase in $\alpha_v\beta_3$ expression on endothelial cell surfaces which may serve for integrin mediated tumor cell binding to endothelial cells, and the third event is the induction of endothelial cell retraction leading to the exposure of underlying subendothelial matrix to which tumor cells preferentially adhere. Consequently, we propose that the balance of various eicosanoids produced by platelets, tumor cells, and endothelial cells, during the interaction of these cell types may be key determinants in the formation, or prevention of a successful metastatic lesion.

ACKNOWLEDGEMENT

This work was supported by NIH grants CA 29997-08 and CA 47115-03.

REFERENCES

1. Weiss L, Orr FW, Honn KV. (1989) Clin Exptl Metastasis 7-127-167.
2. Grossi IM, Hatfield JS, Fitzgerald LA, Newcombe M, Taylor JD, and Honn KV. (1988) FASEB J 2: 2382-2395.
3. Chopra H, Fitzgerald LA, Chang YS, Grossi IM, Taylor JD, and Honn KV. (1988) Cancer Res 48: 3787-3800.
4. Honn KV, Grossi IM, Steinert BW, Chopra H, Onoda JM, Nelson KK, and Taylor JD. (1988) In: P Wong, B Samuelsson, and F Sun (eds), Advances in Prostaglandin, Thromboxane, and Leukotriene Research, Vol 18 pp 439-443, New York, Raven Press.
5. Chopra HJ, Timar J, Rong X, Fitzgerald LA, Taylor JD, and Honn KV. The Lipoxygenase Metabolite 12(S)-HETE Induces Cytoskeleton-Dependent Increase in Integrin $\alpha IIb\beta 3$ Surface Expression on Melanoma Cells (submitted).
6. Charo IF, Bekeart LS, and Phillips DR. (1987) J Biol Chem 262: 9935-9938.
7. Ruoslahti E, and Pierschbacher MD. (1987) SCIENCE 238: 491-497.
8. Grossi IM, Fitzgerald LA, Umbarger LA, Nelson KK, Diglio CA, Taylor JD, and Honn KV. (1989) Cancer Res 49: 1029-1037.
9. Honn KV, Grossi IM, Nelson KK, Umbarger LA, Fitzgerald LA, Hatfield JS, Fligiel SEG, Steinert BW, Diglio CA, Taylor JD, and Onoda JM. (Submitted) Cancer Res.
10. Varani J. (1982) Cancer Metastasis Rev 1: 17-28.
11. Honn KV, Bockman RS, and Marnett LJ. (1981) Prostaglandins 21: 833-864.
12. Honn Kv, Busse WD, and Sloane BF. (1983) Biochem Pharmacol 32: 1-11.
13. Batchev AC, Reser BL, Hellner EG, Fligiel SEG, and Varani J. (1986) Clin Exptl Metastasis 4: 51-61.

14. Honn KV, and Dunn JR. (1982) FEBS Letters 139: 65-68.
15. Dunn JR, Ohannesian DW, Malik D, Kendall A, Taylor JD, Sloane BF, and Honn KV. (1987) In: ES Garaci, R Paoletti, and MG Santoro (eds), Prostaglandins in Cancer Research, pp 257-260, Berlin: Springer-Verlag.
16. Marnett LJ, Leithauser, MT, Richards, KM, Blair I, Honn KV, Yamamoto S, and Yoshimoto, T. (1991) In: Advances in Prostaglandin Thromboxane and Leukotriene Research, Vol. 19 (B. Samuelsson, R. Paoletti, and P. Ramwell, eds). Raven Press, New York, Vol. 21B, 895-900.
17. Buchanan MR, Butt RW, Magas Z, Van Ryn J, Hirsh J, and Nazir PJ. (1985) Thromb Haemost 53: 306-311.
18. Buchanan MR, Hass TA, Lagarde M, and Guichardant M. (1985) J Biol Chem 260: 16056-16059.
19. Setty BNY, Berger M, and Stuart MJ. (1987) Biochem Biophys Res Commun 146: 502-509.
20. Niitsu Y, Ishigaki S, Kogawa K, Mogi Y, Watanabe N, Kohgo Y, and Urushizaki, I. (1988) Invasion Metastasis 8: 57-72.
21. Mahalingam M, Ugen KE, Kao K-J, and Klein PA. (1988) Cancer Res 88: 1460-1464.
22. Menter DG, Onoda JM, Moilanen D, Sloane BF, Taylor JD, and Honn KV. (1987) J. Natl. Cancer Inst. 78: 961-989.
23. Menter DG, Harkins C, Onoda JM, Riorden W, Sloane BF, Taylor JD, and Honn KV. (1987) Invasion Metastasis 7: 109-128.
24. Honn KV, Menter DG, Onoda JM, Taylor KD, and Sloane BF. (1984) In: GL Nicloson , L Milas (eds), Cancer Invasion and Metastasis: Biologic and Therapeutic Aspects, pp 361-388, New York, Raven Press.
25. Kramer AH, Gonzalez R, and Nicolson GL. (1980) Int J Cancer 26: 639-645.
26. Kramer AH, and Nicolson GL. (1979) Proc Natl Acad Sci USA 76: 5704-5708.
27. Honn KV, Onoda JM, Pampaloma K, Battaglia M, Neagos G, Taylor JD, Diglio CA, and Sloane BF. (1985) Biochem Pharmacol 34: 235-241.
28. Crissman JD, Hatfield JS, Schaldenbrand J, Sloane BF, and Honn KV. (1985) Lab Invest 53: 470-478.
29. Crissman JD, Hatfield JS, Menter DG, Sloane BF, and Honn KV. (1988) Cancer Res 48: 4065-4072.
30. Buchanan MR, Vazquez MJ and Gimbrone MA, Jr. Blood, 62:889-895, 1983.
31. Chopra H, Marzouq L, Taylor JD, and Honn KV. (1989) Proc Amer Assoc Cancer Res Vol 30: 88A.
32. Schafer AI, Takayama H, Farrell S, and Gimbrone MA. (1986) Blood 67: 373-378.
33. Honn KV, Grossi IM, Diglio CA, Wojtukiewicz M, and Taylor JD. (1989) FASEB J 3:2285-2293.
34. Honn KV, Steinert BW, Moin K, Onoda JM, Taylor JD, and Sloane BF. (1987) Biochem Biophys Res Commun 145: 384-389.

THE LIPOXYGENASE METABOLITE OF ARACHIDONIC ACID, 12-(S)-HETE, INDUCES CYTOSKELETON DEPENDENT UPREGULATION OF INTEGRIN $\alpha_{IIb}\beta_3$ IN MELANOMA CELLS

J. TIMAR[1], H. CHOPRA[1], I.M. GROSSI[1], J.D. TAYLOR[2] and K.V. HONN[1]

[1]Departments of Radiation Oncology, [2]Biological Sciences, Wayne State University, Detroit, MI 48202; Gershenson Radiation Oncology Center, Detroit, MI 48201

INTRODUCTION

Cell-extracellular matrix interactions are essential prerequisites of normal cell function mediated by specific receptors including integrins (1). This family of transmembrane proteins are characterized by α and β heterodimers linked with S-S bonds. There are a limited number of β subunits and a large number of a units which can combine to form at least 16 unique heterodimers (1).

Tumor cell extracellular matrix interactions are critical steps in tumor progression (2) and a target for experimental chemotherapy for control tumor dissemination. Initially attention was directed to tumor cell - basement membrane interaction and the integrins involved in these interactions (2,3). Tumor cells with higher invasive capacity frequently adhere to, spread and migrate on certain components of basement membrane with greater efficiency. The principal receptors involved in such interactions are β_1 integrin complexes with affinities to fibronectin, laminin or collagen type IV (3). However the involvement of the $\alpha_v\beta_3$ complex in the melanoma - extracellular matrix interaction has been described (4).

In platelets the major matrix and cell-adhesion molecule is the integrin $\alpha_{IIb}\beta_3$ which recognizes a wide variety of matrix molecules as well as mediating fibrinogen-dependent platelet aggregation (6). Recently we observed that malignant cells express epitopes of the $\alpha_{IIb}\beta_3$ integrin which are involved in matrix recognition (7,8) as well as mediating adhesion of platelets to the tumor cell surface (7,13). However it was not clear whether these tumor cells express authentic $\alpha_{IIb}\beta_3$ or only related epitopes. Therefore in the present work we compared the protein from B16a cells carrying $\alpha_{IIb}\beta_3$ epitopes to authentic $\alpha_{IIb}\beta_3$ isolated from platelets.

The mechanism for regulation of integrin expression is unknown. TGFβ increases expression of several integrins and is thought to be a physiological mediator (9). The tumor promoter PMA, among other effects, also serves as an activator of integrin expression in several normal and malignant cells (8,10). We observed that PMA-effect is mediated through LOX metabolites of arachidonic acid (8). and in fact we demonstrated that expression of integrin $\alpha_{IIb}\beta_3$ in 3LL tumor cells is under the control of LOX metabolites (8).

In the present paper we examined the effect of exogenous 12-(S)-HETE on the expression and function of integrin $\alpha_{IIb}\beta_3$ in B16a melanoma cells.

MATERIALS AND METHODS

Tumor cell culture.

The B16a tumor cell line and culturing conditions were as previously described (11).

Washed mouse and human platelets.

Washed mouse and human platelets used as positive controls for $\alpha_{IIb}\beta_3$ in immunoblotting studies were isolated and prepared as previously described (12).

Cytoskeletal inhibitors .

The three inhibitors used in this study were colchicine (CL) (Sigma, St. Louis,MO), a microtubule inhibitor (15 min at 50 μM), cytochalasin D (CD) (Sigma) a microfilament inhibitor (15 min at 50 μM) and cycloheximide (CX) (Sigma), an intermediate filament inhibitor (8 hrs at 50 μM). They were solubilized in distilled water, DMSO or ethanol respectively and used as previously described (13). Effects were monitored by immunocytochemistry of cytoskeletal elements.

Eicosanoid treatment.

The following monohydroxylated fatty acids; 12(S)-HETE, 12(R)-HETE, 5(S)-HETE, and 15(S)-HETE (Cayman Chemical Company Inc, Ann Arbor, MI) were dissolved initially in absolute ethanol, diluted with the appropriate buffer and used at a concentration of 0.1 μM . Cells in suspension or after 48 h culturing on glass were treated in serum-free medium for 5 min at 37°C.

Antibodies

Cytoskeletal Proteins. Rabbit antisera to tubulin, goat IgG-fluorescein isothiocyanate (FITC) or -rhodamine ; goat antibody to vimentin, rabbit IgG-FITC or -rhodamine were obtained from ICN Immunobiologicals, (Lisle, IL). Rhodamine labeled phalloidin (Molecular Probes, Eugene, OR) was used to label polymerized actin .

Platelet $\alpha_{IIb}\beta_3$. Monoclonal antibody 10E5 -IgG1a(14) raised in mouse against human platelet $\alpha_{IIb}\beta_3$, a generous gift from Dr. B.S. Coller (Stony Brook, NY) (affinity purified from ascites; stock solution 1 mg/ml), was used to probe B16a cells for the presence of $\alpha_{IIb}\beta_3$ at a concentration of 20 μg/ml. The specificity of this antiserum for human platelet $\alpha_{IIb}\beta_3$ was reported previously (14). Goat whole serum (34-37 mg/ml total protein; Cooper Biomedical, Malvern, PA) or mouse IgG (40 μg/ml, Jackson Immunoreserach Labs, West Grove, PA) was used as a blocking sera for Fc receptors in immunofluorescent studies. Mouse monoclonal IgG_{1a} MOPC21 (Sigma, St.Louis, MO) with no affinity to integrins was used as a control monoclonal antibody for non-specific inhibition of adhesion.

Rabbit antibody to $\alpha_{IIb}\beta_3$ was prepared as reported previously (8). Monoclonal antibody against platelet Gplb was obtained from Dakopacts (Glostrup, Denmark) and used as an additional control for non-specific inhibition in adhesion studies. Mouse monoclonal antibody Ab-1 against the α_5 component of the fibronectin receptor was obtained from Oncogene Science Inc., Manhasset, NY. and used to asses the role of $\alpha_5\beta_1$ in B16a cell adhesion to fibronectin.

Immunoblotting of $\alpha_{IIb}\beta_3$.

Mouse platelets (1X10^9), human platelets (1 X 10^9) or B16a cells (2 X 10^7) were lysed in buffer containing Ca++ and Mg++ free PBS, 0.5% NP-40, 1 mM EDTA 2mM PMSF (30min, at 4°C). Samples were then centrifuged (11,000 x g), supernatants were separated on 8% non- denaturing acrylamide gels and were transferred electrophoretically to nitrocellulose paper (Schleicher and Schuell Inc. Munich, Germany) utilizing a Bio-Rad Mini-Transfer cassette. Non-denaturing gels were used to separate the native protein-complex for immunoblot analysis, since mAb 10E5 will only recognize the intact $\alpha_{IIb}\beta_3$ complex and not the individual monomeric glycoproteins (14). After transfer, the nitrocellulose paper was placed in quench solution containing 1.15% casein in PBS and azide for a minimum of 2h at 4°C. After quenching, the nitrocellulose paper was incubated with mAb10E5 (1:200) for 1h at 24°C, washed with the quench solution, and then incubated with quench solution containing approximately 2µCi of ^{125}I labelled secondary antibody for 1-1 1/2 h at 24°C. The nitrocellulose paper was then washed with the quench solution containing 0.1% Tween 20, blotted between 2 sheets of Whatman 3 MM paper, dried and exposed to X-Ray film for 1-10 days at -70°C. Murine IgG was used as a non immune serum control.

Immunofluorescence

Localization of Cytoskeletal Components. B16a cells grown on coverslips were fixed, permeabilized and labeled with the appropriate antibodies as previously described (13). In negative controls, the primary antibodies were replaced with PBS. No background staining was observed .

Localization of F actin. B16a cells were fixed with 3.7% formaldehyde/PBS (10min), washed in PBS (3x), permeabilized with acetone (-20°C;10min), incubated with rhodamine labeled phalloidin (1:200) washed with PBS and mounted in glycerol on glass slides.

Localization of Membrane Glycoprotein $\alpha_{IIb}\beta_3$. B16a cells grown on coverslips were fixed and labeled with mAb 10E5 and anti-mouse IgG-FITC as previously described (6,14). In negative controls, the primary antibody was omitted or replaced by mouse IgG. No background staining was observed .

Localization of Intracellular $\alpha_{IIb}\beta_3$. B16a cells were grown on coverslips as described above, washed (3X) with PBS (pH 7.2) to remove serum proteins, fixed in 1% paraformaldehyde/PBS for 10 min, permeabilized with 50% ethanol (4°C for 30 min.). These cells were then processed for immunofluorescent microscopy as described (13). In negative controls the primary antibody was omitted or replaced with mouse IgG.

Double Immunofluorescent Labeling to Localize Intracellular $\alpha_{IIb}\beta_3$, Actin, Tubulin and Vimentin. Cells grown on coverslips as described above, were fixed with 2% paraformaldehyde and washed extensively for 1h using six, 10min changes of PBS with Ca++ and Mg++. For intracellular localization of $\alpha_{IIb}\beta_3$, cells were permeabilized as for cytoskeleton labelings, washed (2X) with PBS containing Ca^{++} and Mg^{+} and processed for mAb10E5 labeling (using goat anti-mouse FITC conjugate) as described (13). Following localization of $\alpha_{IIb}\beta_3$, cells were processed further to localize actin, vimentin, or tubulin as described above but instead of FITC-secondary antibody conjugates, Rhodamine-conjugated antibodies were used. In negative controls the primary antibodies (or the Rhodamine labeled phalloidin) were replaced with PBS. No significant background fluorescence was observed.

Whole-mount and transmission electron microscopic immunocytochemistry.

B16a cells were seeded on carbon coated Formvar-gold grids for 4 h in serum containing medium and were fixed in 1% paraformaldehyde/0.1% glutaraldehyde/HBSS for 10 min at room temperature. After washing in HBSS (3x10 min) the FC receptors were blocked by incubating the cells in normal goat serum diluted 1:10. Surface $\alpha_{IIb}\beta_3$was detected by incubating the grids in mAb10E5 (5 μg/ml in HBSS) for 1 h, washed (3x10 min in HBSS) and reincubated in goat anti-mouse IgG-G15 conjugate diluted 1:10 in HBSS (Amersham) for 1 h. After washing in buffer the cells were refixed in 2% glutaraldehyde/HBSS for 1 h, dehydrated in ethanol and critical point dried using Freon TC113. Samples were analyzed in Philips 301 transmission electron microscope at an accelerating voltage of 80 kV.

Adhesion.

Tumor cell adhesion to fibronectin-coated 24 well plates (Falcon, Becton Dickinson Labs., Lincoln Park, NJ) were studied as described (8). Cells, treated with antibodies (40 μg/ml,15 min at 25°C) or cytoskeleton inhibitors, were stimulated with 12(S)-HETE (5 min at 37°C) before adhesion. Each experimental condition was measured in four wells and each experiment was repeated a minimum of 3 times.

Flow Cytometric Analysis.

Flow cytometric studies were performed to quantitate the surface expression of $\alpha_{IIb}\beta_3$ as previously described (8). The fluorescent signal for each measurement was converted from log based to linear data as previously described and expressed as relative fluorescent intensity (8).

Statistics.

Adhesion data were analyzed by the ANOVA test and the Scheffe's test using the STATA VIEW 512 + software (Brain Power, Inc., Calabasas, CA), on a Macintosh Plus computer (Apple Computer, Cupertino, CA). Differences were considered significant when $p < 0.05$. Linear regression analysis was performed by Cricket Graph software (Cricket Software Inc., Malvean,PA).

RESULTS

Mab 10E5 immunoprecipitated mouse and human platelet $\alpha_{IIb}\beta_3$ which appeared as a 265 kD band running on a non-reducing gel (Figures1a, b). An identical molecular mass band was immunoprecipitated from cellular proteins of B16a cells (Figure1c). Murine IgG did not reveal proteins in human or mouse platelets (data not shown).

Integrin receptor $\alpha_{IIb}\beta_3$ was localized diffusely at the apical plasma membrane of adherent B16a cells by immunofluorescence using mAb10E5 (Figure 2a). Five min treatment of B16a cells with 0.1 μM 12-(S)-HETE at 37°C resulted in an increased fluorescence of the plasma membrane and appearance of focal receptor aggregates mostly at the cell margins (Figure 2b). Whole mount electron microscopy and immunostaining with mAb10E5 showed rare $\alpha_{IIb}\beta_3$ epitopes at the plasma membrane, sometimes on or at cell processes (Figure 2c - arrows). 12-(S)-HETE treatment (0.1 μM, 15 min,37°C) resulted in a dramatic increase in surface labeling as indicated by colloidal gold labeling (Figure 2d - arrows). The receptor

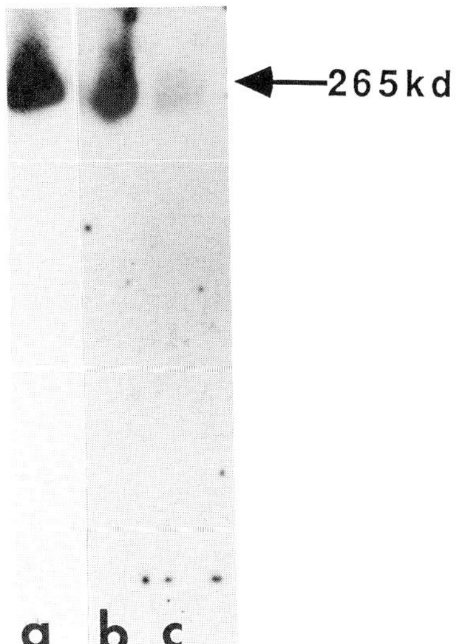

Figure 1a, b, c. Immunoprecipitation of $\alpha IIb\beta 3$ Receptor in B16a Cells

aggregated at the surface and concentrated at the cell margins as well as on filopodia - similar to the findings using immunofluorescence.

Integrins, involved in matrix adhesion are present in adhesion structures, which contain the matrix ligand, the receptor as well as cytoskeletal components. In permeabilized cells, integrin $\alpha_{IIb}\beta_3$ could be rarely detected in the adhesion plaques in unstimulated cells kept on fibronectin (Figure 2e.- arrow). However, after 5 min 12-(S)-HETE stimulation, $\alpha_{IIb}\beta_3$ was present in cell-body- as well as peripheral adhesion structures at high frequency (Figure 2f - arrow). Using stronger permeabilization, an intracellular $\alpha_{IIb}\beta_3$ pool was visualized in the perinuclear zone of unstimulated cells (Figure 2g - arrow). Upon 12-(S)-HETE stimulation $\alpha_{IIb}\beta_3$ carrying cytoplasmic vesicles dispersed throughout the cytoplasm and the clear perinuclear ring disappeared (Figure 2h - arrow).

The dose dependency of 12-(S)-HETE effect on surface expression of $\alpha_{IIb}\beta_3$ in B16a cells was measured using flow cytometry and immunofluorescence. Five min treatment of B16a cells with increasing concentrations of 12-(S)-HETE (0.001-1 µM) resulted in a dose dependent increase in the expression of $\alpha_{IIb}\beta_3$ approaching a plateau at 1 µM (Figure 3a). The effect of 12-(S)-HETE treatment (0.1 µM) on adhesion of B16a cells to fibronectin was also tested. A significant increase was observed (Figure 3b). This increased adhesion to fibronectin can be inhibited by pretreating the tumor cells with mAb10E5 (50 µg/ml, 15 min) indicating, that stimulated adhesion is due to the increased involvement of $\alpha_{IIb}\beta_3$ in fibronectin binding. Studies of integrin expression in B16a cells at the mRNA level demonstrated that the major integrin expressed is the fibronectin receptor $\alpha_5\beta_1$ (J.Q.Chen, K.V.Honn - unpublished observation). However, basal adhesion of B16a cells is inhibited by only 30% and 12-(S)-HETE-stimulated adhesion is not inhibited at all by monoclonal antibody against the $\alpha 5$ domain (data not shown). These results suggest that $\alpha 5\beta 1$ is not functionally the dominant integrin mediating B16a cell adhesion to fibronectin.

The $\alpha_{IIb}\beta_3$ integrin in platelet is connected with cytoskeletal elements (6) but the existence of such associations in the case of other cell types especially tumor cells is not known. Therefore we have performed double labeling immunocytochemistry on unstimulated B16a cells to compare localization of microfilaments and intermediate filaments with $\alpha_{IIb}\beta_3$. It is reported that B16a cells do not have well established microtubular network (11). The diffuse cytoplasmic tubulin staining (Figure 4b) does not

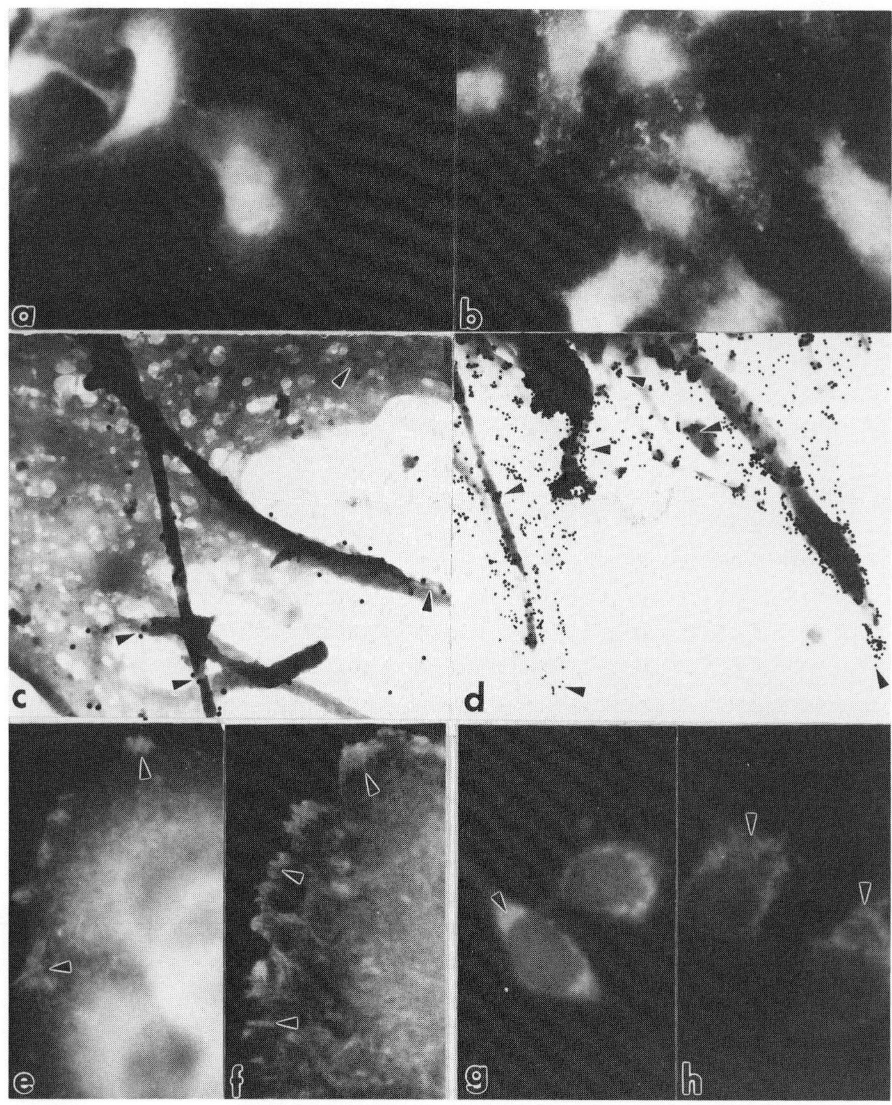

Figure 2. Immunocytochemical Localization of $\alpha_{IIb}\beta_3$ Receptor in B16a Cells

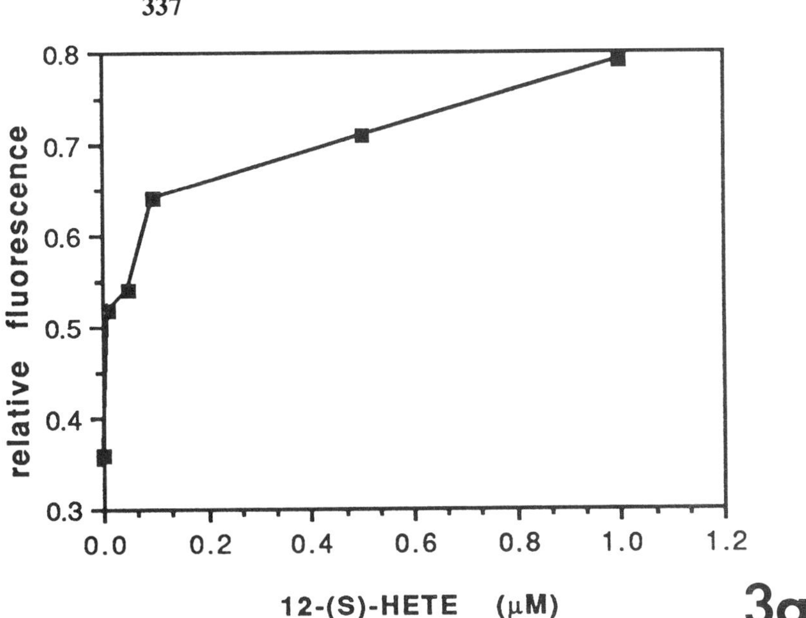

Figure 3a. Effect of 12(S)-HETE on the Surface Expression of $\alpha_{IIb}\beta_3$ in B16a Cells (Flow Cytometry)

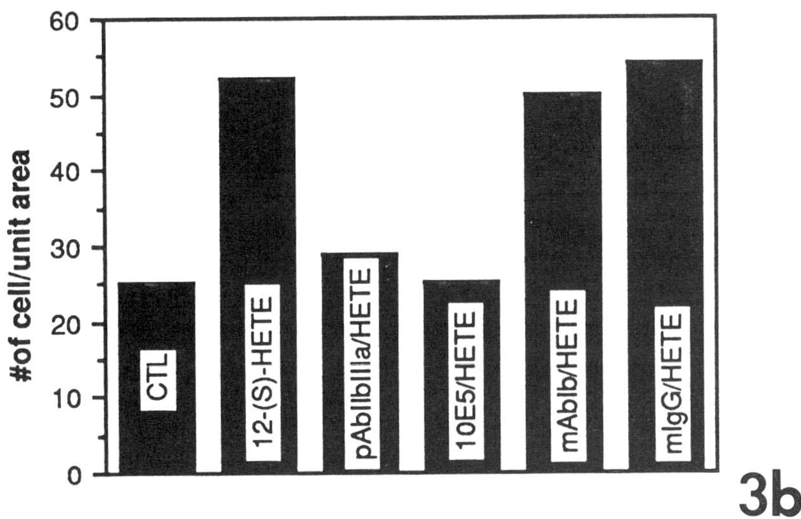

Figure 3b. Effect of 12(S)-HETE on the Adhesion of B16a Cells to Fibronectin (90 min. 37°C)

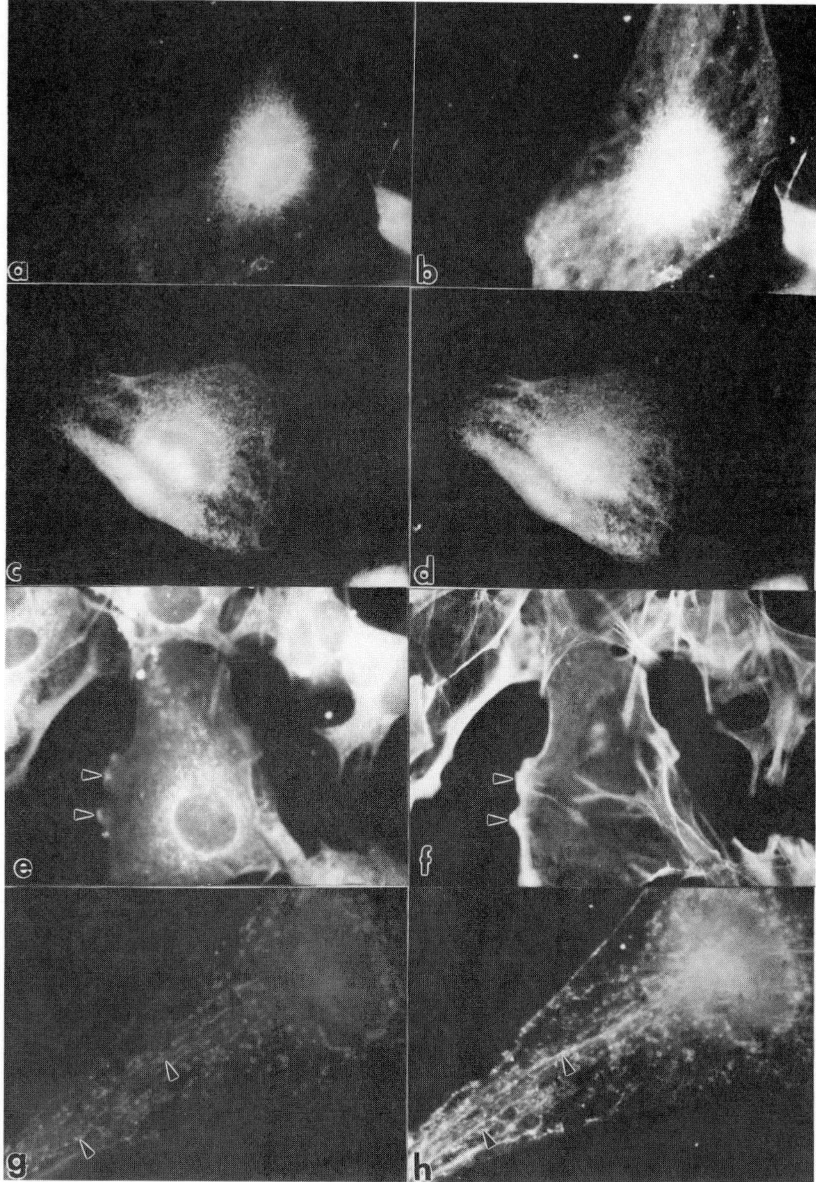

Figure 4. Localization of $\alpha_{IIb}\beta_3$ and Cytoskeletal Components in B16a Cells (Immunofluorescent Microscopy).

corresponds to intracellular $\alpha_{IIb}\beta_3$ (Figure 4a). Staining for actin using anti-actin antibody revealed a relatively diffuse cytoplasmic staining and some labeling at the plasma membrane (Figure 4d). The cytoplasmic $\alpha_{IIb}\beta_3$-containing vesicles and some $\alpha_{IIb}\beta_3$ staining at the plasma membrane (Figure 4c) colocalized with actin. Staining of F-actin in B16a cells revealed few stress fibers and some rare accumulation of F-actin at the plasma membrane probably corresponding to focal contact areas (Figure 4f - arrows). Plasma membrane $\alpha_{IIb}\beta_3$ showed clear colocalization with F-actin in these focal contacts (Figure 4e - arrows). B16a cells exhibited a fine intermediate filament network (vimentin) in the perinuclear zone and throughout the cytoplasm (Figure 4h - arrows). The cytoplasmic vimentin filaments showed clear colocalization with $\alpha_{IIb}\beta_3$ containing vesicles (Figure 4g - arrows).

12-(S)-HETE treatment of B16a cells induced alterations in F-actin staining (Figure 5a). The frequency of stress fibers increased in the cytoplasm and F-actin containing filopodia appeared. Interestingly $\alpha_{IIb}\beta_3$ frequently colocalized with F-actin at the plasma membrane in the newly formed filopodia (Figure 5b). When anti-actin antibody was used to stain cytoplasmic actin (both F- and G-actin) in stimulated cells, beside the plasma membrane colocalization of actin and $\alpha_{IIb}\beta_3$ (Figures 5c,d), colocalization was observed in the cytoplasm as well. 12-(S)-HETE stimulation induced bundling of vimentin filaments in the cytoplasm (Figure 5e) and these bundles remained in close association with $\alpha_{IIb}\beta_3$-containing cytoplasmic vesicles (Figure 5f).

To study further the role of cytoskeleton in 12-(S)-HETE induced upregulation of $\alpha_{IIb}\beta_3$ in B16a cells we have applied agents known to disrupt specifically cytoskeletal components. Tubulin staining (Figure 6a) became more diffuse after 15 min treatment of B16a cells with 50 μM colchicine (Figure 6b). The F-actin-containing microfilament network (Figure 6c) was disrupted by 15 min treatment with cytochalasin D (50 μM), resulting in fragmented, collapsed F-actin network (Figure 6d). The detailed intermediate filament network (vimentin) (Figure 6e) was disrupted by 8 hrs treatment with cyclohexamide (50 μM) when the vimentin filament became fragmented and more diffuse (Figure 6f). As cytoskeletal components are in close association with each other, we tested whether there is any effect of disruption of one component on the integrity of others. Colchicine treatment (disruption of microtubules) does not alter intermediate filament network (Figure 6g,h). Similarly, colchicine treatment had no effect on the F-actin network as well (data not shown) indicating a specific effect of colchicine. We examined the cytochalasin D effect on intermediate filaments and detected the collapse of this network besides the collapse of microfilaments (data not shown). However, cyclohexamide treatment had no effect on microfilaments or microtubules (data not shown) indicating high specificity of this treatment regiment for disruption of intermediate filaments.

Next we studied the effect of the above mentioned pretreatments on the 12-(S)-HETE-induced upregulation of $\alpha_{IIb}\beta_3$ on the surface of B16a cells. We have measured the surface expression of $\alpha_{IIb}\beta_3$ by flow cytometry after immunolabeling with mAb10E5. It was clear, that colchicine (CL) pretreatment does not affect the stimulatory effect of 12-(S)-HETE (Figure 7a), while both cytochalasin D (CD) and

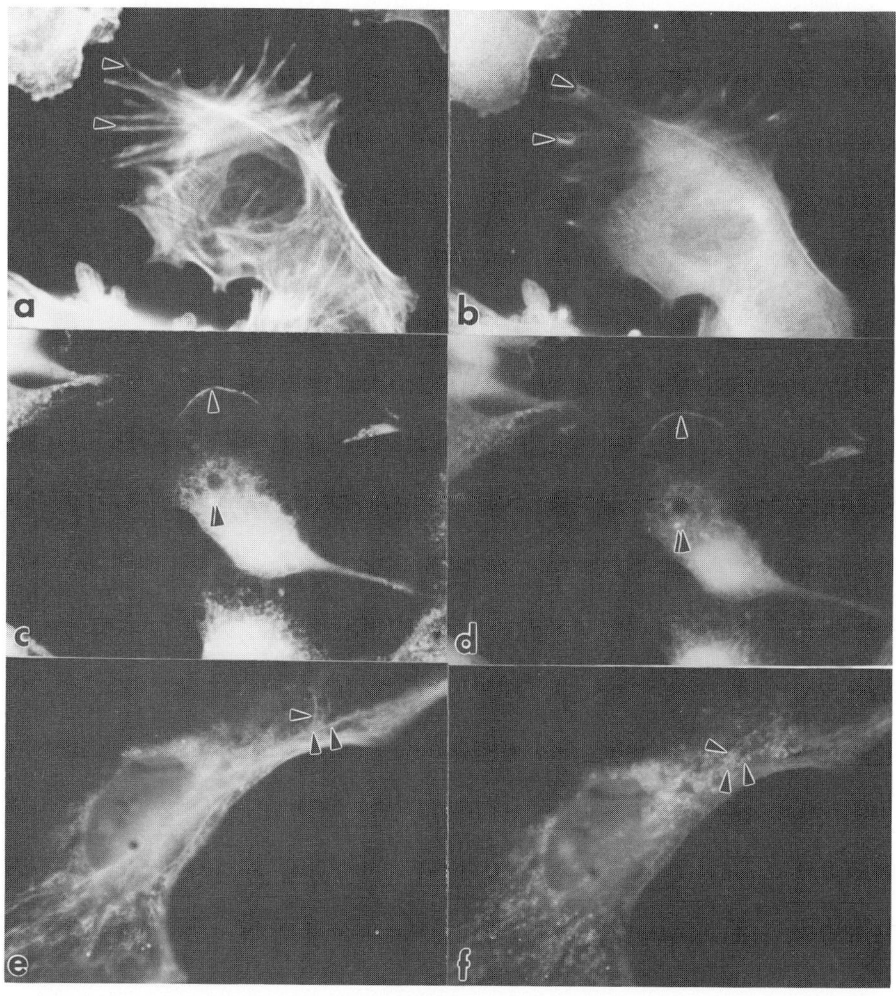

Figure 5. Effect of 12(S)-HETE Treatment on the Cytoskeleton and $\alpha_{IIb}\beta_3$ Distribution in B16a Cells (Immunofluorescent Microscopy).

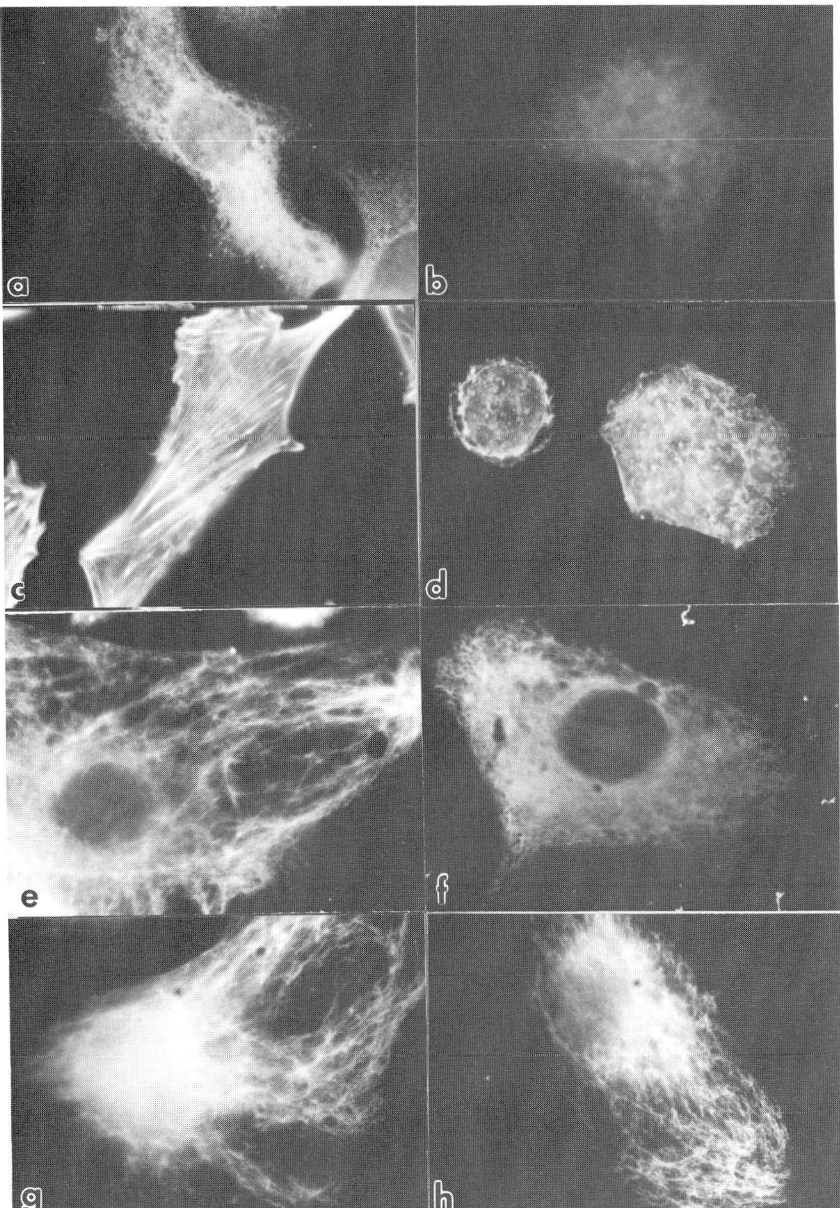

Figure 6. Effect of Cytoskeleton Disrupting Agents on B16a Cells. (Immunofluorescent Microscopy)

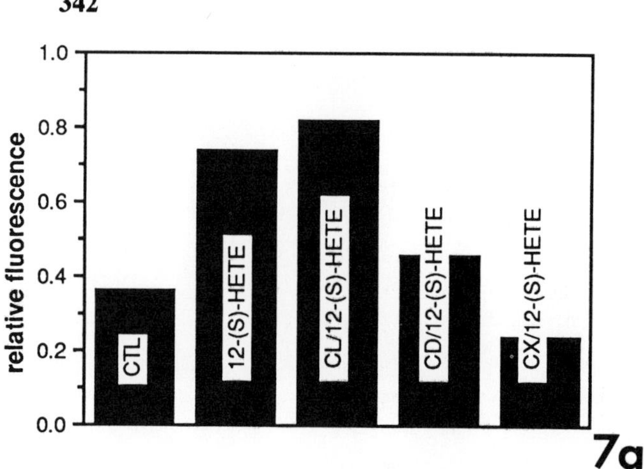

Figure 7a. Effect of Cytoskeleton Disruption on the Surface Expression of $\alpha_{IIb}\beta_3$ on B16a Cells. (Flow Cytometry)

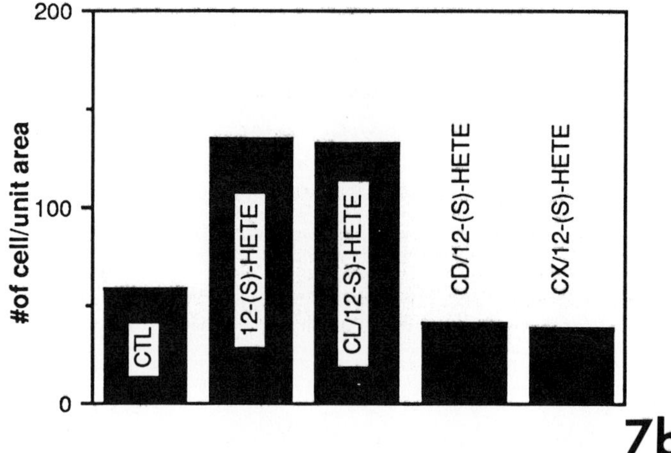

Figure 7b. Effect of Cytoskeleton Disruption on the Adhesion of B16a Cells to Fibronectin In Vitro (90 min, 37°C)

cyclohexamide (CX) pretreatments inhibited the 12-(S)-HETE-induced upregulation of $\alpha_{IIb}\beta_3$ (Figure 7a). The lower level of surface $\alpha_{IIb}\beta_3$-expression in cyclohexamide-treated cells compraed to controls may be due to inhibition of newly synthesized receptors. Finally we studied the effect of cytoskeleton disruptions on the 12-(S)-HETE induced adhesion of B16a cells to fibronectin (90 min). Similarly to the observation for $\alpha_{IIb}\beta_3$ expression, colchicine (CL) had no effect on 12-(S)-HETE-induced adhesion (Figure 7b), but both cytochalasin D (CD) and cyclohexamide (CX) pretreatments prevented the stimulatory effect of 12-(S)-HETE (Figure 7b), further supporting the importance of cytoskeleton (micro- and intermediate filaments) and $\alpha_{IIb}\beta_3$ -epitopes in stimulated adhesion to fibronectin.

DISCUSSION

The mechanism in control of integrin expression and function is relatively unknown. TGFβ (9) and tumor promoter PMA (10) were shown to increase expression and enhance function of different integrins in normal and tumor cells. Recently it was shown that some integrin-mediated functions, such as migration, can be inhibited by G-protein inhibitors suggesting that matrix-ligand initiated signal mechanisms involve G proteins. The subcellular target of PMA is PKC, a key effector element in signal transduction pathways. PMA-induced PKC activation involves both membrane receptor (15) and cytoskeletal protein (16) phosphorylations preceeded by enzyme translocation. The fact that certain PKC isozymes were detected in adhesion plaques (15), where integrins are concentrated suggest involvement of PKC activity in integrin mediated cellular functions.

Arachidonic acid can be considered as second messenger, the metabolites of which serve as components of different signaling pathways (17). It was shown, that LOX metabolites of arachidonic acid are involved in stimulated adhesion of tumor cells to different extracellular matrices (8). In 3LL cells, expression of $\alpha_{IIb}\beta_3$ integrin is under control of LOX metabolites of arachidonic acid and as a result $\alpha_{IIb}\beta_3$ mediated adhesion to fibronectin, subendothelial matrix and endothelial cells can be inhibited by LOX inhibitors (8). During these studies it became evident that 12-lipoxygenase metabolite of arachidonic acid, 12-(S)-HETE, is most probably responsible for the above described alterations in integrin $\alpha_{IIb}\beta_3$ expression and functions (8).

We show here that exogenous 12-(S)-HETE stimulates tumor cell surface expression of $\alpha_{IIb}\beta_3$ in a dose dependent manner between concentrations of 0.001-1 μM. Upon stimulation, we observed a diffuse appearance of $\alpha_{IIb}\beta_3$ epitopes on the apical membrane, as well as concentration of those epitopes at focal adhesions. Exogenous 12-(S)-HETE stimulates adhesion of B16a cells to fibronectin exclusively via an $\alpha_{IIb}\beta_3$-mediated mechanism. B16a cells contain a significant intracellular pool of the $\alpha_{IIb}\beta_3$ complex in the perinuclear zone. Upon 12-(S)-HETE stimulation $\alpha_{IIb}\beta_3$ -containing cytoplasmic vesicles disperse throughout the cytoplasm to the plasma membrane suggesting, that 12-(S)-HETE stimulation involves integrin translocation to the plasma membrane as well. On the contrary B16a cells contain and express integrin $\alpha_5\beta_1$ as well (J.Q.Chen, J. Timar, K.V.Honn - unpublished data). However, these epitopes are not the dominant integrin involved in basal fibronectin adhesion of B16a cells and they are not involved in stimulated adhesion either.

Integrins are transmembrane proteins providing a link between matrix ligand(s) and cytoskeleton. Integrin functions (adhesion, spreading and migration) involve extensive cytoskeletal rearrangements (18). 12-(S)-HETE stimulate adhesion and spreading therefore it was conceivable to study its effect on various cytoskeletal elements in B16a cells. We have shown, that exogenous 12-(S)-HETE increases the occurence of stress fibers, increases accumulation of F-actin in filo- and lamellopodia, where microfilaments colocalize with the upregulated $\alpha_{IIb}\beta_3$. Interestingly, another cytoskeletal component; i.e. intermediate filaments, are also involved in 12-(S)-HETE stimulation. We observed pronounced bundling of intermediate filaments upon 12-(S)-HETE stimulation. It is interesting, that intracellular $\alpha_{IIb}\beta_3$ frequently colocalized with intermediate filaments suggesting a role for intermediate filaments in the translocation process. These data suggest, that $\alpha_{IIb}\beta_3$ expression and function may be linked to the integrity of microfilaments and intermediate filaments. This hypothesis was further supported by the fact that disruption of microfilaments and intermediate filaments prevent 12-(S)-HETE -induced upregulation of $\alpha_{IIb}\beta_3$ and $\alpha_{IIb}\beta_3$-mediated adhesion of B16a cells. We suggest, that intermediate filaments are responsible for translocation of intracellular $\alpha_{IIb}\beta_3$-carrying vesicles to the plasma membrane, where the receptor becomes associated with microfilaments, most probably through actin-binding proteins. PMA and 12-(S)-HETE share strikingly similar effects on integrin expression (10) and cytoskeleton rearrangement (19), suggesting that the 12-(S)-HETE effect may also involve PKC activation and phosphorylation of membrane receptor(s) and/or cytoskeletal proteins.

The in vivo role of endogenous LOX metabolites of arachidonic acid - among them 12-(S)-HETE- is still questionable. However it is known, that several cells types, including tumor cells, produce 12-(S)-HETE (20,21). It is worth mentioning, that upon tumor cell-platelet interaction the production of 12-(S)-HETE is increased in platelets (22). Tumor cell-platelet interaction may be one rate limiting factor during hematogenous dissemination (5). The in vivo activation of platelets during this process is well documented (23). Therefore it is resonable to propose a transitory increase in local concentration of 12-(S)-HETE in the tumor cell micromilieu in the microvasculature after platelet aggregation which could affect tumor cell expression of $\alpha_{IIb}\beta_3$ and their adhesion to the vessel wall. Based on these data we consider 12-(S)-HETE as a physiological promoter of tumor dissemination and the mechanisms leading to 12-(S)-HETE production may well serve as attractive targets for new experimental protocols to control tumor dissemination.

ACKNOWLEDGEMENT

This work was supported by NIH grants CA 29997-08 and CA 47115-03.

REFERENCES

1. Akaiyama, S.K., Kagata, K., Yamada, K.M. Biochem. Biophys. Acta, 1031:91-110, 1990.
2. Liotta, LA. Cancer Res. 46:1-7, 1986.
3. Kramer, R.H., McDonald, K.A., Crowley, E., Ramos, D.M., Damsky, C.H. Cancer. Res., 49:393-402, 1989.
4. Albeda, S.M., Mette, S.A., Elder, D.E., Stewart, R.M., Damjanovich, L., Herlyn, M., Buck, C.A.. Cancer Res. 50:6757-6764, 1990.
5. Weiss, L., Orr, F.W., Honn, K.V. Clin. Expl. Metast. 7:127-167, 1989.
6. Fitzgerald, L.A., Phillips, D.R. In: Platelet Immunology: Molecular and Clinical Aspects (Kunicki, T.J. and Goerge, J.N., eds) J.B. Lippinocott Company, pgs. 9-30, 1989.
7. Grossi, I.M., Hatfield, J.S., Fitzgerald, L.A., Newcombe, M., Taylor, J.D., and Honn, K.V. FASEB J., 2:2385-2395, 1988.
8. Grossi, I.M., Fitzgerald, L.A., Umbarger, L.A., Nelson, K.K., Diglio, C.A., Taylor, J.D., and Honn,

K.V. Cancer Res., 49:1029-1037, 1989.
9. Yamada, K.M. Current Opinion in Cell Biology, 1:956-963, 1989.
10. Singer, I.J., Scott, S., Kawka, D.W., Kazazis, D.M. J. Cell Biol., 109:3169-3182, 1989.
11. Chopra, H., Fligiel, S.E.G., Hatfield, J.S., Nelson, K.K., Diglio, C.A., Taylor, J.D., Honn, K.V., Cancer Res, 50:7686-7696, 1990.
12. Menter, D.G., Steinert, B.W., Sloane, B.F., Gundlach, N., O'Gara, C.Y., Marnett, L.J., Diglio, C., Walz, D., Taylor, J.D., Honn, K.V. Cancer Res. 47:6751-6762, 1987.
13. Chopra, H., Hatfield, J.S., Chang, Y.S., Grossi, I.M., Fitzgerald, L.A., O'Gara, C.Y., Marnett, L.J., Diglio, C.A., Taylor, J.D., Honn, K.V. Cancer Res. 48:3787-3800, 1988.
14. Coller, B.S., Peerschkee, E.V., Scudder, L.E., Sullivan, C.A. J. Clin. Inv. 72:326-338, 1983.
15. Jaken, S., Leach, K., Klauch, T. J. Cell Biol. 109:697-704, 1989.
16. Mochly-Rosen, D., Henrich, C.J., Cheever, L., Khaner, H., Simpson, P.C. Cell Reg., 1:693-706, 1990.
17. Axelrod, J., Biochem. Soc. Transact. 18:503-507, 1990.
18. Hynes, R.O., Cell, 48:549-554, 1987.
19. Hass, R., Bartels, H., Topley, N., Hadam, M., Kohler, L., Goppelt-Strube, M., Resch, K., Eur. J. Cell Biol. 48:282-293, 1989.
20. Marnett, L.J., Leithauser, M.T., Richards, K.M., Blair, I., Honn, K.V., Yamamoto, S., Yoshimoto, T., In: Advances in Prostacyclin, Thromboxane and Leukotriene Research, (Samuelsson, B., Paoletti, R., and Ramwell, P., eds.) Vol. 19, Raven Press, NY (in press).
21. Hamberg, M., Svensson, J., Samuelsson, B. Proc. Natl. Acad. Sci, US, 72:2988-2994, 1975.
22. Honn, K.V., Steinert, B.W., Moin, K., Onoda, J.M., Taylor, J.D. and Sloane, B.F. Biochem Biophys Res Communic, 145:384-389, 1987.
23. Menter, D.G., Hatfield, J.S., Harkins, C.J., Sloane, B.F., Taylor, J.D., Crissman, J.D., and Honn, K.V. Clin. Exp. Metastasis, 5:65-78, 1987.

EICOSANOID METABOLISM AND TUMOR CELL ENDOTHELIAL CELL ADHESION

M.R. BUCHANAN[1], M.C. BERTOMEU[1], E. BASTIDA[2], F.W. ORR[1] and S. GALLO[1]

[1]Department of Pathology, McMaster University, Hamilton, Canada, and [2]Hospital Clinico, Universidad de Barcelona, Barcelona, Spain

INTRODUCTION

The intravascular transport of tumor cells and their attachment to the vessel wall are important steps in metastasis. However, little is known about the intracellular mechanisms which regulate tumor cell adhesion to the vessel wall, particularly, to intact endothelial cells. A number of studies have suggested that circulating tumor cells preferentially adhere to the exposed underlying extracellular matrix rather than to intact endothelial cells (1,2). However, other studies suggest that tumor cells can also adhere to endothelial cells, and that this adherence is dependant upon specific characteristics of the endothelium. It has also been suggested that the metabolic characteristics of tumor cells themselves influence their own adhesion to the vessel wall (3-4). Finally, a number of recent studies suggest that adhesion receptor molecules are expressed following cell stimulation, facilitating cell/cell adhesion (5-7). In this paper we will focus on the possible intracellular regulation of expression of these adhesion molecules by two lipoxygenase derived fatty acid metabolites synthesized from arachidonic and linoleic acids. In particular, we will review the relationship between 13-hydroxyoctadecadienoic acid (13-HODE) derived from linoleic acid and 15-hydroxyeicosatetraenoic acid (15-HETE) derived from arachidonic acid, and tumor cell endothelial cell adhesion.

13-HODE and 15-HETE Synthesis and Tumor Cell/Endothelial Cell Adhesion.

A number of recent studies suggest that the intracellular levels of 13-HODE in endothelial cells, and the intracellular ratio of 13-HODE:15-HETE in tumor cells, regulate the expression of adhesion molecules on their extracellular surfaces. When 13-HODE synthesis is increased in the resting endothelial cell, (eg. by adding exogenous dbcAMP, or by growing the cells in the presence of a phosphodiesterase inhibitor, dipyridamole), there is a corresponding dose-related decrease in the ability of tumor cells to adhere to the endothelial cell surface (8,9). In contrast, when endothelial cells are stimulated with a cytokines, eg. Interleukin-1, tumor necrosis factor, or the synthetic peptide fMLP, endothelial cell 13-HODE synthesis decreases and tumor cell/endothelial cell adhesion increases. Similarly, when tumor cells are grown in the presence of the phosphodiesterase inhibitor, tumor cell cAMP levels are also increased, and the increase in cAMP is associated with increased intracellular 13-HODE synthesis and a dose-related decrease in the ability of these tumor cells to adhere to intact endothelial cells. Furthermore, the decrease in 13-HODE synthesis in tumor cells following stimulation, is associated with an increased synthesis of 15-HETE (9-11). It should be noted that under these conditions, there is no detectable 13-HODE nor 15-HETE released into the ambient surroundings. Thus, studies using a variety of human and murine tumor cell lines, indicate that the ratio of 13-HODE:15-HETE in tumor cells correlates significantly with their adhesive ability; the more the 13-HODE and the less the 15-HETE, the less adhesive the tumor cell, under resting conditions. Upon stimulation, 13-HODE synthesis decreases and there is a corresponding increase in 15-HETE synthesis, and the ability of the tumor cells to adhere.

13-HODE and PGI_2 Synthesis and Tumor Cell/Endothelial Cell Adhesion.

We also explored the relationship between the intracellular levels of 13-HODE in either tumor cells or endothelial cells and prostacyclin (PGI_2) synthesis, in relation to the ability of tumor cells to adhere to endothelial cells. It was interesting to note that increased tumor cell adhesion following endothelial cell stimulation, was paralleled by increased endothelial cell PGI_2 synthesis (8,10), suggesting that elevated PGI_2 synthesis does not impair the adhesion step in metastasis. This is consistant with the observation of Laekeman et al. (12) and challenges the concept that PGI_2 and TxA_2 play important roles in the adhesion step of metastasis (13,14). Furthermore, specific inhibitors of the lipoxygenase and cyclo-oxygenase enzymes provide additional evidence that metabolites from the lipoxygenase pathway rather than from the cyclo-oxygenase pathway, play a more important role in the regulation of tumor cell endothelial cell adhesion. For example when PGI_2 in endothelial cells is inhibited by low dose aspirin, tumor cell adhesion to the endothelial cell surface is uneffected. In contrast, when inhibitors of the lipoxygenase pathway are used (to block 13-HODE synthesis), tumor cell adhesion to the endothelial cell surface is increased (10). These observations have lead us to postulate that the intracellular levels of 13-HODE and 15-HETE influence tumor cell endothelial cell adhesion. The most likely mechanism by which these metabolites achieve this effect is, by regulating the expression of adhesion molecules on the external cell surfaces.

Tumor Cell/Endothelial Cell Adhesion: Role of Integrins.

The rapid development in molecular biology techniques has lead to the identification of a host of adhesion molecules, in particular, the integrins, which are expressed on the surface of various cells following stimulation (7). Many of these molecules have a common amino acid sequence i.e. Arginine-GlycineAspartic acid, known as the RGD sequence. This sequence is necessary for their adhesive property (7). However, little is known about the biochemical regulators inside the cells which influences the expression of these molecules on the external cell surfaces.

We examined the relationship between 13-HODE synthesis in endothelial cells, expression of RGD-recognizing molecules, and tumor cell/endothelial cell adhesion. Our studies demonstrated that there is an inverse relationship between 13-HODE synthesis and expression of adhesion molecules on endothelial cell surfaces. When endothelial cells are exposed to Interleukin-1, or to plasmas obtained from cancer patients undergoing chemotherapy, endothelial cell adhesivity is enhanced (6,15). The enhanced adhesivity of endothelial cells exposed to the chemotherapy-treated patient plasma, was attributed to chemotherapy drug-induced Interleukin-1 release (15). Thus, in both studies, the adhesion following Interleukin-1 stimulation, was abolished by an RGD-containing peptide, suggesting that an integrin-like adhesion molecule was expressed on the endothelial cell surface. Further studies, using specific antibodies to a number of integrins, suggest that the adhesion molecule most likely involved, is the vitronectin receptor (16). Finally, the enhanced expression of this RGD recognizing adhesion molecule is associated with decreased 13-HODE synthesis in endothelial cells (10,11).

Tumor Cell/Endothelial Cell Interactions: Effects of Radiation.

While radiation is beneficial in the treatment of many cancer types other studies suggest that radiation treatment can be detrimental to the normal vasculature (17). The explanations for these adverse effects are multiple. Recent studies in our laboratory suggest that part of these adverse effects of radiation are related to damage to the endothelial cell 13-HODE pathway. Thus, when endothelial cells are irradiated in vitro (1 Gy/min for 10 min), intracellular 13-HODE is destroyed and released to the ambient surrounding (18), and endothelial cell adhesivity is markedly increased. When C57B/6 mice were irradiated (1000 rads/ 5 min) and then injected with tumor cells (B16F10 melanoma cells), the number of tumor cells trapped within the lungs 24 hours later was significantly increased (Figure 1). Increased tumor cell entrapment correlated with increased tumor cell metastasis (19). While extrapolation of these experimental observations to the clinical setting must be made with caution, our observations provide an additional explanation for the adverse effects of radiation treatment . Namely, excessive or

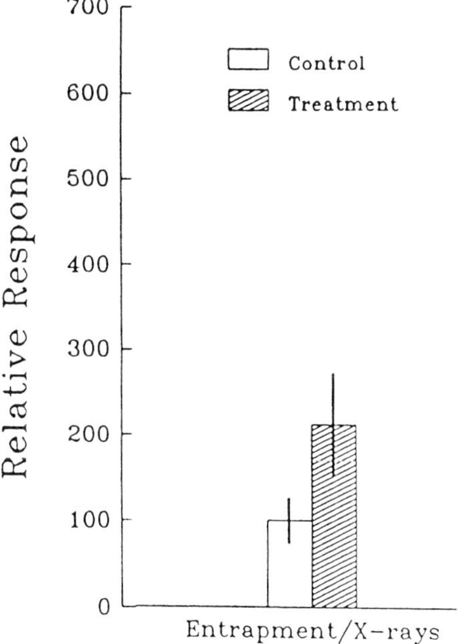

Figure 1. Effect of Irradiation on Tumor Cell Entrapment in Mice

misdirected radiation may inhibit vessel wall 13-HODE synthesis and consequently enhance the expression of adhesion molecules on the endothelial cell surface, which in turn influence tumor adhesion to and migration through the vascular wall barrier.

CONCLUSIONS

The majority of studies on fatty acid metabolism and cell/cell interactions has focussed predominately on arachidonic acid metabolites produced via the cyclo-oxygenase pathway. However, recent studies which have considered metabolites derived via the lipoxygenase pathway, from both arachidonic and linoleic acids, suggest that 13-HODE and 15-HETE regulate tumor cell/endothelial cell adhesion. In particular, these studies raise the possibility that intracellular 13-HODE and 15-HETE, modulate the expression of adhesion receptor molecules on the surface of both tumor cells and endothelial cells, thus facilitating tumor cell adhesion to and migration through the vascular wall barrier. 13-HODE appears to down-regulate adhesion both in tumor cells and in endothelial cells, while 15-HETE appears to up-regulate adhesion. This possibility is supported by the recent works of Grossi et al (20) who demonstrated that exogenous 12-HETE (the platelet arachidonic acid lipoxygenase metabolite), facilitates the expression of a IRGpIIb/IIIa like molecule on tumor cells, increasing their adhesion, whereas exogenous 13-HODE blocks this adhesion event.

REFERENCES

1. Liotta, L.A. Am. J. Pathol. 117:339-348, 1984.
2. Weiss, L. Principles in Metastasis (New York, Academic Press) 1985.
3. Auerbach, R., Wei, C.L., Pardon, E., Gumkowski, F., Raminska, G. Cancer Res. 47:1492-1496, 1987.
4. Nicolson, G.L. Biochem. Biophys. Acta. 695:113-116, 1982.
5. Rice, G.E., Gimbrone Jr., M.A., Bevilacqua, M.P. Am. J. Pathol 133:204-210, 1988.
6. Lauri, D., Bertomeu, M.C., Orr, F.W., Bastida, E., Sauder, D., Buchanan, M.R. Clin. Exp. Met. In Press, 1989.
7. Ruoslahti, E., Pierschbacher, M.D. Cell 44:517-518, 1986.
8. Haas, T.A., Bertomeu, M.C., Bastida, E., Buchanan, M.R. Clin. Invest. Med. 12:B9, 1989.
9. Bastida, E., Almirall, L., Buchanan, M.R., Haas, T.A., Lauri, D., Orr, F.W. Thromb. Haemost. 58:315, 1987.
10. Bastida, E., Almirall, L., Alonso, A., Ordinas, A., Buchanan, M.R., Bertomeu, M.C., Haas, T.A. Thromb. Haemost. 62:138, 1989.
11. Buchanan, M.R., Bastida, E., Med. Hypoth. 27:317-325, 1988.
12. Laekeman, G.M., Vergote, I.B., Keersmaekers, G.M., Heiremans, J., Haensch, G.F., de Roy, G., Uyttenbroeck, F.L., Herman, A.G., Br. J. Canc. 54:431-437, 1986.
13. Karmali, R., Welt, S., Thaler, H., Lefevre, F., Br. J. Cancer 48:689-695, 1983.
14. Honn, K.V., Cicone, B., Skoff, A. Sci 212:1270-1272, 1981.
15. Bertomeu, M.C., Levine, M., Lauri, D, Goodyear, M., Buchanan, M.R. Am. Assoc Canc Res May, 1989.
16. Lafrenie, R.M., Poder, T.J., Buchanan, M.R., Orr, F.W. Proc 1st Int'l Conf. Eicosanoids Bioactive Lipids in Cancer & Radiation Injury. Book of Abst. Detroit USA, Oct 11-14, 1989.
17. Law, M.P., Advances in Radiation Biology 9:37-73, 1981.
18. Matznery, Y., Cohn, M., Hyam, E., Razin, E., Fuks, Z., Buchanan, M.R., Haas, T.A., Vlodavsky, I., Eldor, A. J. Immun. 140-2681-2685, 1988.
19. Bertomeu, M.C., Whybourne, K., Orr, F.W., Buchanan, M.R., Proc 1st Int'l Conf. Eicosanoids Bioactive Lipids in Cancer & Radiation Injury. Book of Abst. Detroit USA, Oct 11-14, 1989.
20. Grossi, I.M., Fitzgerald, L.A., Umbarger, L.A., Nelson, K.K., Diglio, C.A., Taylor, J.D., Honn, K.V., Cancer Res. 49:1029-1037, 1989.

TUMOR GROWTH INVASION AND DIFFERENTIATION

LEVELS OF PHOSPHOSERINE, PHOSPHOTHREONINE AND PROSTAGLANDINS IN A RAT TRANSPLANTABLE HEPATOMA AND PROSTATIC TUMOR

L. LEVINE and H. VAN VUNAKIS

Department of Biochemistry, Brandeis University, Waltham, MA 02254, U.S.A.

Phosphorylation and dephosphorylation of proteins have been associated with regulatory mechanisms in many biological processes (1). In eukaryotic cells, tyrosine, threonine and/or serine residues represent the main substrates for phosphorylation by protein kinases. Many of the compounds that we have found to affect metabolism of arachidonic acid are associated with phosphorylation reactions (2). These include growth factors, diacylglycerol analogs and uncouplers of oxidative phosphorylation (Table 1). In addition, most tumor promoters stimulate arachidonic acid metabolism in a dose-dependent manner, but they vary in the capacity to induce ornithine decarboxylase, to irritate skin, to induce HL-60 cell adhesion, to inhibit [^{3}H] TPA binding, and to activate protein kinase C (3). Based on the capacity to activate protein kinase C, the tumor promoters, TPA, teleocidin and aplysiatoxin were classified as TPA-types; okadaic acid, thapsigargin and palytoxin were classified as non-TPA type tumor promoters (3). Okadaic acid is an inhibitor of a phosphatase active on serine (threonine)-phosphate (4). It could be functioning as a tumor promoter and stimulator of arachidonic acid metabolism by preventing dephosphorylation of a serine (threonine)-phosphate that regulates a pathway leading to both tumor formation and prostaglandin production. Thapsigargin activates entry into cells of Ca^{2+} (5), an intracellular messenger whose manifold activities include phosphorylation reactions. The third of the non-TPA type tumor promoters, palytoxin, is thought to interact with the Na^+, K^+-ATPase, transforming this ion pump into a nonspecific cation channel (6).

Table 1.
Compounds whose biological properties, and/or agonist-receptor interactions probably include phosphorylating or dephosphorylating activities as well as stimulation of arachidonic acid metabolism.

Insulin (7-9)	12-O-tetradecanoylphorbol-13-acetate (17)
Insulin growth factor-1 (10)	Okadaic Acid (2)
Platelet derived growth factor (11)	Duramycin (18)
Epidermal growth factor (12)	Oligomycin (19)
1-Oleoyl-2-acetyl-glycerol (13)	Antimycin (19)
Transforming growth factor-α (14)	Ouabain (19)
Dexamethasone (15,16)	Vanadate (20,21)

The regulatory roles of phosphorylated amino acids were originally based upon detection of kinase-generated [^{32}P]-proteins and identification of the phosphoamino acids either by differential base lability of phosphotyrosine *vs* phosphoserine and phosphothreonine and/or by chromatography of the amino acids generated by chemical or proteolytic digestion. We, however, have prepared specific antibodies directed toward phosphotyrosine, as well as phosphothreonine and phosphoserine, and have developed RIAs for them (22). (An immunization procedure was used that, in rabbits, had elicited the production of antibodies directed toward adenosine-5'-phosphate, uridine-5'-phosphate, and ribose-5-phosphate [23].) With all three immune systems, the antibodies are directed to the N-acyl-phosphoamino acids. The serologic specificity for the phosphotyrosine immune system is shown in Table 2. Each antiserum is specific for its homologous phosphoamino acid and the requirement for the phosphate moiety is essentially absolute. The limits of detection for N-acyl-tyrosine(PO_3), N-acyl-threonine(PO_3) and N-acyl-serine(PO_3) are approximately 0.008, 0.03 and 0.07 pmoles respectively. The serologic specificities of the immune systems are such that dephosphorylation or deacylation would decrease and phosphorylation would increase the immunologically determined levels of the phosphoamino acids in proteins. In order to eliminate the activities of phosphatases, kinases, and/or deacylases in our analyses, extractions of tissues are carried out under conditions that denature the enzymes. The frozen tissues (frozen immediately after collection) are extracted in 8 M urea, 1 mM 2-mercaptoethanol and incubated at 60° for 60 min. However, the possibility that phosphatases, kinases and/or deacylases are active prior to the extraction cannot be excluded.

Table 2
Serologic specificity of the N-succinyl-[^{3}H]-phosphotyrosine-anti-phosphotyrosine reaction. (from 22)

Ligand	Quantities required for 50% inhibition (pmoles)
N-Succinyl-phosphotyrosine	0.06
N-Acetyl-phosphotyrosine	0.08
Phosphotyrosine	8.0
Phenylphosphate	7×10^3
N-Succinyl-phosphothreonine	4×10^3
Phosphate	2×10^5
N-Succinyl-phosphoserine	a
N-Succinyl-tyrosine	b
N-Succinyl-tyrosinesulfate	c
Adenosine-5'-phosphate	d

a. Inhibition with 1.7×10^4 pmoles was 7%
b. Inhibition with 1.8×10^5 pmoles was 8%
c. Inhibition with 1.3×10^5 pmoles was 31%.
d. Inhibition with 2.9×10^5 pmoles was 0%.

The phosphoamino acids and the prostaglandins are stable to the extraction conditions. Fifty μl of such extracts can be assayed directly in the RIA under our conditions (total volume of 400 μl) without interfering with the antigen-antibody reaction. Dose-response curves of inhibition generated with the homologous N-succinyl-phosphoamino acids in the presence or absence of 50 μl of the urea, 2-mercaptoethanol solvent and under the same incubation conditions gave identical results. Inhibition of immune binding by N-succinyl-phosphoamino acids incubated with the urea, 2-mercaptoethanol solvents and heated at 60° for 60 min also was not affected. N-succinyl-phosphoamino acids were quantitatively recovered when added to crude tissue extracts and carried through the extraction procedure. However, in the absence of denaturing agents or enzyme inhibitors, loss in serologic activity occurred. The extent of the loss of serologic activity, presumably by phosphatase activities but possibly by deacylases as well, varied among extracts obtained from different tissues. The N-succinyl-phosphotyrosine was usually affected the most, and its loss of serologic activity could be inhibited completely by addition of 500 μM Na_3 orthovanadate. In experiments in which the three phosphoamino acids were determined by RIA, cytoplasmic fractions of normal rat tissues showed that, on a protein basis, levels of phosphoserine were much greater than those of phosphothreonine in most tissues (Table 3). The content of phosphotyrosine in cytoplasmic fractions of the normal tissues is extremely low (analyses of membrane fractions may yield higher levels). Levels of phosphoserine and phosphothreonine in normal cells are together reported to be three orders of magnitude greater than those of phosphotyrosine (24).

The LC-18 hepatoma transplants in Fischer 344 rats and the R-3327AT-3 prostatic tumor transplants in Copenhagen rats have been studied. Tumors were excised from the implantation site. At the same time, the livers or the prostates of the recipient rats were collected. The tumors and control organs were immediately frozen (-70°C). For extraction, the frozen tumors organs were suspended in 8 M urea, 1 mM 2-mercaptoethanol (about 10-50 mg wet weight per ml), cut into small fragments and homogenized in a Sorvall Omni-Mixer. The extracts were incubated in a 60° water bath for 60 min and clarified by centrifugation at 50,000 rpm in a Beckman 70.1 rotor for 60 min at 5°. The cytoplasmic fractions were assayed for phosphoamino acids, prostaglandins, leukotrienes and protein. Even though the hepatomas and prostatic tumors were excised and trimmed carefully, several areas of each tumor were extracted and analyzed in order to minimize contributions from extra-hepatic or extra-prostatic tissue.

The levels of threonine (PO_3) and serine (PO_3) (pmoles per mg protein) in the hepatomas and serine(PO_3) in the prostatic tumors were significantly less ($P < 0.05$) than those found in the control organs. The levels of PGE_2, $PGF_{2\alpha}$,PGI_2 and PGD_2 (pg/mg protein) were also less in the tumors than in the control organs. The decreased levels of PGE_2 and $PGF_{2\alpha}$ did not reflect increased metabolic activities in the tumors - they did not contain increased levels of the 13,14-H2-15-keto-metabolites. Of importance was the finding that in the control prostates, but not in the tumors, the levels of serine (PO_3) were associated positively with the levels of PGE_2, $PGF_{2\alpha}$, PGD_2 and PGI_2, suggesting that a phosphor-

Table 3
Range of levels of phosphoamino acids in rat organ extracts.* (from 22)

Organ	Number of Rats	pmoles/mg Protein		
		Phosphotyrosine	Phosphothreonine	Phosphoserine
Lung	(3)	<0.008 - <0.01	0.04 - 0.06	0.34 - 0.89
Liver	(4)	<0.004 - 0.01	0.08 - 0.18	0.24 - 0.82
Pancreas	(3)	<0.016 - 0.03	0.13 - 1.6**	0.7 - 1.2
Brain	(3)	<0.004	0.04 - 0.06	0.34 - 0.59
Heart	(3)	<0.005 - 0.003	0.03 - 0.05	0.4 - 0.7
Uteri	Pool	<0.008	0.3	0.5
Thyroid	Pool	<0.005	0.02	0.2
Thymus	Pool	<0.005	0.02	0.1
Spleen	(3)	<0.003 - <0.004	0.09 - 0.14	0.87 - 1.1
Kidney	(4)	<0.004 - <0.007	0.84 - 0.95	0.97 - 1.9
Pituitaries	Pool	<0.01	0.16	0.87
Ovaries	Pool	0.013	2.5	2.3
Prostates	Pool	0.018	0.25	3.3

* Organs were collected and immediately immersed in liquid nitrogen and stored frozen until extracted. Organs, designated in the table as pool, were obtained from Pel-Freeze on dry ice and stored frozen. The organs were extracted in a Sorvall "omni-mixer" for 2 min at 0° in 8 M urea containing 1 mM 2-mercaptoethanol. The extract was incubated at 60° for 60 min and the cytosol collected by ultracentrifugation at 50,000 rpm for 60 min in a Beckman 70.1 rotor.

** Individual levels were 0.13, 0.19 and 1.57 pmoles/mg protein.

ylated serine residue, directly or indirectly, regulates either cyclooxygenase activity or deesterification of cellular lipids. The lower levels of threonine (PO_3) and serine (PO_3) in the hepatomas and serine (PO_3) in the prostatic tumors could reflect (1) increased phosphatase activity, possibly resulting from decreased phosphatase-inhibitor activity or (2) decreased kinase activities. Decreased synthesis of a protein that is a substrate for kinases would also account for the lower levels of serologically determined serine (PO_3) and threonine (PO_3) in the hepatoma or serine (PO_3) in the prostatic tumors.

The evidence is strong that tumor promotion and progression reflect anomolous expression of oncogenes. Several of the oncogene products are structurally related to growth factors or growth factor receptors and most of the oncogene products have functions related to growth. Many of these oncogene products and growth factor-receptor interactions have or generate kinase activities (25). Prostaglandin production is associated with tumor promotion and regulation of prostaglandin production may be associated with phosphorylation. Thus, any one of the reactions listed that can explain the decreased levels of the phosphoamino acid in the tumors would link tumor formation and prostaglandin production.

ACKNOWLEDGEMENTS

This work was supported by BRSG S07 RR07044 awarded by the Biomedical Research Support Grant Program, Division of Research Resources, National Institutes of Health. H.V.V. is the recipient of a Research Career Award (5K6-A12372) from the National Institute of Allergy and Infectious Disease. We wish to thank Hilda B. Gjika, Nancy Worth, Jing Zhang, and Ron Carroll for their technical assistance and Inez Zimmerman for preparation of the manuscript.

REFERENCES

1. Hunter, T., Cooper, J.A. (1985) Ann. Rev. Biochem. 54, 897-930.
2. Levine, L. (1987). In Prostaglandins in Cancer Research, E. Garaci, R. Paoletti, and M.G. Santoro, eds. Springer-Verlag, Berlin Heidelberg, pp. 6273.
3. Fujiki, H., Sugimura, T. (1987) Adv. Cancer Res. 49:223-264.
4. Bialojan, C., Takai, A. (1988) Biochem. J. 256:283-290.
5. Takemura, H., Hughes, A.H., Thastrup, O, Putney, J.W. Jr. (1989) J. Biol. Chem. 264:12266-12271 .
6. Chhatwal, G.S., Hessler, H.J., Habermann, E. (1983) Naunyn-Schmiedeberg's Arch Pharmacol. 323:261-268.
7. Benjamin, W.B., Singer, I. (1974) Biochim. Biophys. Acta 351:28-41.
8. Kasuga, M., Karlsson, F.A., Kahn, C.R. (1982) Science. 215:185-187.
9. Rosen, O.M., Herrera, R., Olowe, Y., Petruzzelli, L.M., Cobb, M.H. (1983) Proc. Natl. Acad. Sci. USA 80:3237-3240.
10. Rubin, J.B., Shia, M.A., Pilch, P.F. (1983) Nature 305:438-440.
11. Ek, B., Westermark, B., Wasteson, A., Heldin, C.H. (1982) Nature 295: 419-420.
12. Ushiro, H., Cohen, S. (1980) J. Biol. Chem. 255:8363-8365.
13. Kaibuchi, K., Takai, Y., Sawamura, M., Hoshijima, M., Fujikura, T., Nishizuka, Y. (1983) J. Biol. Chem. 258:6701-6704.
14. Pike, L.J., Marquardt, H., Todaro, G.J., Gallis, B., Casnellie, T., Bornstein, P., Krebs, E.G. (1982) J. Biol. Chem. 257:14628-14631.
15. Hirata, F. (1981) J. Biol. Chem. 256:7730-7733.
16. Touqui, L., Rothwi, B., Shaw, A.M., Fradin, A., Vargaftig, B.B., Russo-Marie, F. (1986) Nature 321:177-180.
17. Nishizuka, T. (1983) Trends Biochem. Sci. 8:13-16.
18. Nakamura, S., Racker, E. (1984) Biochemistry 23:385-389.
19. Lehninger, A.L. (1982) Principles of Biochemistry, Worth, New York.
20. Tamura, S., Brown, T.A., Whipple, J.H., Fujita-Yamaguchi, Y., Dubler, R.E., Cheng, K., Lamer, J. (1984) J. Biol. Chem. 259:6650-6658.
21. Rosen, O.M., Herrera, R., Olowe, Y., Petruzzelli, L.M., Cobb, M.H. (1983) Proc. Natl. Acad. Sci. USA 80:3237-3240.
22. Levine, L., Gjika, H.B., Van Vunakis, H. J. Immunol. Methods. 124:239-249, 1989.
23. Van Vunakis, H., Seaman, E., Setlow, P., Levine, L. (1968) Biochemistry 7:1265-1270.
24. Sefton, B.M., Hunter, T., Beemon, K., Eckhart, W. (1980) Cell 20:807-816.
25. Hunter, T. (1987). In NATO ASI SER. SER. A 329-344. "Signal Transduction Protein Phosphorylation."

ROLE OF ARACHIDONIC AND LINOLEIC ACID METABOLITES IN GROWTH REGULATION OF SYRIAN HAMSTER EMBRYO FIBROBLASTS: STUDIES WITH TUMOR SUPPRESSOR GENE (+) AND SUPPRESSOR GENE (-) PHENOTYPES

W.C. GLASGOW, J.C. BARRETT*, and T.E. ELING

Laboratory of Molecular Biophysics and *Molecular Carcinogenesis, National Instutite of Environmental Health Sciences, Research Triangle Park, North Carolina 27709

INTRODUCTION

The binding of polypeptide mitogens like epidermal growth factor (EGF) to specific cell surface receptors activates a variety of biochemical processess that ultimately result in quiescent cells undergoing cell cycle traverse and initiating DNA synthesis (1). The role of each of these pathways in transducing the growth factor proliferation signal remains to be fully characterized.

Several lines of evidence suggest that the release and subsequent metabolism of arachidonic acid is an important part of the mitogenic response of cells to growth factors (2-5). Our laboratory reported that prostaglandins act as key intracellular mediators in transducing the mitogenic signal of EGF-stimulated BALB/c 3T3 fibroblasts (5). Moreover, we have recently observed that EGF treatment of quiescent BALB/c 3T3 cells stimulates lipoxygenase-mediated oxygenation of linoleic acid; the monohydroxy linoleate derivatives formed in the cell are very active in potentiating EGF-induced DNA synthesis.

To examine whether these pathways are involved in the mitogenic response of other cell lines, we have utilized carcinogen-induced Syrian Hamster Embryo (SHE) fibroblast clones which were selected for their ability to suppress (sup^+) or not suppress (sup^-) the tumorigenic phenotype of neoplastic cells in cell-cell hybrids. The loss of tumor suppressor gene function is essential in the multistep process of neoplastic progression of SHE cells transformed by chemical carcinogens or by oncogenic transfection (6-8). The goals of the studies described here were to (1) characterize the role of arachidonic and linoleic acid metabolism in the EGF signal transduction pathway of SHE cells; and (2) determine if alterations in these biochemical processes are related to loss of tumor suppressor gene function.

RESULTS AND DISCUSSION

SHE cells fibroblasts arrested at subconfluence by serum-depletion are induced by EGF(optimal dose: 10 ng/ml) to initiate DNA synthesis as measured by [^{3}H] thymidine incorporation. Thus, in all subsequent experiments EGF at 10 ng/ml was used to elicit a mitogenic response. When SHE cells were incubated with 1μM arachidonic acid (with 1 μCi [^{3}H]-AA as tracer), the fatty acid was actively metabolized to two products that were isolated on reverse phase-HPLC (HPLC method described in reference 9). Chemical characterization of this material (as described in reference 5) resulted in the identification of the arachidonate metabolites as PGE_2 and $PGF_{2\alpha}$ (derived via the cyclooxygenase pathway). The sup^+ SHE cells appeared to produce more PGE_2 than the sup^- cells.

The effects of prostaglandins on DNA synthesis in SHE cells were assessed by measuring incorporation of radioactive thymidine into trichloroacetic acid-insoluble material after 24 hrs. PGE_2 at concentrations as low as 10^{-8}M was found to attenuate the response of both sup^+ and sup^- to EGF (Table I). $PGF_{2\alpha}$ (10^{-8} M to 10^{-5} M) did not significantly alter EGF-stimulated DNA synthesis in SHE cells (both sup^+ and sup^-). The cyclooxygenase inhibitor indomethacin at 10^{-6} M (a concentration which blocks PG biosynthesis) also did not affect the EGF response. In contrast, the lipoxygenase inhibitor nordihydroguaiaretic acid (NDGA) at 10^{-6} M blocked 80% of EGF-dependent [^{3}H] thymidine incorporation (Table I). These results suggest the possible involvement of lipoxygenase products in the EGF response; however, only low levels of lipoxygenase-derived arachidonate products were detected.

Compound + EGF (10 ng/ml)		[^{3}H] Thymidine Incorporation (expressed as % of EGF response)	
		sup^+	sup^-
EGF (alone)		100 ± 2	100 ± 2
PGH_2	10^{-8} M	103 ± 3	110 ± 3
PGE_2	10^{-8} M	30 ± 2	38 ± 2
$PGF_{2\alpha}$	10^{-8} M	118 ± 10	119 ± 5
13-HPODD	10^{-8} M	360 ± 30	100 ± 3
13-HODD	10^{-8} M	300 ± 40	95 ± 2
9-HPODD	10^{-8} M	540 ± 60	97 ± 3
9-HODD	10^{-8} M	350 ± 20	95 ± 5
Indomethacin	10^{-6} M	95 ± 5	108 ± 3
NDGA	10^{-6} M	16 ± 4	19 ± 5

Table I

Effects of Linoleic and Arachidonic Acid Metabolites on EGF-induced DNA Synthesis in SHE Cells. Cells were grown to near confluence in 96-well plates and then were serum-depleted for 16 hrs. Test compounds and EGF were added simultaneously and DNA synthesis was measured by [^{3}H] thymidine incorporation after 24 hrs. Data (mean ± standard deviation, five determinations) are expressed relative to stimulation by EGF alone (designated 100%).

As observed with BALB/c 3T3 fibroblasts, EGF was found to activate lipoxygenase metabolism of linoleic acid in SHE cells. Quiescent SHE cells were stimulated by EGF (10 ng/ml) to convert 10-15% of exogenous linoleic acid (10 μM) to hydroxy fatty acids that were isolated on reverse phase-HPLC (Figure 1). No linoleate metabolites were detected in the absence of EGF. The isolated compounds were characterized further by straight phase-HPLC, UV spectroscopy, and GC-MS analyses; they were identified as 13-hydroxyoctadecadienoic acid (13-HODD) and 9-hydroxyoctadecadienoic acid (9-HODD).

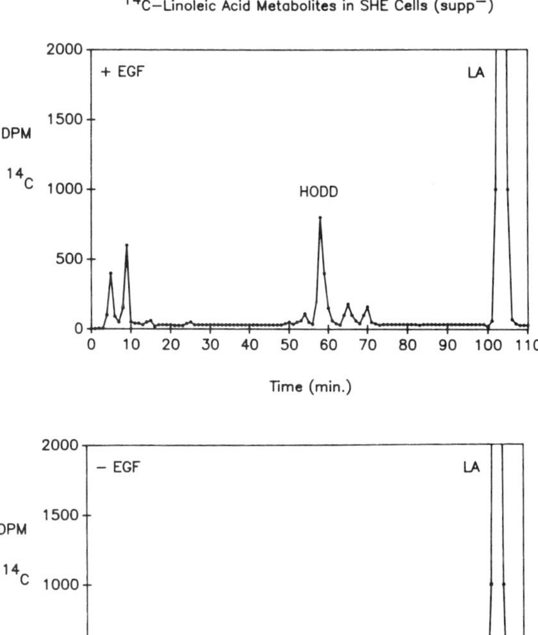

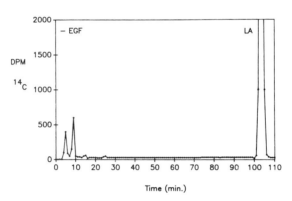

Figure 1. RP-HPLC radiochromatograms of products formed in the incubation of [^{14}C] linoleic acid (10 µM) with SHE cells (sup$^-$). Cells were incubated for 4 hr in serum-free Dulbeccos' medium (BOTTOM); or in serum-free medium containing EGF, 10 ng/ml (TOP). Media were extracted and chromatographed on a C_{18} Ultrasphere column eluted with methanol/water/acetic acid (70:30:0.01, v/v) at 1 ml/min. The results are representative of triplicate incubations in several experiments. Identical results were obtained with sup$^+$ cells.

The production of these compounds was inhibited by NDGA (1 µM), but not by indomethacin (1µM); indicating a lipoxygenase mechanism of biosynthesis. When the linoleate metabolites were added alone to quiescent SHE cells, they stimulated [^{3}H] thymidine incorporation to a very small extent. However, when added in the presence of EGF, the hydroxy metabolies and their hydroperoxy presursors greatly potentiated the growth factor-induced cellular response in sup$^+$ clones (Table I). Both 13- and 9-H(P)ODD were able to act synergistically with EGF and produce a 3-5 fold enhancement of [^{3}H]-thymidine incorporation in the sup$^+$ cells. These linoleate derivatives did not alter EGF-mediated DNA synthesis in sup$^-$ cells.

These results indicate that activation of SHE cells with EGF results in the formation of arachidonic and linoleic acid metabolites. Oxygenation of these unsaturated fatty acids must now be examined further as an important element in the cascade of biochemical events mediated by EGF in fibroblasts. The metabolic products of the cyclooxygenase and lipoxygenase pathways appear to play a regulatory role in growth factor-dependent mitogenesis and may be related to differences in phenotypic properties which correlate to tumor suppressor function.

REFERENCES

1. Carpenter, G. (1987) Annu. Rev. Biochem. 56: 881-914.
2. Shier, W.T., and Durkin, J.P. (1982) J. Cell Physiol. 112: 171-181.
3. Habenicht, A.J.R. Goerig, M., Grulich, J., Roth, D., Gronwald, R., Loth, U., Schettler, G., Kommerall, B., and Ross, D. (1985) J. Clin. Invest. 75: 1381-1387.
4. Habenicht, A.J.R., Glomset, J.A., Goerig, M., Gronwald, R., Grulich, J., Loth, U., and Schettler, G. (1985) J. Biol. Chem. 260: 1370-1373.
5. Nolan, R.D., Danilowicz, R.M., and Eling, T.E. (1988) Mol. Pharm. 33: 650-656.
6. Koi, M., and Barrett, J.C. (1986) Proc. Natl. Acad. Sci. USA 83: 5992-5996.
7. Thomassen, D.G., Gilmer, T.M., Annab, L.A., and Barrett, J.C. (1985) Cancer Res. 45: 726-732.
8. Oshimura, M., Gilmer, T.M., and Barrett, J.C. (1985) Nature 313: 636-639.
9. Henke, D.C., Kouzan, S., and Eling, T.E. (1984) Anal. Biochem. 140: 87-94.

INTERCELLULAR COMMUNICATION AMONG SV40-TRANSFORMED RAT GRANULOSA CELLS MAY BE AN INDEX OF DIFFERENTIATION

T.A. FITZ,[1] R.C. BURGHARDT,[2] M.M. MARR,[1] T.L. WALDEN, JR.,[3] and C.A. WINKEL[4]

[1]OB/GYN, Uniformed Services University of the Health Sciences, Bethesda MD 20814; [2]Texas A&M University, College Station TX 77843; [3]AFFRI, Bethesda MD 20814; [4]Jefferson Medical College, Philadelphia PA 19107

INTRODUCTION

Ovarian Granulosa cells serve critical functions related to steroidogenesis, follicular development and selection, ovum maturation, ovulation and corpus luteum formation by undergoing changes in structural and functional status during development and maturation of the ovarian follicle.[1,2,3,4] Because of their many activities, granulosa cells have become among the most intensively investigated endocrine tissues.

We have conducted studies to develop a cell model for the study of granulosa cell functions, using a clonal derivative of SV40-transformed rat granulosa (DC3) cells. DC3 cells have been shown to retain a variety of characteristics that would be expected of normal granulosa cells in an intermediate stage of differentiation; DC3 cells are steroidogenic, responsive to physiologically relevant secretagogues, and capable of intercellular communication via gap junctions.

Unlike normal granulosa cells, which readily differentiate in vitro to the terminal, luteinized state, DC3 cells appear capable of only limited differentiation. In response to all regimens (short of toxic measures) which we have attempted thus far, DC3 cells continued to proliferate, exhibited morphology typical of an "immature" cell, and produced significant amounts of estrogen, none of which are characteristic of luteinized granulosa cells. However, it appears possible to induce at least some features of differentiation in DC3 cells. We have developed treatment regimens that resulted in marked increases in steroidogenesis, morphological changes, retarded proliferation, and induction of gonadotropin receptors. We believe that DC3 cells may serve as a unique model for the analysis of transformation in a cell with epithelial properties, as well as for the study of cellular differentiation in a transformed cell line derived from a highly plastic cell type.

MATERIALS AND METHODS

DC3 cells were derived from SV40-infected rat granulosa cells. The parent line was passaged through rats, and a clonal derivative was selected from tumors in which growth was modulated hormonally[5]. The techniques for DC3 cell culture, gonadotropin receptor assays, and treatment regimens have been described[6]. More recently, we assessed morphological features and intercellular communication of DC3 cells[7]. Intercellular communication was monitored employing transmission electron microscopic examination, and by assessing transfer of carboxyfluorescein between abutting cells, using the Meridian ACAS 470 Workstation. The fluorescence transfer methodology we used was described initially for human cancer cells by Wade et al[8]. In our studies of carboxyfluorescein transfer among abutting cells, we have defined intercellular communication abundance as the proportion of abutting cells within the entire population of cells examined that exhibited carboxyfluorescein transfer. Intercellular communication efficiency was defined as the rate of carboxyfluorescein transfer among communicating cells.

To determine if proliferation could be attenuated and associated with irradiation, DC3 cells were irradiated with 4 or 20 Gy at 37°C in a bilateral ^{60}Co gamma-irradiation field at a dose rate of 1 Gy/min.

RESULTS

The effectiveness of various treatments to promote differentiation in DC3 cells was assessed on the basis of proliferation, morphology, steroid secretion patterns, gonadotropin receptor expression, and intercellular communication. We demonstrated previously that steroidogenesis on a per cell basis was augmented if cultures were serum-starved and confluent, and that treatments that included substrates for steroid biosynthesis and agents stimulating cAMP secretion resulted in up to l00-fold elevation of progesterone secretion over basal rates[6].

Gonadotropin receptors were scarce on unstimulated DC3 cells; specific binding of FSH was demonstrable but specific binding of LH was minimal[6]. However, incubation of DC3 cells in culture medium that contained pregnant mare serum gonadotropin (PMSG; a long-acting FSH analog) resulted in elevated binding of human FSH and LH (Table I). Interestingly, cells incubated in media that contained human chorionic gonadotropin (hCG; a long-acting LH analog) proliferated at a slower rate, and hCG appeared to negate the stimulatory effect of PMSG upon receptor induction (Table I). Proliferation of DC3 cells was also inhibited by estrogen; incubation in medium that contained 100 nM estradiol-17β for 96 hr resulted in a 10-fold decrease in cell numbers compared with control cultures lacking estrogen (data not shown).

Table I. Induction of Gonadotropin Specific Binding to DC3 Cells.

	Specific	Binding
Treatment	hFSH[a]	hLH[b]
None (basal level)	0.28	21.0
PMSG (1.4 IU/ml)	2.19	107.0
PMSG + hCG (1.8 IU/ml)	0.86	11.8

[a]hFSH binding in pmol/mg membrane protein
[b]hLH binding in fmol/mg membrane protein

Characteristic morphological changes were induced in DC3 cells using the treatment regimens summarized in the legend to Figure 1. Cholera toxin, which potently stimulates cAMP secretion and steroidogenesis, caused cells to become spindle-shaped and elongated. 25-Hydroxycholesterol, which serves effectively as a steroidogenic substrate, caused cell rounding and aggregation. Irradiation from a ^{60}Co source resulted in a large increase in cell volume.

The status of intercellular communication appeared to serve as an index of differentiation. While the incidence of intercellular communication appeared to be 100% in luteinized rat granulosa cells, only 35-40% of abutting DC3 cells exhibited carboxyfluorescein transfer, and this proportion was not altered markedly by any treatment attempted thus far (Table II). Furthermore, untreated DC3 cells exhibited relatively poor communication efficiency relative to normal granulosa cells (Figure 2). However, chronic treatment with dbcAMP (as an analog of cAMP) caused increased areal fraction of gap junctions in DC3 and normal granulosa cells[7]. Communication efficiency among DC3 cells was increased by chronic treatment with cholera toxin (Figure 3) or transiently by treatment with phorbol myristate acetate (an activator of protein kinase C; Figure 4).

Gamma irradiation reduced the rate of cell proliferation and appeared to have a slight inhibitor effect upon communication incidence (Table II), but due possibly to the low number of replicates, this effect was not significant (p=0.6). The effect of irradiation upon communication efficiency was not interpretable.

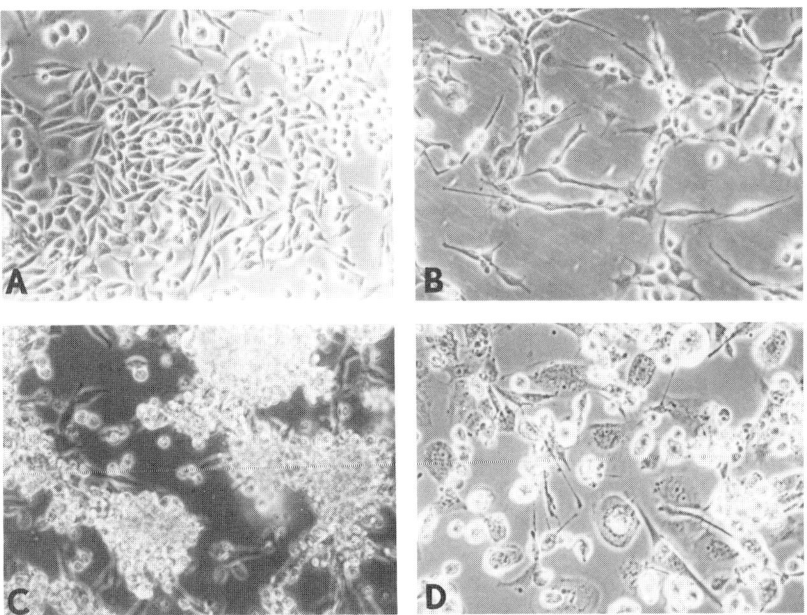

Figure 1. Appearance of DC3 cells following treatments. (A) untreated; (B) treated for 48 hr with 10 ng/ml cholera toxin; (C) treated with 10 µg/ml 25-hydroxycholesterol; (D) 72 hr after 20 Gy ^{60}Co irradiation.

Table II. Incidence of Carboxyfluorescein Transfer Among Abutting Cells

Cells/Treatment	pairs communicating total # pairs	cells (%)
Nontransformed rat granulosa cells	19/19	100
DC3 cells		
basal control	49/130	38
defined medium	6/15	40
100 uM dbcAMP	8/25	32
10 uM FSK	12/33	36
10 ng/ml CT	14/44	32
10 ug/ml 25-OHC	13/37	35
100 ng/ml 25-OHC	3/25	12
4 hr post 5 Gy	4/9	44
96 hr post 5 Gy[1]	1/9	11
4 hr post 20 Gy	7/18	39
96 hr post 20 Gy[2]	3/16	19

[1] proliferation rate inhibited by 40%
[2] proliferation rate inhibited by 72%

An extreme variability of carboxyfluorescein transfer among abutting irradiation cells was apparent, due possibly to the effects of radiation upon cell wall integrity. Some DC3 cell cultures were treated with 1 µg/ml PGE_2 before and after irradiation.

DISCUSSION

A number of properties of DC3 cells make them useful as models for the study of ovarian carcinogenesis and elements of granulosa cell differentiation[5,6]. This report emphasized those properties which might be exploited for further analyses of cellular differentiation. DC3 cells are immortalized and do not spontaneously luteinize. Under the influence of physiologically relevant stimuli, they undergo morphological alterations associated with secretion of steroids, induction of gonadotropin receptors, and exhibit modulation of intercellular communication. Each

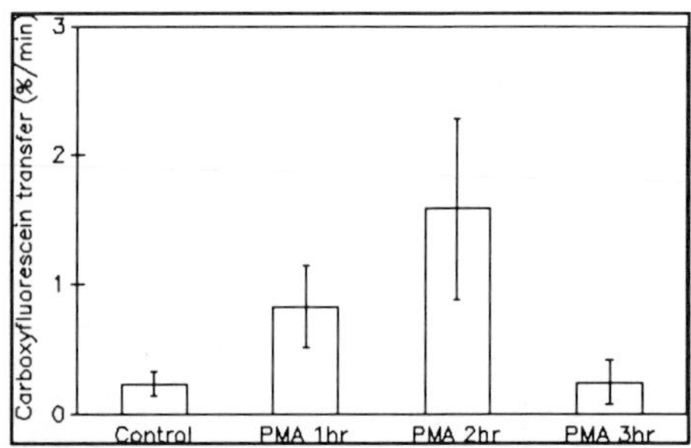

Figure 2. Effect of Phorbol Myristate Acetate (100 ng/ml) on Intercellular Communication Efficiency among DC3 Cells (mean ± sd).

of these properties correlates with properties of normal granulosa cells during differentiation.[2]

In these investigations, particular attention has been directed towards an analysis of the permeability properties of cell-cell channels which are thought to mediate the exchange of regulatory and informational molecules between cells in contact[9]. Both the incidence and efficiency of cell-cell communication in DC3 cells is considerably less than that measured in primary cultures of rat granulosa cells. This may reflect the fact that DC3 cells are less differentiated than the luteinized primary cultures but could also result as consequence of the transformation process.

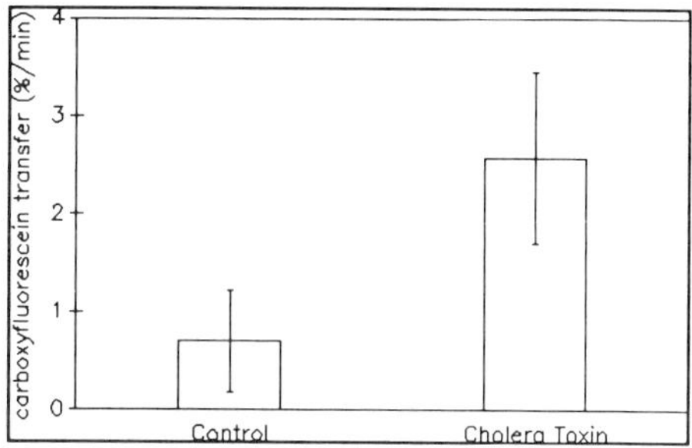

Figure 3. Effect of Cholera Toxin (0.1 ng/ml for 48 hr) on Intercellular Communication Efficiency among DC3 Cells (mean ± sd).

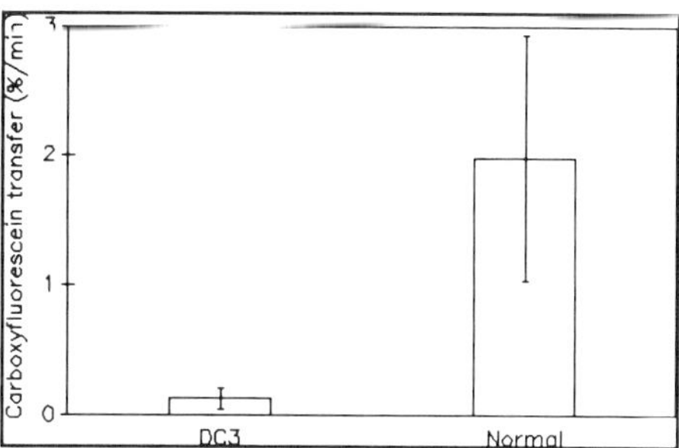

Figure 4. Intercellular Communication Efficiency; Untreated DC3 vs. Normal Granulosa Cells (mean ± sd).

Since DC3 cells retain at least a subset of the features exhibited by ovarian granulosa cells, they may prove useful for further studies of cellular differentiation in a steroid hormone-producing cell type. Furthermore, the epithelial properties of DC3 cells are particularly attractive as a model for the analysis of ovarian cancer because most in vitro model systems for multistep carcinogenesis are of fibroblast origin, yet most human cancers are derived from epithelial cells[10]. Studies are underway to examine further the roles of DC3 cells in relation both to granulosa cell functions and to tumor cell biology.

REFERENCES

1. Hsueh AJW, Adashi EY, Jones PBC, Welsh Jr TH. Endo Rev 5:76,1984.
2. Amsterdam A, Rotmensch S. Endocr Rev 8:309,1987.
3. Ying S-Y. Endocr Rev 9:267,1988.
4. Franchimont P, Demoulin A, Valcke JC. Horm Metab Res 20:193,1988.
5. Schmidt WA. In:Hirshfield AN (ed), Growth Factors and the Ovary. New York:Plenum Press, 33, 1989.
6. Fitz TA, Wah RM, Schmidt WA, Winkel CA. Biol Reprod 40:250,1989.
7. Fitz TA, Winkel CA, Marr MM, Schmidt WA, Stein LS, Burghardt RC. Manuscript submitted.
8. Wade MH, Trosko JE, Schindler M. Science 232:525,1986.
9. Loewenstein WR. Physiol Rev 61:829,1981.
10. Grunert DC. BioTechniques 8:740,1987.

EFFECTS OF THE IMMUNOSTIMULATOR CORYNEBACTERIUM PARVUM ON MOUSE NC TUMOUR GROWTH, SPREAD AND PROSTANOID FORMATION

A. BENNETT, P.B. MELHUISH and I.F. STAMFORD

Department of Surgery, King's College School of Medicine and Dentistry, London SE5 8RX, England

INTRODUCTION

The cyclo-oxygenase inhibitor indomethacin exerts an anticancer effect on mouse NC tumours (1). Since prostaglandins (PGs) can depress the immune response (2), indomethacin might act by suppressing a PG-mediated depression of the host response. We therefore examined the effect of the immunostimulant Corynebacterium parvum (C parvum) (3) on NC tumour growth and prostanoid formation. The NC tumour arose spontaneously in the mammary region of a WHT/Ht mouse, and has been transplanted continuously in the same strain (4).

MATERIALS AND METHODS

There were two separate experiments each with 9 or 10 WHT/Ht female mice (average weight 27 g) per group. Body weights were measured twice weekly from three weeks prior to the start of the experiment until death. The mice were injected sc on day 0 with 10^6NC cancer cells (1,5). On day 10 each had a palpable solid tumour into which was injected C parvum 0.5 mg as a killed vaccine (Wellcome) or 0.1 ml vehicle (methiolate in saline). The tumours were excised on day 17 under ether anaesthesia, weighed, homogenised in acidified ethanol, and extracted for prostanoids. Each mouse was examined twice daily for tumour recurrence in the excision scar and spread to lymph nodes. The mice were killed humanely if they had advanced cancer, or on day 58, and examined at postmortem.

Mouse survival time was measured from the day of inoculation with tumour cells. At postmortem the incidence of recurrence in the excision scar, lymph node involvement and distant metastases were noted. Some sections of tumours stained with haematoxylin and eosin were examined by a pathologist unaware of treatment, and specific cell types and features were scored to allow comparisons of treatments.

Prostanoid contents of the tumour extracts were determined by RIA using antisera whose cross-reactivities and sources were reported in reference (6). Since the PGE antiserum does not distinguish between PGE_1 and PGE_2, these results are expressed as PGE.

Survival was analysed by the method of Lee and Desu (7), and other data were analysed using the Mann-Whitney U-test or Fisher's exact test. All the values are medians, with semiquartile ranges in parentheses.

RESULTS

Mouse survival.

Mice treated with C parvum appeared to have a slightly (14%) longer median disease-free survival of 33 days compared with 29 days in the controls (Table 1; P=0.03). However, there was no significant difference in overall survival. The only mouse that survived to the end of the experiment was in the control group. Tumour weights seemed to be unaffected, being 450(310-540) mg in the test group compared with 400(300-470) mg in the controls (P=0.8).

Table 1

Time to the first detected spread to lymph nodes or scar recurrence, and disease-free and overall survival. C parvum or its vehicle were injected on day 10, and the tumours excised on day 17. All values are days from time of tumour transplantation.

Survival (days)	Scar Recurrence (days)	Spread to Lymph Nodes (days)	Disease-free Survival	Overall Survival
Controls 38 (37-41)	31 (24-34) n = 3	28 (27-29) n = 19	29 (27-29) n = 20	38 (37-41) n = 20
C Parvum 41 (38-45)	36 (34-39) n = 7	33 (29-35) n = 20	33 (29-35) n = 20	41 (38-45) n = 20
	P =0.15	P = 0.14	P = 0.03	P = 0.2

Tumour histology.

Generally the tumour sections showed tumour nodules composed of cells in which the nuclear cytoplasmic ratio was increased; the nuclei were pleomorphic and hyperchromatic. Several foci of necrosis were seen within the tumours, but there was no evidence of increased cellular infiltration or immune stimulation. The findings were similar in the treated and untreated groups.

Postmortem findings.

Postmortem findings were also similar in the test and control groups (Table 2). However, even though death was slightly delayed by C parvum, the spread of cancer in the two groups would be expected to be similar at the time that it killed the mice.

Tumour prostanoids.

The results are shown in Table 3. Median amounts of tumour PGE and TXB_2 from the mice given C parvum were respectively 42%, and 79% higher than controls (P=0.1 and P<0.2). The tumour 6-keto-$PGF_{1\alpha}$ was similar in the two groups (P=0.7).

Table 2

Postmortem data showed no influence of C parvum on the incidence of lymph node involvement, tumour recurrence at the excision site or lung metastasis. The results are the numbers of mice affected.

	+ve Lymph Nodes	Scar Recurrence	Lung Metastasis
Controls	19/20	5/20	17/20
C Parvum	19/20	8/20	18/20

Table 3

Effect of C parvum on tumour prostanoid formation. C parvum was injected on day 10, and the tumours were excised on day 17. The results are medians with semiquartiles in parentheses.

	PGE	6-keto-$PGF_{1\alpha}$	TXB_2
Controls	169 (154-293) n = 19	117 (59-142) n = 19	29 (20-56) n = 18
C parvum	240 (191-287) n = 20 P = 0.1	97 (56-133) n = 20 P = 0.7	52 (26-67) n = 18 P<0.2

DISCUSSION

Woodruff and Boak (3) first demonstrated the effectiveness of C parvum against an established syngeneic tumour. Since then various experimental animal models have been found to vary in their response to C parvum. Lasting regression of a mammary adenocarcinoma was demonstrated (8), and a single dose of C parvum prior to tumour excision reduced the incidence of lung metastases from transplants of Lewis lung carcinoma in C57 B1 mice (9). However, Hewitt and Blake (10) using two nonimmunogenic mouse tumours (one being the NC tumour used in the present study) showed that C parvum given prior to tumour transplantation did not modify secondary disease. Furthermore, in humans the use of C parvum is often disappointing (11-14).

Our results on the NC tumour showing only a small increase in the mouse disease-free survival with C parvum, and no significant effect on overall survival, therefore mainly agree with the findings in human cancer and those of Hewitt and Blake (10). The latter authors found that the NC tumour in WHT/Ht mice is not immunogenic, and they therefore did not expect any effect with immunostimulation. They considered that isotransplants of spontaneously arising tumours are the only appropriate models of human cancer. The contrasting results obtained with C parvum in other experimental tumours might be due to artefactual immunogenicity, a problem associated with viral or chemical induction of tumours and their allogenic transplantation. If the small increase of disease-free survival we obtained with C parvum is genuine, perhaps some immunogenicity has developed in the NC tumour during the last decade. Furthermore, any increase of the tumour PGE yield by C parvum might somewhat counteract any stimulation of the immune response with C parvum. If so, a PG synthesis inhibitor might aid an anticancer effect.

REFERENCES

1. Bennett, A., Berstock, D.A. and Carroll, M.A. Br. J. Cancer. 45: 762-768, 1982 .
2. Goodwin, J.S. J. Immunopharmac 2:397-424, 1980.
3. Woodruff, M.F.A. and Boak, J.L. Br. J. Cancer 20: 345-355, 1966.
4. Hewitt, H.B., Blake, E.R. and Walder, A.S. Br. J. Cancer 33:241-259, 1976.
5. Bennett, A., Houghton, J., Leaper, D.J. and Stamford, I.F. Prostaglandins 17:179-191, 1979.
6. Bennett, A., Melhuish, P.B. and Stamford, I.F. Br. J. Pharmac. 86:693-695, 1985.
7. Lee, E. and Desu, M. Computer Programmes in Biomedicine 2:315-321, 1972.
8. Likhite, V.V. and Halpern, B.N. Cancer Research 34:341-344, 1974.
9. Sadler, T.E. and Castro, J.E. Br. J. Surg. 63:292-296, 1976.
10. Hewitt, H.B. and Blake, E.R. Br. J. Cancer 38:219-223, 1978.
11. Von Blomberg, B.H.E., Glerum, J., Croles, J.J., Stam, J. and Drexhage, H.A. Br. J. Cancer 41:609-617, 1980.
12. Souter, R.G., Gill, P.G., Gunning, A.J. and Morriss, P.J. Br. J. Cancer 44:496-501, 1981.
13. Haskell, C.M., Sarna, G.P. and Liu, P.Y. Br. J. Cancer 45:794-795, 1982.
14. Ludwig Lung Cancer Study Group. J. Thorac. Cardiovasc. Surg. 89:842-847, 1985.

EFFECTS OF 12-HYDROXYEICOSATETRAENOIC ACID ON RELEASE OF CATHEPSIN B AND CYSTEINE PROTEINASE INHIBITORS FROM MALIGNANT MELANOMA CELLS

B.F. SLOANE, J. ROZHIN, A.P. GOMEZ, I.M. GROSSI and K.V. HONN

Departments of Pharmacology, Radiation Oncology and Chemistry, Wayne State University and Gershenson Radiation Oncology Center, Harper/Grace Hospitals, Detroit, MI 48201, USA

INTRODUCTION

The cysteine proteinase cathepsin B as well as the endogenous inhibitors of this enzyme have been implicated in the progression of tumors from a premalignant to a malignant state (for review see 1,2). Activity of cathepsin B has been shown to be elevated in parallel with malignancy or metastatic potential of both human and rodent tumors. These increases in cathepsin B activity correspond in part to increases in mRNA for cathepsin B and in part to reduced regulation by the endogenous low M_r cysteine proteinase inhibitors (CPIs). The inhibition constants for the interaction between stefin A purified from human tumors and cysteine proteinases are an order of magnitude greater than those for stefin A purified from human liver. Most properties of tumor cathepsin B appear to be similar to those of cathepsin B from normal tissues. However, the subcellular distribution of cathepsin B and CPIs is altered in tumors, resulting in association of cathepsin B and CPIs with plasma membrane fractions or in release of CPIs and of high M_r forms of cathepsin B (native and latent) into the extracellular mileau.

Many of the studies in our laboratory have used a highly malignant, spontaneously metastatic variant of the murine B16 melanoma: the B16 amelanotic melanoma (B16a). Cathepsin B activity in the B16a melanoma is high and this corresponds to high levels of cathepsin B mRNA in this tumor. A significant proportion (37%) of cathepsin B activity in the B16a melanoma is associated with plasma membrane fractions isolated by sequential differential and Percoll density gradient centrifugation. In addition, B16a cells in culture release both native and latent (pepsin activatable) forms of cathepsin B into their culture media. Cathepsin B can degrade laminin, fibronectin and type IV collagen, three components of the basement membrane. Therefore, we suggest that the presence of cathepsin B activity in the vicinity of the tumor cell surface may contribute to the local dissolution of basement membrane observed during tumor cell extravasation.

The lipoxygenase product 12(S)-hydroxyeicosatetraenoic acid, 12(S)-HETE, has been shown to modify the membrane and microfilament network of B16a cells such that surface expression of integrin receptors in B16a cells is increased (for review see 3,4 and Chapters 48, 49, and 61 this volume). Since cathepsin B and CPIs are also expressed at the surface and/or released from tumor cells, we have determined whether 12(S)-HETE alters the release of cathepsin B and CPIs from B16a cells.

MATERIALS AND METHODS

Tissue culture.

B16 amelanotic melanoma cells (Human and Animal Tumor Bank, Division of Cancer Treatment, National Cancer Institute) were obtained from primary subcutaneous tumors grown in the left axillary region of male C57Bl/6J mice (Jackson Laboratory, Bar Harbor, ME). Tumor brei was aliquoted into T75 flasks (Corning Glass, Corning, NY) containing Earle's minimal essential medium (MEM) supplemented with 5% (w/v) fetal bovine serum (Gibco, Grand Island, NY). Cells which had not adhered to the flasks at the end of 24 h (primarily host cells and cellular debris) were washed off using culture medium; adherent cells were grown to confluency as primary cultures. Confluent cultures were routinely passaged every 4th day; only cultures at passage #3 were used for these studies. Briefly, cultures grown to 80-85% confluency were washed free of serum proteins with serum-free MEM and then incubated overnight in serum-free MEM. The day of the experiment the cultures were washed once again in fresh serum-free MEM and treated (15-60 min, 37°C) with 0.1 μM (final concentration) of 12(R)- or 12(S)-hydroxyeicosatetraneonic acid diluted in 5 ml of serum-free MEM. The culture medium was collected, centrifuged at 100,000 x *g* for 60 min to remove cellular debris and concentrated 5- to 10-fold by ultrafiltration in Centricon 10 Microconcentrators (Amicon, Danvers, MA) or Millipore Centrifugal Ultrafree 10,000 NMWL UltraFilters (Millipore, Bedford, MA).

Cathepsin B assay.

Cathepsin B (EC 3.4.22.1) is released from B16a tumor cells in both active and latent (pepsin activatable) forms (1). We, therefore, assayed the culture media for native cathepsin B activity, total (pepsin activatable) cathepsin B activity and latent (total minus native) cathepsin B activity. Native cathepsin B activity was measured using a modification of our published procedure (5) in which aliquots of the media were incubated in triplicate at 37° C and pH 6.2 for 30 min with the substrate Z-Arg-Arg-NHMec (5 μM, final concentration; Enzyme Systems Products, Livermore, CA). To determine total cathepsin B activity the aliquots of media were preincubated for 60 min at pH 3.0 with pepsin (0.5 mg/ml; Sigma, St. Louis, MO) prior to assaying as above. Corrections were made for quenching by the sample.

Inhibitor assays.

To determine the levels of endogenous CPIs, we dissociated CPI-cysteine proteinase complexes by taking advantage of differences in stability of cysteine proteinases and their inhibitors (6). We tested two methods: 1) exposure to pH 11.5 for 2 h at 37° C and 2) heating at 100° C for 5 min. Since the results were similar, the data presented in this study used the simpler procedure of heating. Denatured proteins were sedimented (12,000 *g* x 10 min) and the supernatant assayed for CPI activity. Thus inhibitory activities reported in this chapter represent only those of heat stable CPIs. Inhibitory activities were determined against the commercially available plant cysteine proteinase papain (Sigma) using our published methodology (7). The activity of the papain used was determined by titration with the active site titrant L-*t*-epoxysuccinylleucylamido (4-guanidino) butane, E-64 (Sigma), as described (8). Activity of the CPIs is expressed as inhibitory units with one unit representing the amount of inhibitory protein which will completely inhibit the release by papain of one μmole of product/min.

RESULTS

B16a cells in culture were shown to release both native and latent forms of cathepsin B (Figure 1) as we had shown previously (1). Release of both native and total cathepsin B activity from B16a cells was significantly increased by incubation with 0.1 μM 12(S)-HETE for 15 min, but not by incubation with the biologically inactive isomer, 12(R)-HETE (Figure 1). In contrast, the release of latent cathepsin B activity from B16a cells was not significantly altered by incubation with either 12(S)- or 12(R)-HETE (Figure 1). The effects of 12(S)-HETE on release of cathepsin B were time dependent; values returned to control levels after 30-60 min of exposure (data not shown).

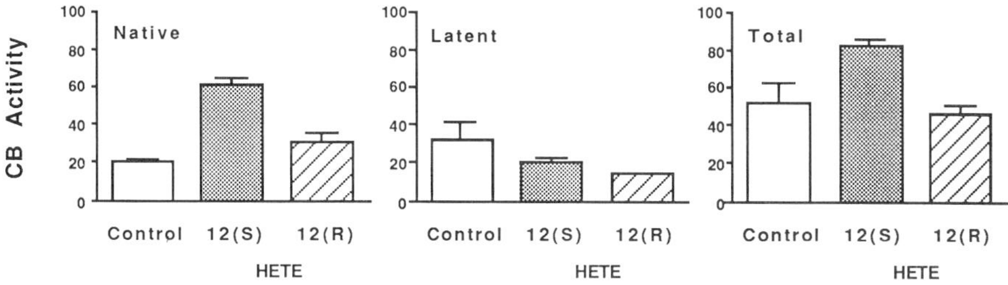

Figure 1. Cathepsin B (CB) activity released from B16 amelanotic melanoma cells after exposure to 12(S)- or 12(R)-HETE for 15 min. The control value was measured 16 h after replacing the culture media with serum-free media. Activity (native, latent or total) is expressed as pmol product per min per 10^6 cells; mean ± SD. See Materials and Methods for experimental details.

Some members of the cystatin superfamily of CPIs are extracellular proteins (for review, see 9). In addition, Nishida et al. (10) have reported that cultured human melanoma cells release CPIs. Therefore, we evaluated the effects of 12-HETE on release of heat stable CPI activities by murine B16a melanoma cells in culture. Incubation with 12(S)-HETE for 15 min resulted in a 40% decrease in the activity of heat stable CPIs in the media of B16a cells (Figure 2). Here again, the effect was time dependent, the decreased release of CPI activity was restored to control with longer times of exposure to 12(S)-HETE (data not shown). The biologically inactive isomer 12(R)-HETE did not affect release of CPI activity (Figure 2).

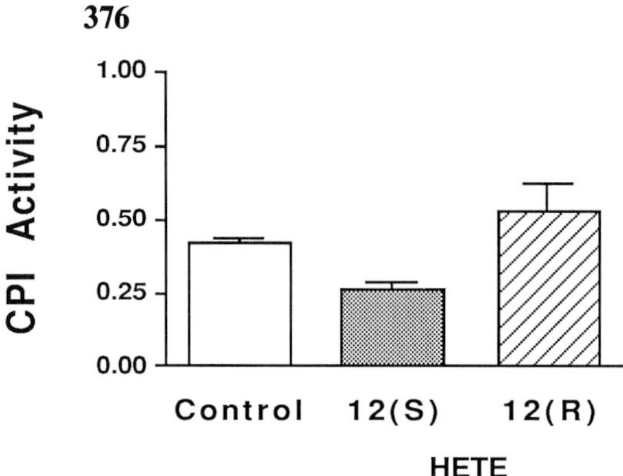

Figure 2. Cysteine proteinase inhibitor activity released from B16 amelanotic melanoma cells after exposure to 12(S)- or 12(R)-HETE for 15 min. The control value was measured 16 h after replacing the culture media with serum-free media. Activity is expressed as units per 10^6 cells; mean $\pm$ SD. See Materials and Methods for experimental details.

The ability of 12(S)-HETE to affect release of both cathepsin B and its endogenous inhibitors from B16a cells in culture could lead to activities of cathepsin B at the surface of B16a tumor cells different than one would predict based on a direct assay of cathepsin B activity in the culture medium, i.e., an assay performed in the presence of various levels of CPIs. Based on a 1:1 binding of cysteine proteinases and their endogenous low M_r CPIs, we have performed an arbitrary calculation of the possible "effective activity" of cathepsin B (i.e., CB/CPI). Exposure to 12(S)-HETE for 15 min significantly increased the "effective activities" of native and total cathepsin B (CB/CPI) above control values, but not the "effective activity" of latent cathepsin B (Figure 3). Exposure to 12(R)-HETE did not result in CB/CPI ratios significantly different from control values (Figure 3).

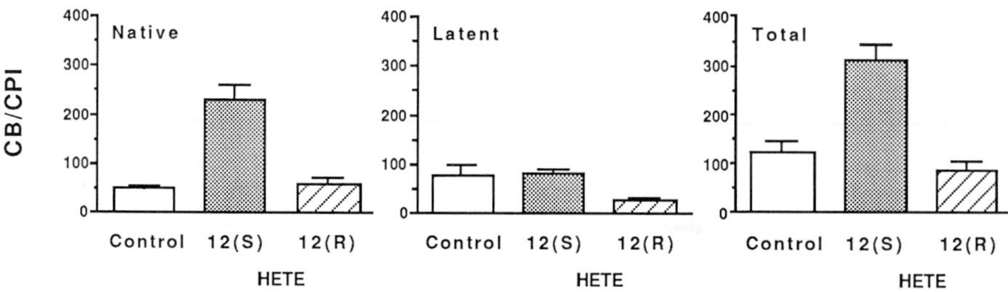

Figure 3. Potential "effective activity" of cathepsin B released from B16 amelanotic melanoma cells after exposure to 12(S)- or 12(R)-HETE for 15 min. "Effective activity" is expressed as an arbitrary ratio between native, latent and total cathepsin B activities and cysteine proteinase inhibitor activity. All values are per 10^6 cells; mean $\pm$ SD. The control value was measured 16 h after replacing the culture media with serum-free media. See Materials and Methods for experimental details.

DISCUSSION

Results from our laboratories suggest that lipoxygenase products may interact in several steps of the metastatic cascade (for review see 3,4 and Chapters 48, 49, and 61 this volume). The results presented in this chapter suggest that by regulating release of the cysteine proteinase cathepsin B and its endogenous inhibitors into the local microenvironment surrounding the tumor cell, 12(S)-HETE may contribute indirectly to the focal dissolution of the basement membrane underlying tumor cells as they undergo extravasation from the vasculature into metastatic sites.

ACKNOWLEDGMENTS

This work was supported in part by Public Health Service grants (CA 36481 and CA 48210) from the National Institutes of Health and grants from Ono Pharmaceuticals (Osaka, Japan) and Harper/Grace Hospitals. BFS is the recipient of Research Career Development Award (CA 00921) from the National Institutes of Health.

REFERENCES

1. Sloane, B.F., Rozhin, J., Hatfield, J.S., Crissman, J.D. and Honn, K.V. Exp. Cell Biol. 55: 209-224, 1987.
2. Sloane, B.F., Moin, K., Krepela, E, and Rozhin, J. Cancer Metastasis Rev. 9:333-352, 1990.
3. Weiss, L., Orr, F.W. and Honn, K.V. FASEB J. 2: 12-21, 1988.
4. Grossi, I.M., Fitzgerald, L.A., Umbarger, L.A., Nelson, K.K., Diglio, C.A., Taylor, J.D. and Honn, K.V. Cancer Res. 49: 1029-1037, 1989.
5. Rozhin, J., Robinson, D., Stevens, M. A., Lah, T. T., Honn, K. V., Ryan, R. E. and Sloane, B. F. Cancer Res. 47: 6620-6628, 1987.
6. Green, G.D.J., Kembhavi, A.A., Davies, M.E. and Barrett, A.J. Biochem. J. 218: 939-946, 1984.
7. Rozhin, J., Wade, R.L., Honn, K.V. and Sloane, B.F. Biochem. Biophys. Res. Commun. 164: 556-561, 1989.
8. Barrett, A. J., Kembhavi, A. A., Brown, M. A., Kirschke, H., Knight, C. J., Tamai, M. and Hanada, K. Biochem. J. 201: 189-198,1982.
9. Barrett, A.J. Trends in Biochem. Sci. 12: 193-196, 1987.
10. Nishida, Y. Sumi, H. and Mihara, H. Cancer Res. 44: 3324-3329, 1984.

ROLE OF ARACHIDONIC ACID IN COLLAGENASE IV PRODUCTION AND MALIGNANT BEHAVIOR OF TUMOR CELLS

R. REICH*[1], L. ROYCE*, S.H. ADLER*, G.R. MARTIN**, R.A. PARTIS***, and R.A. MUELLER***

Laboratory of Developmental Biology and Anomalies, NIDR, NIH Bethesda, MD 20892, **Gerontology Research Center, NIA, NIH Baltimore, MD 21224, ***Molecular and Cellular Biology Department, G.D.Searle, Co. Skokie, IL 60077

The spread of cancer from the original lesion is a critical event in cancer etiology, placing the tumor beyond conventional modes of treatment. Indeed, metastasis is the major cause of death in cancer (1). The actual success of a given tumor cell to metastasize depends on numerous factors including the invasiveness of the tumor cell, the host's immune system and local factors which support the growth of the tumor at different sites (2-4). During metastasis the cells must breach numerous barriers to their invasion and dissemination. These barriers include stromal matrix, basement membranes and cellular layers. Because of the diversity of these barriers, the penetration of the cells must involve proteolytic enzymes.

Basement membranes are ubiquitous structures which provide structural support to all epithelial tissues, they act as a molecular filter preventing the passage of proteins, and they also act as barriers to the passage of most cells. The breaching of basement membranes by malignant tumor cells is thought to be a critical step in metastasis (5). Various studies have concentrated on the enzymatic mechanisms used by the metastatic cells (6-8). Initially, the tumor cells adhere to the matrix via a variety of surface receptors. Once anchored, tumor cells secrete proteolytic enzymes or induce host cells to do so and cause a local[0] degradation of the extracellular matrix. Degradation of basement membranes requires a specific collagenase because the structural protein in the matrix is a unique collagen (type IV) which is not susceptible to interstitial collagenases (9).

Little is known of the biochemical mechanisms or the regulation involved in the initiation of specific proteinase secretion (10-12). Recently we have found that metabolites of arachidonic acid are required for tumor cell invasion through basement membranes in vitro and for their metastasis (13). The cyclooxgenase and the lipoxygenase pathways were found to be involved in the regulation of collagenase IV production and when inhibited, tumor cells become non-invasive. We have shown that specific metabolites of cyclooxygenase and 5-lipoxygenase pathways are required for the expression of

---

[1]Present address- Dept of Pharmacology, Faculty of Medicine, Hebrew Univ. of Jerusalem, Jerusalem 91010, Israel

the malignant activity of tumor cells, but do not induce malignant characteristics by themselves. In this study, we show that a highly specific 5-lipoxygenase inhibitor given to the tumor cells or given orally to mice, prevents the invasion of basement membranes in vitro and metastasis formation in vivo, respectively.

MATERIALS AND METHODS

Cell Lines and Culture Conditions.

Human fibrosarcoma, (HT-1080 cells) (CCL 121), derived from a metastatic lesion, were obtained from the American Type Culture Collection, Rockville, MD. Murine melanoma B16F10 cells were provided by Dr. I.J. Fidler, M.D. Anderson Hospital, Houston, TX. The cells were maintained under an atmosphere of 5% CO_2, Dulbecco's Minimal Essential Medium (DMEM) and MEM respectively, supplemented with 10% fetal calf serum, glutamine, vitamins, non-essential amino acids and antibiotics.

Chemoinvasion Assay.

The chemoinvasion assay was performed as previously described (14). Briefly, polyvinylpyrrolidone-free polycarbonate filters, 8 μm pore size (Nucleopore, Pleasanton, CA), were coated with a mixture of basement membrane components (Matrigel) (25 μg/filter) and placed in modified Boyden chambers. The cells (2×10^5) were released from their culture dishes by short exposure to EDTA (1mM), centrifuged, re-suspended in 0.1% BSA/DMEM, and placed in the upper compartment of the Boyden chamber. Fibroblast conditioned medium was placed in the lower compartment as a source of chemoattractants (14). After incubation for 6 h at 37°C the cells on the lower surface of the filter were stained with Diff-Quick (American Scientific Products, McGaw, IL) and were quantified with an image analyzer (Optomax V) attached to a Olympus CK2 microscope. The data are expressed as the area in μm^2 per field occupied by the cells on the lower surface of the filter, a value proportional to the number of cells.

Collagenase Assay.

The proteolytic degradation of collagen IV by collagenase IV was measured using a modified solid phase radioassay (8). Briefly, collagen IV was purified from EHS tumor tissue (gift from Dr. Roy Ogle, LDBA) and was labelled with [^{125}I] by the Bolton-Hunter method. A solution of the labelled collagen (10,000-20,000 cpm) was applied to microtiter plates (Removawell, Dynatech, Chantilly, VA) and allowed to bind overnight. Aliquots of media taken from the Boyden chamber after the termination of the assay were added to the collagen-coated microtiter plates for 24 h at 37°C and the amount of radioactivity released from the solid phase in the presence of a serine proteinase inhibitor (ε-aminocaproic acid) was measured.

Experimental Metastasis.

B16F10 tumor cells (2×10^5 in 0.2ml), some of which had been treated in culture with various inhibitors and metabolites, were injected into the tail vein of mice (C57BL/6). Three weeks later, the mice were sacrificed by cervical dislocation and the number of melanotic lesions on the surface of the lungs was counted. Each experiment was repeated twice and each group of animals in these experiments included 10 mice.

RESULTS

In vitro systems have been developed that allow the individual steps, in particularly invasion to be analyzed. This chemoinvasion system allowed us to study the enzymatic mechanisms involved in the invasion of basement membranes by tumor cells and screen for inhibitors of metastasis.

Invasion in vitro.

Previous studies have shown that metastatic tumor cells readily penetrate through the reconstituted basement membrane used in our experiments while benign tumors or normal cells do not. When inhibitors of cyclooxygenase or mixed inhibitors of lipoxygenase and cyclooxygenase were added to the cells in culture, the ability of the cells to invade through reconstituted basement membrane was significantly reduced (13). Our studies showed that specific prostanoid, $PGF_{2\alpha}$, and a product of 5-lipoxygenase were required for collagenase IV production, invasiveness and metastasis. In the present study, we used a novel, highly specific 5-lipoxygenase inhibitor (SC-41661) and tested its effect on the invasive potential of malignant tumor cells. Cells when exposed to different doses of the inhibitor for 18 h prior to the assay, showed reduced invasiveness. SC-41661 is a selective 5-lipoxygenase inhibitor in vitro (15). The IC_{50} is 0.15 μM against RBL-1 derived 5-lipoxygenase. The compound also inhibits the production of LTC_4/D_4 by RBL-1 cells in culture (IC_{50} 1.6 μM). SC-41661 does not inhibit ram seminal vesicle cyclooxygenase, soybean 15-lipoxygenase or human platelet 12-lipoxygenase at doses up to 100 μM.

Collagenase production.

Production of collagen IV degrading enzymes has been found to be correlated with metastatic potential and collagenase IV is required for cells to invade through basement membranes. We have investigated both extracellular events and intracellular reactions involved in invasion. Our previous studies have shown that inhibitors of both cyclooxygenase and lipoxygenase pathways reduce the production of collagenase IV in a dose-dependent manner (13). In the present study, we measured the effect of a specific 5-lipoxygenase inhibitor on induction of collagenase IV activity in vitro. The drug reduced the collagenase IV activity in a dose dependent manner.

Metastasis formation.

Since collagenase IV activity is essential for metastasis formation and the lipoxygenase inhibitor reduced collagenase IV activity in vitro, we tested its effect on lung colonization using the experimental metastasis model (Figure 1). Since the drug has high bioavilability, we tested its effect in several ways: a) pretreatent in vitro- the tumor cells were treated with different doses of the drug for 18 h and injected into syngeneic mice; b) treatment in vivo- the mice were fed with different doses of the drug starting day'-1' (one day before the injection of the tumor cells) and treated daily for 21 days (end of the experiment); c)

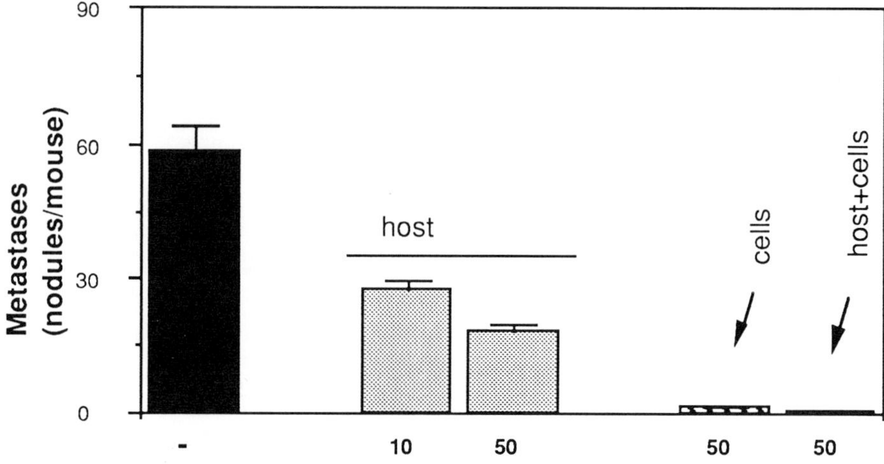

Figure1. The effect of SC-41661 on the formation of melanotic lung lesions 21 days post injection of the tumor cells.

combination of a and b- namely, the tumor cells were treated in vitro before injection and the mice were fed for the whole period of the experiment.

Our results show that the drug was effective in reducing colony formation in the lungs in all treatments. The combined treatment was found to be the most effective.

SUMMARY

Several studies have shown that the growth of certain tumors is altered in animals treated with cyclooxygenase inhibitors such as aspirin, flurbiprofen and indomethacin. In recent studies, we treated tumor cells in vitro with either cyclooxygenase or mixed lipoxygenase-cyclooxygenase inhibitors and then injected those cells into mice. These studies showed that the invasive activity of the cells required both pathways of arachidonic acid metabolism through $PGF_{2\alpha}$ and lipoxygenase dependent reactions. In the present studies, we tested the effect of a highly specific 5-lipoxygenase inhibitor, SC-41661, on metastasis formation in experimental models. The advantage of this drug besides its high specificity as 5-lipoxygenase inhibitors, is in its high oral bioavailability and lack of toxicity at the concentrations tested for long period of time.

It should be noted that the manner in which the metabolites of arachidonic acid function in the production of collagenase IV is not known but may involve cellular receptors that modulate gene transcription. Further, it is not known what additional cellular function may be altered by inhibition of 5-lipoxygenase. One should not rule out an effect on the immune system which is known to be modulated by metabolites of arachidonic acid.

REFERENCES

1. Sugarbaker, E.V., Weingarg, D.N., Roseman, J.M. (1982). Observations on cancer metastases in Cancer Invasion and Metastasis. ed LA Liotta, IR Hart Boston, Martinuf Nighoff pp. 427-465.
2. Fidler, I.J. Gersten, D.M., Hart, I.R. (1978). The biology of cancer invasion and metastasis. Adv Cancer Res 28,149-250.
3. Weiss, L., Ward, P.M. (1983). Cell detachment and metastasis. Cancer Metastasis Rev. 2, 111-123.
4. Liotta, L.A., Mandler, R., Murano, G., Katz, D.A., Gordon, R.K., Chiang, P.K., Schiffmann E (1986). Tumor cell autocrine motility factor. Proc. Natl. Acad. Sci USA 83, 3302-3306.
5. Terranova, V.P., Hujanen, E.S., Martin, G.R. (1986). Basement membrane and the invasive activity of metastatic tumor cells. JNCI 77, 311-316.
6. Mullins, D.E., Rohrlich, S.T. (1983). The role of proteinases in cellular invasiveness. Biochim. Biophys. Acta 695,177-214.
7. Mignatti, P., Robbins, E., Rifkin, D.B. (1986). Tumor invasion through the human amniotic membrane: requirement for a proteinase cascade. Cell 67, 687-698.
8. Reich, R., Thompson, E., Iwamoto, Y., Martin, G.R., Deason, J.R., Fuller, G.C., Miskin, R. (1988) . Inhibition of plasminogen activator, serine proteinases and collagenase IV prevents the invasion of basement membranes by metastatic cells. Cancer Research 48, 3307-3312.
9. Liotta, L.A., Abe, S., Gehron-Robey, P., Martin, G.R. (1979). Preferential digestion of basement membrane collagen by an enzyme derived from a metastatic murine tumor. Proc. Natl. Acad. Sci USA 76, 2268-2272.
10. Turpeenniemi-Hujanen, T., Thorgeirsson, U.P., Rao, C.N., Liotta, L.A. (1986). Laminin increases the release of type IV collagenase from malignant cells. J Biol.Chem 4 1883-1889.
11. Iwamoto, Y., Robey, F.A., Graf, J., Sasaki, M., Kleinman, H.K., Yamada, Y., Martin, G.R. (1987) Science 238,1132-1134.
12. Kleinman, H.K., McGarvey, M.L., Hassell, J.R., Star, V.L., Cannon, F.B., Laurie, G.W., Martin, G.R. (1986). Basement membrane complexes with biological activities. Biochemistry 25, 312-318.
13. Reich, R., Martin, G.R. Identification of arachidonic acid pathways required for the invasive and metastatic activity of malignant tumor cells. Cancer Research (in press).
14. Albini, A., Iwamoto, Y., Kleinman, H.K., Martin, G.R., Aaronson, S.A., Kozlowski, J.M., McEwan, R.N. (1987). A rapid in vitro assay for quantitating the invasive potential of tumor cells Cancer Research 47, 3239-3245.
15. Nakao, A., Yang, D-C, Jungi, G., Partis, R.A., Mueller, R.A. in preparation, USA patent 4,663,333.

EFFECTS OF EICOSANOID ANALOGS ON TUMOR GROWTH AND METASTASIS

EICOSANOIDS AND RADIOPROTECTION OF CULTURED CELLS

D.B. RUBIN*, E.A. DRAB*, T.L. WALDEN, JR.[t], and W.R. HANSON[tt]

*Departments of Medicine and Therapeutic Radiology, Rush-Presbyterian-St. Luke's Medical Center, Chicago, IL 60612, [t]Armed Forces Radiobiology Research Institute, Biochemistry Division, Bethesda MD, [tt]Loyola University, Department of Radiotherapy, Hines IL

INTRODUCTION

A number of studies have shown in vivo that many eicosanoids are cytoprotective to cell renewal systems of the intestine (1) and bone marrow (2) when given before irradiation. Also, pretreatment with certain eicosanoids have enhanced survival of irradiated mice (3). Although evidence suggests that the eicosanoids protect by first binding to specific receptors (4), the subsequent events that lead to radiation protection by the eicosanoids is not known.

Prior Studies In Vitro: the role of cyclic AMP.

Reports of in vitro studies on radiation protection by eicosanoids have been less consistant in their results and conclusions than those in vivo. In the earliest reports on the prostaglandin effect, both Prasad (5) and Lehnert (6) reported in vitro radiation protection of CHO cells and V-79 cells respectively by PGE_1. Ironically, this is the one compound that has been shown to have no radioprotective activity in vivo in the mouse intestine (7). Both investigators speculated that the protective mechanism of PGE_1 was due to an elevation of cyclic AMP. Prasad noted that a phosphodiesterase inhibitor enhanced reproductive integrity following irradiation but he did not measure cyclic AMP. Lehnert did document by radioimmunoassay an elevation of cyclic AMP one hour after PGE_1 exposure. However, radioprotection by the prostaglandin was noted only at lower doses while prostaglandin-induced radiosensitization was observed above 12 Gy. Similar to Prasad's observation, Lehnert noted radioprotection after phosphodiesterase inhibition which she associated with an elevation of cyclic AMP.

In contrast, later investigations by Millar and Jinks (8) were unable to demonstrate radiation protection in V-79 cell lines using PGE_1 and PGA. Their methods differed from the two earlier studies by using both a lower concentration of PGE_1 (1 vs 10 ug/ml) and a more prolonged drug exposure prior to irradiation (overnight to 3 days versus 1 to 3 hours). Millar et al. (9) also could not modify survival curves of irradiated cell lines following treatments non-steroidal anti-inflammatory agents.

Lastly, Walden et al. (10) reported slight radiation protection by pretreating V-79 cells with LTC_4. However, their later investigations with PGE_2 (11) failed to demonstrate radioprotection in vitro in cell lines from transformed rat granulosa and mouse fibrosarcoma. Similar to our investigations cited below, the cell lines lacked specific binding for PGE_2.

Prior Studies In Vitro: other mechanisms.

The controversy of eicosanoid-induced radioprotection in vitro has been further fueled by more recent studies. Holahan and co-workers (12) failed to find protection induced by 16-16 dimethyl PGE_2 in V-79 cells; however, if these cells were first depleted of glutathione by glutathione synthetase inhibition, prostaglandin-induced radiation protection could then be shown.

Other mechanisms related to eicosanoid-induced radioprotection in vitro have been suggested by the studies of Hanson et al. (13). M-1 melanoma cells were not protected from radiation by 16-16-dimethyl-PGE_2 when the cells were grown as a monolayer. However, when grown as spheroids, these cells were radioprotected by the prostaglandin. This observation suggests the possible importance of cell to cell contact or the possibility of an interaction of the growth media when in direct contact with cells on eicosanoid-induced production.

Eicosanoids and Radioprotection of Vascular Endothelial Cell In Vitro.

Vascular endothelial cells are important clinical targets of radiation (14). Indeed, the radiation response of vascular endothelial cells may be critical to the response of vascularized tumors as well as the dose-limiting factor for normal tissues in radiation therapy. Based on evidence that the eicosanoids are radioprotective in vivo, in vitro studies were done to investigate radioprotection by several eicosanoids in cultures of bovine aortic endothelial cells.

The cells were irradiated (0-500 cGy, ^{137}Cs) one hour after the addition of the following eicosanoids: PGD_2, PGE_1, PGI_2, misoprostol (PGE_1-analog), 16-16-dimethyl-PGE_2, PGA_1 and LTC_4. All prostaglandins were added at a concentration of 10 ug/ml and the leukotriene at 1 ug/ml. Radiation protection was assayed using indexes of cell loss and inhibition of DNA synthesis 4 to 24 hrs after irradiation. In addiation, radiation protection was assessed using clonogenicity as a measure of cell survival. Reduced [^3H] thymidine incorporation followed by cell loss from the irradiated cell monolayers 24 hours post exposure could be demonstrated. Clonogenic capability as a measure of reproductive death was also reduced. In contrast to in vivo radioprotection, the eicosanoids did not attenuate the radiation-induced damage in these cultured cells. One eicosanoid, PGD_2, appeared to be toxic, but all other compounds tested had no apparent effect.

In order to determine why eicosanoid treatments failed to be radioprotective, we looked for evidence of an eicosanoid-receptor by measuring radioligand binding of [^3H] PGE_2 and [^3H] LTC_4 and by measuring levels of endothelial cyclic AMP. Evidence for specific receptors was not found, although non-specific endothelial cell binding of LTC_4 and metabolism of LTC_4 to LTD_4 was observed. Cyclic AMP was elevated by 16-16 dimethyl PGE_2 in the presence of isobutylmethylxanthine. However, a combination of the PG and methylxanthine was not radioprotective. These investigations suggest that an elevation of cAMP levels does not reflect a radioprotective mechanism of eicosanoids and that there might be a link between the radioprotective effect of eicosanoids and the expression of eicosanoid receptors in cultured endothelial cells.

CONCLUSIONS AND SPECULATIONS

Despite well documented radioprotection in vivo, the cell biology of enhanced survival following eicosanoid treatment remains unclear. The bulk of evidence indicates that cells in vitro are not readily protected from radiation damage by eicosanoids. Inability to express eicosanoid receptors, perhaps either due to their absence or masking, appears to be an important explanation for this lack of an effect. Our investigations and those of Millar et al. (9) suggest that a boost of cyclic AMP levels is not key to radioprotection by the eicosanoids; however, studies by Holahan et al. (12) imply involvement of glutathione metabolism. Future work on the cell biology of this phenomenon will focus on the expression of eicosanoid receptors in vitro and on the effect of eicosanoids in anti-oxident defenses.

ACKNOWLEDGMENTS

This work was supported by, NIH HL-41155-02, The American Cancer Society, Illinois Division, Inc., The Upjohn Company, Rush University, and the Department of Defense.

REFERENCES

1. Hanson, W.R., and Thomas, C. Radiat. Res. 96:393-398, 1983.
2. Hanson, W.R., Jarnagin, W., DeLaurentiis, K., and Malkinson, F.D. In: Prostaglandin and Lipid Metabolism in Radiation Injury (Eds. Walden, Jr., T.L., and Hughes, H.M.), Plenum Press, New York, 1987, pp. 331-338.
3. Walden, Jr., T.L., Patchen, L., and Snyder, S.L., Radiat. Res. 109:540-549, 1987.
4. Hanson, W.R., Houseman, K.A., Nelson, A.K., and Collins, P.W. Prostaglandins Leukotrienes and Essential Fatty Acids, 32:101-105, 1988.
5. Prasad, K.N. Int. J. Radiat. Biol. 22:187-189, 1972.
6. Lehnert, S. Radiat. Res. 62:107-116, 1975.
7. Hanson, W.R., DeLaurentiis, K. Prostaglandins. 33 (suppl.):93-104, 1987.
8. Millar, B.C., and Jinks, S. Int. J. Radiat. Biol. 46:367-373, 1984.
9. Millar, B.C., Jinks, S., and Powles, T.J. Br. J. Cancer, 44:733-740, 1981.
10. Walden, Jr., T.L., Holahan, E.V., and Catravas, G.N. Prog. Lipid Res. 25:587-590, 1986.
11. Farzaneh, N.K., Speicher, J.M., Fitz, T., and Walden, Jr., T.L., 37th Radiation Research Society Meeting. p. 186a, 1989.
12. Holahan, Jr., E.V., Blakely, W.F., Walden, Jr., T.L. In: Prostaglandin and Lipid Metabolism in Radiation Injury (Eds. Walden, Jr., T.L., and Hughes, H.M.), Plenum Press, New York, 1987, pp. 253-262.
13. Hanson, W.R., DeLaurentiis, K. Proceedings of the American Association for Cancer Research. 26:68a, 1985.
14. Hopewell, J.W., In: Radiation Biology in Cancer Research (Eds. Meyn, R.E., and Withers, H.R.) Raven, New York, 1980, pp. 449-459).

INCREASED MOUSE SURVIVAL BY 16,16-DIMETHYL PROSTAGLANDIN E2 PRETREATMENT AND/OR BONE MARROW TRANSPLANTATION AFTER SUPRA-LETHAL WHOLE BODY IRRADIATION

L. BERK*, K. PATRENE and S. BOGGS

Department of Radiation Oncology, University of Pittsburgh School of Medicine, University of Pittsburgh, Pittsburgh, PA 15261 *now at the Department of Radiation Oncology, University of Pennsylvania, Philadelphia, PA 19104

INTRODUCTION

There is increasing interest in treating tumors with higher doses of radiation or chemotherapy than normal tissues can withstand. The two organs at the highest risk for acute toxicity during systemic treatment are the hematopoietic system and the intestinal mucosa (1). Several studies have shown that many leukotrienes and prostaglandins, including 16,16-dimethyl prostaglandin E2 (dmPGE2), are radioprotective (2). DmPGE2 has been shown to protect the intestinal mucosa as measured by microcolony assays (3), the hematopoietic system as measured by endogenous spleen colony assays (4) and increase overall survival after total body irradiation (TBI) (5). Several intensive treatment protocols for cancer therapy utilize autologous bone marrow transplantation (BMT) to allow otherwise lethal doses of chemotherapy or radiation to be given. It was therefore of interest to see if the combination of prostaglandins and BMT could protect mice from even higher doses of TBI.

METHOD

Mice used for all experiments were 12-26 wk old, 23-25 gm female C57BL-6J x DBA/2JF1 (BDF1) from Jackson Laboratories (Bar Harbor, Maine). They were housed 5-6/cage with acidified water and food ad libitum.

The dmPGE2 (Upjohn, Kalamazoo, MI) was received dissolved in methyl acetate at 10 mg/ml. The solvent was removed with flowing nitrogen and then the dmPGE2 was resuspended in absolute methanol at 4 mg/ml. This was diluted with normal saline to 0.2 mg/ml. All solutions were prepared within one hr of use. Twenty micrograms (0.1 ml) of the dmPGE2 was injected subcutaneously at the nape of the neck 10 to 20 mins before irradiation. This allowed an interval of less than 30 mlns between injection and the midpoint of the irradiation.

The mice were irradiated in batches of 20 in a rotating lucite container. They received 0.97 Gy/min form a Model 68 ^{137}cS Irradiator (J.L. Sheppard and Associates, San Fernando, CA). Two to three hrs after irradiation the mice received tail vein injections of 0.2 ml Hanks' solution with or without 2 x 10^{6} freshly harvested syngeneic bone marrow cells.

After treatment the mice were monitored for survival twice a day. All mice which died during the first

7 days had heart punctures, and their blood was cultured on blood agar for Pseudomonas. No Pseudomonas was found.

Peripheral cell counts were obtained by retroorbital puncture. Samples were lysed with Zap-oglobin II and counted. Iron uptake was determined to measure erythropoiesis. Seventeen hrs after intraperitoneal injection of 0.1 uCi of ^{59}Fe (Amersham, England) the mice were killed, spleens were harvested, weighed, fixed in Bouin's solution and counted to determine ^{59}Fe uptake.

RESULT

Figure 1A shows that animals not given any treatment died within 10 days at all the radiation doses used. As the TBI dose was decreased from 18 to 14 Gy there was a slight extension of time of death from a median of 5 days to a median of 7.5 days. Death rate in those groups with BMT as their only treatment (Figure 1B) decreased markedly as the radiation dose was decreased. All of the deaths in these animals occurred within 10 days, except one which occurred on day 11. In those groups treated with only dmPGE2 (Figure 1C) and given 18 or 16 Gy TBI the animals died in a pattern similar to BMT alone in that death occurred within 10 days. However, as the radiation dose was decreased to 15 Gy the pattern changed, and a large fraction of mice died after 10 days. At 14 Gy these mice suffered a very small percentage of deaths during the first 10 days but then died between 10 and 20 days. These later deaths were largely absent in mice given both BMT and dmPGE2 (Figure 1D).

Table 1 shows the peripheral white blood cell (WBC) count on days 1, 2, 7, and 9 after 14 Gy. It can be seen that there was a marked rise in the WBC count for the group with BT alone and a more subdued increased in the group given combined BMT and prostaglandin. There was no rise in the peripheral WBC count for the untreated mice. On day 7 the prostaglandin treated mice showed a significant decrease from control and on day 9 the counts were even lower but not significantly lower than the controls.

Table 2 shows data for the marrow cellularity and for spleen wt and iron uptake 5 days after 14 Gy TBI. Only the BMT group had significant increases in these values.

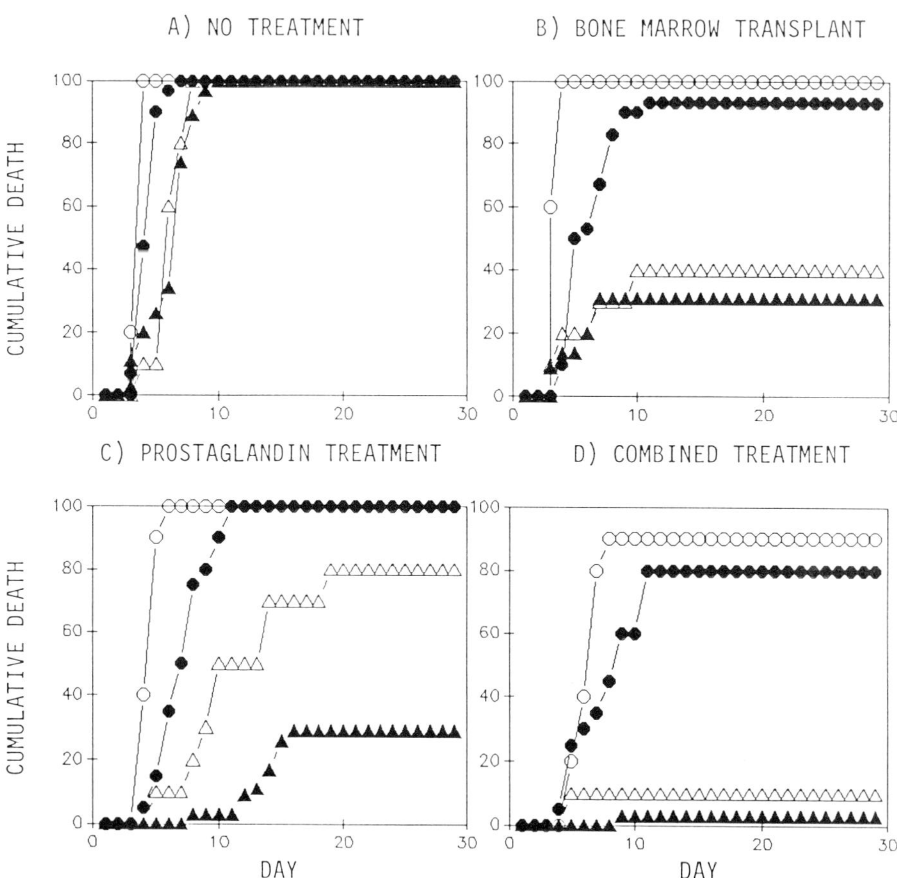

Figure 1. Death rates in mice given no treatment (A), BMT (B), dmPGE2 (C) and dmPGE2 plus BMT (D). The TBI doses used were 18 Gy (open circles), 16 Gy (closed circles), 15 Gy (open triangles) and 14 Gy (closed triangles). The numbers of mice were 35 for 14 Gy, 10 for 15 Gy, 20 for 16 Gy groups given dmPGE2, 30 for 16 Gy groups given no treatment or BMT and 10 for the 18 Gy groups. The mice were given TBI alone or 20 ug dmPGE2 was given subcutaneously 10-20 min before TBI with or without intravenous injection of 2 x 10^6 bone marrow cells 3 hrs after TBI. Generalized Wilcoxon p values for treatment groups comparad to nontreated controls are $\leq$ 0.05 for all groups given dmPGE2 plus BMT, for all but the 18 Gy group given dmPGE2 alone, all but the 16 Gy group given BMT alone and the combined treatment exceeds dmPGE2 alone for 15 and 18 Gy and BMT alone for 16 and 18 Gy.

Table 1. Effect of treatment on blood leukocytes after 14 Gy TBI.

Day	1	3	7	9
none	1166 ± 120	678 ± 400	835 ± 166	526 ± 282
BMT	1098 ± 57	577 ± 57	1662 + 588	6164 + 4148
dmPGE2	1148 ± 111	726 ± 172	363 + 52	269 + 83
dmPGE2 + BMT	1128 ± 97	1041 ± 179	2861 + 708	2843 + 1880

values are geometric means ± 1 SE
underlined values differ from controls at $p \leq 0.05$
groups contained 5 mice at the beginning but because of deaths control and BMT groups only had 4 mice on day 9

Table 2. Effect of treatment on marrow cellularity, spleen wt and splenic erythropoiesis 5 days after 14 Gy TBI.

Treatment	Nucleated cells/humerus (thousands)	Spleen wt (mg)	Spleen ^{59}Fe uptake (cpm)
none	792 ± 143	17 ± 1	650 ± 33
BMT	1087 + 60	26 + 2	856 ± 56
dmPGE2	633 ± 58	18 ± 1	513 ± 44
dmPGE2 + BMT	914 ± 108	28 ± 5	699 ± 114

values are mean ± 1 SE
underlined values differ from controls at $p \leq 0.01$
4-5 mice/group

DISCUSSION

Mice were protected by both BMT and by dmPGE2 treatment. The protection by BMT may be mediated by the earlier repopulation of the peripheral WBC. The timing of the rise in counts correlates well with the 5-10 day phase of death. This early phase is thought to be due to a combination of lowered blood cell defenses and bacterial leakage into the blood as well as metabolic losses due to denuding of the intestinal epithelium (3). Previous studies have shown accelerated regeneration of the intestinal mucosa with prostaglandin pretreatment (4). Therefore one can postulate that the protection from death seen in dmPGE2 treated animals could be due to earlier repopulation or delayed denuding of the intestinal mucosa and that protection by BMT could be due to earlier recovery of the peripheral WBC count. If this is true then it would be expected that the combination of the two would have an additive or supra-additive effect, and that the dmPGE2 treated mice would be more susceptible to late death due to failure of the marrow to continue to repopulate. Both of these predictions were seen to be true. It should be noted that the dmPGE2 treated mice have significant survival at doses which are lethal to the hematopoietic system (the LD_{99} for these mice is approximately 9.5 Gy). This is consistent with the radioprotective effects on hematopoietic spleen colonies (4) which are usually erythroid, but our data suggest that WBC recovery was suppressed by dmPGE2.

CONCLUSIONS

The results presented confirm that pretreatment with dmPGE2 or BMT protects mice from otherwise lethal TBI doses. Further, the combination of BMT with dmPGE2 pretreatment increased the survival after TBI doses beyond that of either individual treatment. The protection due to BMT seems to arise from the earlier repopulation of peripheral WBC as well as repopulation of the marrow. Protection by dmPGE2 probably arises from a combination of protection of the intestinal mucosa and some protection of the marrow. These data suggest that prostaglandin treatment of patients before TBI and BMT may increase the dose of TBI which can be given without unacceptable toxicity.

REFERENCES

1. Bond, V.P., Fliedner, T.M., Archambeau, J.O. In: Mammalian Radiation Lethality: A Disturbance in Cellular Kinetics. Academic Press New York, 1965.
2. Steel, L.K., Catravas, G.N. In: Eicosanoids and Radiation (Eds. P. Polgar), Kluwer Academic Publishers, Boston, 1985, pp 79-88.
3. Withers, H.R., Elkind, M.M. Int. J. Radiat. Biol. 17(3): 261-267, 1970.
4. Hanson, W.R., Ainsworth E.J. Rad. Res. 103: 196-203, 1985.
5. Walden, T.L., Patchen, M.L., Snyder, S.L. Rad. Res. 109: 440-448, 1987.

NOVEL 5-LIPOXYGENASE INHIBITOR (SC-41661) REDUCES HUMAN OVARIAN CANCER CELL INVASION AND ASCITIC TUMOR GROWTH

R. FRIDMAN*, T. KANEMOTO*, G. R. MARTIN**, T. HAMILTON***, R. A. PARTIS#, and R. A. MUELLER#

*Lab. Devel. Biol. and Anomalies, NIDR, NIH, Bethesda, MD 20892. **Gerontology Research Ctr., NIA, NIH, Baltimore, MD 21224. ***Med. Oncology, Fox Chase Cancer Ctr., Philadelphia, PA 19111. #Molec. and Cell. Biol. Dept., G.D. Searle & Co., Skokie, IL 60077

INTRODUCTION

Ovarian cancer, the fourth leading cause of cancer-related deaths in American women, accounts for nearly 15,000 deaths annually (1). The tumor arises from the epithelial cells covering the surface of the ovary. These cells proliferate, escape from the primary tumor, and spread into the peritoneal cavity where multiple secondary tumors form that are difficult to remove or to treat. The obstruction of peritoneal lymphatics by the tumor cells further results in the development of ascites. The formation of ascites can then further facilitate the spread of malignant cells to other sites within the peritoneal cavity. The most common form of treatment for ovarian cancer involves the surgical excision of intraperitoneal tumors, followed by chemotherapy. Small tumor masses cannot be easily removed. Furthermore, ovarian cancer is clinically noted for the rapid development of primary drug resistance and a broad cross resistance to conventional chemotherapy which makes this tumor particularly difficult to treat.

Previous studies have suggested a role for arachidonic acid metabolites and prostaglandins in malignant diseases (2), particularly in metastasis formation (3,4). Little is known about the role of 5-lipoxygenase (5-LO) products in malignancy. Recently, it has been shown that 5-HETE may be involved in tumor cell invasion of basement membranes, the principal barrier for the dissemination of malignant cells to distant sites (5). A novel inhibitor of 5-LO has been recently developed by the G.D. Searle & Co. (Skokie, IL) (6). This synthetic inhibitor, designated SC-41661, shows a high degree of specificity for 5-LO and at concentrations of 0.3 μM it blocks 50% of the activity of semi-purified 5-LO from rat basophilic leukemia cells (RBL-1). Table 1 summarizes the in vitro properties of SC-41661 (7).

In the present study, we have examined the effects of SC-41661 on the in vitro invasiveness and on the tumorigenicity of a human ovarian carcinoma cell line, NIH-OVCAR-3.

Table 1. SC-41661 Inhibitory Activity In Vitro

Test	Result
RBL-1* 5-lipoxygenase	IC_{50} = 0.3 μM
RBL-1 LTC_4 /D_4 synthesis	IC_{50} = 1.6 μM
Cyclooxygenase (seminal vesicle)	44% Inhibition (@100 μM)
12-lipoxygenase (platelets)	33% Inhibition (@ 100 μM)
15-lipoxygenase (soybean)	No Inhibition

*Rat basophilic leukemia cells

MATERIALS AND METHODS

Cell line.

OVCAR-3 cells were isolated from a patient with an adenocarcinoma of the ovary (8). The cells were grown in RPMI 1640 supplemented with 10% fetal calf serum, insulin (10 μg/ml), and antibiotics and were maintained in a 5% CO_2 incubator at 37°C.

Chemicals and proteins.

The SC-41661 5-LO inhibitor was obtained from G.D. Searle & Co. (Skokie, IL) (6). Matrigel, an extract of basement membrane proteins, was prepared from the EHS tumor as previously described (9).

Invasion and migration assays.

The invasive activity of OVCAR-3 cells was studied in vitro using modified Boyden chambers in which the filters were coated with Matrigel (10). For migration assays, a similar assay was employed except that the filters were not coated with Matrigel (10). The area covered by the cells on the lower surface of the filter was measured by image analysis (Optomax). In vitro invasion was also studied in cells seeded between two layers of Matrigel as previously described (11).

In vivo studies.

OVCAR-3 cells were injected (3 x 10^7 cells/mouse) intraperitoneally (i.p.) into 4-8 week-old female athymic NIH nude mice (Nu/Nu). Intraperitoneal administration of SC-41661 was initiated one day prior to the injection of the tumor cells and was given on a daily basis thereafter.

RESULTS AND DISCUSSION

SC-41661 inhibits invasion of basement membranes in vitro.

The metastatic potential of malignant tumor cells correlates well with their ability to invade a reconstituted basement membrane (Matrigel) in vitro (5,10,11,12). This ability appears to depend upon a number of cellular activities, including adhesion of the cells to the matrix components, cell motility, and secretion of proteolytic enzymes such as collagenase IV (5,10,11,12). To test the effect of SC-41661 on ovarian tumor cell invasion two different approaches were utilized. First, cells were seeded between two layers of Matrigel and their morphology was observed after 1-4 days. We have shown previously that metastatic cells seeded on Matrigel form branched colonies in contrast to non-malignant cells which remain as aggregates (5,10,11,12). We have found that OVCAR-3 cells on Matrigel show an invasive morphology (branched colonies) similar to that observed with a metastatic human fibrosarcoma cell line (HT-1080), but different from that observed with a non-malignant human lung fibroblast cell line (WI-38) (12). The 5-LO inhibitor inhibited the invasive morphology of OVCAR-3 cells in culture. At concentrations of 25 and 100 μM, the 5-LO inhibitor significantly reduced the size of OVCAR-3 colonies in Matrigel (Table 2) such that they resembled the non-invasive phenotype. We further explored the effect of the 5-LO inhibitor on invasiveness using polycarbonate filters coated with Matrigel in modified Boyden chambers (8). The presence of SC-41661 inhibited ovarian tumor cell invasion of Matrigel (Table 2) . A 50% inhibition of invasion was observed at concentrations of 50 uM. In contrast, the inhibitor had no effect on OVCAR-3 migration when tested using uncoated filters (Table 2). Thus, SC-41661 inhibited basement membrane invasion in vitro presumably by an effect on cell adhesion and/or production of proteolytic enzymes.

Table 2. Effect of SC-41661 on the in vitro invasiveness of OVCAR-3 cells

SC-41661 (μM)	Invasive Colonies*	Invasion Assays* (Boyden Chambers)	Chemotaxis*
0	100	100	100
10	NT	95 ± 2	100
25	70 ± 5	72 ± 8	98 ± 10
50	NT	48 ± 5	95 ± 7
100	45 ± 7	35 ± 7	82 ± 9

NT: Not Tested
*Data are expressed as percentage (%) of invasion/chemotaxis from untreated samples.

Effect of SC-41661 on human ovarian tumors in nude mice.

To test the effects of SC-41661 in vivo, OVCAR-3 cells were injected i.p. into nude mice. Daily i.p. injections of the 5-LO inhibitor prevented the formation of ovarian peritoneal tumors and significantly prolonged the survival of the mice. Injection of 1.25 mg/mouse (n=6) of the inhibitor resulted in 80% survival after 90 days. In contrast, the untreated mice had a median survival of 51 days. Similar results were obtained with lower doses of SC-41661 (0.62 mg/mouse, n=8). The treated mice did not have abdominal enlargement observed in the untreated mice (Figure 1) nor did they manifest any signs of over toxicity to SC-41661. Discontinuation of the treatment did not result in tumor recurrence within a period

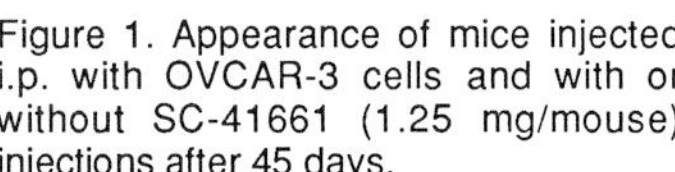

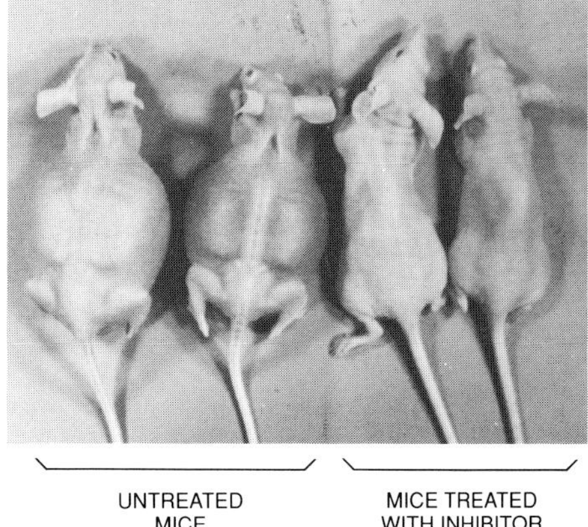

Figure 1. Appearance of mice injected i.p. with OVCAR-3 cells and with or without SC-41661 (1.25 mg/mouse) injections after 45 days.

of 3 months after the last doses. These studies suggested that the presence of SC-41661 inhibited almost completely the establishment of ovarian ascitic tumors.

At the present time, the precise mechanism of action of the 5-LO inhibitor is not known. SC-41661 exhibits an antiproliferative effect in OVCAR-3 cells, as measured by [^{3}H]-thymidine incorporation, with 50% inhibition at concentrations of 15 μM. Thus, inhibition of tumor cell growth in vivo is a possible explanation for the antitumor activity of SC-41661. Since formation of ascites may occur as a consequence of tumor cell obstruction of lymphatics and since SC-41661 inhibits invasion in vitro, it is possible that the 5-LO inhibitor prevents the invasion of malignant ovarian cells from the peritoneal cavity into the lymphatics. An effect on vascular permeability cannot be excluded. In summary, our studies have shown that a novel and relatively specific 5-LO inhibitor inhibits the in vitro invasiveness of human ovarian cancer cells and reduces the formation of ascites induced by peritoneal human ovarian tumors in nude mice.

REFERENCES

1. Richardson, G.S., Scully, R.E., Nikrui, N., and Nelson, J.H. N. Eng. J. Med. 312:415-424, 1985.
2. Powles, T.J., Bockman, R.S., Honn, K.V., and Ramwell, P.W. (eds.) Prostaglandins and Cancer, New York, Alan R. Liss, Inc., 1984.
3. Young, M.R., Young, M.E., and Wepsic, H.T. Cancer Res. 47:3679-3683, 1987.
4. Kort, W.J. Hulsman, L.O.M., van Schalkwijk, W.P., Wejima, I.M., Zondervan, P.E., and Westbroek, D.L. J. Nat'l. Cancer Inst. 76:711-720, 1986.
5. Reich, R., and Martin, G.R. Cancer Res., submitted, 1989.
6. Mueller, R.A., and Partis, R.A., US Patent 4,663,333, 1988.
7. Nakao, A., Yang, O-C., Jung, G., Partis, R.A., and Mueller, R.A., in preparation.
8. Hamilton, T.C., Young, R.C., Laurie, K.G., Bephens, B.C., McKoy, W.M., Grotzinger, K.R., and Ozols, R.F. Cancer Res. 44:5286-5290, 1984.
9. Kleinman, H.K., McGarvey, M.L., Hassell, J.R., Star, V.L., Cannon, F.B., Laurie, G.W., and Martin, G.R. Biochem. 25:312-318, 1986.
10. Albini, A., Iwamoto, Y., Kleinman, H.K., Martin, G.R., Aaronson, S.A., Kozlowski, J.M., and

McEwan, R.N. Cancer Res., 47:3239-3245, 1989.
11. Kramer, R.H., Bensch, K.G., and Wong, J. Cancer Res. 46:1980-1989, 1986.
12. Fridman, R. Lacal, J.C., Reich, R., Bonfil, R.D., and Ahn, C. J. Cell. Physiol., in press, 1989.

NSAID INDOMETHACIN ENHANCED CYTOSTATIC EFFECT OF CIS-PLATINUM OF THE PROLIFERATION OF PROSTAGLANDIN PRODUCING AND NON-PRODUCING CANCERS IN CELL LINE

M. OGINO, S. OKINAGA, M. KAIBARA, and I. ISHIWATA*

Department of Obstetrics & Gynecology, Teikyo University, School of Medicine, Ichihara Hospital and Ishiwata Hospital*

INTRODUCTION

Non-steroidal anti-inflammatory drug, INDOMETHACIN, a potent cyclooxygenase inhibitor, has been recently regarded as biological response modifier in that it inhibits the production of immunosuppressing prostaglandins, among which prostaglandin E_2 has been shown to play a clear role in the regulation of lymphokine production and considered as being involved in the suppression of immune response system (1). Therefore, indomethacin has been thought to exert its anti-tumor effect through stimulating cellular immune function by inhibiting the formation of immunosuppressing prostaglandins (2). In the early 80's, some papers have reported the anti-tumor effect of indomethacin by in vivo studies (3) (4). Furthermore, in the other works, indomethacin has been revealed to enhance the immunocompetence (5) (6). In this way, most of these documents attributed to the anti-tumor effect of indomethacin to the inhibition of increased formation of immunosuppressing prostaglandin E_2 by the cancer per se and/or as a result of paraneoplastic manifestation. However, there have been a very few number of papers issued reporting direct cytostatic effect of indomethacin. In the present study, we obtained prostaglandin producing and non-producing cell lines of the uterine cervical cancer, then we assessed the changes in cell growth of the cancer when indomethacin was added to the culture medium. Moreover, we investigated whether or not additional cytostatic effect would be expected if indomethacin was used in combination with cis-platinum.

MATERIALS AND METHODS

Cell lines of the uterine cervical cancer.

SKG-II (large cell non-keratinizing squamous cell carcinoma of the uterine cervix) and HKUS (small cell non-keratinizing squamous cell carcinoma of the uterine cervix) have been established (7) (8).

Culture medium and incubation study.

Culture medium consisted of F-10 supplemented with 10% heat inactivated fetal bovine serum and kanamycin sulfate. Incubation study for the measurement of prostaglandins generated by the cancer cells was carried out using serum free F-10 as an incubation medium.

In vitro biosynthesis of prostaglandins by the cancer cells.

Four fractions of prostaglandins, i.e. PGE_2, TXB_2 (a stable metabolite of TXA_2), $PGF_{2\alpha}$ and 6-keto-$PGF_{1\alpha}$ (a stable end product of prostacyclin) generated by the cancer cells were determined by radioimmunoassay as previously reported (9). Confirmation of the production of these prostaglandins was performed by gas-chromatogram selected ion monitoring as previously reported (10).

Chemicals and agents.

Indomethacin crystalline was purchased from SIGMA and cis-platinum was the kind gift from Nippon Kayaku Co. Ltd. Indomethacin was dissolved in 99.5% ethanol (1:1, w/vol) and cis-platinum was dissolved in normal saline (1:2, w/vol). An aliquot of each solution was added to the culture medium at the given concentrations according to the experimental schedule. The culture media thus prepared were treated through sonication just prior to use for 15 min.

Experimental schedule.

Cell suspension containing x 10^5 cells were dispersed in the culture dishes (35 mm in diameter) and preincubated for 48 hr, then experiment was started. Experimental regimen was prepared at the given concentrations of each and/or both agents as follows: a) untreated control b) indomethacin only (1.0 mg/ml) c) cis-platinum only (0.1 µg/ml and 1.0 µg/ml) d) indomethacin plus cis-platinum (1.0 µg/ml and 0.01 µg/ml) and e) indomethacin plus cis-platinum (1.0 µg/ml and 0.1 µg/ml) respectively. Medium change was performed at 48 hr interval in a), b), d) and e), while medium change was carried out every day in c). Number of the viable cells in the culture dishes was counted every day up to 5 culture days following 48 hr preincubation and expressed as mean $\pm$ s.e. in pentaplicate dishes.

RESULTS

In vitro biosynthesis of prostaglandins by the cancer cells.

SKG-II was definitely shown to generate prostaglandins, ie PGE_2, TXA_2 and $PGF_{2\alpha}$, among which PGE_2 was a major product. In contrast to this, HKUS was revealed not to form any of these prostaglandins (Figure 1). Gas-chromatogram selected ion monitoring has shown single ion peaks of derivatized samples corresponding to basal ion peaks of derivatized preparation for each authentic prostaglandin (Figures 2 and 3).

Inhibition of prostaglandin production by indomethacin.

Addition of indomethacin at a concentration of 1.0 µg/ml was shown enough to completely inhibit the formation of each prostaglandin by SKG-II.

Cytostatic effect of indomethacin and/or indomethacin plus cis-platinum on cell growth of both cancer cell lines (Figures 4 and 5).

Indomethacin was clearly demonstrated to suppress the cell growth of both prostaglandin producing and non-producing cancer in cell line significantly compared with that of the untreated control. Furthermore, indomethacin, as used in combination with cis-platinum, enhanced 100 fold cytostatic effect of cis-platinum in SKG-II and 10 fold cytostatic effect of cis-platinum in HKUS. Thus, synergistic

	PGE_2	TXB_2	$PGF_{2\alpha}$	6-keto-$PGF_{1\alpha}$
Blank value	UD	UD	UD	23.7*
SKG-Ⅱ	289.7±9.5 (n=30)	161.3±9.4 (n=24)	164.1±6.4 (n=10)	4.0±1.3** (n=10)
HKUS	UD	UD	UD	UD

* Mean blank value (pg/mℓ, n=3)

** Corrected by mean blank value

Amount of prostaglandins formed by the cancer cells : pg/mℓ/x 10^6 cells/30 min

UD : undetectable (less than the lower limit of RIA)

Fig. 1 Biosynthesis of prostaglandins by the cancer in cell line. The amount of each prostaglandin was corrected by recovery rate obtained during the entire course of preparation.

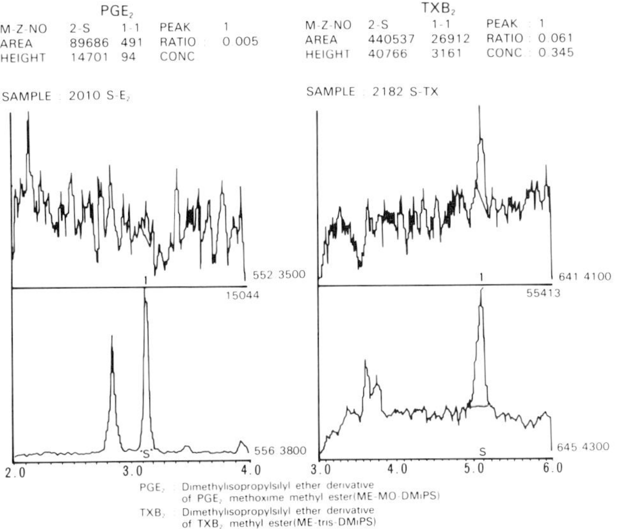

Fig.2 Gas-chromatogram selected ion monitoring. Evaluable ion peak of derivatized samples corresponding to authentic prostaglandin derivatives was indicated by "peak 1".

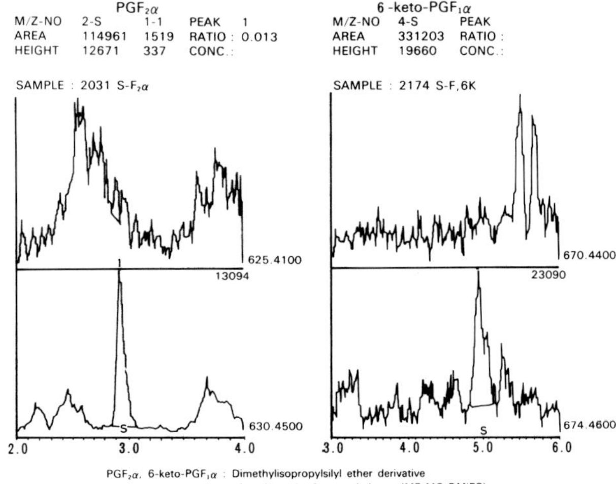

Fig.3 Gas-chromatogram selected ion monitoring. Evaluable ion peak of derivatized samples corresponding to authentic prostaglandin derivatives was indicated by "peak 1".

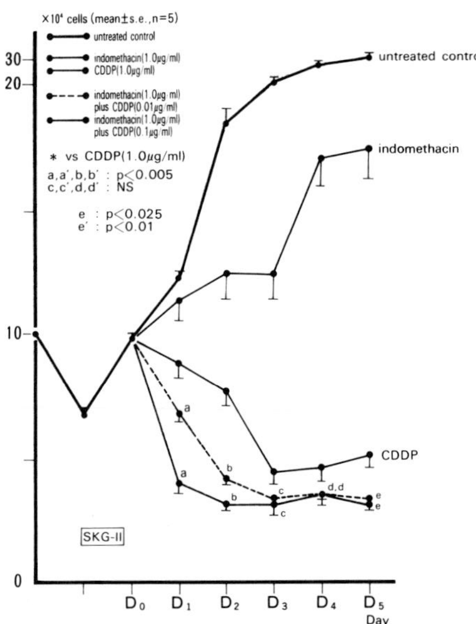

Fig.4 Cell growth: untreated control, indomethacin treated, cis-platinum(CDDP) treated and combined treatment of indomethacin with CDDP.

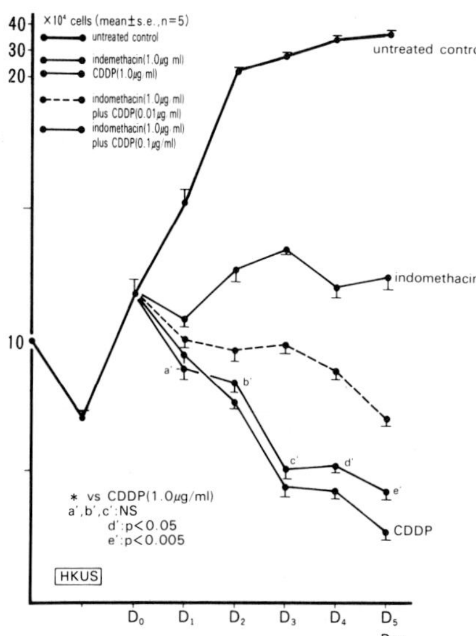

Fig.5 Cell growth: untreated control, indomethacin treated, cis-platinum(CDDP) treated and combined treatment of indomethacin with CDDP.

effect of indomethacin in combination with cis-platinum on the cell growth of both cell lines was definitely ascertained.

CONCLUSION AND DISCUSSION

It is generally thought that PGE_2 (considered as an immunosuppressing factor) and TXA_2 (regarded as an accelerating factor for cancer metastasis and/or cancer proliferation) play a possible role in modifying the prognosis of the cancer bearing patients. On the other hand, it is widely accepted that small cell type of the uterine cervical cancer has poor prognosis compared with that of large cell type of the uterine cervical cancer (11). In the present work, it became clear that large cell type of the cancer was shown to produce both prostaglandins, whereas small cell type of the cancer was revealed not to form any of these prostaglandins. Thus, it still remains further to be investigated to explain the discrepancy between the clinical surveillance data and the results so far obtained by basic studies.

The evidence that indomethacin suppressed the cell growth of both prostaglandin producing and non-producing cancers in cell line might suggest that direct cytostatic effect of indomethacin was thought to be exerted via prostaglandin unrelated pathway rather than via prostaglandin depending pathway.

In the present work, it was also demonstrated that combined regimen of indomethacin with cis-platinum at subnormal concentrations strikingly enhanced cytostatic effect of cis-platinum which was comparable to that obtained by conventional concentration of cis-platinum. However, it seems very difficult to verify the so far unknown mechanism by which indomethacin enhanced cytostatic effect of cis-platinum. There are various factors thought to be involved in that mechanism and some related data are accumulating at our laboratory, but they could not always clarify such mechanism in detail.

In any way, the results obtained in the present work, when they are reinforced also by in vivo study, would encourage us to apply indomethacin in the practical aspect for the cancer bearing patients who are situated away from medical rescue.

REFERENCES

1. Rappaport, R.S. and Dodge, G.R. J. Exp. Med. 155:943-948, 1982.
2. Goodwin, J.S. and Ceuppens, J. J. Clin. Immunol. 3:295-315, 1983.
3. Weppelmann, B. and Monkemeier, D. Gynecol. Oncol. 17:196-199, 1984
4. Bennet, A., Carroll, M.A. Melhuish, P.B. and Stamford, I.F. Br. J. Cancer. 52:245-249, 1985.
5. Foldgren, P. and Sjogren, H.O. Cancer Immunol. Immunother. 19:28-34, 1985.
6. Maca, R.D., Burford, J.G. and Taylor, R.T. J. Clin. Immunol. 5:158-165, 1985.
7. Ishiwata, I., Nozawa, S., Kiguchi, K., Kurihara, S. and Okumura, H. Acta Obst Gynaec Jpn. 30:731-738, 1978.
8. Ishiwata, I., Ishiwata, C., Ishikawa, H., Nozawa, S. and Iizuka, R. Acta Obst Gynaec Jpn. 40:616-620, 1988.
9. Ogino, M., Abe, Y., Jimbo, T. and Okahara, T. Endocrinol. Japan. 33:197-202, 1986.
10. Miyazaki, H., Ishibashi, M., Yamashita, K., Nishikawa, Y. and Katori, M. Biomed. Mass. Spectrom. 5:521-526, 1981.
11. Wentz, W.B. and Reagan, J.W. Cancer. 12:384-388, 1959.

CONTROL OF TUMOR CELL INDUCED ENDOTHELIAL CELL RETRACTION BY LIPOXYGENASE METABOLITES, PROSTACYCLIN AND PROSTACYCLIN ANALOGUES

I.M. GROSSI[*], C.A. DIGLIO[#], and K.V. HONN[*¥]

Wayne State University, Depts. Radiation Oncology[*¥], Chemistry[*¥], and Pathology[#].

The primary element responsible for the morbidity and mortality of malignant cancers is tumor metastasis. During hematogenous metastasis the vascular endothelium forms the primary barrier between the circulatory system and extravascular tissues. Circulating tumor cells have the potential to interact with a variety of circulating host cells and the vascular wall, however only a small fraction of these tumor cells survive hemodynamic forces and host defence mechanisms to form distant metastases (1,2). Specific interactions between circulating tumor cells and a variety of host cells (i.e., platelets, leukocytes, and endothelial cells) is believed to affect tumor cell arrest and extravasation from the circulation (3,4). These types of cell-cell interactions generally occur in the microcirculation where the blood flow rate is low and the vascular surface area to blood volume ratio is high, allowing increased cell-cell contact in the microvascular space.

Tumor cell adhesion to the microvasculature involves multiple interactions which are mediated by cell adhesion molecules. The families of adhesion molecules involved in this process include cadherins (5), intercellular adhesion molecules (ICAM's; 6), endothelial cell-leukocyte adhesion molecules (ELAM's; 7), and integrins (8). Studies of tumor cell adhesion to endothelial cells, subendothelial matirx, and components of the subendothelial matrix demonstrate that these adhesion molecule-directed interactions are an important mechanism by which tumor cells can metastasize (9).

Recently we reported that tumor cell adhesion to endothelial cell monolayers and fibronectin was increased following pretreatment of tumor cells with 12(S)-hydroxyeicosatetraenoic acid [12(S)-HETE], a lipoxygenase metabolite of arachidonic acid (10). Ultrastructural analysis of early in vivo events associated with tumor cell arrest indicate that initial tumor cell host cell interaction occurs with the endothelial cell, followed by the initiation of platelet aggregation (11). Morphological evidence suggests that platelets involved during initial tumor cell arrest possibly facilitate tumor cell adhesion to endothelium and subendothelial matrix (11), however, the mechanism is unknown.

Kramer et al. (12) first reported that tumor cell adhesion to endothelial cell monolayers in vitro is followed by endothelial cell retraction and tumor cell migration to the underlying subendothelial matrix. In vivo, endothelial cell retraction is evident 4 hours after tumor cell arrest, a time coincident with maximum platelet activation by the arrested tumor cells (11). These observations suggested that the tumor cell or

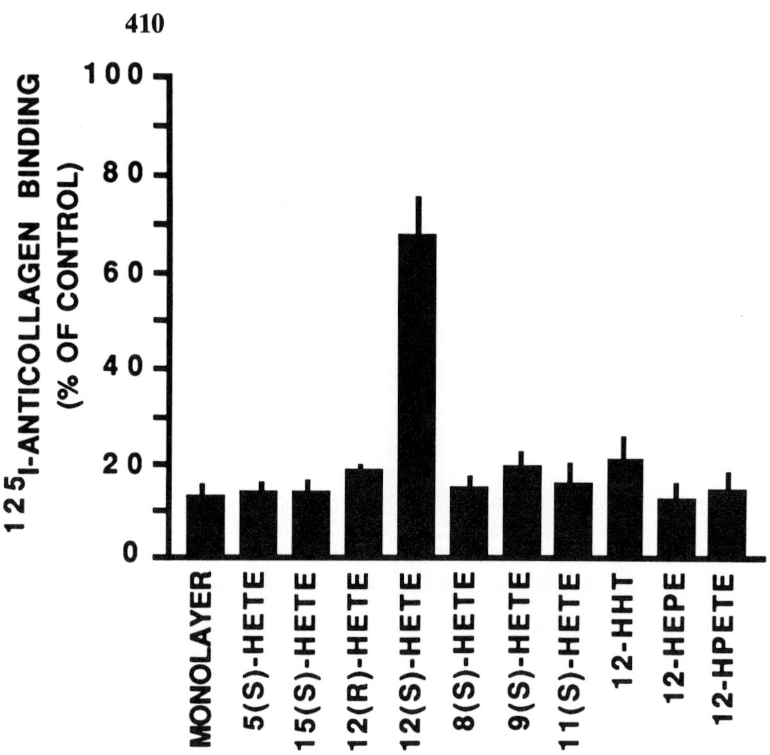

Figure 1. Eicosanoid induced murine pulmonary microvessel endothelial cell retraction. Only the 12(S)-HETE (E) was demonstrated to induce endothelial cell retraction while other eicosanoids tested were ineffective. Endothelial cell monolayers were grown upon Collagen IV (25μg) to confluency and probed with ^{125}I-anticollagen Iv antibody (10μg/ml) 60 min post eicosanoid treatment. Results expressed as mean±S.D. [A, endothelial monolayer; B, 5(S)-HETE; C, 15(S)-HETE, D, 12(R)-HETE; E, 12(S)-HETE; F, 8(S)-HETE; G, 9(S)-HETE; H, 11(S)-HETE; I, 12-HHT; J, 12-HEPE; K, 12-HPETE].

platelet [or factor(s) derived from these cells] may enhance endothelial cell retraction during tumor cell-platelet-endothelial cell interactions.

Several lines of evidence suggest that 12(S)-HETE may be the key mediator in the induction of endothelial cell retraction, as 12(S)-HETE is the principle lipoxygenase metabolite of arachidonic acid in platelets as well as in murine Lewis lung carcinoma (3LL) cells (13). Furthermore, 12(S)-HETE treatment of tumor cells increases tumor cell expression of an integrin receptor and subsequent tumor cell adhesion to biologically relevant substrata (14), as well as increases lung colonization by pretreated tumor cells (unpublished observation). Lastly, 12(S)-HETE may transfer from cell types (i.e., platelet to endothelial cell), termed transcellular metabolism (15).

We have previously proposed that lipoxygenase products of arachidonic acid produced by the platelet, tumor cell, and endothelial cell affect the interactions of these three cell types, possibly by altering vessel wall prostacyclin biosynthesis (16). We now propose that platelet derived 12(S)-HETE [as well as tumor cell derived 12(S)-HETE] may be transcellularly metabolized and influence both tumor cells and endothelial cells during the interaction of platelets with those two cell types following arrest in the microcirculation. 12(S)-HETE has been demonstrated to inhibit endothelial cell biosynthesis of prostacyclin, a cyclooxygenase metabolite of arachidonic acid (17). Prostacyclin is a potent inhibitor of tumor cell-platelet-endothelial cell interactions and tumor cell metastasis (16). We therefore investigated the role of prostacyclin (and prostacyclin analogues) on 12(S)-HETE mediated tumor cell adhesion to endothelial cells and platelet enhanced tumor cell induced endothelial cell retraction.

We have previously demonstrated that 12(S)-HETE induced integrin receptor expression on tumor cells correlates with increased tumor cell adhesion to endothelial cells (10). Pretreatment of tumor cells with prostacyclin, iloprost, or ZK96.480 prior to 12(S)-HETE stimulation reduced receptor expression and subsequent enhanced tumor cell adhesion to basal levels (data not shown). Exogenous 12(S)-HETE can induce nondestructive, reversible endothelial cell retraction, a phenomena specific for the 12(S)- enantiomere (Figure 1). Tumor cell derived 12(S)-HETE can also induce nondestructive, reversible endothelial cell retraction, and this retraction can be enhanced in a dose dependent manner with an increasing concentration of platelets (Figure 2). Both tumor cell- and platelet enhanced tumor cell

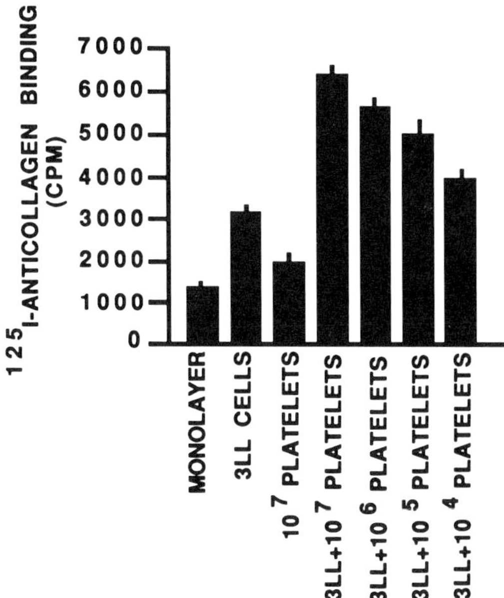

Figure 2. Quantitation of tumor cell- or platelet enhanced tumor cell induced endothelial cell retraction. Platelets are demonstrated to enhance tumor cell induced endothelial cell retraction in a dose dependent manner. Results expressed as mean ± S.D.

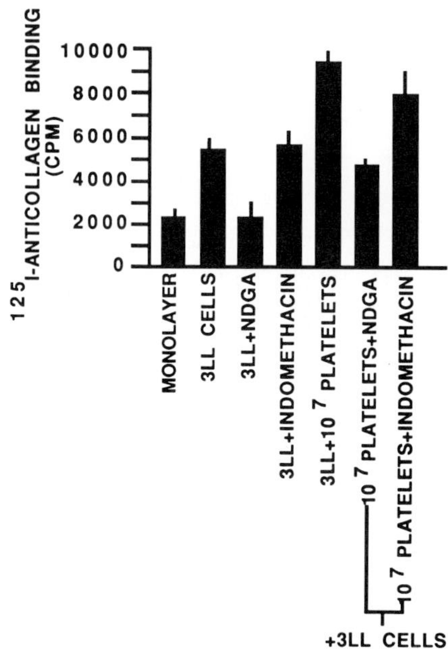

Figure 3. A general lipoxygenase inhibitor such as NDGA (10 μM) is shown to inhibit both tumor cell- and platelet enhanced tumor cell induced endothelial cell retraction whereas the cyclooxygenase inhibitor indomethacin (10 μM) does not. Results expressed as mean±S.D.

induced endothelial cell retraction can be inhibited by treatment of the tumor cells or platelets with lipoxygenase inhibitors, but not by cyclooxygenase inhibitors (Figure 3). In addition, if platelets are pretreated with prostacyclin or analogues (i.e., iloprost or ZK96.480), the extent of retraction is reduced to that of the intact monolayer (Figure 4)

From previous studies we know that 12(S)-HETE acts directly on tumor cells to promote their attachment to endothelial cells, a rate limiting step in the metastatic cascade. We therefore promote the concept that activated platelets may be the primary contributors of 12(S)-HETE to tumor cells and endothelial cells during their interaction in the microcirculation, and thus enhance tumor cell metastasis by accelerating the process of tumor cell induced endothelial cell retraction. Furthermore, we suggest two sites of action for the antimetastatic effects of prostacyclin and prostacyclin analogues, namely the inhibition of 12(S)-HETE enhanced expression of integrin receptors by tumor cells, reducing the interaction of tumor cells with platelets and endothelial cells, and, the inhibition of platelet enhanced tumor cell induced endothelial cell retraction by 12(S)-HETE. These results suggest a bidirectional regulation of tumor cell adhesion and subsequent metastasis is at the level of cyclooxygenase and lipoxygenase metabolites of arachidonic acid.

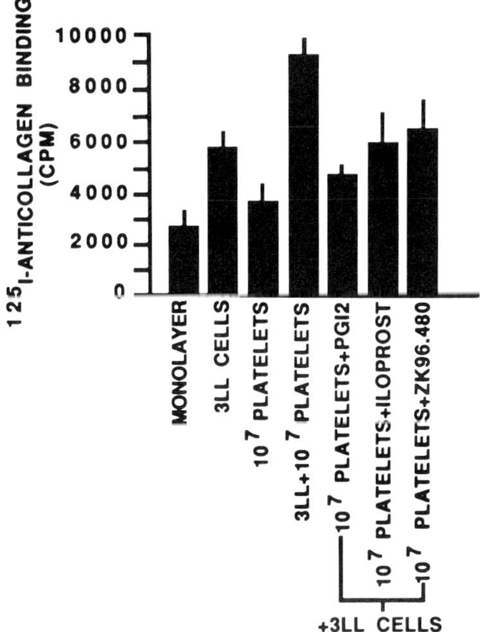

Figure 4. Inhibition of platelet enhanced tumor cell induced endothelial cell retraction by prostacyclin and prostacyclin analogues, iloprost and ZK96.480. Results expressed as mean±S.D.

ACKNOWLEDGEMENT

This work was supported by NIH grant CA 29997-08.

REFERENCES

1. Fidler IJ, and Nicolson GL. (1981) Cancer Biol Rev 2: 171-234.
2. Fidler IJ, and Nicolson GL. (1976) J Natl Cancer Inst 57: 1100-1210.
3. Nicolson GL. (1988) Cancer Met Rev 7: 143-188.
4. Weiss L, Orr FW, and Honn KV. (1988) FASEB J 2: 12-21.
5. Dustin ML, Rothlein R, Bhan AK, Dinarello CA, and Springer TA. (1986) J Immunol 37: 245-254.
6. Bevilacqua MP, Pober JS, Mendrick DL, Cotran RS, and Gimbrone MA. (1987) Proc Natl Acad Sci USA 84: 9238-9242.
7. Crossin KL, Chuong CM, and Edelman GM. (1985) Proc Natl Acad Sci USA 82: 6942-6946.
8. Hynes RO. (1987) Cell 48: 549-554.
9. Knudsen DA, Smith L, Smith S, Karczewski J, and Tuszynski GP. (1988) J Cell Physiol 136: 471-478.
10. Honn KV, Grossi IM, Fitzgerald LA, Umbarger LA, Diglio CA, and Taylor JD. (1988) Proc Soc Exptl Biol Med 189: 130-135.

11. Crissman JD, Hatfield J, Menter DG, Sloane BF, and Honn KV. (1988) Cancer Res 48: 4065-4073.
12. Kramer AH, Gonzales R, and Nicolson GL. (1980) Int J Cancer 26: 639-645.
13. Marnett LJ, Leithauser MT, Richards KM, Blair I. Honn KV, Yamamoto S, and Yoshimoto T. (1990) In: B. Samuelsson, R. Paoletti and P. Ramwell (eds) Prostaglandins and Related Compounds; for the 7th International Conference on Prostaglandins and Related Compounds, Florence, Italy, (in press).
14. Grossi IM, Fitzgerald LA, Umbarger LA, Nelson KK, Diglio CA, Taylor JD, and Honn KV. (1989) Cancer Res. 49: 1029-1037.
15. Schafer AI, Takayama H, Farrell S, and Gimbrone MA. (1986) Blood 67: 373-378.
16. Honn KV, Cicone B, and Skoff A. (1981) SCIENCE (Washington DC) 212: 1270-1272.

ANTIMETASTATIC ACTION IN MICE OF PGI_2 ANALOG ILOPROST

T. GIRALDI, V.RAPOZZI, L. PERISSIN and S. ZORZET

Istituto di Farmacologia, Universita di Trieste I-34100 Trieste, Italy

INTRODUCTION

The process of hematogenous metastasis formation for solid malignant tumors has been shown to require effective interactions between the circulating tumor cells and the hemostatic system of the host (1,2). Correspondingly, drugs affecting the blood clotting mechanism, including prostacyclin (PGI_2) (3), have been demostrated to produce antimetastatic effects in experimental animal-tumor systems (4-6). In particular, the administration of exogenous PGI_2 shortly before intravenous injection of B16 melanoma cells was found to reduce the number of tumor lung colonies in the treated mice (7), and this effect was attributed to the inhibition of platelet aggregation caused by PGI_2 (4,8,9).

The aim of the present investigation has been therefore that of examining in mice bearing Lewis lung carcinoma (3LL) the antimetastatic properties of Iloprost, a chemically stable analog of PGI_2, endowed with platelet anti-aggregatory activity equivalent to that of PGI_2 (3,10). The time- and dose-dependency of the effects of Iloprost on artificial lung metastasis have been determined in comparison with PGI_2, together with the effects of Iloprost on spontaneous metastasis formation, in terms of metastasis number and survival time of the hosts after surgical removal of the primary tumor. The effects of *in vivo* treatment of mice with Iloprost have been examined on *in vitro* platelet aggregation, in relation to the antimetastatic action of the drug. Finally, the effects of Iloprost on spontaneous metastasis have been determined also in mice pretreated with immunomodifiers; the results obtained are hereafter reported.

MATERIALS AND METHODS

Tumor transplantation and evaluation.

The animals used for this investigation are female mice, weighing 18-20 g, purchased from Charles River, Calco Como, Italy. The Lewis lung carcinoma line was originally provided by DCT-Tumor Repository, NCI-Frederick Cancer Research Facility, MD, USA. Tumor implantation (10^6 cells) was performed i.m. and 10 days later the tumor bearing leg was amputated after anesthesia with ketalar (125 mg/Kg i.p.) (11). The procedures employed for tumor transplantation, and for the evaluation of tumor growth and metastasis formation have been described in detail elesewhere (12).

Drug treatment.

Iloprost, kindly supplied by Schering SpA, Milan, Italy, was administered i.v. in 0.1 ml/animal of 0.05

M Tris buffer (pH 9.4). Cyclophosphamide (200 or 240 mg/kg), silica (10 mg/mouse) or carrageenan (5 mg/mouse) were administered i.p. in 0.1 ml of isotonic saline. Treatment schedules are indicated in the Tables.

Clot retraction inhibition assay.

The aggregation of platelets obtained from *in vivo* treated mice was determined indirectly by means of inhibition of clot retraction, as described by De Gaetano et al. (13). Blood was collected by intracardiac puncture in mice anesthetized with ethyl uretane (1.5 g/Kg i.p.); 9 volumes of blood were mixed directly in the syringe with 1 volume of 0.126 M trisodium citrate. Platelet rich plasma (PRP) samples were obtained, prepared and pooled from groups of 3 donor mice, as described by Gasic et al. (14). Clot retraction was evaluated on PRP by adding 0.2 ml of 0.05 $MCaCl_2$ to a mixture of 0.32 ml PRP + 0.08 ml PBS containing $4x10^5$ 3LL viable tumor cells. The measure of inhibition of clot retraction is calculated as the percent ratio of the volumes of serum extruded in the presence of the aggregating agent (tumor cells) over PRP samples obtained from drug untreated mice in the absence of the aggregating agent.

RESULTS AND DISCUSSION

The treatment of mice bearing 3LL with Iloprost reduces the formation of artificial metastasis; this effect is comparable in magnitude with that caused by PGI_2, but is obtained with remarkably smaller dosages (0.2 vs. 10 mg/kg), and has a significantly longer duration (24 hr vs. 30 min.). The treatment with Iloprost significantly reduces also spontaneous metastasis, con-comitantly increasing the survival time of the hosts when combined with surgical tumor removal (15) (Table 1, Figure 1). The combination of the

Table 1. Effects on metastasis formation of the preoperative treatment with Iloprost combined with cyclophosphamide administered after surgery.

Treatment	Lung metastases		Animal
	Number	Weight	free
–	21.4 ± 0.3	211.2 ± 29.0	0/10
Iloprost	19.1 ± 0.1	133.2 ± 16.8*	0/10
Cy	2.1 ± 0.6**	6.7 ± 0.7**	4/10
Iloprost + Cy	-	-	10/10

Groups of 10 mice were implanted i.m. with 10^6 tumor cells on day 0, and treated with Iloprost (200 µg/kg i.v.) 1 hr before surgery on day 12, and/or with cyclophosphamide (Cy, 240 mg/kg i.p.) 24 hr after tumor removal. Sacrifice and lung examination for metastases were performed on day 21. * and **: means significantly different from untreated controls ($p \leq 0.05$ and $p \leq 0.01$ respectively, Student-Newmann-Keuls test) (22).

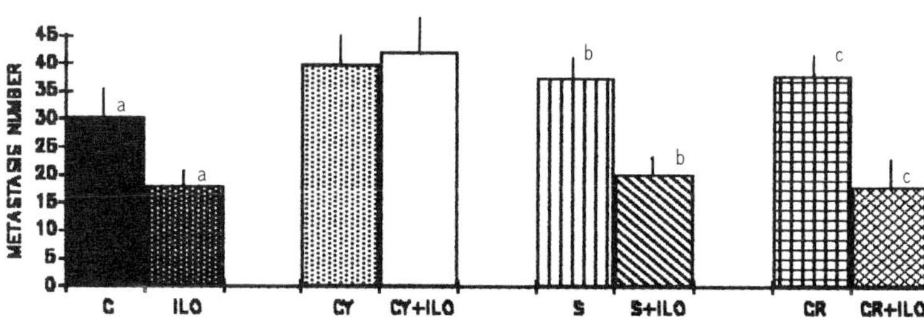

Figure 1. Effects of the pretreatment of the hosts with immunomodifiers on the antimetastatic action of Iloprost

Groups of 10 mice were treated i.p. with cyclophosphamide (Cy), silica (S) or carrageenan (Cr) 24 hr before i.m. tumor implantation (day 0). The animals received Iloprost (Ilo:200 µg/kg i.v.) on day 10, and the tumor bearing leg was amputated 1 hr after treatment with Iloprost; sacrifice and lung examination for metastasis were performed on day 21. Means with the same letter are significantly different, $p \leq 0.05$, Student-Newmann-Koulc test (22).

preoperative treatment with Iloprost followed by surgical tumor removal is synergistic with the post-operative treatment with cyclophosphamide (Table 1). The aggregation by tumor cells of platelets obtained from mice 24 hr after treatment *in vivo* with Iloprost is not reduced. A significant inhibition of artificial metastasis is still evident at 24 hr from treatment (15) (Table 2), and this finding indicates a dissociation of the effects on metastasis from those on hemostasis. When the effects of Iloprost on spontaneous metastasis are examined in mice pretreated with immunomodifiers, the antimetastatic action of Iloprost is not modified by silica and carrageenan, whereas it is abolished by cyclophosphamide. This finding is in agreement with the reported inhibition of B16 melanoma and 3LL artificial metastasis by the anticoagulant drugs warfarin and heparin, which required an intact functionality of NK immune effectors (16).

Table 2. Inhibition of clot retraction after *in vivo* treatment with Iloprost of platelet donor mice.

Treatment	Treatment before blood collection	Clot retraction inhibition, %
-	-	37.9 ± 4.0
Iloprost	1 hr	6.8 ± 3.7*
Iloprost	24 hr	*38.4 ± 3.7

Groups of 15 normal mice were treated with 200 µg/kg i.v. Iloprost at the time indicated before platelet collection. 3LL cells have been used as the aggregating agent in the clot retraction inhibition assay. *: means significantly different from drug untreated controls, t-test for grouped data (22).

These results show that Iloprost inhibits artificial metastasis of 3LL, as reported by other investigators for B16 melanoma (17), with a long lasting action. Correspondingly, Iloprost reduces also spontaneous metastasis of 3LL, increasing the survival time of hosts treated before surgical tumor removal. The examination of platelets obtained from mice treated *in vivo* with Iloprost indicates a lack of correlation between platelet aggregation and antimetastatic effects, in contrast with data obtained using *in vitro* treated human platelets (17-19). At the same time, the inhibition by cyclophosphamide of cellular T and NK immune effectors (20,21) suppresses the antimetastatic action of Iloprost, indicating a participation of immune mechanism(s) in the action of Iloprost. A potential therapeutic indication thus results for the use of Iloprost as an adjuvant for reducing intraoperative tumor cell dissemination, with the limitation of the exclusion of hosts with impaired immune functions.

ACKNOWLEDGMENTS

This work was supported by the Italian National Research Council, Special Project Oncology, contract n. 88.00691.44, and by grants from the Ministry of Education (MPI 40% and 60%).

REFERENCES

1. Donati, M.B., Davidson, J.F., and Garattini, S. Malignancy and the Hemostatic System. Raven Press, New York, 1981.
2. Donati, M.B., Poggi, A., Mussoni, L., de Gaetano,G., and Garattini, S. In: Cancer Invasion and Metastasis: Biological Mechanism and Therapy (Eds. S.B. Day, W.P.L. Myers, P. Stansley, S. Garattini and M.G. Lewis), Raven Press, New York, 1977, pp. 151-160.
3. Gryglewski, R.J., and Stock, G. Prostacyclin and its stable analogue iloprost. Springer-Verlag, Berlin, 1987.
4. Honn, K.V., Cicone, B., and Skoff, A. Science 212: 1270-1272, 1981.
5. Hilgard, P., and Thornes, R.D. Eur. J. Cancer 12: 755-762, 1976.
6. Maat, B., and Hilgard, P. J. Cancer Res. Clin. Oncol. 101: 275-283, 1981.
7. Karpatkin, S., Ambrogio, C., and Pearlsten, E. Cancer Res. 44: 3880-3884, 1984.
8. Honn, K.V. Clin. Expl. Metastasis 1: 103-114, 1983.
9. Menter, D.G., Onoda, J.M, Taylor, J.D., and Honn, K.V. Cancer Res. 44: 450-456, 1987.
10. Krause, W., and Krais, T. Eur. J. Clin. Pharmacol. 30: 61-68, 1986.
11. Sava, G., Giraldi, T., Lassiani, L. and Nisi, C. Cancer Res. 44: 64-68, 1984.
12. Sava, G., Giraldi, T., Zupi, G. and Sacchi, A. Invasion Metastasis 4: 171-178, 1984.
13. De Gaetano, G., Vermylen, J., and Verstraete, M. Thromb. Diath. Haemorragica (Stuttg.) 29: 661-670, 1973.
14. Gasic, G., Gasic, T.B., and Steward, C.C. Proc. Nat. Acad. Sci. USA 61: 46-52, 1968.
15. Sava, G., Perissin, L., Zorzet, S., Piccini, P. and Giraldi, T. Clin. Expl. Metastasis, in press.
16. Gorelik, E. Cancer Res. 47: 809-815, 1987.
17. Costantini, V., Fuschiotti, P., Allegrucci, M., Agnelli, G., Nenci, G.G. and Fioretti, M.C. Cancer Chemother. Pharmacol. 22: 289-293, 1988.
18. Belch, J.J.F., Greer, I., McLaren, M., Saniabadi, A.R., Miller S., Sturrock, R.D. and Forbes, C.D. Prostaglandins 28: 67-77, 1984.
19. Schror, K., Darius, H., Matzky, R. and Ohlendorf, R. Naunyn Schriedeberg's Archive Pharmacology 316: 252-255, 1981.
20. Hilgard, P., Pohl, J., Stekar, J. and Voegeli, R. Cancer Treat. Rev. 12: 155-162, 1985.
21. Fazioli, F., Sironi, M., Vecchi, A., Sozzani, S. and Spreafico, F. Meth. Find. Expl. Clin. Pharmacol. 9: 595-604, 1987.
22. Tallarida, R.J., and Murray, R.B. Manual of pharmacologic calculation with computer programs. Springer-Verlag, New York, 1987.

ANTIMETASTATIC ACTIVITY OF A STABLE PROSTACYCLIN ANALOGUE: EFFECT ON PLATELET AGGREGATION AND HOST IMMUNOCOMPETENCE IN THE MOUSE

V. COSTANTINI, P. FUSCHIOTTI*, G. STINCARELLI*, A. GIAMPIETRI*, M. ALLEGRUCCI*, G. AGNELLI, G.G. NENCI, and M.C. FIORETTI*

Istituto di Semeiotica Medica ed *Istituto di Farmacologia, Universita' di Perugia, 06100 Perugia, Italy

INTRODUCTION

The stable prostacyclin (PGI_2) analogue, iloprost is a potent inhibitor of platelet function and antithrombotic agent (1). Because it has been postulated that platelet-tumor cell interactions are involved in the pathogenesis of tumor metastasis (2,3), we tested the effect of iloprost treatment in a murine model of experimental metastasis. In this model iloprost showed far more potent and persistent antimetastatic activity than PGI_2 (4). Unlike PGI_2, the antimetastatic effect of a single dose of iloprost remained detectable for up to 6 hours after tumor cell challenge (4).

However the mechanism of its antimetastatic effect is still poorly defined. We have observed previously that iloprost was a potent inhibitor of *in vitro* human platelet aggregation induced by murine melanoma $B_{16}BL_6$ tumor cells (4) and hypothesized that the antimetastatic activity of the drug might be related to its capacity to inhibited platelet-tumor cell interaction *in vivo*. In order to further test this hypothesis, we have now evaluated the antiaggregant effect of iloprost on murine platelets. In addition, we have explored the effect of iloprost on certain parameters of mouse immunocompetence, particularly natural killer (NK), macrophage and T-cell mediated antitumor activities, that are thought to influence tumor growth and metastasis formation (5). This study appeared to be justified because, of all the arachidonic acid metabolites, only prostaglandins (PG) of the E series have been extensively investigated in term of regulation of cellular and humoral immune response (6).

MATERIALS AND METHODS

<u>Platelet aggregometry studies.</u>

Effects of iloprost on mouse platelet aggregation were evaluated both *in vivo* and *ex vivo*, following intravenous injection of mice with the drug (0.2 mg/kg). Platelet aggregation was performed by the turbidometric techinique described by Born (7). Aggregation was induced using a mixture of collagen and epinephrine. The aggregating agents were used in threshold aggregating concentrations (TAC) defined as the minimal amount of aggregant which induced irreversible platelet aggregation exceeding 60%.

<u>*In vivo* effect of iloprost on tumor cell-induced thrombocytopenia</u>.

Male $C_{57}BL_6$ mice were pretreated with iloprost (0.2 mg/kg i.v.) at different times with respect to tumor challenge. Fifteen min after $B_{16}BL_6$ melanoma cell injection (10^5 cells, i.v.) the blood was drawn to evaluate the tumor induced thrombocytopenia.

Evaluation of immunomodulating activity in mice.

For this purpose, iloprost dissolved in saline was injected into mice according to following different treatment schedules: 0.2 mg/kg i.v.; 0.2 mg/kg s.c. for 5 days and 2 mg/kg s.c. for 5 days. Control groups were injected with vehicle alone. At different times after drug treatment, standard parameters of the immune response involved in the control of tumor cell growth and metastatic dissemination were examined. These tests included macrophages-mediated tumor cell cytostasis (growth inhibition) (8); NK cell activity assay *in vitro* (9); *in vivo* clearance of tumor cells by the lungs (9); T-cell mediated immune response *in vitro* (10).

Statistical analysis.

The analysis of data was performed by Student's t-test. Differences were considered significant when P values were <0.05.

RESULTS

Antiplatelet activity of iloprost in mice.

Platelet aggregation generated by subthreshold concentration of collagen plus epinephrine was completely and irreversibly inhibited by $4x10^{-8}$ M iloprost added *in vitro* two min before introduction of the aggregating agents. The inhibitory effect of iloprost on platelet aggregation remained throughout the entire 180 min of observation.

In *ex vivo* experiments we found that 0.2 mg/kg of iloprost completely inhibited platelet aggregation induced by collagen plus epinephrine for as long as 90 min after single i.v. dose. However the antiplatelet effect declined rapidly thereafter and was gone at 120 min after injection.

The *in vivo* antiplatelet activity of iloprost was compared to the tumor cell-induced thrombocytopenic effect. These results are shown in Figure 1.

Immunomodulating activity of iloprost in mice.

Macrophages collected from iloprost-treated mice induced about 30% (with 0.2 mg/kg) and 40% (with 2 mg/kg) inhibition of P815 tumor cell growth compared to the maximum cytostatic activity of macrophages collected from Poly I:C-treated mice, used as positive control. By contrast macrophages collected from vehicle-treated mice showed no detectable cytostatic activity.

Furthermore NK lytic activity of spleen cells obtained from mice treated with different doses of iloprost was significantly boosted compared to activity of splenocytes obtained from vehicle-treated mice. These results are shown in figure 2.

In addition, the effect of iloprost on *in vivo* pulmonary clearance of tumor cells was evaluated. For this purpose, mice treated with different doses of drug were injected with labelled YAC-I cells and the radioactivity retained within the lung was determined 4 hr later. We found that the radioactivity retained in the lungs was less in iloprost-treated mice than in mice treated with vehicle alone. However, this

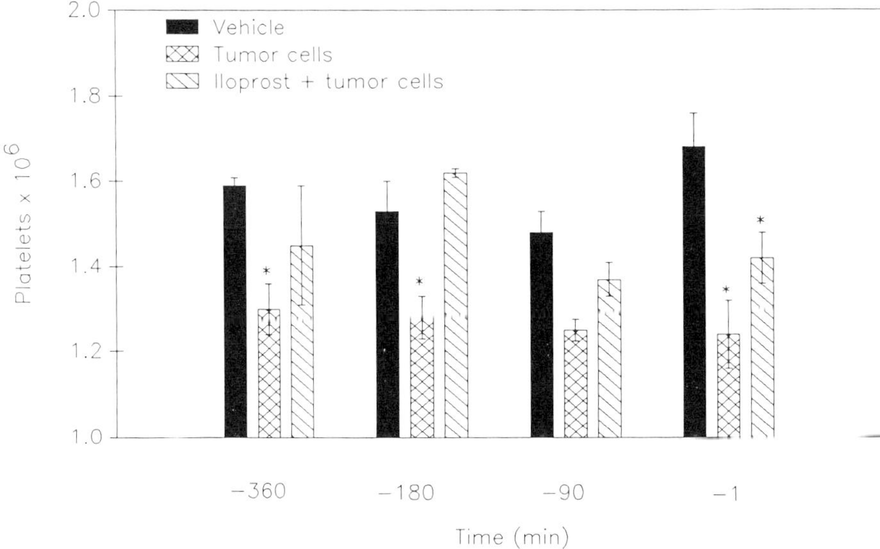

Figure 1 *In vivo* effect of iloprost (0.2 mg/kg, i.v.) on tumor cell-induced thrombocytopenia. Mice were injected with melanoma $B_{16}BL_6$ cells (10^5) at the indicated times after drug injection and platelet count was performed fifteen min after tumor cell challenge. *$p < 0.05$ with respect to vehicle alone.

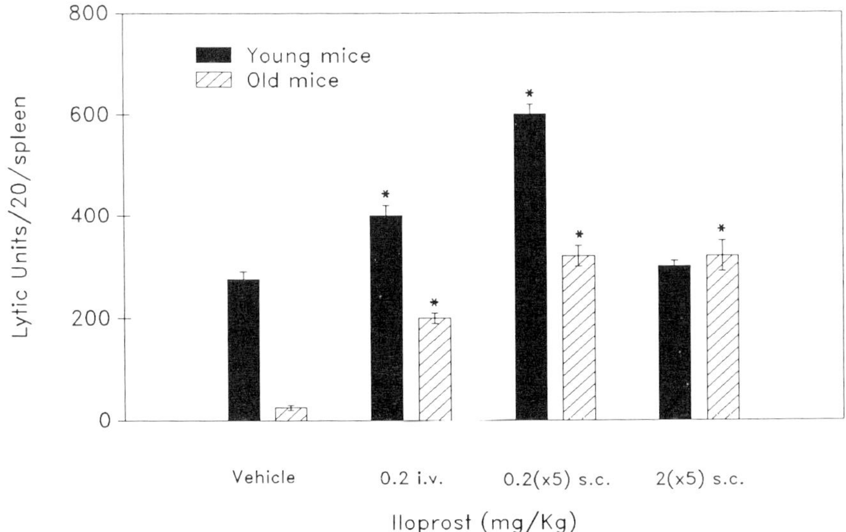

Figure 2 Effect of iloprost treatment on NK cell activity *in vitro*. Mice (8 or 32 weeks old) treated with different doses of iloprost, were used as donors of lymphocytes to be reacted *in vitro* with radiolabelled YAC-1 cells. *$p < 0.05$ with respect to vehicle alone.

reduction reached statistical significance only in younger mice treated with 0.2 mg/kg i.v. iloprost.

Finally we evaluated the effect of iloprost treatment on generation of cytoxic T-lymphocytes. Mice treated with different doses of iloprost were used as donors of lymphocytes to be sensitized *in vitro* with allogenic spleen cells and then assayed for cytoxic activity to radiolabelled RBL-5 tumor target cells. We found that iloprost treatment increased significantly the lymphocyte cytotoxicity.

DISCUSSION

The present results indicate that the effects of iloprost, both *in vitro* and *ex vivo*, on mouse platelets are similar to the effects on human and rat platelets reported previously (1). In addition, iloprost pretreatment prevented the *in vivo* interaction between platelets and $B_{16}BL_6$ tumor cells even when the drug was injected 360 min before tumor challenge.

Because the dosage and duration of effects of iloprost on mouse platelet aggregation correspond to those that inhibit metastasis (4), it is conceivable that the antimetastatic activity of the drug may be due, at least in part, to its platelet antiaggregating effects.

However, because our tumor cell line showed a relatively small capacity to aggregates platelet *in vivo,* as demonstrated by the small reduction (about 20%) in platelet count after tumor cell injection, we postulated that the profound inhibitory effect of iloprost in metastasis might be only partially ascribed to its interference with the platelet aggregation process.

In order to better define the mechanism of antimetastatic activity of iloprost we also have obtained evidence that iloprost treatment is able to modulate host immunocompetence. In particular, the efficacy of the some standard parameters of the immune response, believed to be involved in the control of tumor cell growth and metastatic dissemination, was increased following iloprost treatment *in vivo* at selected doses.

A lot of data are now available about the regulation of the immune response by PGs (6). Nevertheless, most of the work reported in literature focuses on the role of PGs of E series in the regulation of cellular and humoral immune response as well on monocyte and NK-cell function (6). In this study we observed that an analogue of PGI_2 induced, both *ex vivo* and *in vivo,* a complex modification of the host immunocompetence of the mice compatible with the antimetastatic capacity of the drug.

In conclusion, our results suggest that the antimetastatic effect of iloprost in the mouse may be attributable to multiple mechanisms inhibition of platelet aggregation and stimulation of certain host immune functions.

ACKNOWLEDGMENTS

We thank Shering SPA, Milano, Italy for the supply of the drug. Work partially supported by CNR, PF "Oncology", grant #88.00489.44, Italy.

REFERENCES

1. Witt, W., Sturzebecher, S. and Muller, B. Thromb. Res. 51:607-616, 1988.
2. Honn, K.V., Busse, W.D. and Sloane, B.F. Biochem. Pharmacol. 32:1-11, 1983.
3. Gasic, J.C. Cancer Metastasis Rev. 3:99-116, 1984.
4. Costantini, V., Fuschiotti, P., Allegrucci, M., Agnelli, G., Nenci, G.G. and Fioretti, M.C. Cancer Chemother. Pharmacol. 22:289-293, 1988.
5. Hanna, N. and Fidler, I.J. J. Natn. Cancer Inst.65:801-809, 1980.
6. Goodwin, J. and Ceuppens, J. J. Clin. Immunol. 3:295-315, 1983.
7. Born, G.V.R. Nature 194:927-909, 1962.
8. Fidler, I.J. In: Cancer Invasion and Metastasis Biologic and Therapeutic Aspects. (Eds. G.L. Nicolson and L. Milas), Raven Press, New York, 1984, pp.421-437.
9. Riccardi, C., Giampietri, A., Migliorati, G., Cannarile, L., D'Adamio, L. and R.B. Herberman. Int. J. Cancer 38:553-562, 1986.
10. Leung, K.H. and Mihich, E. Nature 288:597-600, 1980

PAF & ETHER LIPIDS - ROLE IN RADIATION INJURY AND TUMOR GROWTH

ROLE OF PLATELET-ACTIVATING FACTOR IN IMMUNE PROCESS

E. PIROTZKY, D. HOSFORD, J.-M. MENCIA-HUERTA, and P. BRAQUET

Institut Henri Beaufour Research Labs., ZA de Courtaboeuf - 1, ave des Tropiques, 91952 Les Ulis Cedex - France

INTRODUCTION

In most instances when the host is asked to mount a specific immune response, the initial event or the subsequent response, or both, are associated with non-specific inflammation. In recent years, with the identification of numerous molecular and cellular components of the inflammatory response, many laboratories have undertaken studies of potential interactions between the latter and the protagonists of more specific immunological reactions. In particular, soluble mediators of inflammation, produced by phagocytes, endothelial cells, skin or nerves have been studied in regard to their possible modulation of lymphocyte and monocyte-macrophage functions. Among them, histamine (1), prostaglandins (2), leukotrienes (3) and neuropeptides (4) have been shown to exert varied immunoregulatory effects.

Platelet-activating factor (PAF) is a potent mediator of inflammation, being released during numerous and varied inflammatory, allergic or immune reactions and participating in their development. The discovery of selective PAF receptor antagonists has contributed immensely to the definition of a role for PAF in many disease processes and identified the mediator a potentially powerful immunoregulatory agent.

Cellular sources of PAF are numerous and include various leukocyte populations (5), endothelial cells and probably other cell types (6). Resting lymphocytes are unable to produce PAF, possibly due to a lack of acetyl transferase (7). However, several T- and B-cell lines (8) and large granular lymphocytes (9) can be activated to produce PAF under certain circumstances. Indeed, many of the cells or tissues which produce PAF are themselves targets of PAF-induced bioactions, with the potential for amplification processes to occur.

EFFECTS ON LYMPHOCYTES

Proliferation.

When PAF was added to cultures of human peripheral blood mononuclear leukocytes (PBML) stimulated with phytohemagglutinin (PHA) or concanavalin A (ConA), a concentration-dependent inhibition of PBML proliferation was observed. The IC_{50} was between 10^{-12} M and 10^{-10} M and PAF needed to be present during the first 3 h of the 72 h culture for suppression to be observed. Lyso-PAF or (S)-PAF were inactive, while a similar effect was seen with the non-hydrolysable PAF analog, enthoxy-

PAF (11). PAF-induced inhibition of PBML proliferation was prevented by the use of the PAF receptor antagonists BN 52020 and BN 52021 indicating that PAF mediated this effect via a class of receptors analogous to that found on platelets. Suppression was also reversed by the cyclo-oxygenase inhibitor indomethacin, suggesting that prostaglandins (PGs) were involved as second messengers in the PAF-induced inhibition of lymphocyte proliferation. Some of these initial findings were confirmed by Dulioust et al., (12) who reported that PAF suppressed CD4+ T-cell proliferation; the effect occurred at high concentrations of PAF and could be seen when PAF was added late during culture. Similarly, Gebhardt et al., (13) reported inhibition by PAF of lymphocyte proliferation in response to allogeneic stimuli in primary or secondary mixed lymphocyte cultures. BN 52021 not only blocked the effects of PAF but had by itself a stimulatory effect on MLC. In contrast, Behrens and Goodwin (14) reported augmented CD4+ T-cell proliferation in response to PAF, which could be blocked by BN 52021.

In a different system, PAF and two non-hydrolysable PAF analogs increased the proliferation of IL-2-stimulated human lymphoblasts, while some PAF receptor antagonists (CV-3988 and L-652731 but not WEB 2086 or BN 52021) inhibited such proliferation (15). This effect of the antagonists was observed even when the drugs were added 48 h after initiation of the 72 h culture, suggesting an interference of the antagonists with later events in proliferation of preactivated T-cells. Furthermore, the possibility that endogenously produced PAF could be involved in some step of IL-2-induced proliferation of human T-lymphoblasts was suggested by inhibition of such proliferation by the PAF synthesis inhibitor, L-648,611 (15).

Interleukin 2 production.

Because lymphocyte proliferation involves, in its early stages, the production of IL-2, the production of this lymphokine by PBML was measured after 24 h of stimulation with PHA, in the presence or absence of PAF. Again, a concentration-dependent inhibition of IL-2 production was observed with an IC_{50} of 10^{-11} M and reversal by the PAF-antagonist, BN 52021 (10). PAF needed to be present during the first hour of the 24 h culture for the effect to be measurable. In contrast, Dulioust et al., (12) reported that PAF suppressed CD4+ T-cell proliferation, but the inhibition was not associated with inhibition of IL-2 production.

In vivo infusion of PAF into rats via osmotic minipumps has allowed the study of PAF effects in the whole animal. After 7 days of infusion, splenocytes from PAF-treated rats showed enhanced IL-2 production in response to Con A (16), indicating that contrary to its direct effects in vitro, PAF could exert a positive effect on T-cells in vivo, potentially via interactions with selected lymphocyte subpopulations or with non lymphoid cells (macrophages, endothelial cells, etc). Both inhibition of lymphocyte proliferation and augmentation of lymphoblast responses to IL-2 in the presence of PAF may be explained by the simultaneous actions of this lipid mediator on separate T-cell subpopulations with divergent immunoregulatory properties.

Induction of suppressor and helper cell activity.

Inhibition of lymphocyte functions may be due to interference with one or more stages of activation. It can also be due to induction or activation of suppressor cells. To test the latter hypothesis in relation to PAF-induced effects, human lymphocytes were preincubated with PAF for 3 - 18 h. The cells were then washed and added to fresh autologous lymphocytes stimulated with mitogens. Using this coculture system, it was observed that PAF-pretreated PBML exerted a significant suppressor effect on proliferation of indicator PBML (17, 18). When PBML were fractionated into selected subsets and purified as monocytes, T-cells or selected T-cell subpopulations before preincubation with PAF, a remarkable spectrum of activities emerged: PAF-preincubated monocytes were induced to express indomethacin-sensitive suppressor cell function. Monocyte-depleted lymphocytes showed a slight helper effect, while CD8+ T-cells were induced to become indomethacin-resistant suppressor cells. CD8+ T-cells required 10 to 100 fold lower concentrations of PAF to exert suppression. CD4+ T-cells, in contrast, were activated to exert a very marked helper effect.

During inflammation, blood lymphocytes cross the wall of blood vessels and infiltrate into the tissues. Endothelial cells, which line the vessels, can thus modulate lymphocyte functions; particularly, some products of endothelial cells, such as PAF, can inhibit the proliferation of lymphocytes. In experiments by Lacasse and Rola-Pleszczynski (19), human endothelial cells (HEC), isolated from the umbilical cord vein, were exposed to PAF for 1 h, the PAF-antagonist, BN 52021 (10^{-4} M), interleukin-1 (IL-1) or to the cyclooxygenase inhibitor indomethacin (10^{-6} M), alone or in combination. The HEC were then treated with mitomycin C, washed and incubated 72 h with lymphocytes and Con A. It was found that the preincubation of HEC with IL-1 alone or with indomethacin induced a significant suppression of lymphocyte proliferation of 20 and 25%, respectively (19). Concomitant use of BN 52021 completely prevented this suppressor activity exerted by HEC, suggesting that endogenous PAF from HEC was mediating the suppressive effect. Preincubation of HEC with exogenous PAF (10^{-12} M - 10^{-8} M) also induced suppressor cell activity and this was blocked by BN 52021. These results suggest that IL-1 and indomethacin together stimulate the production of PAF by HEC, which in turn suppresses lymphocyte proliferation. This effect of PAF is blocked by BN 52021 which can thus restore normal lymphocyte proliferation.

Immunoregulation by endothelial cell-derived PAF and its prevention by a PAF-antagonist may have important implications in the numerous disease states where vascular inflammation is a prominent component.

Membrane antigen expression.

The induction of suppressor lymphocytes was accompanied, in the above studies, by an increase in CD8+ T-cell numbers and a slight decrease in CD4+ T-cells (18), as assessed by indirect immunofluorescence and flow cytometry. CD2+ (sheep erythrocyte receptor-positive) T-cells also increased in numbers, but the most striking increase was seen in T-cells bearing DR antigens. No effect was seen on numbers of IL-2 receptor (Tac)-positive T-cells. In contrast, Vivier et al., (20) reported partial down-regulation of CD2 and CD3 antigen expression by PAF following incubation with PAF in a time and concentration-dependent manner. HLA class I antigen expression was not affected. Differences in the concentrations of PAF used in the different experimental systems may account for the contradictory results.

Cytotoxic cell functions.

Cytotoxic cells and their various effector mechanisms are thought to play an important role in host defenses against a whole array of foreign invaders, including parasites, viruses, neoplastic and grafted cells. Many effector cell types (T-cells, NK-cells and other natural cytotoxic lymphocytes, macrophages, polymorphonuclear leukocytes, etc) participate in these functions and most of the effector mechanisms involved appear distinct but are still largely undefined.

Preliminary data from several laboratories suggest that PAF may play a role during certain cytotoxic activities, as PAF receptor antagonists have been shown to inhibit them. For example, BN 52021 can inhibit rat splenic lymphocyte-mediated lysis of Langerhans islet cells (21). In other non-lymphocyte systems, keratinocyte killing of Candida albicans (22) and eosinophilmediated cytotoxicity against Schistosoma mansoni (23) were also found to be blocked by the PAF-antagonist.

Several lines of evidence indicate that NK-cell activation involves membrane phospholipid metabolism and modulation of NK function by the arachidonic acid metabolites, leukotriene B_4 (24, 25) and thromboxane A_2 (26) has previously been described. When human monocyte-depleted lymphocytes were cultured with the NK-sensitive K562 target cells in a standard 4 h 51 Cr release assay, in the presence of graded concentrations of PAF, NK activity was significantly enhanced (32 to 110 %) at all effector target cell ratios, but predominantly so at lower ratios (27, 28). Maximum activity was found at PAF concentrations of 10^{-13} M to 10^{-11} M, and this was not blocked by the PAF-antagonists, BN 52021 and WEB 2086. In contrast, PAF concentrations of 10^{-7} M or greater were often associated with inhibition of NK activity, an effect which could be reversed by PAF-antagonists. While optimal enhancement was observed when PAF was added at the initiation of the cytotoxicity coculture, or within the first 30 min, significant enhancement was also seen when PAF was added as late as 1 h to the culture. Lymphocytes could also be preincubated for 1 to 18 h with PAF, followed by washing to avoid interaction of PAF with target cells, and significant enhancement of NK activity still ensued. Both binding of lymphocytes to K562 cells and post-binding single cell lytic efficiency were augmented by PAF (28).

Although it is impossible to verify at the present time, the above findings could be explained by the presence of two PAF receptors on NK-cells, one with a lower affinity, which could be linked with inhibition of cell function, and another with high affinity, linked with augmentation of cell function. Mandi et al., (29) reported a marked inhibition of both rat and human NK-cell function by BN 52021 and other structurally non-related PAF-antagonists such as BN 52111 and 52115. Conversely, data concerning allospecific cytotoxic T-lymphocytes (CTL) suggest that PAF may have inhibitory effects, since BN 52021 enhances the generation of CTL when included in the mixed lymphocyte culture (13).

In several transplantation models, however, PAF appears to act as a prorejection mediator (30). BN 52021 increases cardiac allograft survival in rats, acting synergistically with azathioprine and cyclosporine A (31).

Analogous findings have also been reported with skin (32), liver (33) and kidney (34) grafts. The mechanism(s) and cells involved in these phenomena in relation to PAF are essentially unknown at this time.

Additional studies have been undertaken to evaluate the possiblity that PAF could modulate NK activity by enhancing the production of cytotoxic cytokines. In these investigations, large granular lymphocytes (LGL) were incubated with various target cell lines (K562, Clone I, MA-160, SK-MEL 109), in the presence or absence of PAF. Supernatants were collected and assayed for cytotoxicity in a 20 h 51 Cr-release assay against WEHI 164 and U-937 target cells which are sensitive to cytotoxic cytokines. The results showed that LGL incubated with several types of target cells, in the presence of PAF, released significantly increased amounts of cytotoxic factors (35). The maximal release was obtained after 8 to 10 h of incubation. Mannose-6-PO_4 (10 mM) which inhibits natural killer cytotoxic factor (NKCF) was not able to block supernatant cytotoxicity against U-937 target cells, while anti-tumor necrosis factor alpha (TNFα) antibody completely abolished supernatant activity. These findings suggest that picomolar concentrations of PAF enhance the release of cytotoxic factor(s), mainly TNFα, by LGL following interaction with target cells.

EFFECTS ON MONOCYTES-MACROPHAGES.

That PAF can activate monocyte or macrophage functions has been known for some time, as shown by Hartung (36). More recently, Ho et al., (37) observed that PAF could modulate the expression of c-fos and c-myc onogenes in human monocytes, indicating that PAF can initiate activation or differentiation of monocytes at the gene level. Studies on the early PAF-induced events of GTPase stimulation, adenylate cyclase inhibiton, phosphoinositide metabolism, calcium mobilization and protein phosphorylation (38, 43) have lead to suggestions that there is more than one class of PAF receptors and that PAF interacts with a GTP-binding (guanine nucleotide regulatory) protein which differs from the classical N_s and N_i proteins by its insensitivity to cholera and pertussis toxins. Elucidation of the molecular events leading to modulation of the various monocyte-macrophage functions is presently the object of numerous studies, in particular as it relates to cytokine synthesis and release.

Interleukin 1 production.

When exogenous PAF is added to monocytes or macrophages, several patterns of responsiveness in terms of IL-1 production can be seen, as reported from different laboratories. Mouse peritoneal macrophages, elicited either with thloglycollate or starch, respond in a varied and irregular manner to PAF (unpublished observations). In contrast, rat splenic macrophages present a biphasic response (44) : low concentrations of PAF (10^{-12} M - 10^{-10} M) significantly enhance IL-1 production while higher concentrations are inhibitory. Continous low rate administration of PAF in vivo, in rats, via osmotic mini-pumps also revealed a biphasic effect on subsequent ex vivo IL-1 production by rat splenic monocytes (16) : cells from rats having received 28 µg of PAF during 7 days showed impaired IL-1 (both released and cell-associated) production in response to LPS stimulation. In contrast, cells from rats having received 1 - 9 μg of PAF showed augmented IL-1 production. These effects were abolished in animals having received a concomitant treatment with BN 52021, given orally.

IL-1 production by human monocytes is also modulated by PAF. Barret et al., (45) initially reported an enhanced production of IL-1 when human monocytes were cultured in the presence of graded concentrations of PAF. Even in the absence of any other stimulus, such as lipopolysaccharide (LPS), (R)PAF and PAF analogs PR 1501 and PR 1502, but not (S)PAF, were capable of inducing IL-1 production. Salem et al., (46) also showed that PAF could increase IL-1 production by human monocytes stimulated with muramyl dipeptide, with higher concentrations of PAF inducing the maximum responses.

Studies also indicate a positive effect of PAF on IL-1 production by human monocytes stimulated with muramyl dipeptide (MDP) or LPS (47). In platelet-free, elutriated human monocytes, PAF augmented IL-1 production in a concentration-dependent manner characterized by 2 peaks, one at high (10^{-8} M - 10^{-6} M) and another at low (10^{-15} M - 10^{-14} M) concentrations. Failure to remove platelets following isolation of monocytes by adherence resulted in varied responses to PAF, with predominant inhibition of IL-1 production at higher concentrations. BN 52021 abrogated the PAF effects, mainly in the higher concentration range. PAF can also synergize with interferon-gamma (IFN) to induce higher levels of IL-1 production by human monocytes (48). This may be part of an amplification loop since various cytokines stimulate a biphasic synthesis of PAF by human monocytes (49). Thus, in addition to directly modulating monocyte activity, at very low concentrations PAF can also "prime" the cells to respond in an enhanced manner to subsequent agonistic stimuli that would otherwise be ineffectual. We have recently shown that PAF can prime (following an 18 h preincubation) monocytes to produce augmented quantities of IL-1. This may be analogous to the observations in polymorphonuclear leukocytes (PMN) where priming with PAF augments their superoxide generation, elastase release and lysis of endothelial cells in response to phrobol ester or formyl-methionyl-phenylalamine (FMLP) (50). Tumor necrosis factor (TNFα) can also prime PMN for enhanced PAF-induced superoxide production (51). When human PMN were incubated for 3 h at 37° C with various concentrations of TNFα (1 - 1000 ng/ml), a significant dose-dependent generation of superoxide was observed. The response was maximal with 10 ng/ml TNFα and after 60 - 90 min of incubation, $O_2^{\cdot-}$ production declining after this time. PAF alone (0.1 fM - 0.1 nM) failed to elicit any superoxide production, however, when PAF was added for 10 min to cells previously incubated for 80 min with 10 ng/ml TNFα, superoxide production was enhanced relative to that induced by TNFα alone. Maximum amplification (+ 30 %) was obtained with 10 fM PAF and the enhancing effect of the mediator was completely abolished by four structurally unrelated PAF-antagonists (BN 52021, kadsurenone, BN 52111 and WEB 2086), added either simultaneously with the TNFα or the PAF (51). In addition, the PAF-antagonists also decreased by 30% the superoxide production elicited solely by TNFα, indicating that TNFα-induced superoxide generation is partially mediated by a mechanism involving endogenous PAF.

Tumor necrosis factor production.

Another major cytokine produced by monocytes and macrophages is TNFα, which has been found to mediate not only cytotoxic activities against various target cells but also inflammatory and immunoregulatory functions.

When rat alveolar macrophages (AM) were cultured with PAF alone, no change in TNFα production was observed. However, the concomitant addition of PAF and MDP to AM cultures markedly enhanced (2 - 3 fold) TNFα production in a concentration-dependent fashion with a maximum effect at 10^{-10} M PAF (53, 54). This enhancement occurred when MDP and PAF were present together at the initiation of the 24 h culture. Stimulation of TNFα production by PAF was blocked by specific PAF receptor antagonists, BN 52020, BN 52021 and WEB 2086 with IC_{50} of respectively, 1 x 10^{-6} M, 2.0 x 10^{-7} M, and 8.0 x 10^{-8} M. Additionally, the stereoisomer of PAF, [S]PAF, used at 10^{-10} M - 10^{-12} M failed to induce significant enhancement in TNFα production. In parallel, addition of PAF to AM triggered leukotriene B_4 (LTB_4) release in a concentration-dependent manner. Inhibition of 5-lipoxygenase by NDGA or AA-861 blocked the PAF-induced augmentation of both TNFα and LTB_4 production. These findings suggest that PAF stimulates TNFα production by interaction with a specific putative receptor and by subsequent induction of endogenous leukotriene production.

The ability of lipoxygenase products, mainly leukotriene B_4, to participate in immunoregulatory processes and to modulate cytokine production has been previously documented (55). Exogenous and endogenous LTB_4 was found to enhance IL-1, IL-2 and IFN production (56, 57). Recently, we observed that exogenous and endogenous LTB_4 can up-regulate TNFα production by rat alveolar macrophages (58) and human monocytes (59). Thus, the findings of a concentration-dependent LTB_4 production by AM stimulated with PAF and the con-comitant inhibition of PAF-induced TNFα production as well as LTB_4 generation by lipoxygenase inhibitors are consistant with the possibility that the action of PAF on AM can be mediated by the generation of endogenous lipoxygenase metabolites, probably LTB_4, which will further act as second messengers to induce TNFα production. Human monocytes-macrophages can also be stimulated by PAF to produce augmented quantities of TNFα (47, 53, 60). It has also been reported that TNFα production is enhanced at two concentration ranges of PAF, 10^{-15} M - 10^{-13} M and 10^{-9} M - 10^{-7} M in LPS-treated monocytes. BN 52021 blocks both effects, while pertussis toxin partially inhibits the effect of higher PAF concentrations, suggesting mediation through a N_i-type guanine nucleotide regulatory protein.

Furthermore, PAF or IL-1 can prime monocytes to respond to LPS with enhanced production of TNFα during a subsequent culture with IL-1 or PAF, respectively. These findings suggest again that a cascade of inflammatory signals may have much greater effects than simultaneous or individual activities.

Cytotoxic activity.

Although several studies are in progress to assess the effects of PAF in monocyte-macrophage-mediated cytotoxicity, relatively little is known at the present time. Bonavida et al., (60) reported that the presence of TNFα inhibitors may be responsible for lack of cytotoxicity when TNFα production by human monocytes was enhanced in response to PAF.

Expression of FcεRII/CD23 receptors.

The demonstration that various cells types can express a receptor for the Fc fragment of IgE distinct from that described on mast cells and basophils (FcεRI) has been obtained by the use of IgE-coated erythrocytes, binding studies with radiolabelled IgE, and more recently by the use of monoclonal anti-Fcε receptor antibodies (61). The expression of this receptor is regulated by various cytokines and, as described recently, by lipids mediators such as PAF and LTB_4 (62, 63). Both animal and human lymphocytes and monocytes/macrophages express FcεRII/CD23 and secrete soluble IgE-binding factor (sCD23), two phenomena now known to play a major role in the regulation of the IgE synthesis (64, 65).

Recent evidence has shown that PAF is involved in the regulation of the expression of FcεRII/CD23. Incubation of monocytes and B lymphocytes, but not T lymphocytes, with PAF induced a dose-dependent increase in FcεRII/CD23 (62, 66). Regarding B-lymphocytes, the possibility that the PAF-dependent FcεRII/CD23 induction might be due to the endogenous production of secondary messengers from contaminating monocytes cannot be excluded. Indeed, PAF has been shown to induce leukotriene synthesis in phagocytes (rev. in 6), and these autacoids, and especially LTB_4 potentiate FcεRII/CD23 expression, the release of the soluble FcεRII/CD23 and the IgE secretion induced by IL-4 (63, 67).

The release of potent pro-inflammatory mediators by IgE-dependent mechanisms suggest that this immunoglobulin class could contribute to allergic and immunological reactions directly by activating FcεRII/CD23-bearing cells. Alveolar macrophages collected from allergic patients release lysosomal enzymes selectively on addition of the specific allergen (rev. in 61). As well, the production of sulfidopeptide leukotriene by alveolar macrophages stimulated with anti-IgE has also been reported (68). The possibility that the cells surface FcεRII/CD23 could play a role in the late phase reaction following antigen or PAF challenge has not been previously considered. Thus, we have investigated the possible modulation of FcεRII/CD23 expression on a alveolar macrophages from sensitized rats, challenged or not with the antigen. In another set of experiments, the FcεRII/CD23 expression on rat alveolar macrophages stimulated by PAF _in vivo_ was also evaluated.

Brown-Norway rats were placed twice at 48 h interval in a plexiglass chamber (30 x 50 x 30 cm) and exposed to aerosols of a saline solution containing 10 mg/ml ovalbumin (OA) for 30 min. A booster administration was performed in the same conditions at day 14. When challenged with antigen at day 21, sensitized rats developed a sustained bronchopulmonary response of about 30%, as calculated over the value obtained by clamping the trachea at the end of the experiment. In contrast, in the absence of the booster administration, rats developed a lower bronchopulmonary response of about 10 - 15%. Fifteen to 20 days after the initial sensitization procedure, the rats were challenged in the plexiglass chamber by exposure to successive solutions of OA, according to the protocol previously described to induce bronchial hyperreactivity in the guinea-pig (62). Histological examination of the lung tissue 4 h and 24 h after the antigen challenge of sensitized rats by aerosol demonstrated an increase in the number of infiltrating eosinophils, predominantly in the peribronchial zones. In addition 24 h after the challenge, alveolar macrophages from sensitized and challenged rats were obtained by 5 successive bronchoalveolar lavages of saline solution (37°C). The expression of FcoRII/CD23 antigen was evaluated by flow cytometry using the BB10 monoclonal antibody. No expression of FcεoII/CD23 on alveolar macrophages from antigen-challenged, non-sensitized rats was observed. In contrast, 74% of the alveolar macrophages expressed FcεRII/CD23 after antigen stimulation by aerosol, compared to 11% following challenge with saline.

In another set of experiments, we observed that aerosolized PAF (500 µg/ml for 30 min) induced the expression of FcεRII/CD23 on 79% of the alveolar macrophages collected from non-sensitized rats, 24 h after the challenge with the autacoid. This is to be compared to the 20% expression of FcεRII/CD23 after administration by aorocol of thc metabolite/precursor of PAF: lyso-PAF (500 µg/ml). These results obtained in animal models strengthen the data obtained in vitro on human monocytes (62, 67) and suggest a role for both FcεRII/CD23 and lipids mediators in the late phase of allergic reaction.

CONCLUSIONS AND PERSPECTIVES

As shown by the results of numerous current studies, PAF appears to exert several potent immunoregulatory functions at various levels of the immune response. Some studies, such as those on NK-cell activity and macrophage production of TNFα suggest that these cells may bear more than one class of receptors for PAF, with different patterns of inhibition by PAF-antagonists and distinct coupling to GTP-binding proteins. The recent demonstration by our laboratory that PAF increases FcεRII/CD23 receptor expression on macrophages further implicates PAF as a crucial mediator of immunological responses in asthma and the late phase allergic response. Further studies on the binding and molecular definition of PAF receptors on cells of the immune system are needed to determine the full extend to which PAF is involved in the modulation of immune responses.

REFERENCES

1. Rocklin RE, Haberek-Davidson A. 1981. J. Clin. Immunol. 1 : 73-79.
2. Goodwin JS, Ceuppens J. 1983. J. Clin. Immunol. 3 : 295-315.
3. Rola-Pleszczynski M. 1985. Immunol. Today. 6 : 302-307.
4. Payan DG, McGillis JP, Goetzl EJ. 1986. Adv. Immunol. 39 : 299-323.
5. Chilton FH, Ellis JM, Olson SC, Wykle RL. 1984. J. Biol. Chem. 259 : 12014-12019.
6. Braquet P, Touqui L, Shen TY, Vargaftig BB. 1987. Pharmacol. Review. 39 : 97-145.
7. Jouvin-Marche E, Ninio E, Beauvain G, Tence M, Niaudet P, Benveniste J. 1984. J. Immunol. 133 : 892-898.
8. Bussolino F, Foa R, Malavasi F, Ferrando ML, Camussi G. 1984. Exp. Haematol. 12 : 688-693.
9. Malvasi F, Tetta C, Funaro A, Bellone G, Ferrero E, Caligaris-Cappio F. 1986. Proc. Natl. Acad. Sci. (USA), 83 : 2443-2447.
10. Rola-Pleszczynski M, Pignol B, Pouliot C, Braquet P. 1987. Biochem. Biophys. Res. Commun. 142 : 754-760.
11. Pignol B, Mencia-Huerta JM, Braquet P, Rola-Pleszczynski M. 1987. Fed. Proc. 46 : 6990.
12. Dulioust A, Vivier E, Salem P, Benveniste J, Thomas Y. 1988. J. Immunol. 140 : 240-245.
13. Gebhardt BM, Braquet P, Bazan HEP, Bazan NG. 1988. Immunopharmacol. 15:11-20.
14. Behrens T, Goodwin JS. 1987. Prostaglandins 34 : 154.
15. Ward SG, Lewis GP, Westwick J. 1987. Prostaglandins 34 : 149.
16. Pignol B, Henane S, Sorlin B, Rola-Pleszczynski M, Mencia-Huerta JM, Braquet P. 1988. New

Trends Lipid Mediator Res. (P. Braquet, Ed.) Karger, Vol. 1 : pp. 38-43.
17. Rola-Pleszczynski M, Turcotte S. 1987. Prostaglandins. 34 : 148.
18. Rola-Pleszczynski M, Pouliot C, Turcotte S, Pignol B, Braquet P, Bouvrette L. 1988. J. Immunol. 104 : 3547-3552.
19. Lacasse C, Rola-Pleszczynski M. 1988. FASEB J. 2 : A1450.
20. Vivier E, Salem P, Dulioust A, Praseuth D, Metezeau P, Benveniste J, Thomas Y. 1988. Eur. J. Immunol. 18 : 425-430.
21. Farkas G, Mandi Y, Koltai M, Braquet P. 1987. Prostagandins. 34:158.
22. Dobozy A, Hunyadi J, Kenderessy A, Csato M, Braquet P. 1988. New Trends Lipid Mediator Res. (Braquet P, ed.) Karger vol. 1 : 168-176.
23. McDonald AJ, Mogbel R, Wardlaw AJ, Kay AB. 1986. J. All. Clin. Immunol. 77 : 227.
24. Rola-Pleszczynski M, Gagnon L, Sirois P. 1983. Biochem. Biophys. Res. Commun. 113 : 531-537.
25. Gagnon L, Girard M, Sullivan AK, Rola-Pleszczynski M. 1987. Cell. Immunol. 110 : 243-252.
26. Rola-Pleszczynski M, Gagnon L, Bolduc D, LeBreton G. 1985. J. Immunol. 135 : 4114-4119.
27. Rola-Pleszczynski M, Turcotte S. 1987. Immunobiol. (Suppl.) 3 : 135.
28. Rola-Pleszczynski M, Turcotte S, Gagnon L, Pignol B, Braquet P, Bolduc D, Bouvrette L. 1988. New Trends Lipid Mediator Res. (Braquet P, Ed.) Karger Vol. 1 : pp. 89-98.
29. Mandi Y, Farkas G, Koltai M, Braquet P, Beladi I. 1988. New Trends Lipid Mediator Res. (Braquet P, ed.) Karger Vol 1. : 76-84.
30. Foegh M, Ramwell P. 1987. Prostaglandins. 34 : 186.
31. Foegh ML, Khirabadi BS, Rowles JR, Braquet P, Ramwell PW. 1986. Transplant. 42 : 86-88.
32. Mulno JC, Ruggieri JP, Ale A, Cejas HA. 1988. Trans. Proc. 20 : 313-315.
33. Filipponi F, Michel A, Guillon JM, Braquet P, Houssin D. 1988. Prostaglandins 35 : 806.
34. Makowaka L, Chapman F, Mazzaferro V, Quian S, Enrichens F, Olivero G, Zerbe A, Sauders R, Starzi T. 1988. Prostaglandins 35 : 806.
35. Bosse J, Turcotte S, Rola-Pleszczynski M. 1988. FASEB J. 2 : A415.
36. Hartung HP. 1983. FEBS Letters 160 : 209-212.
37. Ho YS, Lee WMF, Snyderman R. 1987. J. Exp. Med. 165 : 1524-1538.
38. Homma H, Hanahan DJ. 1988. Arch. Biochem. Biophys. 262 : 32-39.
39. Bachelet M, Adolfs MJP, Masliah J, Bereziat G, Vargaftig BB, Bonta IL. 1988. Eur. J. Pharmacol. 149 : 73-78.
40. Barzaghi G, Mong S. 1988. Prostaglandins 35 : 819.
41. Hopple S, Meurer R, Westwick J, Macintyre DE. 1988. FASEB J. 2 : A415.
42. Prpic V, Uhing RJ, Weiel JE, Jakol L, Gawdi G, Herman B, Adams DO. 1988. J. Cell. Biol. 107 : 363-372.
43. Bussolino F, Turrini F, Fischer E, Alessi D, Karzatchline MD, Arese, P. 1988. Prostaglandins 35 : 803.
44. Pignol B, Henane S, Mencia-Huerta JM, Rola-Pleszczynski M, Braquet P. 1987. Prostaglandins 33:931-939.
45. Barret ML, Lewis GP, Ward S, Westwick J. 1987. Br. J. Pharmacol. 90 : 113P.
46. Salem P, Dulioust A, Derickz S, Vivier E, Benveniste J, Thomas Y. 1987. Fed. Proc. 46 : 922.
47. Rola-Pleszczynski M, Gingras D, Poubelle P. 1988. Submitted.
48. Barthelson R, Valone FH, Debs R, Philip R. 1988. FASEB J. 2 : A1228.
49. Valone FH, Epstein LB. 1988. FASEB J. 2:A878.
50. Vercellotti GM, Yin HQ, Gustabson KS, Nelson RD, Jacob HS. 1988. Blood 71:1100-1107.
51. Paubert-Braquet M, Lonchampt MO, Klotz P, Guilbaud J. 1988. Prostaglandins 35 : 803.
52. Worthen GS, Seccombe JF, Clay KL, Guthrie LA, Johnston RB Jr. 1988. J. Immunol. 140 : 3553-3559.
53. Rola-Pleszczynski M, Bosse J, Bissonnette E, Dubois C. 1988. Prostaglandins 35 : 802.
54. Dubois C, Bissonnette E, Rola-Pleszczynski M. 1988. Submitted.
55. Rola-Pleszczynski M. 1985. Today. 10 : 302-307.
56. Rola-Pleszczynski M, Lemaire I. 1985. J. Immunol. 135 : 3958-3961.
57. Rola-Pleszczynski M, Chavaillaz PA, Lemaire M. 1986. Prostagl. Leuk. Med. 23 : 207-210.
58. Dubois C, Bissonnette E, Rola-Pleszczynski M. 1988. J. Immunol. Submitted.
59. Gagnon L, Fillon LG, Rola-Pleszczynski M. 1988. J. Leuk. Biol. Submitted.
60. Bonavida B, Braquet P. 1988. Prostaglandins 35 : 802.
61. Dessaint JP, Capron A. 1988. Triangle 27 : 95-101.
62. Dugas B, Paul-Eugene N, Mencia-Huerta JM, Braquet P. 1989a. Taipei proceedings, Experta Medica Asia, Hong Kong, in press.
63. Dugas B, Paul-Eugene N, Gordon J, Spur BW, Braquet P, Mencia-Huerta JM. 1989b. Submitted.
64. Pene J, Rousset F, Briere F, Chretien I, Wideman J, Bonnefoy JY, De Vries JE. 1988. Eur. J.

Immunol. 18 : 929-935.
65. Delespesse G, Sarfati M, Hofstetter H, Frost H, Kilcher E, Suter U. 1989. Int. Arch. Allergy Appl. Immunol. 88 : 18- 22.
66. Paul-Eugene N, Dugas B, Gordon J, Yamaoka K, Spur BW, Kolb JP, Mencia-Huerta JM, Braquet P. 1989. Submitted.
67. Paul-Eugene N, Dugas B, Picquot S, Lagente V, Mencia-Huerta JM, Braquet P. 1989. Submitted.
68. Rankin JA, Hitchcock M, Merrill W, Bach MK, Brashler JR, Askenase PW. 1982. Nature 297 : 329-331.

CYCLOPENTENONE PROSTAGLANDINS: ANTI-PROLIFERATIVE AND ANTI-VIRAL ACTIONS AND THEIR MOLECULAR MECHANISM

S. NARUMIYA and M. FUKUSHIMA

Department of Pharmacology, Kyoto University Faculty of Medicine, Sakyo-ku, Kyoto 606, Japan, and Department of Internal Medicine, Aichi Cancer Center, Chikusa-ku, Nagoya 464, Japan

PERSPECTIVE AND SUMMARY

PGs of A and J series are active compounds exerting anti-proliferative and anti-viral activities of PGs. They are a group of PGs having a reactive α, β-unsaturated ketone group in their cyclopentane ring and thus named cyclopentenone PGs. Some cyclopentenone PGs occur in nature. Clavulones and punaglandins, acetoxy and halogenated derivatives of PGA, are isolated from octocoral, and Δ^{12}-PGJ_2 was identified as a PGD_2 metabolite in human urine. These PGs dose-dependently inhibit growth of cultured cells. The structure activity relationship of these PGs is quite different from those of other PGs, and unlike other PGs, they do not express their actions by acting on a cell surface receptor. They are actively transported into cells, and accumulate in nuclei. These cellular uptake and nuclear accumulation correlate well with their anti-proliferative actions. Flow cytometric analysis revealed that they block cell cycle progression at a specifc point in the G1 phase. Concurrent with this block, the PGs induce and suppress expression of several proteins. In addition to the anti-proliferative actions, these PGs show anti-viral activity at concentrations not toxic to host cells. The structure activity relationship for this activity is similar to that for the anti-proliferative activity, and studies have suggested that the PGs suppress expression of some viral genes to prevent virus replication. Thus, there are accumulating evidences that the cyclopentenone PGs exert their actions by regulating specific genes in nuclei. Based on these _in vitro_ studies, pre-clinical trials are in progress using synthetic analogues of these PGs on their anti-tumor and anti-viral activities.

PROSTAGLANDINS A AND J AND THEIR ANTI-PROLIFERATIVE ACTIONS

Cyclopentenone PGs as active compounds.

It is well known from 1970s that PGs of E and A series show potent growth inhibition in cultured cells (1). In early 80s we showed that PGs of D series have similar _in vitro_ anti-proliferative activity (2). Growth inhibition by these PGs is not limited to cells of special lineage, but seen in a variety of cultured cells. For example, more than 40 cultured cell lines from different source and species are now known to be sensitive to PGD_2 (3). This spectrum of PGD_2-sensitive cells had no relation to those for other PGD_2 actions such as stimulation of adenylate cyclase. In 1982 we found that dehydration derivative of PGD_2, 9-deoxy-Δ^9-PGD_2, shows growth inhibitory activity several times more potent than PGD_2 itself, whereas a potent PGD_2 agonist, BW245C, has no such activity on cultured cells (4). This finding led us to speculate that such dehydration type compounds are the ultimate form of PGs exerting growth inhibition. In the following years we found that PGD_2 actually undergoes such dehydration in plasma or in culture medium containing serum to form a new compound, 9-deoxy-Δ^9, ^{12}-PGD_2 (Figure 1) (5,6).

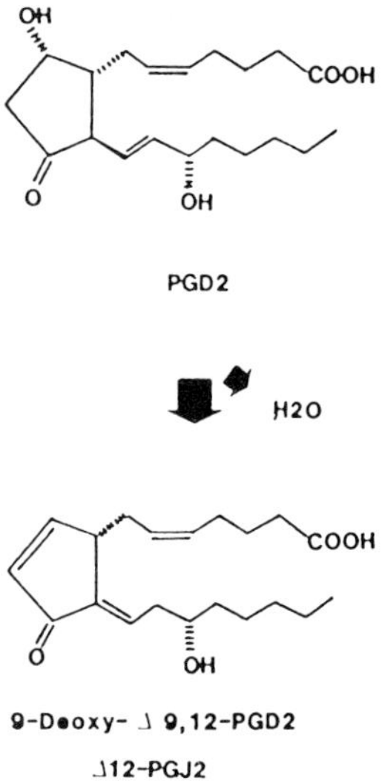

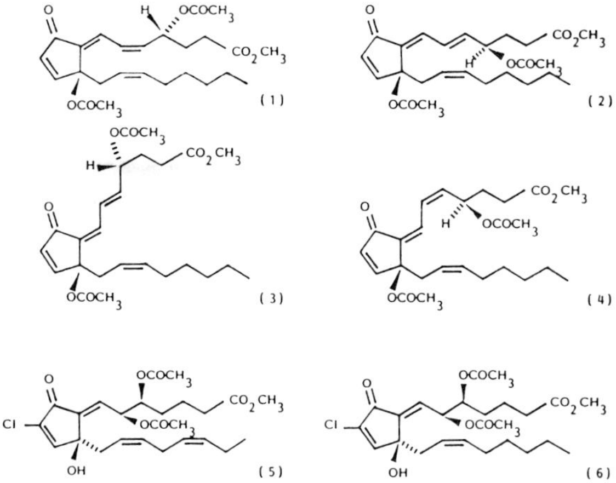

PGD2

H2O

9-Deoxy-Δ 9,12-PGD2

Δ12-PGJ2

Figure 1 (left) Metabolic activation of PGD_2 to a Δ^{12}-PGJ_2 in culture medium. Figure 2 (right) Structures of marine cyclopentenone PGs. 1-4: clavulones I, II, III and IV. 5,6: punaglandin-3 and -4.

We further found that this compound is the active compound exerting growth inhibition and PGD_2 serves only as a precursor to this compound (6). Since 9-deoxy-Δ^9-PGD_2 and 9-deoxy-Δ^9, ^{12}-PGD_2 have a novel cyclopentane structure with a 9,10-double bond and a 11-carbonyl group and a unique growth inhibitory activity, we named them PGJ_2 and Δ^{12}-PGJ_2, respectively (4,5). Similar study was carried out on the actions of PGE_2 on cultured cells and found that enzymatic dehydration occurs also on PGE_2, and that the dehydration metabolite, PGA_2, is the active compound (7). PGA and J have a conjugated enone structure in common in their cyclopentane ring, and are, therefore, called together cyclopentenone PGs. Concurrent with these findings, naturally occuring cyclopentenone PGs were isolated from octocoral (8,9). They are clavulones and punaglandins (Figure 2). These compounds showed more potent growth inhibitory activity than PGA and J. The in vitro potency of punaglandins is almost equivalent to those of vinka alkaloids and cis-platin and they suppress the growth of cultured cells at ng/ml concentrations (8).

Structure-activity relationship.

Based on the structure of PGA, clavulones and punaglandins, many structural analogues have been synthesized, and the structure-activity relationship for anti-proliferative action has been extensively studied (8,10). Several points were drawn from these studies (Figure 3). First, insertion of a double bond

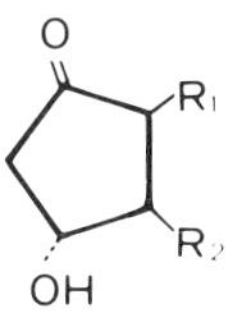 PGE, D	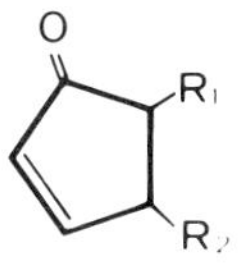 PGA, J	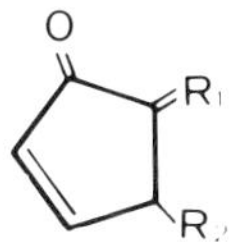 Δ^7-PGA, Δ^{12}-PGJ	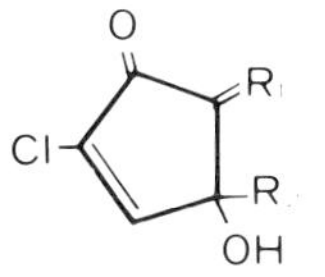 Punaglandin
IC 50 (µg/ml)			
2~5	0.7	0.3	0.03
Relative cytotoxicity			
1	5	10	100

Figure 3. Structure-activity relationship for the anti-proliferative activity of prostaglandins.

to the 7th position and increasing conjugation to cyclopentenone enhanced the activity several fold. This compound, Δ^7-PGA_1 is of about equivalent potency to clavulones but still much weaker than punaglandins. Chemical synthesis of punaglandins and related compounds revealed that the simultaneous presence of 12-hydroxy group and 10-chloride group is essential for its strong potency (8). Thus, increasing reactivity of α, β-unsaturated ketone in the ring structure appears most important for the growth inhibitory activity. Secondly, these studies revealed that the 15 hydroxy group is not required for the anti-proliferative action. Nor the streochemistry of the two side chains are not necessarily of natural configuration, because 12-epi-derivatives of PGA show equivalent potency. These structural requirements are in sharp contrast with those for other PG actions, and suggested that the anti-proliferative actions are mediated by a mechanism quite different from other PG actions.

Cellular uptake and nuclear accumulation as the mechanism for anti-proliferative action.

In 1986 we found that the cyclopentenone PGs such as PGA_2 and Δ^{12}-PGJ_2 are transported into cells by a carrier-mediated mechanism (11,12). This uptake was carried out by a cell membrane carrier specific for the cyclopentenone PGs. No incorporation of other PGs was observed. This uptake ocurrs in a temperature-dependent manner and concentrates the PGs about 20-fold over the medium, suggesting that it is an active transport. The PGs transported into the cytoplasm are further transferred to nuclei and accumulate there by binding to some nuclear proteins. We have shown that these processes, particularly nuclear accumulation, correlate well with expression of anti-proliferative actions. For example, growth inhibition by the PGs correlates well with the amount of the PGs taken up by the cells (11).

Moreover, when pharmacodynamics and actions of Δ^{12}-PGJ_2 was compared with those of PGA_2, we found that Δ^{12}-PGJ_2 forms irreversible binding to nuclear proteins, while that of PGA_2 is reversible. Consistently, the growth inhibition by Δ^{12}-PGJ_2 is irreversible and persistent, but that by PGA_2 was reversed by cell wash (13). Thus, evidences now accumulate to suggest that cell nuclei is a primary target for the cyclopentenone PGs. Then, what kind of actions do these PGs exert in nuclei and how do these lead to growth inhibition in cells? Before discussing them, we review the nature of PG-induced growth inhibition.

Induction of G1-block in cell cycle progression.

Dependent on concentrations used, the cyclopentenone PGs exerts either cytostatic or cytotoxic actions on cultured cells (3). Hughes-Fulford et al. (14) using flow cytometric analysis first showed that dimethyl-PGA_1 blocked cell cycle at G1 phase in randomly growing S-49 cyc^- cultured lymphoma cells. Following this report, Bhuyan et al. (15) reported that PGs A_1, A_2 and D_2 exerted similar action on several lines of human and murine melanoma cells. This G_1 block is now regarded as the major basis for anti-proliferative actions of cyclopentenone PGs at the cytostatic concentrations. However, the cell cycle analysis reported in the above studies were done using exponentially growing cells, and could not identify the PG-induced arresting point in the G1 phase. In order to clarify this, we (16) used HeLa S3 cells of synchronized growth, and analyzed the effect of these PGs. We found that the PGs arrested cell cycle progression at a point in the G1 phase which lies several hours before G1/S boundary. We also found that the arrest caused by PGA_2 is reversible, while that by Δ^{12}-PGJ_2 is irreversible, which is consistent with the behaviours of these two PGs in cell nuclei as discussed above. The most important observation in this study is that the PGs have to act specifically on the G1 phase cells to induce this G1 arrest. This strongly suggests the presence of specific target in the nuclei of G1 phase cells. The identity of this target is the focus of current study in this area. This target appears to be a minute component in nuclear proteins reacting with the PGs, because about the same amounts of the PGs are incorporated into nuclei in either phases of cell cycle (17).

Induction and suppression of specific genes.

In 1982 Santoro et al. (18) reported the induction by PGA of a specific protein of about 74 KDa in cultured African Green Monkey Kidney cells. Induction of proteins of similar molecular weight by PGA and J was also reported by other groups in other cultured cell lines, and correlation of this induction with the expression of anti-proliferative activity was suggested (19,20). We confirmed these findings in HeLa S3 cells of synchronized growth, and further found that this induction was associated with the G1 block of cell cycle progression caused by these PGs (17). From the properties of the induced protein(s), we suspected that they are so called HSPs (heat shock proteins), and confirmed this by identification on the two dimensional gel electrophoresis as well as peptide mapping (17). Although HSPs are induced in cells at high temperature or by other stress and such induction is associated with growth arrest in some systems, the causative relation of HSP induction with growth arrest has not been established yet, and the role of HSPs induction in the anti-proliferative actions of the cyclopentenone PGs remains unknown.

In addition to such induction, the PGs also suppress the synthesis of several proteins. Ishioka et al. (21) examined if the cyclopentenone PGs affect the expression of some oncogenes known to regulate the cell cycle progression. They were interested particularly in c-myc, because its suppression is reported to be associated with the G1 block. Using Northern hybridization method, they found that PGA_2 treatment completely suppressed transcription of c-myc gene after 3 and 6 h of incubation. Like other actions of PGA, this suppression then gradually disappeared during next 24 and 48 h. Suppression of c-myc appears specific, because expression of one of the constitutive gene HLA-B was not affected with the PG treatment at any time of the incubation. The above results suggest that c-myc suppression may be involved in the mechanism of PG-induced growth arrest. Whether the c-myc expression is the primary target for the PG action, again, remains to be elucidated (see below).

In relation to these studies on induction and suppression of specifc genes by the PGs, several groups showed that some protein synthesis inhibitors such as cycloheximide protected cells from the growth inhibition and cytotoxicity induced by the cyclopentenone PGs (20,22). Indeed, we have found that protein synthesis inhibitors such as cycloheximide and emetine attenuated the PG-induced G1 arrest of cell cycle (16). These results can be interpreted in two different ways. One interpretation is that the PG-induced G1 block is mediated by some proteins synthesized *de novo* and cycloheximide suppressed its synthesis and resumed growth. However, cycloheximide inhibits not only actions of the cyclopentenone PGs but also those of other anti-cancer agents such as cytosine arabinoside, methotrexate and vincristine. Since no protein induction was found in cells treated with the latter agents, inhibition of specific protein synthesis is difficult to conceive as a general mechanism of cycloheximide action. A more plausible explanation is that cycloheximide stops progression of the cells on the cell cycle at a point in the G1 phase before the PG can attack them. It is known that protein synthesis inhibitors can stop cell cycle progression in the G1 phase at a specific point named restriction point, or simply R point. As discussed above, the cyclopentenone PGs exert their action by acting on some target appearing specifically in the G1 phase. If this target appears after the R point in G1, the PGs cannot exert their action in cells arresting at the R point. Such relations can be mapped as shown in Figure 4. Suppression of c-

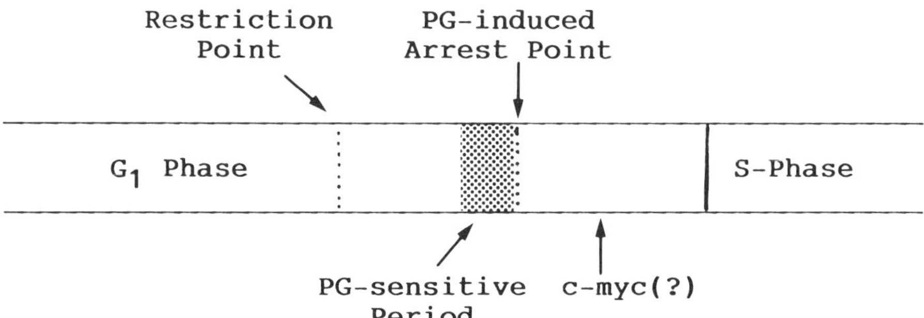

Figure 4. Presumed positions of the PG-sensitive period and the PG-induced arresting point in the G_1 phase.

myc described above could be explained also in this context, because this proto-oncogene is transiently expressed in the G1 phase. If the position of c-myc expression lies after the arresting point by the PGs, its suppression is the results of the PG-induced G1 arrest and not the mechanism. If the relative positions of the PG-sensitive period and the PG-induced arresting point with other G1 phase markers could be known by analogous analyses, we will be able to pin-point their positions at specific times in the G1 phase and identify the primary target and event for the PG actions.

PRECLINICAL TRIALS AS ANTI-TUMOR AGENT

Because of the potent in vitro anti-proliferative activity of the cyclopentenone PGs, several attempts have been made to develop clinically useful anti-tumor agents from these PGs. Δ^7-PGA_1 and its analogues are now under preclinical investigations in nude mice bearing tumors such as ovarian cancer, osteosarcoma, neuroblastoma, breast cancer and melanoma. These tumors are tested because they can be treated intra-cavitally or intra-arterially. Topical application in vivo of the PGs has already been shown quite effective. For example, local application of PGA_1 effectively inhibited tumor growth of human melanoma inoculated subcutaneously into nude mice (23). However, treatment of tumors by systemic administration have some difficulties because of systemic toxicity of the PG compounds. Several trials are being carried out to overcome this side effect. One is to develop drug delivery system for the PGs. Mizushima et al. (24) used lipid microsphere-integrated Δ^7-PGA_1 and observed improved efficacy in the treatment of several tumors. Another is drug design of PG molecules. Preliminary experiments showed that increased hydrophilicity of the PG molecules by modification of their side chains leads to improvement in in vivo efficacy. From this point, several analogues including sugar-conjugated PGA have been synthesized, and are now under trials (25).

Another approach in the preclinical trials is combination therapy of the synthetic PGs with other agents. One is the combination of Δ^7-PGA_1 with α-interferon (26). This combination reduced the colony-forming units of human melanoma cells on soft agar to only 20% of the control, whereas almost 90% recovered after treatment of either agent alone. The other is combination of PGD_2 and cisplatin (27). This combination significantly inhibited the growth of human ovarian cancer transplanted in nude mice when compared to those treated with either cisplatin or PGD_2 alone.

ANTI-VIRAL ACTIONS

Cyclopentenone PGs also have potent anti-viral activity. Table 1 summarizes reports on the anti-viral activities of prostaglandins. Since Luczak et al. (28) first reported in 1975 that PGs of E series inhibit the production of parainfluenza 3 virus in WISH cells, twelve species of viruses are known sensitive to PG actions. They include RNA viruses such as measles, polio and vesiclular stomatitis viruses as well as DNA viruses such as vaccinia and herpes simplex. Santoro et al. (29) are the first to show the antiviral activity of cyclopentenone PGs. They showed in 1980 that PGA has potent inhibitory activity on multiplication of Sendai virus in AGMK cells. Recently they also reported that PGJ_2 has similar inhibitory activity against

Table 1. Summary of reported anti-viral activity of prostaglandins.

Virus	Host Cell	PG ID90 (ug/ml)			References
RNA virus					
Parainfluenza 3	WISH[a]	PGE_2	>1	(48h)	28
		PGF_2	>1	(48h)	
Sendai	AGMK[b]	PGAs	4	(72h)	29
Measles	VERO (AGMK)	PGEs	>0.35	(48h)	36
Mengo	L929 fibroblast	PGE_1	>10	(96h)	37
MM	"	"	>10		
Polio	"	"	>10		
VSV[c]	mouse L-fibroblast	PGA	4	(24h)	32
EMC[d]	mouse L-fibroblast	"	4	(6h)	38
Sendai	AGMK	PGJ_2	4	(48h)	30
DNA virus					
Vaccinia	mouse L-fibroblast	PGAs	4	(24h)	39
HSV[d] I	Human amnion FL cell	PGD_2	5	(24h)	40
HSV II	AGMK	PGJ_2	4	(48)	30
HSV II	Human embroyonic fibroblast	Δ^{12}-PGJ_2	4	(24h)	31
HSV II	"	Δ^{7}-PGA_1	1	(24h)	31

a: Human amnion cell (WISH Inst) b:African green monkey kidney cell c:Vesicular stomatitis virus
d: Encephalomyocariditis
e: Herpes simplex virus

not only Sendai but also herpes simplex II (30). However, relative anti-viral potencies had not been examined for various PGs until Yamamoto et al. (31) examined the activities of PGs of E, A, D and J in human embryonic fibroblasts infected with Herpes simplex II. They found that all of PGD, E, A and J showed the antiviral activity. The potencies of PGD and E are much lower than PGA and J. PGJ and A, in turn, are weaker than their alkylidene derivative, Δ^{12}-PGJ and Δ^{7}-PGA, respectively. Thus, the structure-activity relationship for anti-viral activity is the same as that found for anti-proliferative activity, suggesting that the anti-viral activity is also associated with conjugated enone of cyclopentenone PGs.

Two mechanisms have been proposed as the molecular mechanism for anti-viral PG actions. Santoro et al. first reported that glycosylation of some virus protein is impaired in PGA-treated cells (32). The same authors later found by the use of the in vitro translation system that transcription of some of viral genes was suppressed in PGA-treated cells (33). More recently Yamamoto et al. demonstrated more directly the impairment of transcription of specific virus gene (31,34). They used human embryonic fibroblasts infected with herpes simplex virus (HSV) II. After virus-infection various concentrations of ^{7}-PGA_1 was added to the cells and incubation was carried out for four hours. Cells were then harvested and total cellular RNA was extracted and used for dot hybridization with a probe encoding immediate early gene of HSV II. They found that the content of the RNA hybridizable with the immediate early gene of HSV II decreased dose-dependently by PGA-treatment. Because the transcription of this immediate early gene of the virus requires the enzymes of the host cells, and this inhibition of transcription occurs in correlation with PG-induced change in protein synthesis as described above, these authors infer that cyclopentenone PGs suppress in host cells aome essential component(s) in transcriptional machinery to induce anti-viral state as well as to cause G1 arrest in cell cycle. Thus, the common mechanism for the anti-proliferative and anti-viral actions of the cyclopentenone PGs is hypothesized as shown in Scheme 1.

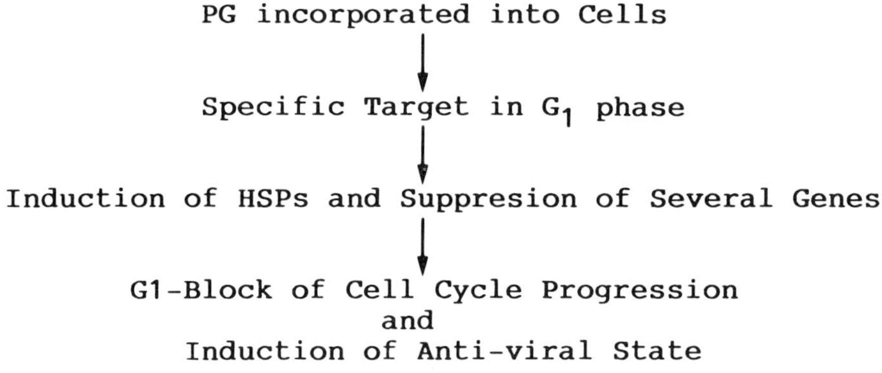

Scheme 1. Current hypothesis for the molecular mechanism for the anti-proliferative and anti-viral actions of the cyclopentenone PGs

The anti-viral activity is seen not only in the in vitro experiments but also in vivo in virus-infected animals. As pointed out by Santoro, one of the characteristics of the anti-viral activity of the PGs is that they do not require pretreatment of cells to exert their effect. That is in contrast with interferon action. Interferon needs to be added to the cells before virus infection. By the use of this property, she and her collaborators examined in vivo therapeutic potential of 16, 16-dimethyl-PGA_2 in Balb/c mice infected with influenza virus (35). They reported that this virus infection caused the death of 50 to 100% depending on the doses inoculated in mice and that dimethyl-PGA2 treatment improved mouse survival by about 40%. It was found that this PG treatment decreased virus titer in the lung, suggesting that the therapeutic action is due to in vivo suppression of virus replication.

PHYSIOLOGICAL SIGNIFICANCE

Although the anti-proliferative and anti-viral actions of cyclo-pentenone PGs are well established, their physiological significance remains unknown. This is partly because the natural occurrence of PGA and J has been questioned. PGA has long been regarded as a degradative metabolite of PGE and believed not to exist in the body. Neither, PGJ-ring metabolites were detected on the extensive analyses of urinary PGD_2 metabolites in humans and monkeys (41,42). Because PGJs are more hydrophobic than PGD and F, we suspected that metabolites containing PGJ ring structure were present in the non-analyzed non-polar fraction in the above studies and failed to be detected. In order to detect PGJ-type compounds in vivo in humans, we developed a sensitive enzyme immunoassay for Δ^{12}-PGJ_2. Using this assay, we purified Δ^{12}-PGJ_2-like immunoreactivity from human urine. This compound was finally identified as Δ^{12}-PGJ_2 by gas chromatography/high resolution-selected ion monitoring (43). We further showed that a single bolus injection of PGD_2 into cynomolous monkeys increased the urinary level of this metabolite 20- to 180-fold over the normal range, suggesting that PGD_2 is metabolized to Δ^{12}-PGJ_2 in the body. Interestingly, the urinary amounts of Δ^{12}-PGJ_2 are consistently higher in males than in females. Although more detailed study is needed to establish Δ^{12}-PGJ_2 as a naturally ocurring PG in the body, this initial report suggests a possibility that cyclopentenone PGs formed in vivo serve as a natural modulator of cell growth and as anti-viral defense mechanism in the body.

REFERENCES

1. Honn, K.V., Bockman, R.S. and Marnett, L.J. Prostaglandins. 21:833-864, 1981.
2. Fukushima, M., Kato, T., Ueda, R., Ota, K., Narumiya, S. and Hayaishi, O. Biochem. Biophys. Res. Commun. 105:956-964, 1982.
3. Fukushima, M. in AOCS Monograph "The Pharmacological Effect of Lipids", in press, 1989.
4. Fukushima, M., Kato, T., Ota, K., Arai, Y., Narumiya, S. and Hayaishi, O. Biochem. Biophys. Res. Commun. 109:626-633, 1982.
5. Kikawa, Y., Narumiya, S., Fukushima, M., Wakatsuka, H. and Hayaishi, O. Proc. Natl. Acad. Sci. U.S.A. 81:1317-1321, 1984.
6. Narumiya, S. and Fukushima, M. Biochem. Biophys. Res. Commun. 127:739-745, 1985.
7. Ohno, K., Fujiwara, M., Fukushima, M. and Narumiya, S. Biochem. Biophys. Res. Commun. 139:808-815, 1986.
8. Fukushima, M. and Kato, T. Adv. Prostaglandin, Thromboxane and Leukotriene Res. 15:415-418, 1985.
9. Honda, A., Yamamoto, Y., Mori, Y., Yamada, Y. and Kikuchi, H. Biochem. Biophys. Res. Commun. 130:515-523, 1985.
10. Kato, T., Fukushima, M., Kurozumi, S. and Noyori, R. Cancer Res. 46:3538-3542, 1986.
11. Narumiya, S. and Fukushima, M. J. Pharmacol. Exp. Ther. 239:500-505, 1986.
12. Narumiya, S., Ohno, K., Fujiwara, M., and Fukushima, M. J. Pharmacol. Exp. Ther. 239:506-511, 1986.
13. Narumiya, S., Ohno, K., Fukushima, M. and Fujiwara, M. J. Pharmacol. Exp. Ther. 242:306-311, 1987.
14. Hughes-Fulford, M., Wu, J., Kato, T. and Fukushima, M. Adv. Prostaglandin, Thromboxane and Leukotriene Res. 15:401-404, 1985.
15. Bhuyan, B.K., Adams, E.G., Badiner, G.T., Li, L.H. and Barden, K. Cancer Res. 46:1688-1693, 1986.
16. Ohno, K., Sakai, T., Fukushima, M., Narumiya, S., and Fujiwara, M. J. Pharmacol. Exp. Ther. 245:294-298, 1988.
17. Ohno, K., Fukushima, M., Fujiwara, M. and Narumiya, S. J. Biol. Chem. 263:19764-19770, 1988.
18. Santoro, M.G., Jaffe, B.M., Elia, G. and Benedetto, A. Biochem. Biophys. Res. Commun. 107:1179-1184, 1982.
19. Shimizu, Y., Todo, S. and Imashuku, S. Prostaglandins. 34:769-781, 1987.
20. Sakai, T., Aoike, A., Marui, N., Kawai, K., Nishino, H. and Fukushima, M. Cancer Res. 49:1193-1196, 1989.
21. Ishioka, C., Kanamaru, R., Sato, T., Dei, T., Konishi, Y., Asamura, M. and Wakui, A. Cancer Res.

48:2813-2818, 1988.
22. Shimizu, Y., Todo, S. and Imashuku, S. Prostaglandins. 32:517-525, 1986.
23. Bregman, M.D., Funk, C. and Fukushima, M. Cancer Res. 46:2740-2744, 1986.
24. Mizushima, Y., Shoji, Y., Kato, T., Fukushima, M. and Kurozumi, S. J. Pharm. Pharmacol. 38:132-134, 1986.
25. Fukushima, M., Kato, T., Narumiya, S., Mizushima, Y., Sasaki, H., Terashima, Y., Nishiyama, Y., and Santoro, M.G. Adv. Prostaglandin, Thromboxane and Leukotriene Res. 19:415-418, 1989.
26. Bregman, M.D. and Fukushima, M. in Cancer Chemotherapy Challenges for the Future II. pp. 82-89, Excerpta Medica, Tokyo, 1987.
27. Kikuchi, Y., Miyauchi, M., Iwano, I., Kita, T., Oomori. K. and Kizawa, I. Eur. J. Cancer Clin. Oncol. 24:1829-1833, 1988.
28. Luczak, M., Gumulka, W., Szmigielski, S. and Korbecki, M. Arch. Virol. 49:377-380, 1975.
29. Santoro, M.G., Benedetto, A., Carruba, G., Garaci, E. and Jaffe, B.M. Science. 209:1032-1034, 1980.
30. Santoro, M.G., Fukushima, M., Benedetto, A. and Amici, C. J. Gen. Virol. 68:1153-1158, 1987.
31. Yamamoto, N., Fukushima, M., Tsurumi, T., Maeno, K. and Nishiyama, Y. Biochem. Biophys. Res. Commun. 146:1425-1431, 1987.
32. Santoro, M.G., Jaffe, B.M. and Esteban, M. J. Gen. Virol. 64:2797-2801, 1983.
33. Benavente, J., Esteban, M., Jaffe, B.M. and Santoro, M.G. J. Gen. Virol. 65:599-608, 1984.
34. Yamamoto, N., Rahman, M.M., Fukushima, M., Maeno, E. and Nishiyama, Y. Biochem. Biophys. Res. Commun. 158:189-194, 1989.
35. Santoro, M.G., Favalli, C., Mastino, A., Jaffe, B.M., Esteban, M. and Garaci, E. Arch. Virol. 99:89-100, 1988.
36. Dore-Duffy, P. Prostaglandins, Leukotrienes and Med. 8:73-82, 1982.
37. Giron, D . J . Proc . Soc . Exp . Biol . Med ., 170: 25-28, 1982.
38. Ankel, H., Mittnacht, S. and Jacobsen, H. J. Gen. Virol. 66:2355-2364, 1985.
39. Santoro, M.G., Jaffe, B.M., Garaci, E. and Esteban, M. J. Gen. Virol. 63:435-440, 1982
40. Tanaka, A., Matsuoka, H., Nishino, H. and Imanishi, J. Prostaglandin, Leukotriene Med. 25:131-138, 1986.
41. Ellis, C. K., Smigel, M.D., Oates, J. A., Oelz, O. and Sweetman, B.J. J. Biol. Chem. 254:4152-4163, 1979.
42. Liston, T. E. and Roberts, L. J. J. Biol. Chem. 260:13172-13180, 1985.
43. Hirata, Y., Hayashi, H., Ito, S., Kikawa, Y., Ishibashi, M., Sudo, M., Miyazaki, H., Fukushima, M., Narumiya, S. and Hayaishi, O . J . Biol . Chem . 263 :16619-16625, 1988.

MEMBRANE-TARGETED BIOCHEMICAL EFFECTS AND THE ROLE OF CELLULAR DIFFERENTIATION IN THE SELECTIVE ANTITUMOR ACTIONS OF ALKYLMETHOXYGLYCEROPHOSPHOCHOLINE

F. SNYDER, D. S. VALLARI, Z. L. SMITH, and M. L. BLANK

Medical Sciences Division, Oak Ridge Associated Universities, Oak Ridge, TN USA

INTRODUCTION

Various studies of the selective antitumor activity of unnatural derivatives of platelet-activating factor (PAF), including clinical trials in Germany, have been reviewed by Berdel and Munder (1) and Berdel et al. (2). The close structural relationship between the antitumor agent, 1-alkyl-2-methoxy-sn-glycero-3-phosphocholine (alkylmethoxy-GPC) and PAF is illustrated in Figure 1. It appears that there is an inverse relationship between phospholipids of similar structure (i.e., those with a short chain aliphatic group at the sn-2 position) that possess PAF biological activities versus those that exhibit selective cytotoxic properties toward sensitive tumor cells. The natural enantiomer of PAF (L form) exhibits no cytotoxicity toward undifferentiated cells, whereas in stark contrast, D-PAF is highly toxic under the same conditions (3).

Our laboratory has utilized the highly sensitive HL-60 cell system as a model in studies directed toward understanding the mechanism responsible for the selective antitumor action of alkylmethoxy-GPC (3-7). Earlier experiments (5) demonstrated that the low activity of the O-alkyl cleavage enzyme (requires Pte • H_4) in tumor cells is not the major factor in explaining the selective antitumor response of the methoxy analog, although it undoubtedly is a contributing cause. Effects of alkylmethoxy-GPC appear to be membrane-targeted since it is associated primarily with the plasma membranes of HL-60 cells (5,7) where it inhibits protein kinase (8,9-11) and severely impairs the transport of small molecules into sensitive cells (6,7). These facts and the ability of the methoxy analog to alter cellular protein phosphorylation patterns (8,12) suggest some type of stimulus/response coupling mechanism might be involved in the biological consequences caused by this type of antitumor agent.

This brief report summarizes and extends some of our recent findings that revealed HL-60 cells become resistant toward the cytotoxic action of alkylmethoxy-GPC after their differentiation into granulocytes by dimethylsulfoxide (Me_2SO) (7). The undifferentiated/differentiated HL-60 cells provides an important system for investigating the biochemical mechanism of the cytotoxic action of the antitumor phospholipid analogs since comparisons can be made between sensitive and control resistant cells of the same origin.

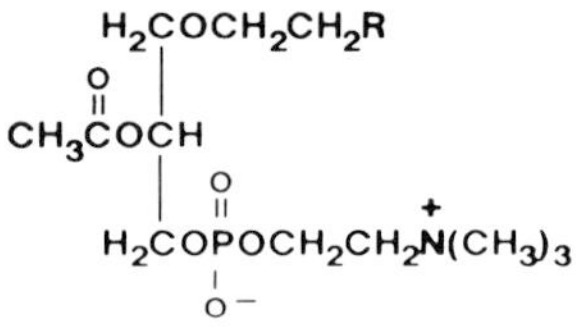

$H_2COCH_2CH_2R$

$CH_3\overset{O}{\overset{\|}{C}}OCH$

$H_2CO\overset{O}{\overset{\|}{P}}OCH_2CH_2\overset{+}{N}(CH_3)_3$

O^-

1-alkyl-2-acetyl-sn-glycero-3-phosphocholine
(platelet activating factor; PAF)

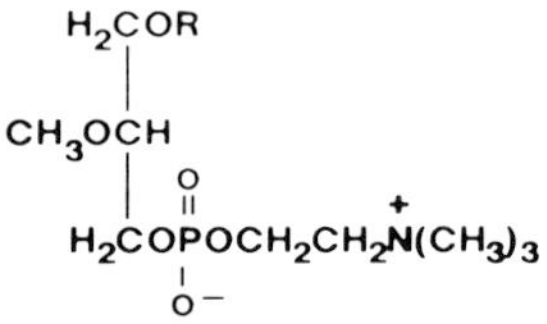

H_2COR

CH_3OCH

$H_2CO\overset{O}{\overset{\|}{P}}OCH_2CH_2\overset{+}{N}(CH_3)_3$

O^-

1-alkyl-2-methoxy-sn-glycero-3-phosphocholine
(PAF antitumor analog)

Figure 1. Structural similarities between PAF and the methoxy antitumor analog.

METHODS

Methodology used for obtaining the results summarized in this report has been described in earlier publications from our laboratory (5,7). Experiments to test the binding of [^{3}H]alkylmethoxy-GPC to undifferentiated HL-60 cells were done essentially according to the techniques described by Valone et al. (13). Binding results were obtained at both 20° and 37°C; approximately 93% of the parent compound remained intact under these experimental conditions.

RESULTS AND DISCUSSION

Undifferentiated HL-60 cells are highly sensitive to the cytotoxicity of alkylmethoxy-GPC, an unnatural analog of PAF (Figure 2).

Surprisingly when HL-60 cells were differentiated into a granulocytic form by Me_2SO, they become resistant to the sn-2 methoxy analog of PAF. Also, of interest is that differentiated HL-60 cells exhibit functionally active specific PAF receptors, whereas the undifferentiated HL-60 cells do not.

[^{3}H]Alkylmethoxyglycerophosphocholine is poorly metabolized (<7%) by both undifferentiated and differentiated HL-60 cells (7) and, therefore, a metabolic product of the analog is unlikely to be a causative factor in the cytotoxic response toward the sensitive form, i.e., undifferentiated HL-60 cells. Nevertheless we did test rac-1-alkyl-2-0-methoxy-glycerol (up to 25 μM), a minor metabolite of the methoxy phospholipid, and found it did not possess any antitumor activity (Figure 3).

As previously reported (7), when the sensitive HL-60 cells (undifferentiated form) were exposed to the alkylmethoxy-GPC (12 μM for 4 hrs.), the initial rate of [methyl-^{3}H] choline uptake was inhibited by

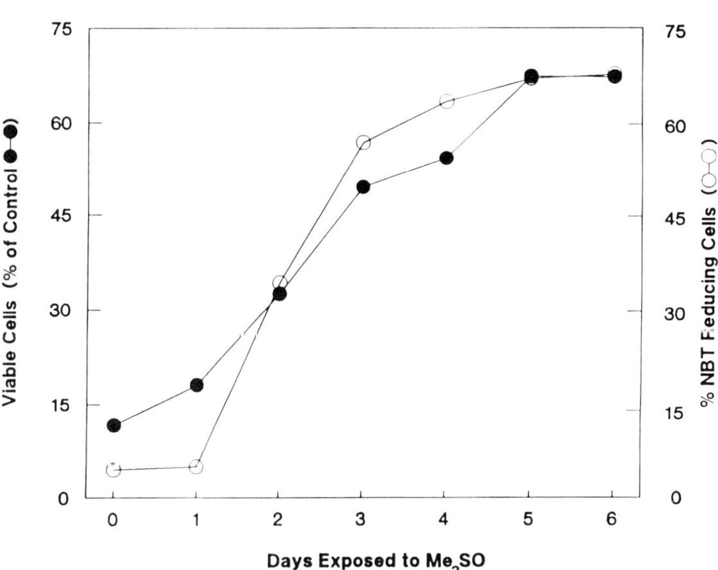

Figure 2. Development of resistance of HL-60 cells toward alkylmethoxy-GPC-mediated cytotoxicity as a function of differentiation to a granulocytic form by Me_2SO (see Ref. 7 for details). Reprinted with permission from Academic Press.

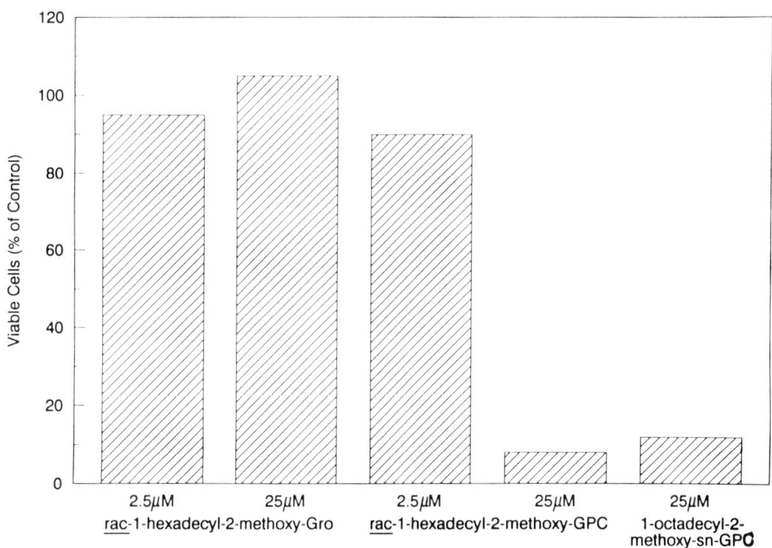

Figure 3. Lack of cytotoxic activity of rac-alkyl-2-methoxy-glycerol towards undifferentiated HL-60 cells.

35%. This is consistent with our earlier findings (6) that indicate sensitive cells exhibit an impaired transport of nutrient molecules across the cell membrane after they are treated with these cytotoxic phospholipids. We do not imply that this is necessarily a direct effect on cell transport systems but instead could possibly be explained by an interference with protein phosphorylation other regulatory factors associated with transport processes.

Based on Scatchard analyses, we were unable to demonstrate the presence of any specific cell surface receptors (at 20° and 37°C) for alkylmethoxy-GPC on cells sensitive (undifferentiated HL-60 cells) to this agent. The undifferentiated cells took up [^{3}H]alkylmethoxy-GPC only by a nonsaturable mechanism. Thus, these results clearly indicate that the antitumor action of alkylmethoxy-GPC does not involve a receptor mediated mechanism. Moreover, in cells exposed to the [^{3}H]methoxy analog for 10 min. at 37°C (63% cellular uptake of the radioactive lipid), we were able to remove 35.9% of the [^{3}H]alkylmethoxy-GPC when the cells were washed six times with 1% bovine serum albumin (in phosphate-buffered saline) as described by Mohandas et al.(14). These results indicate that approximately two thirds of the methoxy analog is inaccessible to the albumin. Thus, it would appear that the labeled compound not removed by the albumin washes is deeply embedded in the internal matrix of the plasma membrane since we have previously shown that the methoxy analog is mainly associated with the cell surface membrane and not within internal organelles of HL-60 cells (5,7).

REFERENCES

1. Berdel, W.E. and Munder, P.G. In: Platelet Activating Factor and Related Lipid Mediators (Ed. Fred Snyder), Plenum Press, 1987, pp. 449-467.
2. Berdel, W.E., Andreesen, R., and Munder, P.G. In: Phospholipids and Cellular Regulation (Ed. J.F. Jo), CRC Press, 1985, pp. 42-74.
3. Hoffman, D.R., Hajdu, J., and Snyder, F. Blood, 63:545-552, 1984.
4. Hoffman, D.R., Stanley, J.D., Berchtold, R., and Snyder, F. Res. Commun. Chem. Pathol. Pharmacol. 44:293-306, 1984.
5. Hoffman, D.R., Hoffman, L.H., and Snyder, F. Cancer Res. 46:5803-5809, 1986.
6. Snyder, F., Record, M., Smith, Z., Blank, M., and Hoffman, D.R. Aktuel. Onkol. 34:19-26, 1987.
7. Vallari, D.S., Smith, Z.L., and Snyder, F. Biochem. Biophys. Res. Comm. 156:1-8, 1988.
8. Parker, J., Daniel, L.W., and Waite, M. J. Biol. Chem. 262:5385-5393, 1987.
9. Helfman, D.M., Barnes, K.C., Kinkade, J.M., Jr., Vogler, W.R., Shoji, M., and Kuo, J.F. Cancer Res. 43:2955-2961, 1983.
10. Daniel, L.W., Etkin, L.A., Morrison, B.T., Parker, J., Morris-Natschke, S., Surles, J., and Piantadosi, C. Lipids, 22:851-855, 1987.
11. Oishi, K., Raynor, R.L., Charp, P.A., and Kuo, J.F. J. Biol. Chem. 263:6865-6871, 1988.
12. Kiss, Z., Deil, E., Vogler, W.R., and Keo, J.F. Biochem. Biophys. Res. Comm. 142:661-666, 1987.
13. Valone, F.H., Coles, E., Reinhold, V.R., and Goetzl, E.J. J. Immunol. 129:1637-1641, 1987.
14. Mohandas, N., Wyatt, J. Mel, S.F., Rossi, M.E., and Shohet, S.B. J. Biol. Chem. 257:6537-6543, 1982.

ANTICANCER ACTIVITY AND EFFECT ON PROTEIN KINASE C (PKC) OF SYNTHETIC PHOSPHOLIPID ANALOGS

W. R. VOGLER[1], A. C. OLSON[1], M. SHOJI[1], J. F. KUO[2], and J. HAJDU[3]

Emory University School of Medicine, Department of Medicine, Division of Hematology/Oncology[1] and Department of Pharmacology[2], Atlanta, GA 30322, and California State University, Northridge[3] Northridge, CA 91330.

The discovery that alkyl-lysophospholipids (ALP), ether analogs of naturally occurring lysophosphatidylcholine (LPC) have antitumor activity has prompted the synthesis of numerous compounds which are cytotoxic to cells by acting on components of membranes (1). These glycerol phospholipids have been shown to have antitumor activity in vitro and in vivo and to be selectively cytotoxic to neoplastic tissues while sparing normal hematopoietic progenitor cells (2-5). Although the exact mechanism of action is unknown and may be multiple, the following observations have been made.

Phosphatidylcholine biosynthesis (PC) is inhibited. Inhibition of the incorporation of radiolabelled choline, LPC and methionine into PC by ALP has been demonstrated (6). This suggests that the salvage pathway and the de novo pathway for PC biosynthesis is impaired. Inhibition of the acylation of LPC to form PC by lysophosphatidylcholine acyltransferase is inhibited (7). Inhibition of choline incorporation suggests that CTP:phosphocholine cytidyltransferase is inhibited (8). Methionine is converted to S-adenosylmethionine which sequentially donates methyl groups to phosphatidylethanolamine (PE) to form PC via methyltransferase I and II (9). This latter reaction is considered a minor pathway and the inhibition is not as dramatic as seen with choline or LPC.

The phorbol ester 12-O-tetradecanoylphorbol-13-acetate (TPA) has been shown to stimulate phospholipid biosynthesis as measured by the uptake of radiolabelled choline by HL60 cells (10). This stimulation is reduced in the presence of ALP (7). Membrane associated enzymes are altered by ALP. Helfman, et al demonstrated that ALP acted competitively with phosphatidylserine to inhibit protein kinase C (PKC) purified from leukemic cells obtained from leukemic patients or human leukemic cell lines (11). Furthermore, ALP inhibited the TPA stimulation of PKC (12) and reduced the TPA induced phosphorylation of some proteins and increased the phosphorylation of another (13). ALP inhibits down regulation of soluble PKC induced by TPA in these HL60 cells (14). Differentiation of HL60 (13) and KG-1 (14) leukemic cells to macrophages after exposure to TPA was inhibited by ALP. Upon stimulation of cells by TPA, there is a translocation of PKC activity from the soluble to the particulate fraction and this correlates with an increase in differentiation to macrophages as measured by cell adherence (15).

ALP has also been shown to inhibit Na,K-ATPase and the sodium pump in brain tissue and HL60 cells in a manner different from that observed with ouabain, the classic inhibitor of ATPase (16). In addition, by using inside-out membranes of human erthyrocytes, Oishi, et al (16) demonstrated that ALP blocked the uptake of radiolabelled sodium, implying that ALP interacted with Na^+,-binding sites of Na,K-ATPase.

Tritiated thymidine incorporation into DNA is also inhibited by ALP (17). This may be a consequence of the observations described above, rather than a direct effect on DNA.

Thus, these compounds are of interest because of their unique site of action and their effect on signal transduction and possible alteration of message transmission within the cell. Because of these observations, efforts have been made to modify the molecule to make it more selectively cytotoxic. To improve the therapeutic index, a series of glycerol phospholipid analogs have been synthesized having 16 or 18 carbon chains in either an ether or a thio linkage at sn-1 and with either methoxy, thio methyl, methyl methoxy, or acetamide substitution at sn-2 and with phosphocholine at sn-3. These compounds have been compared to an earlier synthesized and most active compound racemic-1-0-stearyl-2-0-methyl-sn-glycero-phosphatidylcholine (ET-18-OCH_3) (1). The assays used were the inhibition of clonogenicity and thymidine incorporation in leukemic cell lines HL60, K562 and Daudi and normal marrow progenitor cells. In addition, their effect on PKC activity was assayed.

METHODS

Figure 1 demonstrates the compounds that were tested. Compounds A, B, C and D were synthesized by one of us. Compound E was provided by Dr. Paul Munder of Freiburg, FRG. Compound F was obtained from Boehringer Mannheim (Mannheim, FRG). The compounds were dissolved in RPMI 1640 medium containing 10% fetal bovine serum (FBS) (GIBCO, Grand Island, NY). The solutions were sterilized by micropore filtration (0.22 μM; Gelman Sciences, Inc., Ann Arbor, MI) and stored at -20°C until used.

Leukemic Cell Lines.

The HL60 myeloblastic cell line was obtained from Dr. Robert Gallo at NIH (Bethesda, MD). The K562 cell line, established from a patient in blast crisis of chronic myelocytic leukemia was obtained from Dr. Bismark Lozzio at the University of Tennessee (Knoxville, TN) and the Daudi leukemic cell line was obtained through the American Type Culture Collection (Rockville, MD).

Normal Bone Marrow Cells.

These cells were obtained by direct aspiration from a donor for allogeneic transplant after obtaining informed consent. Bone marrow mononuclear cells were separated by Ficoll-Hypaque (Histopaque-1077, Sigma Chemical Co., St. Louis, MO).

Treatment.

Cells were incubated at 37°C in 5% CO_2 for 4 hours with various concentrations of compounds. Incubations were performed in plastic culture tubes in RPMI 1640 medium containing 10% fetal bovine serum (FBS) and 1 to 5 X 10^6 cells per ml.

PHOSPHOLIPID ANALOGS

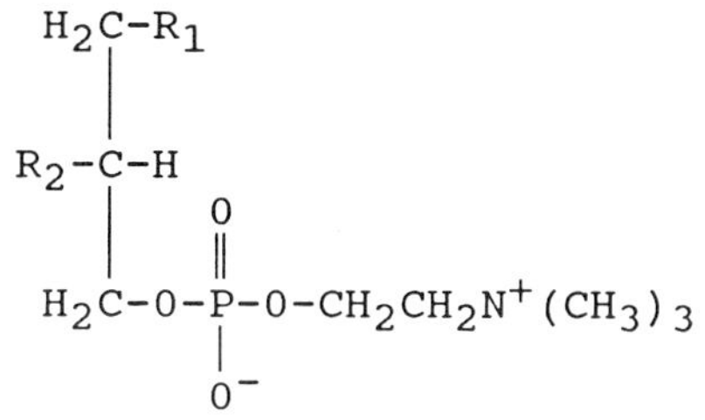

$$
\begin{array}{l}
H_2C-R_1 \\
\quad | \\
R_2-C-H \\
\quad | \qquad\quad O \\
\quad | \qquad\quad \| \\
H_2C-O-P-O-CH_2CH_2N^+(CH_3)_3 \\
\qquad\qquad\ | \\
\qquad\qquad O^-
\end{array}
$$

COMPOUND	R_1	R_2
A	$O-(CH_2)_{15}CH_3$	H_3C-S
B	$S-(CH_2)_{15}CH_3$	$H_3C-C(=O)-HN$
C	$O-(CH_2)_{15}CH_3$	H_3C-O
D	$O-(CH_2)_{15}CH_3$	$H_3C-C(=O)-HN$
E	$O-(CH_2)_{17}CH_3$	H_3C-O
F	$S-(CH_2)_{15}CH_3$	$H_3C-O-CH_2$

Figure 1. Phospholipid analogs. Compounds A-D were synthesized by one of the authors (J.H.).

Cell Viability.

After incubation, the cells were checked for viability by Trypan blue dye exclusion.

Clonogenic Assay.

Normal hematopoietic progenitor cells were assayed by a modification of the method of Fauser and Messner as previously described (5,18). One ml aliquots containing 1 X 10^5 cells were cultured in triplicate in 35-mm culture dishes (Lux; Miles Scientific, Naperville, IL) at 37°C in 5% CO_2 humidified air. The growth of colonies on each plate was scored at day 14 of culture and defined as the sum of CFU-GEMM, CFU-E, BFU-E, CFU-GM and GM clusters. Leukemic cell lines, after adequate dilution of the cell suspension, were cultured in the medium used for the assay of normal hematopoietic progenitor cells without stimulators. Cell aggregates consisting of more than 40 cells were scored as colonies on day 7 (HL60 and K562) or on day 14 (Daudi).

Tritiated Thymidine Incorporation.

Tritiated thymidine incorporation was carried out in triplicate as previously described (19). After 1 hour exposure to high specific activity tritiated thymidine (80-90 Ci/mmol), the cells were harvested in a mini-mash harvester and the isotope incorporation counted in a liquid scintillation counter.

PKC Assay.

PKC was assayed using purified PKC from brain tissue as previously described (15).

Statistical Methods.

The IC_{50} was defined as the concentration of compound that caused a 50% inhibition of the control value for the particular assay. Because of some variability in growth patterns of the cell culture assays, the means of repeated experiments were averaged and plotted as percent of control. The IC_{50} was calculated by the least-squares method.

RESULTS

Viability remained above 60% for all cell lines at concentrations of 75 μM for all of the compounds tested over the 4 hours of incubation (data not shown).

Table 1 compares the IC_{50}'s as determined by clonogenic assay and thymidine incorporation for the various compounds. By the clonogenic assay, the HL60 cell line is the most sensitive, compounds B and D were less active than the others. K562 was the most resistant and Daudi was intermediate. Compounds E and F appeared to be the most active. This was also observed when assayed by tritiated thymidine incorporation.

Table 1

IC_{50} (μM)

	CLONOGENIC ASSAY			THYMIDINE INCORPORATION		
COMPOUNDS	HL60	K562	DAUDI	HL60	K562	DAUDI
A	22	96	103	55	211	140
B	40	NI*	134	50	NI*	148
C	19	285	39	60	NI*	80
D	32	73	55	49	150	28
E	24	72	40	48	120	17
F	23	50	NT**	30	64	NT**

*NI = No Inhibition

**NT = Not Tested

Table 2 shows the effect of the compounds on PKC activity. Compounds D, E and F are more active than A or B (C has not been tested).

Table 2

PKC ACTIVITY (pmol P/min/mg/protein)

Compounds	IC_{50} (μM)
A	14
B	47
C	NT
D	5
E	7
F	5

NT = not tested

Table 3 shows the IC_{50} for normal bone marrow progenitor cells. As can be seen, normal cells are relatively resistant to these agents. We have previously reported that compounds D, E and F had no significant effect on normal marrow progenitor cells at concentrations that inhibited leukemic cells (20). Furthermore, there was no significant shift in the types of colonies formed. Preliminary results here (data from 1 donor) suggest that compounds A, B and C are more toxic to normal cells, but more studies are needed. The IC_{50}'s for GEMM were lower than the other types of colonies.

Table 3

EFFECT ON NORMAL BONE MARROW PROGENITOR CELLS

COMPOUNDS	IC_{50} (μM)	FRACTION SURVIVING 100 μM (%)
A	97	46
B	120	54
C	113	37
D	261	98
E	146	105
F	386	87

Table 4 gives the computed therapeutic indices for the clonogenic assays. This was obtained by dividing the IC_{50} for normal marrow progenitors by the IC_{50} for each of the compounds in each cell line. As shown, compound F gave the highest therapeutic index.

Table 4

THEREAPEUTIC INDICES*

	HL60	K562	DAUDI
A	4.41	1.01	0.94
B	2.99	NI**	0.90
C	5.95	0.40	2.91
D	8.15	3.57	4.75
E	6.08	2.03	3.65
F	16.08	7.72	NT***

*Calculated by dividing IC_{50} for total marrow progenitor cells by IC_{50} for each compound for each cell line

**NI = No Inhibition

***NT = not tested

DISCUSSION

Compound F which has a thio linkage in sn-1 and methyl-methoxy in the sn-2 position appears to have the highest therapeutic index, although it has not yet been tested on the Daudi cell line. Compound B which differs from F in that acetamide replaces the methyl-methoxy group in compound F has less activity. However, when there is an ether linkage at sn-1 and acetamide at sn-2 (compound D), the therapeutic index is improved. Compound C, which has a 16 carbon chain in sn-1 is just as active as the 18 carbon compound E against HL60 cells, but significantly less active against K562 and somewhat less active against Daudi.

It is of interest that compound B demonstrated less PKC activity than the others tested. How this is linked to the lesser cytotoxic effects and inhibition of thymidine incorporation at the molecular level remains unknown.

Thus, varying the substitution in sn-1 and sn-2 of glycerophospholipids alters the selective cytotoxicity of these analogs.

ACKNOWLEDGMENT

Supported in part by grants from The National Institutes of Health (CA-29850) and by the Beat Leukemia! Celebrity Classic. The authors are grateful to Dixon Lackey, Robert Raynor and Winnie Long for technical assistance and Barbara Adair for typing the manuscript.

REFERENCES

1. Berdel, W.E., Andreesen, R., Munder, P.G. In: Phospholipids and Cellular Regulation II (Ed. J. F. Kuo), CRC Press, Boca Raton, FL, 1985, pp. 41-73.
2. Andreesen, R., Modolell, M., Weltzien, H.U., Eibl, H., Common, H.H., Lohr, G.W., Munder, P.G. Cancer Res. 38:3894-3899, 1978.
3. Berdel, W. E., Fromm, M., Fink, U., Pahlke, W., Bicker, U., Reichert, A., Rastetter, J. Cancer Res. 43:5538-5543, 1983.
4. Muschiol, C., Berger, M.R., Schuler, B., Scherf, H.R., Garzon, F.T., Zeller, W.J., Unger, C., Eibl, H.J., Schmaehl, D. Lipids. 22:930-934, 1987.
5. Okamoto, S., Olson, A.C., Vogler, W.R., Winton, E.F. Blood. 69:1381-1387, 1987.
6. Vogler, W.R., Whigham, E., Bennett, W., Olson, A.C. Exp. Hematol. 13:629-633, 1985.
7. Vogler, W.R., Olson, A.C., Shoji, M., Li, H., Kiss, Z., Kuo, J.F. In: Pharmacological Effect of Lipids 3, in press.
8. Pelech, S.L., Cook, H.W., Paddon, H.B., Vance, D.E. Biochimica et Biophysica Acta. pp. 433-440, 1984.
9. Hirata, F., Viveros, O.H., Diliberto, E.J. Jr., Axelrod, J. Proc. Natl. Acad. Sci. 75:1718-1721, 1978.
10. Cassileth, P.A., Suholet, D., Cooper, R.A. Blood. 58:237-243, 1981.
11. Helfman, D.M., Barnes, K.C., Kinkade, J.M. Jr., Vogler, W.R., Shoji, M., Kuo, J.F. Cancer Res. 43:2955-2961, 1983.
12. Kuo, J.F., Shoji, M., Girard, P.R., Mazzei, G.J., Turner, R.S., Su, H.-D. In: Advances in Enzyme Regulation 25 (Ed. G. Weber), Pergamon Press, l986, pp 387-400.
13. Kiss, Z., Deli, E., Vogler, W.R., and Kuo, J.F. Biochem. Biophys. Res. Comm. 142:661-666, 1987.
14. Shoji, M., Raynor, R.L., Berdel, W.E., Vogler, W. R., and Kuo, J. F. Cancer Res 48:6669-6673, 1988.
15. Shoji, M., Girard, P.R., Charp, P.A., Koeffler, P., Vogler, W.R., Kuo, J.F. Cancer Res. 47:6363-6370, 1987.
16. Oishi, K., Zheng, B., White, J.F., Vogler, W.R., Kuo, J.F. Biochem Biophys. Res. Comm. 157:1000-1006, 1988.
17. Vogler, W.R., Whigham, E.A., Somberg, L.B., Long, R.C. Jr., Winton, E.F. Exp. Hematol. 12:569-574, 1984.
18. Fauser, A.A., Messner, H.A. Blood. 52:1243-1248, 1978.
19. Vogler, W.R., Olson, A.C., Okamoto, S., Shoji, M., Raynor, R.L., Kuo, J.F., Berdel, W.E., Eibl, H., Hajdu, J., Nomura, H. Lipids, in press.
20. Okamoto, S., Olson, A.C., Vogler, W.R. Cancer Res. 47:2599-2603, 1987.

RELATIONSHIP BETWEEN TRANSFORMED PHENOTYPE AND ETHER-LINKED LIPIDS

A. FALLANI, L. CALORINI, G. MANNORI, O. CECCONI, D. TOMBACCINI, E. BARLETTA, G. MUGNAI and S. RUGGIERI

Institute of General Pathology, School of Medicine, University of Florence, 1-50134 Florence, Italy.

INTRODUCTION

Interest in the structure and biochemistry of ether-linked glycerolipids has been stimulated by the finding that large amounts of ether-linked lipids are present in a variety of neoplasms (1,2). Intensive study of the biosynthesis of ether-linked lipids has led to the discovery that ether-linked lipids are the final products of the dihydroxyacetone-phosphate pathway (3) and that this pathway is prominent in tumors (4). It has been recently demonstrated that ether-linked lipids are precursors of PAF (5) and represent the major source of arachidonic acid for the biosynthesis of eicosanoids (6-8). However, our knowledge of the physiological significance of ether-linked lipids is still limited and, consequently, their role in malignant transformation remains obscure.

There are few investigations that correlate the level of ether-linked lipids to specific biological parameters in malignant cells. Howard et al. (9) found in a series of hepatomas that the highest levels of ether-linked lipids corresponded directly to a high growth rate. Moreover, the metastatic potential has been correlated with the level of alkyl-linked lipids in a series of mammary carcinomas (10). A high content of alkyldiacylglycerols was found to be associated with a high tumorigenicity and metastatic potential in polyethyleneglycol-resistant variants derived from mouse L cells (11) .

As a part of a long-term research program focused on the biological significance of the variations of lipid structure in malignant cells, we are currently investigating, by using appropriate model systems, the possible involvement of ether-linked lipids in specific aspects of the transformed phenotype, such as the loss of contact inhibition of growth, anomalous differentiation, and metastatic capacity.

MATERIALS AND METHODS

Cell Lines and Culture Conditions.

The following cell systems were used in the present study: the Balb/c3T3, SV3T3, and Concanavalin A-selected SV3T3 revertant cells (12); the B77-3T3 and B77-AA6 cells (13); the Friend erythroleukemia cells (14); the B16-F1 and B16-F10 melanoma cells (15); and the T3 cells (16) and subclones isolated in our laboratory by growing T3 cells in agar or in plastic.

The various fibroblastic and melanoma cell lines were grown in a monolayer using DMEM supplemented with 10% fetal calf serum (FCS), while FEL cells were grown in a suspension culture using RPMI 1640 medium supplemented with 5% FCS. FEL cells were induced to erythroid differentiation by growth in media supplemented with 280 mM DMSO or 5 mM HMBA (17). The metastatic potentials of the various metastatic cell lines were routinely checked by counting the lung nodules after injecting intravenously $5x10^4$ cells of the B16 and T3 cell systems, or subcutaneously $5x10^5$ cells of the B77-3T3 and B77-AA6 cell system into syngeneic animals.

Analysis of ether-linked lipids.

Total lipids were extracted from the sonicated cell suspensions and fractionated into individual lipid classes as described in a previous paper (12). Alkyldiacylglycerols, and alkyl-acyl- and alkenyl-acyl subfractions of phosphatidylethanolamine (PE) and phosphatidylcholine (PC) were determined following the method of Su and Schmid (18). This procedure involves the conversion of the alkenyl-groups of alkenyl-linked lipids into the cyclic acetals derivatives and the release of the alkylglycerols from alkyl-linked lipids by Vitride-mediated hydrogenolysis. The cyclic acetals and the isopropylidene derivatives (19) of alkylglycerols are then analyzed by quantitative gas-liquid chromatography using appropriate internal standards.

RESULTS AND DISCUSSION

We explored whether ether-linked lipids play a role in the loss of contact inhibition of growth by studying the following system of virally-transformed and revertant lines: the Balb/c3T3 cells transformed by the B77 strain of RSV (B77-3T3 cells) or by SV40 virus (SV3T3 cells), and the Concanavalin A-selected SV3T3 revertant cells. These latter exhibit a normal morphology and maintain contact inhibition of growth, although they contain the complete viral genome (20).

As shown in Table 1, Balb/c3T3 cells contain a high percentage of an alkenyl-acyl subfraction in PE and an appreciable amount of an alkyl-acyl subfraction in PC. Compared to untransformed Balb/c 3T3 cells, B77-3T3 and SV3T3 had a significantly ($P < 0.001$) higher levels of alkenyl-acyl PC. This level reverted to a normal value in Concanavalin A-selected SV3T3 revertant cells. Therefore, the behavior of alkenyl-acyl PC in transformed cells represents one of the several molecular changes characteristic of transformation.

In order to investigate whether ether-linked lipid changes in malignant cells are caused by a blockage of differentiation, we examined the changes of ether-linked lipids of Friend erythroleukemia (FEL) cells differentiated by dimethylsulfoxide (DMSO) or hexamethylene-bis-acetamide (HMBA). We also examined the ether-linked pattern of syngeneic DBA/2 mouse erythrocytes as a model of terminal differentiation in erythroid lineage.

FEL cells are virally-transformed cells blocked at an early stage of differentiation (21). When FEL cells are treated with specific chemical agents, they express several characteristics of normal erythropoiesis (22). Therefore, implicit in this model is the expectation that, once the differentiation process is completed, some of the aspects of the transformed phenotype revert to a normal pattern.

Table 1
Ether-linked (Alkenyl-Acyl and Alkyl-Acyl) Subfractions of Phosphatidylethanolamine (PE) and Phosphatidylcholine (PC) From BALB/C3T3, B77-3T3 and SV3T3 Cells, and Concanavalin A-Selected SV3T3 Revertant Cells

Values are expressed as percentages of the total phospholipid class which were calculated as previously reported (12).

Subfraction	Balb/c3T3	B77-3T3	SV3T3	SV3T3 Rev.
Alkenyl-acyl PE	33.0	46.7	40.4	29.3
Alkyl-acyl PE	12.0	12.0	8.9	5.9
Diacyl PE	55.0	41.3	50.7	64.8
Alkenyl-acyl PC	3.8	8.0	13.3	1.7
Alkyl-acyl PC	12.0	8.4	9.9	8.0
Diacyl PC	84.2	83.6	76.8	90.3

Table 2 shows that the undifferentiated FEL cells contained a high proportion of alkenyl-acyl molecules and an appreciable amount of alkyl-acyl molecules in PE . A high proportion of PC in FEL cells consisted of alkyl-acyl molecules, while alkenyl-acyl PC was scarcely represented. DBA/2 mouse erythrocytes had only limited proportions of ether-linked subfractions in PE and PC, mainly alkenyl-acyl PE. The levels of alkyl-acyl PE and PC tended to decrease ($P<0.01$) when FEL cells were induced to erythroid differentiation by either DMSO or HMBA. Their values, however, still exceeded the very low levels in the DBA/2 mouse erythrocytes; this behavior may be related to the incomplete stage of maturation reached by the differentiated FEL cells.

Table 2.
Changes of Ether-Linked (Alkenyl-Acyl and Alkyl-Acyl) Subfractions of Phosphatidylethanolamine (PE) and Phosphatidyl-Choline (PC) From FEL Cells Upon Differentiation With DMSO or HMBA

Values are expressed as percentages of the total phospholipid class which were calculated as previously reported (12).

	FEL cells			
Subfraction	Control	DMSO	HMBA	DBA/2 mouse erythrocytes
Alkenyl-acyl PE	34.0	35.9	49.5	13.0
Alkyl-acyl PE	10.1	6.9	4.7	1.0
Diacyl PE	55.9	57.2	45.8	86.0
Alkenyl-acyl PC	2.5	2.1	4.1	N.D.
Alkyl-acyl PC	21.9	11.4	7.7	2.3
Diacyl PC	75.6	86.5	88.2	97.7

To determine whether a metastatic phenotype may be correlated with a characteristic ether-linked lipid pattern, we examined the following systems of metastatic cells: a) the B16-F1 and B16-F10 melanoma cells with different lung-colonizing potentials (23); b) a high spontaneously-metastasizing subclone (B77-AA6 cells) isolated from the low metastatic B77-3T3 cells by growth in 0.6% agar (24); c) a high lung-colonizing line derived from a murine fibrosarcoma, the T3 cells (16), and a series of subclones with a different metastatic potential which have been isolated in our laboratory by growing T3 cells in agar or in plastic.

As shown in Table 3, all the cell lines, both metastatic and non-metastatic, contained high proportions of alkenyl-acyl molecules in PE and appreciable amounts of alkyl-acyl molecules in PC; these latter molecules were also present in PE of B77-3T3 and B77-AA6 cells. However, compared to their corresponding low metastatic counterparts, B16-F10 cells had a higher level of alkyl-acyl PC ($P< 0.05$), while B77-AA6 cells showed higher proportions of both alkyl-acyl PC and PE ($P<0.001$). Moreover, a low metastatic subclone (T3A), isolated from the high metastatic T3 cells, showed a level of alkyl-acyl PC lower than that of the parental cells ($P<0.01$). On the other hand, a high metastatic variant (T3C) of subclone T3A exhibited a percentage of alkyl-acyl PC similar to that found in the original T3 cells, while a low metastatic variant (T3B) had the same low level of alkyl-acyl PC as that found in the parental subclone.

All cell lines we examined also contained alkyldiacylglycerols in an amount not exceeding 1-2 % of total lipids, a value previously reported for LM cells (25). There was no significant difference in the alkyldiacylglycerol content between the cell lines which constituted the various model systems we examined (data not reported in table).

Table 3.
Ether-Linked (Alkenyl-Acyl and Alkyl-Acyl) Subfractions of PE and PC From Murine Cell Lines With Different Metastatic Potential.

Values are expressed as percentages of the total phospholipid class which were calculated as previously reported (12).

Subfraction	F1	F10	B77-3T3	B77-AA6	T3	T3A*	T3Bδ	T3Cδ
Alkenyl-acyl PE	13.0	12.8	46.7	54.6	43.5	42.8	37.9	49.0
Alkyl-acyl PE	N.D.	N.D.	12.0	21.3	0.2	0.3	N.D.	N.D.
Diacyl PE	87.0	87.2	41.3	24.1	56.3	56.9	62.1	51.0
Alkenyl-acyl PC	N.D.	N.D.	8.0	4.3	3.4	1.6	2.7	2.5
Alkyl-acyl PC	2.5	4.7	8.4	20.3	8.9	3.9	4.9	8.0
Diacyl PC	97.5	95.3	83.5	75.4	76.7	94.5	92.4	89.5

* T3A is a low metastatic subclone isolated by subclonation in plastic of a high metastatic clone derived from T3 cells.

δ T3B is a low and T3C is a high metastatic subclone, both of which have been isolated from T3A subclone.

CONCLUSIONS

All the cell lines which constituted the model systems used in this study contained high percentages of ether-linked molecules in their phospholipids. Indeed, adaptation to culture conditions has been shown to raise the ether-linked lipid levels in various types of cells both transformed and untransformed (9, 26, 27). However, the overall results of our study proved that there are peculiarities in the ether-linked lipid patterns that may be related to the biological characteristics of the various cell systems we examined. In particular, the behavior of alkenyl-acyl phospholipids in our system of normal, virally-transformed and revertant cells indicates that a high level of alkenyl-acyl phospholipids represents a molecular characteristic of transformation by oncogenic viruses. Moreover, the reduction of alkyl-acyl PC and PE which paralleled the erythroid differentiation of FEL cells suggests that the high levels of alkyl-linked lipids in tumor cells represent a molecular trait of their anaplasia. A higher level of alkyl-acyl phospholipids is also a characteristic of a metastatic phenotype in malignant cells. Alkyl-linked lipids might be involved in the metastatic process since they are known to generate bioactive molecules (5-8) which have been shown to influence different steps of metastatic diffusion (28).

ACKNOWLEDGMENTS

This work has been supported by the Consiglio Nazionale delle Ricerche (Special Project: Oncologia), by the Associazione Italiana per la Ricerca sul Cancro, and by the Ministero della Pubblica Istruzione.

REFERENCES

1. Snyder, F. and Snyder, C. (1975) Prog. Biochem. Pharmacol. 10, 2-41.
2. Spener, F. In: Ether Lipids - Biochemical and Biomedical Aspects (Eds. Mangold, H.K. and Paltauf, F.) Academic Press New York, 1983, pp. 239-259
3. Hajra, A.K. (1968) J. Biol. Chem. 243, 3458-3465.
4. Hajra, A.K. In: Tumor Lipids: Biochemistry and Metabolism (Ed. Wood, R.) Amer. Oil Chem. Soc. Champaign, 111. 1973, pp.183-199.
5. Hanahan, D.J., (1986) Ann. Rev. Biochem. 55, 483-509.
6. Swenden, C.L., Ellis, J. M., Chilton, F.H., O'Flaherty, J.T. and Wykle, R.L. (1983) Biochem. Biophys. Res. Comm. 113, 72-79.
7. Chilton, F.H., Ellis, J.M., Olson, S.O. and Wykle, R.L. (1984) J. Biol. Chem. 259, 12014-12019.
8. Kramer, R.M., Jakubowski, J.A. and Deykin, D. (1988) Biochim. Biophys. Acta 959, 269-279.
9. Howard, B.V., Morris, H.P. and Bailey, J.M. (1972) Cancer Res. 32, 1523-1538.
10. Friedberg, S.J., Smajdek, J. and Anderson, K. (1986) Cancer Res. 46, 845-849.
11. Roos, D.S., and Choppin, P.W. (1984) Proc. Natl. Acad. Sci. U.S.A. 81, 7622-7626.
12. Fallani, A., Bracco, M., Tombaccini, D., Mugnai, G.and Ruggieri, S. (1982) Biochim. Biophys. Acta 711, 208-212
13. Calorini, L., Fallani, A., Tombaccini, D., Barletta, E., Mugnai, G., Di Renzo, M.F., Comoglio, P.A. and Ruggieri, S. (1989) Lipids, 24, 685-690.
14. Fallani, A., Arcangeli, A. and Ruggieri, S. (1988) Biochem. J. 255, 731-736.
15. Calorini, L., Fallani, A., Tombaccini, D., Mugnai, G. and Ruggieri, S.(1987) Lipids, 22, 651-656.
16. Bomford, R. and Olivotto, M. (1974) Inter. J. Cancer, 14, 226-235.
17. Fallani, A., Arcangeli, A. and Ruggieri, S. (1988) Biochem. J. 252, 918-920.
18. Su, K.L. and Schmid, H.H.O. (1974) Lipids, 9, 208-213.
19. Oswald, E.O., Piantadosi, Anderson, C.E. and Snyder, F. (1966) Lipids, 1, 241-246.
20. Culp, L.A. and Black, P.H. (1972) J. Virol. 9, 611-620.
21. Friend, C., Scher, W., Holland, J.G. and Sato, T. (1971) Proc. Natl. Acad. Sci. USA, 68, 378-382.

22. Marks, P.A. and Rifkind, R.A. (1978) Ann. Rev. Biochem. 47, 419-448.
23. Fidler, I.J. (1973) Nature New Biol. 242,148-149.
24. Di Renzo, M.F. and Bretti, S. (1982) Inter. J. Cancer, 30, 751-757.
25. Anderson, R.E., Cumming, R.B., Walton, M. and Snyder, F. (1969) Biochim. Biophys. Acta 176, 491-501.
26. Scott, C.C., Heckman, C.A., Nettesheim, P. and Snyder, F. (1979) Cancer Res. 39, 207-210.
27 Tombaccini, D., Fallani, A. and Ruggieri, S. (1988) Biochem. Arch. 4, 219-229.
28. Honn, K. V. In: Basic Mechanisms and Clinical Treatment of Tumor Metastases (Eds. Torisu, M. and Yoshida, T.) Academic Press, New York, 1985, pp. 311-334.

MECHANISM OF THE CYTOTOXIC INTERACTION BETWEEN ET-18-OMe AND HEAT

K. FUJIWARA, C. FLETCHER, E. J. MODEST, and C. A. WALLEN

Departments of Radiology and Biochemistry, Bowman Gray School of Medicine of Wake Forest University, Winston-Salem, NC 27103

INTRODUCTION

Ether lipid analogues of platelet-activating factor have been shown to kill cancer cells either alone or in combination with other cancer chemotherapeutic agents (1-3). Recently, we have shown that one of the ether lipid analogues, ET-18-OMe[1], and 44°C hyperthermia interact supra-additively to kill BG-1 human ovarian carcinoma cells at concentration ≤0.5 μM of ET-18-OMe and additively at higher concentrations (0.5 to 2.0 μM) of ET-18-OMe (4). The mechanism of this cytotoxic interaction of ET-18-OMe and heat is presently unknown. In this study, we examine flow cytometrically two parameters, cell cycle distribution and nuclear protein content, that are altered after heat treatment to determine if they are involved in the mechanism governing the interaction of heat and ET-18-OMe.

MATERIALS AND METHODS

Cells.

BG-1 cells, derived from a human ovarian carcinoma (5), were maintained in McCoy's Medium 5A supplemented with 10% fetal bovine serum, 0.05% L-glutamine, 1% BME nonessential amino acids, 100 U/ml penicillin G, 100 μg/ml streptomycin sulfate and 0.1 U/ml semilente insulin. Exponentially growing BG-1 cells (day 2) were plated at 1×10^6 in 25 cm^2 culture flasks with 5 ml of medium. The cells were incubated for 3 days in a 7% CO_2, 100% humidified, 37°C incubator and then treated with either ET-18-OMe, 44°C heat or both.

ET-18-OMe Treatments.

The ET-18-OMe (provided by Dr. Wolfgang Berdel, Technical University of Munich, Federal Republic of Germany) was dissolved in ethanol and diluted to 10 times the desired concentration by phosphate buffered saline. The final concentration of ET-18-OMe used in this study was either 2 μM or 8 μM. The maximum concentration of ethanol in the medium during treatment was 0.02%. No killing or enhanced heat sensitivity was observed at this ethanol concentration. The ET-18-OMe (0.55 ml) was added to each flask and incubated at 37°C for various lengths of time (1-48 hr). The drugs were added shortly (5 to 10 min.) before heating in the combination treatments.

---

[1] 1-octadecyl-2-methyl-*rac*-glycero-3-phosphocholine

Heat Treatment.

The culture flasks were sealed and submersed in a temperature-controlled (±0.02°C) water bath for 60 min at 44°C. After heating, the flasks were removed to a 37°C water bath for equilibration and then placed in a 37°C incubator for recovery (0-48 hr).

Nuclear Isolation.

After removing the cells from the flasks by trypsin (0.1%), nuclei were isolated by a modification of the procedure of Roti Roti *et al.* (6). Briefly, the cells were washed three times with spinner salts (5.4 mM KCl, 0.4 mM $MgSO_4$, 0.12 M NaCl, 26 mM $NaHCO_3$, 10 mM NaH_2PO_4, 5.5 mM D-glucose). The cells were resuspended in a Triton X-100 solution (1% Triton X-100 in 0.08 M NaCl, 0.02 M EDTA) and incubated for 10 min to remove the cytoplasm. The isolated nuclei were then visually inspected for cytoplasmic contamination. If there was no significant contamination, the nuclei were then washed once with 0.15 M NaCl and resuspended with propidium iodide (PI) and fluorescein isothiocyanate (FITC) solution. The entire isolation procedure was performed at 4°C.

DNA and Protein Analysis.

The nuclei (≈2 x 10^6/ml) were stained with 50 μg/ml PI to determine DNA content and 0.03 μg/ml FITC to determine protein content. The stained nuclei were held overnight at 4°C. Analysis was performed on a FACS 440 flow cytometer (Becton-Dickinson) with a 488 nm excitation beam. Four parameters were measured: a) forward angle light scatter, b) FITC fluorescence (green, 530 ± 30 nm), c) PI fluorescence (red, 630 ± 22 nm), and d) pulse width of the PI fluorescence. The samples were gated on the intensity and pulse width of the PI fluorescence to eliminate debris and doublets from the analysis. All PI fluorescence data were input into the COTFIT program of the VAX consort 40 software (Becton-Dickinson) and the proportion of the cells in the G_1/G_0, S and G_2/M phases of the cell cycle was calculated. To determine if cells with multiple nuclei occurred in the populations treated with ET-18-OMe (7), the DNA analysis was repeated on BG-1 cells fixed in 70% ethanol and then stained with 35 μg/ml PI.

The relative nuclear protein content was determined by dividing the median channel number for the FITC fluorescence of the nuclei from treated cells by that of the untreated nuclei analyzed at the same incubation time. Since both 60 min at 44°C heat and 8 μM ET-18-OMe alter the cell cycle distribution of BG-1 cells, and the protein content of the nuclei doubles as cells progress from G_1 to G_2, the protein analysis was performed separately for the nuclei having a G_1 DNA content. To obtain nuclei from the G_1 fraction, the samples were gated on the computer to include only cells with a DNA fluorescence of ± 3 channels from the G_1 peak.

RESULTS

DNA Analysis.

The cell cycle distributions of BG-1 cells heated at 44°C for 60 min, 8 μM ET-18-OMe and 2 and 8 μM ET-18-OMe in combination with heat changed from that observed for untreated BG-1 cells (Figure 1). During the 48 hr period, the percentage of untreated cells in S and G_2/M phases decreased with a concomitant increase in the proportion of cells in G_1. Treatment of BG-1 cells with 2 μM ET-18-OMe did not significantly alter the cell cycle distribution from that observed for untreated cells. However, 8 μM ET-18-OMe induced several changes in the cell cycle distribution: a) a significant G_2 block that started to appear 4-6 hr after initiation of treatment and b) a fraction of cells with a hypodiploid DNA peak (8-20% by 24 hr). A heat treatment of 60 min at 44°C also induced a marked G_2 block that began to appear 12-16 hr after heating and continued to increase during the 48 hr period after heating (Figure 1). No hypodiploid fraction was observed after this treatment. The alterations in the cell cycle distributions after the combination treatment of heat and 2 μM ET-18-OMe were indistinguishable from those of cells that were only heated (Figure 1). When cells were treated with 8 μM ET-18-OMe and 44°C heat for 60 min, a larger hypodiploid population (40-60% at 24 hr) was measured that appeared earlier (by 10 hr) than in cells treated with ET-18-OMe alone.

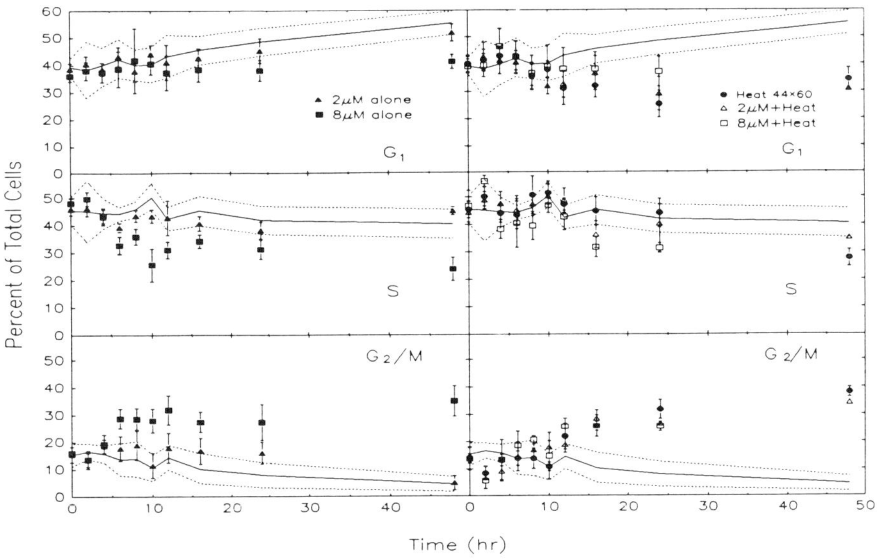

Figure 1. Percentage of cells in the cell cycle phases as a function of time after initiation of experiments: G_1 (top), S (middle), or G_2/M (bottom). The percentage of untreated BG-1 cells in each phase is indicated by the solid line. The dashed lines are ±2 SEM of the untreated value. The cell cycle distributions are shown for treated BG-1 cell: ether lipid alone (left panels) and heat with or without ether lipid (right panels). The error bars are 1 SEM of at least 3 independent experiments and are smaller than the data points when not shown.

Nuclear Protein Analysis.

The protein content, measured flow cytometrically, was approximately 4 times higher in G_1 nuclei isolated from BG-1 cells heated for 60 min at 44°C than in unheated cells (Figure 2). Removal of excess nuclear protein began immediately after heating and was complete within 12 hr (Figure 2). Exposure to either 2 or 8 μM ET-18-OMe induced no alteration in nuclear protein content. Similarly, the addition of ET-18-OMe prior to heating did not alter the removal of the excess nuclear protein. Identical results were obtained when nuclei from S and G_2/M were analyzed (data not shown).

DISCUSSION

Recently, we have shown that heat and ET-18-OMe are an effective combination of agents in killing cancer cells (4). ET-18-OMe has several characteristics that make it unusual when compared to other membrane active agents that interact with heat to kill cells: a) it is cytotoxic at 37°C (3,4), b) its sensitization of BG-1 cells to heat is not dose dependent (4), and c) it does not appear to induce tolerance to either ET-18-OMe or heat (8). To discover the mechanism by which ET-18-OMe and heat interact, we have chosen to investigate alterations that either correlate with cell kill in heated cells or have been implicated in heat-induced cell kill to determine if they are changed (enhanced, inhibited, accelerated, or retarded) in the presence of ET-18-OMe. In this study, we examined two parameters that are altered after heat treatment: cell cycle distribution and nuclear protein content.

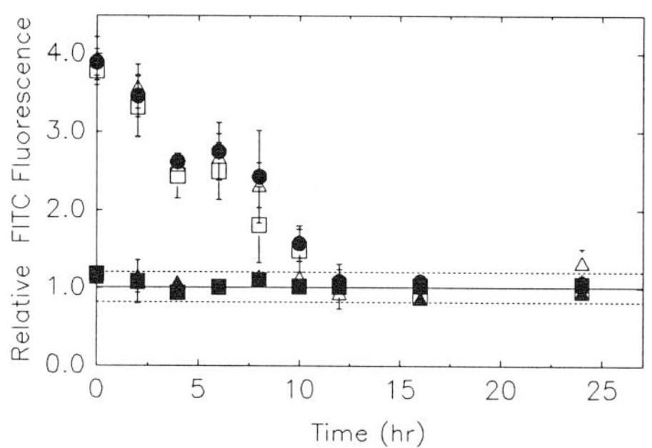

Figure 2: Relative nuclear protein fluorescence of G_1 BG-1 cells as function of time. The solid and dashed lines represent the value for untreated cells ±2 SEM. The BG-1 cells were treated with 2 (triangles) or 8 μM (squares) ET-18-OMe either alone (solid symbols) or in combination with heat at 44°C for 60 min heat (open symbols). Cells that were only heated are represented by the closed circles. The error bars are 1 SEM of at least 3 independent experiments and are smaller than the data point when not shown.

The cell cycle distribution of BG-1 cells was not perturbed by continuous exposure to 2 μM ET-18-OMe. However, exposure to a high concentration (8 μM) of ET-18-OMe (Figure 1) induced a substantial G_2 block. Furthermore, continuous exposure to 8 μM ET-18-OMe for as little as 16 hr also induced a substantial hypodiploid DNA peak. The majority of cells in this hypodiploid peak had normal forward angle light scatter for BG-I nuclei indicating that the DNA in these nuclei were probably more condensed so that the stain bound or fluoresced differently. It is likely that these cells are committed to death.

A 60 min heat treatment at 44°C also induced a substantial G_2 block that first appeared 12 hr after the treatment and continued to increase in magnitude for at least 48 hr. The combination of heat (44°C for 60 min) and 8μM ET-18-OMe resulted in changes that were not identical to those observed with either agent alone: a) an increase in the percentage of nuclei in the hypodiploid peak, b) an accelerated appearance of hypodiploid cells, and c) a reduction in the number of cells in G_2. However, combinations of heat with 2 μM ET-18-OMe induced no greater alterations in the cell cycle distribution than those observed when the BG-1 cells were heated alone. Because the latter combination increases cell kill substantially, it is unlikely that the mechanism by which heat and ET-18-OMe interact to kill BG-1 cells involves cell cycle alterations.

Roos and Berdel (7) had previously observed in several human hematopoietic cell lines that exposure to ET-18-OMe induced a subpopulation of cells with 2 or more nuclei. In our experiments, no cells with more than a 4C DNA content were observed after exposure to ET-18-OMe (data not shown). These data support their finding that the induction of multi-nucleation is a cell line dependent phenomenon (7).

One of the primary effects of a heat treatment is to increase the non-histone protein content of nuclei (9,10). In our recent studies (11) and those of Kampinga *et. al* (12), it has been shown that survival after a heat treatment is directly related to the length of time required to remove the excess nuclear proteins. In this study, we examined the influence of ET-18-OMe on the quantity of proteins added during a specific heat treatment (44°C for 60 min) and the kinetics of excess nuclear protein removal. As shown in Figure 2, the addition of 2 or 8 μM ET-18-OMe prior to heat had no influence on either the quantity of proteins added to the nucleus or the protein removal. Therefore, alterations in nuclear protein content are unlikely to be involved in the enhancement of heat-induced cell kill by ET-18-OMe.

In conclusion, the cell cycle distribution and alterations in nuclear protein content observed after treatment with heat and a moderate concentration of ET-18-OMe were not different from those observed after heat treatment alone. Therefore, additional investigations are needed to determine the mechanism by which heat and ET-18-OMe interact to kill cancer cells.

ACKNOWLEDGEMENTS

This research was supported by Grant CA44105 from the National Cancer Institute. The FCM analysis was performed in the FCM Facility of the Cancer Center of Wake Forest University which is supported in part by NIH grant 12197 from the National Cancer Institute. Authors thank Angie Brendle for preparation of this manuscript.

REFERENCES

1. Modest, E.J., Daniel, L.W., Wykle, R.L., Berens, M.E., Piantadosi, C., Surles, J.R., and Morris Natschke, S. In: New Avenues in Developmental Cancer Chemotherapy (Eds. K.R. Harrap and T.A. Connors), Academic Press, London, 1987, pp. 387-400.
2. Berdel, W.E., Andressen, R., and Munder, P.G. In: Phospholipids and Cellular Regulation. (Ed. J.F. Kuo), CRC Press, Vol. 2, Boca Raton, 1985, pp. 41-73.
3. Noseda, A., Berens, M.E., White, J.G. and Modest, E.J. Cancer Res. 48:1788-1719, 1988.

4. Fujiwara, K, Modest, E.J., Welander, C.E., and Wallen, C.A. Cancer Res. 49:6285-6289,1989.
5. Geisinger, K.R., Kute, T.E., Pettenati, M.J., Welander, C.E., Dennard, Y., Collins, L.A., and Berens, M.E. Cancer, 63:280-288, 1989.
6. Roti Roti, J.L., Higashikubo, R., Blair, O.C. and Uygur, N. Cytometry. 3:91-96, 1982.
7. Roos, G. and Berdel, W.E. Leukemia Res. 10:195-202, 1986.
8. Fujiwara, K, Modest, E.J., and Wallen, C.A. Proc. AACR 30:578, 1989.
9. Roti Roti, J.L., and Winward, R.T. Radiat. Res. 74:159-169, 1978.
10. Tomasovic, S.P., Turner, G.N. and Dewey, W.L. Radiat. Res. 73:535-552. 1978.
11. Wallen, C.A. and Landis, M. Int. J. Hyperthermia 1990, 6:87-95.
12. Kampinga, H.H., Turkel-Uygur, N., Roti Roti, J.L., and Konnings, AW.T. Radiat. Res. 117:511-522, 1989.

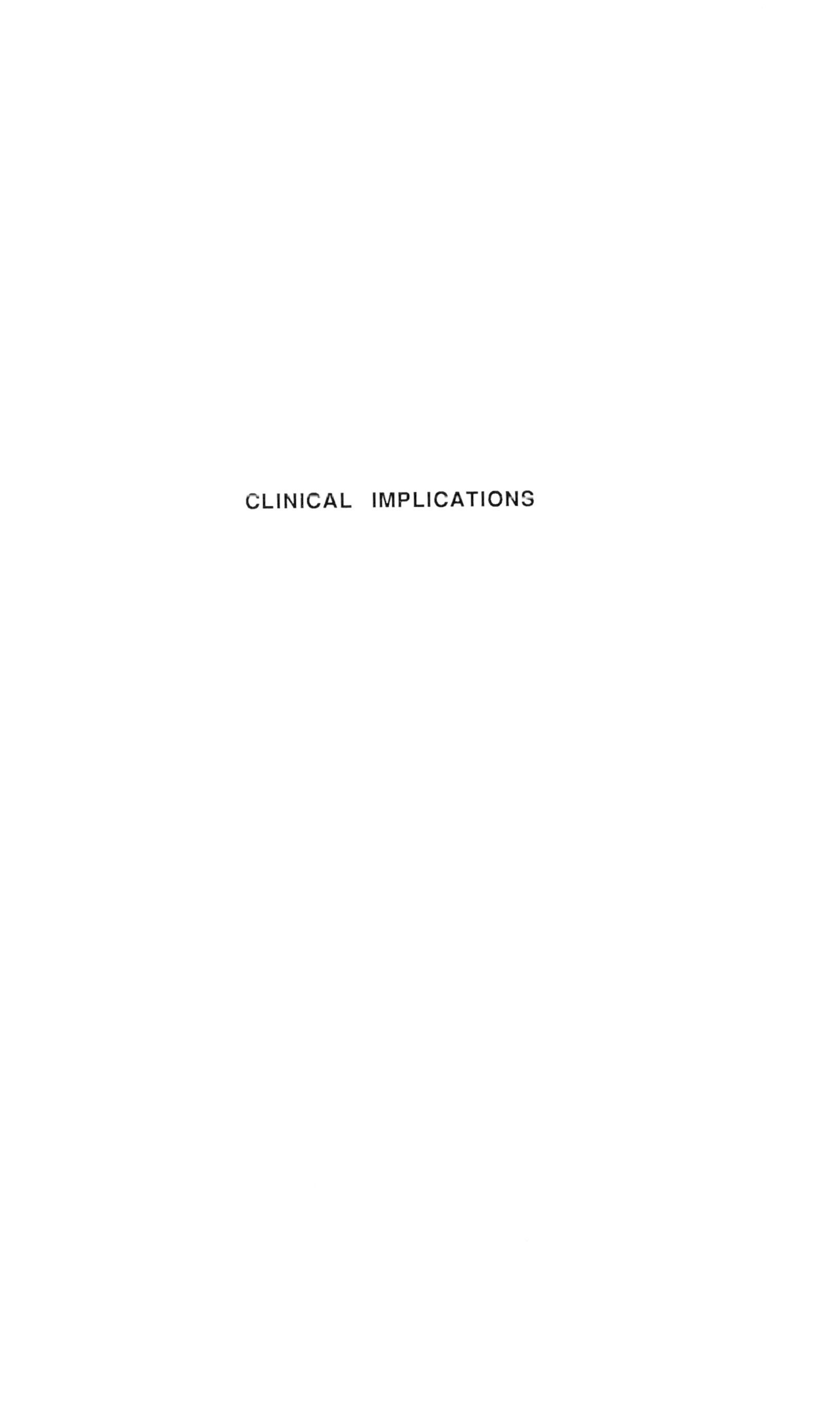

CLINICAL IMPLICATIONS

INHIBITION OF PROSTAGLANDIN PRODUCTION IN MALIGNANT TUMORS: IMPLICATIONS TO RADIOTHERAPY

L. MILAS

Department of Experimental Radiotherapy, The University of Texas M. D. Anderson Cancer Center, 1515 Holcombe Boulevard, Houston, Texas 77030

INTRODUCTION

It is a predominant view that prostaglandins (PGs) stimulate tumor growth and spread, and that they do this through their immunosuppressive actions (1). Treatment of tumor hosts with PG-inhibiting agents, such as indomethacin (INDO), has frequently been reported to result in tumor growth retardation and inhibition of tumor spread. This activity of PG-inhibiting agents has commonly been attributed to the increased antitumor immune resistance due to inhibition of immunosuppressive PGs. Tumor response to INDO treatment is variable, with only a fraction of tumors showing a good response, evidenced usually as retardation of tumor growth. Hence, the therapeutic potential of INDO and other PG-inhibiting agents can be expected to be achieved only when these agents are combined with other treatment modalities.

The above consideration, and the recent reports that PGs act as potent radioprotectors (2,3), suggest that a particularly effective tumor treatment could be achieved by combining INDO with radiotherapy. If PGs act as radioprotective agents, one can anticipate that they would regulate tumor radioresponse more than that of normal tissues because tumors produce high levels of PGs. Consequently, treatment of tumor hosts with INDO would be expected to increase radioresponse of both tumors and normal tissues, but that the augmentation of tumor radioresponse should be greater than that of normal tissues. We have investigated the effect of INDO on radioresponse of tumors and normal tissues in mice (4-7) and here we review our major findings.

MATERIALS AND METHODS

The studies used 5 murine tumors, of which 3 were sarcomas designated FSA, NFSA, and SA-NH and 2 were carcinomas, designated MCA-K and HCA-I. The tumors are syngeneic to C_3Hf/Kam mice and were grown as transplants in the right thighs. They were exposed to single or fractionated doses of γ-rays when 8 mm in diameter, and their radioresponse was assessed by tumor growth delay and TCD_{50} assays. (TCD_{50} designates the radiation dose required to control 50% of irradiated tumors). Treatment with INDO (usually in drinking water at 35 μg/ml) was initiated when tumors grew to 6 mm in diameter and was given daily for 10 consecutive days. Tumors were irradiated 3 to 4 days after INDO treatment was started. The effect of INDO on radioresponse of hematopoietic tissue, lung, esophagus, colon, jejunum, hair follicles, and tissues involved in the development of radiation-induced leg contractures was also studied. Endogenous spleen colony formation and mouse lethality ($LD_{50/30}$) were used to evaluate the radioresponse of hematopoietic tissue. PGs and other arachidonic acid metabolites produced by tumors were analyzed by HPLC or radioimmunoassay. These and other assays used in this study were described in detail elsewhere (4,5).

RESULTS

PG production by tumors and its relevance to tumor response to indomethacin.

FSA, NFSA, SA-NH, MCA-K, and HCA-I tumors were analyzed for production of eicosanoids (PGs, leukotrienes and HETEs). Of these five tumors, FSA, NFSA and HCA-I produced PGs, whereas SA-NH and MCA-K did not. Especially good producers of PGs were FSA and NFSA tumors. The three tumors that produced PGs demonstrated quantitative and qualitative differences in their profiles of individual PGs (4). Production of leukotrienes and HETEs by these tumors is described elsewhere (4).

These tumors responded to the treatment with INDO differently, depending on PGs production. Only tumors that produced PGs responded to INDO by slowing their growth. The level of PGs in INDO-treated tumors was greatly reduced compared to that of untreated tumors. INDO was not directly cytotoxic or cytostatic for tumor cells, as assayed both in vitro and in vivo, but it perturbed cell cycle in tumors causing reduction in the proportion of S-phase cells. Furthermore, its antitumor activity did not depend on tumor immunogenicity (FSA and MCA-K are immunogenic, whereas NFSA, SA-NH and HCA-I are nonimmunogenic tumors), and was not reduced in immunosuppressed mice (4).

Potentiation of tumor radioresponse.

Tumor growth delay and TCD_{50} were used to assess the effect of INDO on tumor radioresponse. The radiation dose-response curves for curability of FSA and NFSA tumors are shown in Figure 1.

INDO greatly reduced the TCD_{50} value for FSA from 38.9 (37.5-40.6) Gy to 27.9 (21.7-33.8) Gy, and for NFSA from 63.1 (57.3-67.8) to 50.2 (44.6-55.6). In parentheses are 95% confidence limits. The enhancement factors were 1.39 for FSA and 1.26 for NFSA. In addition to the increased radiocurability, INDO significantly delayed the time to recurrence of tumors which were not controlled by the combined treatment. INDO was somewhat more effective when, instead of TCD_{50}, the tumor growth delay was the response endpoint. Here, the enhancement factors were 1.55 for FSA and 1.4 for NFSA. More recently, we have established that INDO was also effective in increasing radioresponse of FSA tumor exposed to fractionated, instead of single dose irradiation. In this setting, the enhancement factor was more than 2. In contrast to this significant increase in tumor radioresponse of FSA and NFSA tumors, INDO caused a negligible increase in radioresponse of the MCA-K tumor, which did not produce PG.

Radioresponse of normal tissues.

The effect of INDO on radioresponse of a number of normal tissues and organs of C_3Hf/Kam mice has been investigated (5-7). These include hematopoietic tissue, lungs, esophagus, jejunum, colon, hair follicles and tissues involved in the development of radiation-induced leg contractures. INDO pro-

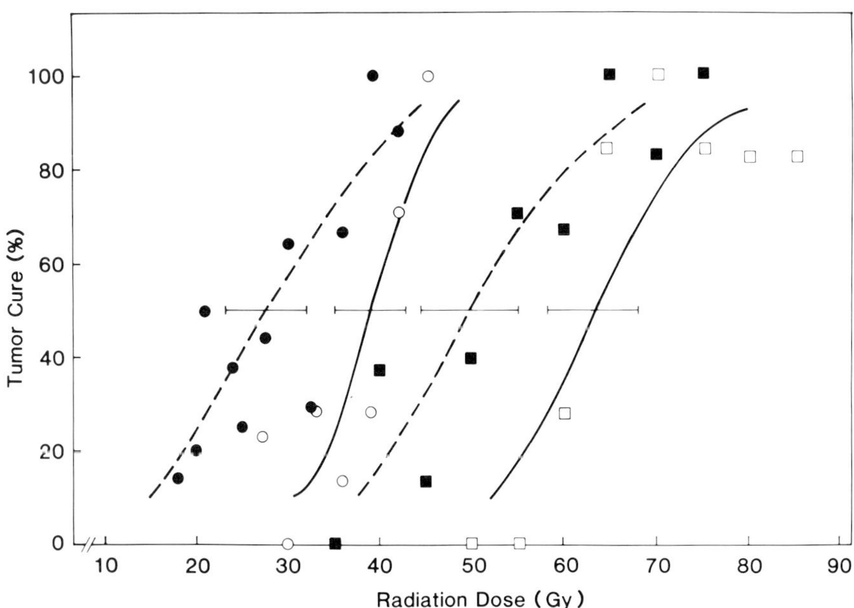

Figure 1. Radiation dose-response curves for local tumor control of FSA (circles) or NFSA tumors (squares). Open symbols represent irradiation only groups, and solid symbols represent INDO plus irradiation groups. Error bars at the TCD_{50} are 95% confidence limits. Treatment with INDO, 35 µg/1 ml in drinking water, was started when tumors grew to 6 mm in diameter and was continued daily for 10 days. Local tumor irradiation was given to 8 mm tumors. Adapted from (5).

tected significantly against radiation damage of hematopoietic tissue (5,7) and lungs (6), but it did not significantly modify radioresponse of the other tissues and organs in either direction.

DISCUSSION

Our investigations show that murine malignant tumors vary greatly in their ability to produce PGs and other eicosanoids. PGs produced by tumors appear to be conducive to tumor growth, since their inhibition by INDO results in slowing of tumor growth. INDO was not cytotoxic for tumor cells, and it did not slow tumor growth through augmentation of antitumor immune responses. This conclusion is based on our observations that INDO is similarly effective in normal and immunocompromised mice, and that its activity did not depend on tumor immunogenicity (4). We recently observed that INDO inhibits tumor angiogenesis in mice, an event associated with retardation of tumor growth (unpublished). Therefore, based on our overall results we hypothesize that the inhibition of tumor neovascularization is a major mechanism by which INDO exerts its antitumor activity.

However, an important observation here, with respect to cancer treatment, is that the effectiveness of INDO was directly related to the ability of tumors to produce PGs. Therefore, analysis of eicosanoids produced by malignant tumors could be used advantageously to screen tumors for treatment with INDO or other PG-inhibiting agents. Only tumors that produce PGs would be good candidates for INDO therapy.

INDO treatment significantly potentiated response of PG-producing tumors (FSA and NFSA) to local tumor irradiation given either in large single doses or as fractionated irradiation. This was evidenced by the increase in tumor growth delay, percentage of mice cured, and time to recurrence of irradiated tumors. Enhancement factors ranged from 1.3 to more than 2, depending on the endpoint of radiation response and treatment settings.

Mechanisms by which INDO increased tumor radioresponse are not clear. A number of them including abolition of radioprotective activities of PGs, cell cycle effect and the role of infiltrating macrophages were considered in our earlier report (5). More recently we observed that the potentiating effect of INDO on tumor radiocurability is greatly suppressed and can even be abolished in nude mice and in mice whose immune system is compromised by whole body irradiation (unpublished). Thus, although antitumor activity of INDO appears to be primarily due to inhibition of angiogenesis (see above), its augmentation of tumor radioresponse appears to be dominantly dependent on normal functioning of the immune system.

To be therapeutically beneficial, agents that increase radiation damage to tumors, including INDO, must be less effective in increasing normal tissue damage by irradiation. Using several normal tissues, we have clearly demonstrated that the radiation response of these tissues was modified much less than that of the tumors studied here, implying that INDO provided a significant therapeutic benefit. In contrast to its effect on tumor radioresponse, INDO caused radioprotection of hematopoietic tissues and the lung, and caused no significant change in radioresponse of esophagus, jejunum, colon, hair follicles and tissues involved in the development of radiation induced leg contractures. INDO is not a true radioprotector for hematopoietic cells, but it acts indirectly through stimulation of hematopoietic stem cell proliferation (7). Mechanisms for INDO-induced radioprotection of the lung have not been investigated yet.

Overall, our data clearly demonstrate that INDO can increase therapeutic gain when combined with tumor radiotherapy. While a significant increase in tumor radioresponse was observed, of 7 normal tissues (or organs) examined, 5 showed no significant change in radioresponse, and 2 exhibited radioprotection. Further studies on the combination of tumor irradiation and INDO or other PG-inhibitory agents are warranted, especially those designed to elucidate how they increase tumor radioresponse and those aimed to define settings under which the greatest therapeutic gain can be achieved.

CONCLUSIONS

Murine tumors vary greatly in their ability to produce PGs. Only PG-producing tumors exhibit growth inhibition when treated with the PG inhibitor INDO. INDO is also capable of significant augmentation of radiocurability of tumors that produce PGs. Because INDO had only minimal effect on radioresponse of normal tissues, it has potential to be successfully used in combination with radiotherapy. Since effectiveness of INDO is directly related to the ability of tumors to produce PGs, the eicosanoid profile of tumors could be valuable in selecting patients likely to respond to INDO, or other PG inhibiting agents, when used alone or in combination with radiotherapy.

REFERENCES

1. Honn, K.V., Bockman, R.S., and Marnett, L.J. Prostaglandins 21:833-864, 1981.
2. Hanson, W.R., and Ainsworth, E.J. Radiat. Res. 103: 196-203, 1985.
3. Walden, T.L. Jr., Patchen, M., and Snyder, S.L. Radiat. Res. 109:440-448, 1987.
4. Furuta, Y., Hall, E.R., Sundja, S., Barkley, T. Jr., and Milas, L. Cancer Res. 48: 3002-3007, 1988.
5. Furuta, Y., Hunter, N., Barkley, T. Jr., Hall, E., and Milas, L. 48:3008-3013, 1988.
6. Fleck, R., and Travis, E.L. 37th Annual Meeting of the Radiation Research Society, Book of Abstracts, p. 78, 1989.
7. Nishiguchi, I., Willingham, V., and Milas, L. J. Radiat. Oncol. Biol. Phys., 18:555-558, 1990.

ENHANCED FORMATION OF LEUKOTRIENE C_4 IN CHRONIC MYELOGENOUS LEUKEMIA LEUKOCYTES

L. STENKE[1,2] and J. Å. LINDGREN[1]

[1]Department of Physiological Chemistry, Karolinska Institutet and [2]Division of Hematology, Department of Medicine, Danderyd Hospital, Stockholm, Sweden

INTRODUCTION

The leukotrienes are established mediators of inflammation and anaphylaxis (1,2) but have also been indicated to modulate e.g. lymphocyte function (3,4) and influence hematopoietic progenitor replication (5,6). Furthermore, a growth factor for these progenitor cells (GM-CSF) has been reported to stimulate the production of LTC_4 in human eosinophils (7). The purpose of the present investigation was to compare the leukotriene producing capacity of peripheral blood leukocytes from patients with CML to that of leukocytes from patients with another myeloproliferative disorder (polycythemia vera), non-malignant leukocytosis patients, and healthy donors. The results indicate an increased LTC_4 formation in CML, but not in PV or non-malignant inflammatory disease (8).

MATERIALS AND METHODS

Peripheral blood samples were collected from 14 CML patients, 10 patients with polycythemia vera (PV) 4 patients with non-malignant inflammatory disease and a total of 25 normal, healthy donors. All CML patients expressed the Philadelphia (Ph') chromosome and were in chronic phase. The white blood cell (WBC) counts at testing were 3.2 - 104 x 10^9/1. Three of the CML patients were previously untreated. The patients with inflammatory disease suffered from appendicitis, cholecystitis, sigmoiditis or polymyalgia rheumatica, respectively. All these four patients had increased WBC counts (range 10.6 - 12.8 x 10^9/1). The control group consisted of healthy students and laboratory staff. No chemotherapy, steroidal or non-steroidal anti-inflammatory drugs were given to any of the patients or the controls at the time of the study. Cell preparation from peripheral blood samples, incubation of cell suspensions with ionophore A23187, sample purification and leukotriene determination using reversed-phase high-performance liquid chromatography (RP-HPLC) were carried out as described (8).

RESULTS

Leukotriene production in WBC suspensions from patients with CML and inflammatory disease.

Suspensions of WBC from CML patients produced significantly more LTC_4 (40.2 $\pm$ 7.9 pmol/10^6 WBC, mean $\pm$ SEM) than the controls (9.0 $\pm$ 1.8 pmol/10^6 WBC, Figure 1). Eight of 14 CML patients synthesized > 28 pmol/10^6 WBC, while this high production was observed in none of the 17 controls.

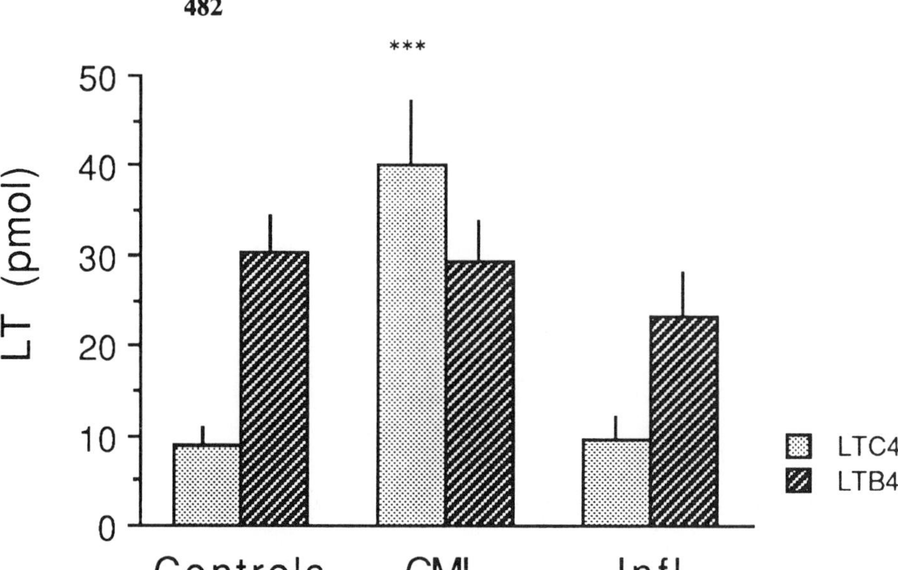

Figure 1. Production of LTC_4 and LTB_4 in A23187 stimulated white blood suspensions from patients with CML and inflammatory disease. Results are expressed as mean values (+SEM) of leukotriene production (pmol /10^6 WBC) . *** = $p<0.001$ when comparing CML with controls.

No statistically significant differences were observed between CML and controls in the production of LTB_4. Furthermore, the total synthesis of leukotrienes was equal in white blood cell suspensions from the two groups. Thus, the sum of LTC_4, LTB_4, 20-OH-LTB_4 and the Δ^6-*trans*-isomers of LTB_4 was 83.5 $\pm$ 24.3 in CML and 81.6 $\pm$ 15.0 pmol/10^6 WBC in controls (Figure 2).

As an indicator of the direction of LTA_4 metabolism, the ratio between the production of LTC_4 and LTB_4 was calculated. Again, highly significant differences between CML and controls were noted. Thus the ratio LTC_4/(LTB_4 + 20-OH-LTB_4) was 0.96 $\pm$ 0.16 for CML versus 0.17 $\pm$ 0.03 for the controls, $p<0.0005$. The production of leukotrienes in WBC preparations from the inflammatory disease patients was comparable to that of the controls (Figures 1,2).

Leukotriene production in purified granulocyte suspensions from patients with CML and PV.

Purified granulocyte suspensions from CML patients (n=5) produced significantly higher levels of LTC_4 than granulocyte suspensions from healthy controls (n=6) (68.3 $\pm$ 17.8 versus 9.1 $\pm$ 3.6 pmol/10^6 granulocytes, p=0.006) after ionophore A23187 stimulation. In contrast, the production of LTB_4 was similar (69.4 $\pm$ 14.0 versus 55.2 $\pm$ 3.7 pmol/10^6 granulocytes, respectively). Granulocyte suspensions from CML patients also showed a significantly elevated LTC_4/LTB_4 ratio as compared to controls (1.06 $\pm$ 0.29 versus 0.18 $\pm$ 0.08, p=0.012). The leukotriene production by granulocyte suspensions was similar in PV patients and controls.

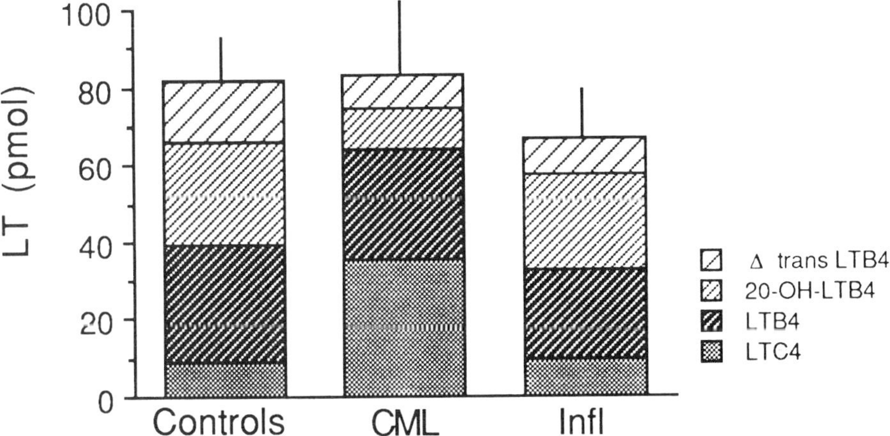

Figure 2. Total leukotriene production in white blood cell suspensions from patients with CML and inflammatory disease. Legend see Figure 1.

Leukotriene formation in CML versus differential cell counts and clinical status.

No significant correlations could be found between the amounts of LTB_4 or LTC_4 produced by the CML leukocytes and the numbers of eosinophilic or basophilic granulocytes, monocytes, myelocytes or myeloblasts in these suspensions. In addition, no correlation was observed between the LTC_4/LTB_4 ratio and the ratio between eosinophils + monocytes (LTC_4 producing cells) and neutrophilic granulocytes (LTB_4 producers). However, there was a significant correlation ($r=0.6$, $p<0.05$) between the levels of LTB_4 and the total number of neutrophils and metamyelocytes in the cell suspensions.

A comparison between leukotriene production and other clinical or laboratory variables (including time from diagnosis to the date of study, time from last chemotherapy treatment, type of previous chemotherapy treatment, post study survival and peripheral white blood cell and platelet counts at the date of study) did not show any significant correlations.

DISCUSSION

In this study we report an increased formation of LTC_4 after calcium ionophore stimulation of white blood cell suspensions and purified granulocyte suspensions from patients with chronic myelogenous leukemia. The production of LTB_4 was normal and the total synthesis of leukotrienes was not elevated in CML. Consequently, the ratio between LTC_4 and LTB_4 was highly increased indicating a shift in the

LTA_4 metabolism towards the formation of LTC_4. No abnormality in leukotriene production could be detected in another myeloproliferative disorder, polycythemia vera (PV). Furthermore, a normal LT production was observed in four patients with non-malignant inflammatory disease. These results indicate a certain degree of specificity of the abnormal leukotriene production observed in CML.

Theoretically, the differential counts of the CML patients may have explained the changed leukotriene formation pattern. Monocytes and eosinophils, e.g., are well-known producers of LTC_4 while neutrophils form predominantly LTB_4 (9,10). However, no correlation was seen between the number of these cell types in the CML white blood cell preparations and the levels of LTC_4 and LTB_4, respectively, although a significant correlation was observed between the LTB_4 production and the sum of neutrophils and metamyelocytes.

We have recently reported that platelets convert granulocyte-derived LTA_4 to LTC_4 and that the presence of platelets leads to increased LTC_4- and decreased LTB_4-formation, i.e. an increased LTC_4/LTB_4 ratio (11). White blood cell preparations contain a large number of platelets and CML platelets could theoretically be more efficient to convert LTA_4 to LTC_4 than normal platelets. However, the elevated LTC_4/LTB_4 ratio was also observed in platelet depleted CML granulocytes suspensions. These findings suggest that the observed abnormality in CML is due to an increased tendency by cells in the granulocyte fraction to produce LTC_4.

Peripheral blood cells of CML patients display obvious morphological abnormalities and immaturities (12-15). This report shows an altered leukotriene production in CML with a highly increased LTC_4 but a normal LTB_4 formation. In addition, we have recently reported deficient lipoxin formation in mixed platelet/granulocyte suspensions in certain patients with CML (16). It is presently not elucidated whether these alterations in the formation of lipoxygenase products is due to cell immaturity or to malignant transformation.

The possible significance of the abnormal leukotriene production observed in CML with regard to the pathogenesis of this disease is still highly speculative. It has been claimed that LTC_4 and LTB_4 can directly stimulate proliferation of granulocyte-monocyte precursors (CFU-GM) *in vitro* (5,17). In addition, the growth factor for these precursor cells (GM-CSF) has been shown to enhance the production of LTC_4 in human eosinophils (7). If the present *in vitro* findings are parallelled by an increased tendency to synthesize LTC_4 *in vivo,* this may suggest an important role for LTC_4 in the pronounced myeloid hypercellularity in CML. Further studies are highly warranted to elucidate the significance of the abnormal LTC_4 production in CML.

ACKNOWLEDGEMENT

We gratefully thank Ms Inger Forsberg and Ms Lillemor Lauren for skillful technical assistance and Ms Susanne Widell for valuable analyses of differential countings. This project was supported by grants from the Swedish Cancer Society, the Swedish Medical Research Council, the Cancer Society of Stockholm, the Swedish Medical Society and the Research Funds of Karolinska Institutet.

REFERENCES

1. Samuelsson, B. Science 220: 568-575, 1983.
2. Samuelsson, B., Dahlen, S-E, Lindgren, J.Å., Rouzer, C.A., Serhan, C.N. Science 237: 1171-1176, 1987.
3. Rola-Pleszczynski, M. Immunol Today 6: 302-307, 1985.
4. Gualde, N., Altura, D., Goodwin, J. J Immunol 134: 1125-1129, 1985.
5. Claesson, H-E, Dahlberg, N., Gahrton, G. Biochem Biophys Res Commun 131: 579-585, 1986.
6. Estrov, Z., Halperin, D., Coceani, F., Freedman, M.H. Br J Haematol 69: 321-327, 1988.
7. Silberstein, D., Owen, W., Gasson, J., DiPersio, J., Golde, D., Bina, J., Soberman, R., Austen, F., David, J. J Immunol 137: 3290-3294, 1986.
8. Stenke, L., Samuelsson, J., Palmblad, J., Dabrowski, L., Reizenstein, P., Lindgren, J.Å. Br J. Haematol 74:257-263, 1990.
9. Lewis, R.A., Austen, K.F. J Clin Invest 73: 889-897, 1984.
10. Verhagen, J., Bruynzeel, P.L., Koedam, J.A., Wassink, G.A., deBoer, M., Terpstra, G.K., Kreukniet, J., Veldink, G., Vliegenhart, J.F. FEBS Lett 168: 23-28, 1984.
11. Edenius, C., Heidvall, K., Lindgren, J.Å. Eur J Biochem 178: 81-86, 1988.
12. Olofsson, T., Odeberg, H., Olsson, I. Blood 48: 581-593, 1976.
13. Chenoweth, D.E., Rowe, J.G., Hyli, T.E. J Immunol Methods 25: 337-353, 1979.
14. El Hallem, H., Fletcher, J., Br. J Haematol 41: 49-55, 1979.
15. Anklesaria, P.N., Advani, S.H., Bhisey, A.N. Leuk Res 9: 641-648, 1985.
16. Stenke, L., Edenius, C., Lindgren, J.Å. Blood Submitted for publication 1989.
17. Miller, A.M., Weiner, R.S., Ziboh, V.A. Exp Hematol 14: 760-765, 1986.

CLINICAL ANTICANCER EFFECTS OF ORAL AND INTRATUMORAL PROSTAGLANDIN INHIBITORS

L. ISRAEL, J.L. BREAU, J.F. MORERE, and C. BOAZIZ

Oncology Unit, Centre Hospitalier Universitaire Avicenne, 93000 Bobigny, France

Although clinical studies are not yet, to our knowledge, available, it is already known from experimental studies that prostaglandin inhibitors can interfere with tumor growth (1) and that PGE2 and PGF2 alpha are involved in the initiation, the growth and the spread of various malignant tumors (2, 3, 4, 5, 6, 7). This is why we started two clinical studies, the preliminary results of which have already been reported (8)(9).

The first study was conducted with piroxicam, given orally daily at a uniform dose of 20 milligrams. 42 patients with various solid tumors, mostly metastatic, were included because conventional therapy had been attempted and failed. All tumors were measurable and their spontaneous doubling time was known. 7 patients could not be evaluated (4 died from early metastatic dissemination, 2 were dropped for cutaneous allergy and 1 for gastric ulceration). Among the 35 evaluable patients all were given piroxicam for at least 3 months. In 8 cases no changes in the doubling time were observed and in 8 cases the slowing down of the growth was minimal. In 10 cases a significant slowing down was obtained (2 to 5 times slower growth rate). In 4 cases we obtained a less than 50% decrease in tumor size (3 bronchial ca, 1 endometrial ca). In 5 cases an objective response was obtained including 4 major (much greater than 50%) regressions and 1 complete disappearance of several lung metastases from a soft tissue sarcoma. The major responses included 2 bronchial ca, 1 endometrial ca with several lung metastases, which is approaching a complete response, and 1 soft tissue sarcoma of the subclavicular area. These 5 responses are being maintained from 3+ to 18+ months. For the minor responses and slowing down of the growth rate, we added retinoic acid and vitamin D3 after 3 months with no escape so far from 2 to 12 months.

The second study used intratumoral, and in 1 case intraarterial indomethacin in a dose of 100 mg to 250 mg daily depending on the volume and 3 times weekly in case of tumor necrosis. We observed 8 major objective responses, 3 soft tissue sarcomas, 4 skin nodules metastatic from breast cancer and 1 very large hepatoma (here indomethacin was given intraarterially for 3 weeks). In addition 1 complete response was obtained in a case of limited Kaposi sarcoma that has not recurred after 32 weeks (Total response rate 75%).

DISCUSSION

Some of our results have been very interesting. We are now considering giving larger doses of oral piroxicam (20 mg/m^2 daily) together with intratumoral or intraarterial indomethacin whenever feasible. It seems that prostaglandin inhibitors show some real promise in the biological management of tumors, and we are also exploring these agents in combination with other antiproliferative drugs. The therapeutic index could also be improved by treating those tumors that synthesize the greatest amounts of prostaglandins. It is speculated that PGE2 and PGF2 alpha produced either by macrophages or by tumor cells themselves act as growth factors in some cases. It would be worth looking at the expression of the genes coding for the enzymes involved in their synthesis.

REFERENCES

1. Goodwin, J.S. J. Immunol. 4: 397-424, 1983.
2. Bockman, R.S. Cancer Invest. 6: 485-493, 1983.
3. Goodwin, J.S. and Ceuppens, J. J. Immunol. 3: 295-315, 1983.
4. Honn, K.V., Bockman, R.S., and Marnett, L.J. Prostaglandins. 21: 833-864.
5. Powles, T.J., Bockman, R.S., Honn, K.V. and Ramwell. L.Prostaglandins and Cancer: First International Conference. Alan R. Liss. Inc., New York, 1982.
6. Bennet, A., Charlier, E.M., McDonald, A.M., Simpson, J.S., Stamford, I.F. and Zebro, T. Lancet. 2: 624-626, 1977.
7. Husby, G., Strickland, R.G., Rigler, G.L., Peake, G.T. and Williams, R.C. Jr. Cancer, 40: 1629-1642, 1977.
8. Breau, J.L., Morere, J.F., Cour, V., Boaziz, C. and Israel, L. International Conference on Advances in Regional Cancer Therapy, Berchtesgaden, West Germany, June 1989 (in press).
9. Breau, J.L., Morere J.F., Israel, L. Bull. Cancer, 76: 321-328, 1989.

PROGNOSTIC IMPORTANCE OF THROMBOXANE IN BREAST CANCER

S. NIGAM*, A. ZAKREZEWICZ, H. LUBBERT, and C. BENEDETTO**

*Dept. of Gynecological Endocrinology, Klinikum Steglitz, Free University Berlin, D-1000 Berlin 45, FRG
**Dept. of Gynecology, University Torino, Via Ventimiglia 3 10126 Torino, Italy

INTRODUCTION

Breast cancer is a major cause of death by cancer worldwide. It is a systemic disease and may recur decades after it has been initially diagnosed (1). It is associated with a high risk of metastasis (2). There is no doubt that breast tumours synthesize high levels of eicosanoids as compared to the normal tissue (3-6). Whether this increased synthesis occurs in response to certain physiological stimuli or in response to intracellular mediators unique to malignant cells or it is contributed by the non-tumerous surrounding cells resident in the tumour tissue in response to the mediators released by malignant cells, is still unknown. Honn et al (7,8) suggested that primary tumours or detached tumour cells may cause the disruption of systemic balance between prostacyclin (PGI_2) and thromboxane (TXA_2) in favour of TXA_2. However, we did not find any alteration in the ratio of TXA_2:PGI_2 in plasma of patients with malignant or benign tumour of the breast (9). Nevertheless, the levels of PGI_2 and TXA_2 in plasma of breast cancer patients were significantly higher than in benign patients. Also, surgical removal of the primary tumour showed no decrease in levels of prostanoids in breast cancer patients (9) .

Recently, we and others showed the significant role of TXA_2 in the tumour cell proliferation (10,11,12), although Honn et al. predicted its modulatory role in the tumour growth in vitro almost a decade ago (7). Since 6-keto-$PGF_{1\alpha}$ and TXB_2, the metabolites of PGI_2 and TXA_2, respectively, have been shown to be unstable compounds in plasma (13), we investigated plasma concentrations of 2,3-dinor-6-keto-$PGF_{1\alpha}$ and 11-dehydro-TXB_2, the stable metabolites of PGI_2 and TXA_2, respectively, in 25 node-negative and 42 node-positive breast cancer patients. For comparison 13 patients with benign tumour of the breast were recruited in our study. The cancer patients were followed up for almost 3 years after the surgery. The aim of our study was to establish the prognostic role of TXA_2 in early recurrence and death in node-negative and node-positive breast cancer.

METHODS

Patients.

Four groups of women have been examined in our study: (a) 42 women with node-positive (>3 nodes) malignant tumour; (b) 25 women with node-negative malignant tumour; (c) 13 women with benign tumour; (d) 9 healthy controls matched for age with other groups. None of these women had taken drugs known to affect eicosanoid biosynthesis.

The clinical records of all the patients were scruitinized and evaluated with respect to smoking habits, contraceptive practice, major diseases, parity, menopausal status, type of surgical operation, therapy as well as the histopathological data, e.g. size and type of the primary tumour, receptor status, the degree of inflammatory reaction etc.

Blood sampling.

Blood samples were taken at the same time of the day commencing before operation (-1) and after 1,3,6,9,12,18,24,30 and 36 months following surgery. The samples were treated as described (9) and stored at -80°C until analysis.

Assay of prostanoids.

11-dehydro-TXB_2 and 2,3-dinor-6-keto-$PGF_{1\alpha}$ were determined by radioimmunoassay (Amersham, FRG) after preseparation on a C_{18} Sep-Pak cartridge (Millipore, USA) and RP-HPLC as described (14,15). Randomly selected samples were analysed by GC-MS (Finnigan, USA) to verify the values obtained by RIA.

Statistics.

Statistical evaluations were made by the Kruskal-Wallis nonparametric procedure. Differences and correlations were considered significant when $p < 0.05$.

RESULTS AND DISCUSSION

Pre- and post-operative concentrations of 11-dehydro-TXB_2 and 2,3-dinor-6-keto-$PGF_{1\alpha}$ were measured for three years in plasma of 42 node-positive and 25 node-negative breast cancer patients. 13 patients with benign tumour of the breast and 9 healthy women served as controls. The data obtained are shown in Tables I and II. It can be seen that the pre-operative concentration of both 11-deydro-TXB_2 and 2,3-dinor-6-keto-$PGF_{1\alpha}$ in plasma of the malignant group (node +ve and node -ve) are significantly different ($p<0.01$) to those found in benign tumour group and healthy women ($p<0.001$). However, the values for the ratio of 11-dehydro-TXB_2:2,3-dinor-6-keto-$PGF_{1\alpha}$ are not significantly different in any of the preoperative groups, except when the node-positive malignant tumour group is compared with benign tumour group or healthy women. The distribution of 11-dehydro-TXB_2 and 2,3-dinor-6-keto-PGFla levels in the malignant tumour group varies over a considerable range (data not shown) and is consistent with our previously reported data (9).

The post-operative follow-up of concentrations of 11-dehydroTXB_2 and 2,3-dinor-6-keto-$PGF_{1\alpha}$ in plasma of malignant tumour patients for 36 months (Tables I and II) shows that the prostanoid concentrations after an initial decrease for approximately 6 months increased gradually till 18 months. This increase was more pronounced in the node-positive breast cancer patients. During the last 18 months of our study period dramatic increases (almost 3 times of pre-operative levels) in plasma levels of both prostanoids were found in node-positive as well as node-negative breast cancer patients. In the

Table I

Pre- and post-operative plasma concentrations of 11-dehydro-TXB_2 during the follow-up period in women with malignant and benign tumour of the breast. The values represent mean ± SEM. Number of patients is indicated in the parenthesis.

Patients	-1 d	OP 1	3	6	9	12	18	24	30	36
	11-Dehydro-TXB_2 (pg/ml) Months									
Node-positive	670 ± 94 (42)	152 ± 28 (42)	210 ± 41 (42)	425 ± 55 (40)	384 ± 32 (39)	484 ± 72 (37)	410 ± 71 (37)	844 ± 185 (31)	1305 ± 270 (31)	1720 ± 210 (30)
Node-negative	545 ± 67 (25)	87 ± 13 (25)	113 ± 20 (24)	104 ± 15 (22)	139 ± 18 (22)	211 ± 24 (20)	280 ± 41 (18)	1115 ± 210 (15)	1420 ± 195 (14)	1630 ± 215 (13)
Benign tumor	210 ± 13 (13)	62 ± 12 (13)	48 ± 9 (13)	-	-	-	-	-	-	-
Healthy pers.	6 ± 2 (9)	-	-	-	-	-	-	-	-	-

Table II

Pre- and post-operative plasma concentrations of 2, 3-dinor-6-keto-PGF$_{1\alpha}$ during the follow-up period in women with malignant and benign tumour of the breast. The values represent mean ± SEM. Number of patients is given in parenthesis.

	2,3-dinor-6-keto-PGF$_{1\alpha}$ (pg/ml) Months										
Patients	-1 d	OP	1	3	6	9	12	18	24	30	36
Node-positive	305 ± 38 (42)		63 ± 11 (42)	95 ± 22 (42)	163 ± 33 (40)	135 ± 22 (39)	147 ± 43 (37)	114 ± 25 (37)	234 ± 72 (31)	343 ± 67 (31)	420 ± 81 (30)
Node-negative	321 ± 23 (25)		58 ± 9 (25)	75 ± 11 (24)	61 ± 8 (22)	77 ± 10 (22)	132 ± 16 (20)	156 ± 17 (18)	743 ± 64 (18)	835 ± 96 (14)	906 ± 112 (13)
Benign tumor	150 ± 25 (13)		44 ± 7 (13)	38 ± 6 (13)	-	-	-	-	-	-	-
Healthy pers.	8 ± 2		-	-	-	-	-	-	-	-	-

Table III

Changes in ratio of 11-dehydro-TXB_2 and 2, 3-dinor-6-keto-$PGF_{1\alpha}$ levels during the follow-up period in womer with malignant and benign tumour of the breast. The values represent mean ± SEM. Numberr of patients is given in parenthesis.

Patients	11-dehydro-TXB_2:2, 3-dinor-6-keto-$PGF_{1\alpha}$ Months									
	-1 d	OP 1	3	6	9	12	18	24	30	36
Node-positive	2.2 ± 0.4 (42)	2.4 ± 0.4 (42)	2.2 ± 0.5 (42)	2.6 ± 0.6 (40)	2.8 ± 0.7 (39)	3.3 ± 0.6 (37)	3.6 ± 0.8 (37)	3.6 ± 0.5 (31)	3.8 ± 0.8 (31)	4.1 ± 0.8 (30)
Node-negative	1.7 ± 0.4 (25)	1.5 ± 0.3 (25)	1.5 ± 0.4 (24)	1.7 ± 0.4 (22)	1.8 ± 0.3 (22)	1.6 ± 0.2 (20)	1.8 ± 0.4 (18)	1.5 ± 0.3 (18)	1.7 ± 0.4 (14)	1.8 ± 0.4 (13)
Benign tumor	1.4 ± 0.3 (13)	1.4 ± 0.2 (13)	1.3 ± 0.2 (13)	-	-	-	-	-	-	-
Healthy pers.	1.3 ± 0.2	-	-	-	-	-	-	-	-	-

benign group, however, no such tendency for the values of prostanoids was observed; rather there is a trend for concentrations of prostanoids to decrease as compared with the pre-operative levels.

Regarding the ratio of 11-dehydro-TXB_2:2,3-dinor-6-keto-$PGF_{1\alpha}$ a clear trend can be observed between groups at corresponding times or within each group at the various times relative to operation (Table III). Moreover, the node-positive malignant group shows a progressive change in the months after operation, pointing to an increasing emphasis on 11-dehydro-TXB_2 relative to 2,3-dinor-6-keto-$PGF_{1\alpha}$. The node-negative patients, however, did not demonstrate such changes.

The data reported above were also evaluated with respect to clinical and histopathological criteria. No significant differences were observed in the pre-operative levels of 11-dehydro-TXB_2 and 2,3-dinor-6-keto-$PGF_{1\alpha}$ in relation to (i) menopausal status; (ii) type and staging of tumour; (iii) estrogen- and progesterone-receptor status; (iv) type of operation and therapy; (v) inflammatory aspects of the tumour. The striking increase in the plasma levels of prostanoids in malignant tumour group, especially node-positive group, during the last 18 months was in most cases coincident with the recurrence of local or distant tumour. We, therefore, evaluated the post-operative levels of 11-dehydro-TXB_2 in malignant and benign tumour groups during the disease-free interval (range 1-24 months) and the period with recurrence of local or distant secondary tumour (range 3-30 months). The data are shown in Table IV. A striking difference can be seen in the values of 11-dehydro-TXB_2 in each group. The relatively high preoperative levels of 11-dehydro-TXB_2 increase even more during the recurrence of local or distant secondary tumour as compared to the values obtained during the disease-free interval ($p<0.01$) .

Table IV
Mean plasma levels of 11-dehydro-TXB_2 post-operative patients with malignant and benign tumour of the breast during the presence of distant or local recurrence of the tumour and disease-free time. The number of patients is indicated in parenthesis.

Patients	Pre-operative (pg/ml)	Post-operative	
		during distant or local recurrence of the tumour (pg/ml)	during disease-free time (pg/ml)
Node-positive	670 ± 94 (42)	1290 ± 222 (31)	344 ± 61 (39)
Node-negative	545 ± 67 (25)	1328 ± 207 (14)	156 ± 22 (22)
Benign tumour	210 ± 13 (13)	-	55 ± 11 (13)

Thus, no firm conclusions can yet be made, although follow-up of plasma levels of 11-dehydro-TXB_2 and 2,3-dinor-6-keto-$PGF_{1\alpha}$ over 36 months revealed higher levels of both prostanoids in patients with recurrence of secondary tumour. However, the data should be interpreted very cautiously, as the number of patients studied is low and urinary levels of stable metabolites of prostacyclin and thromboxane have not been measured. Nevertheless, TXA_2 is potentially interesting in breast cancer, because it has been shown to play a part in the metastatic process (7). Moreover, it acts as an autocrine mitogen on certain cancer cells, including breast cancer cells (10,11). Recently, the presence of TXA_2-synthetase has been shown in the breast cancer tissue (16). We believe TXA_2 plays a role in mediating the effect of estrogen on the tumour growth and invasion. Although somewhat higher levels of 11-dehydro-TXB_2 in node-positive breast cancer group suggest the metastatic potential of thromboxane, no prediction of the clinical outcome of the patients could be made on the basis of 11-dehydro-TXB_2. The reason for this is still unclear. Furthermore, our data could not confirm the generally accepted good prognosis for node-negative breast cancer patients. Moreover, the recurrence of local or distant tumour was not observed in most of the patients after the operation.

Nevertheless, looking at the data on 2,3-dinor-6-keto-$PGF_{1\alpha}$ in the node-positive malignant group, it can be predicted that prostacyclin has a protective action against metastasis in the breast cancer. In the node-negative group, prostacyclin demonstrated its incapability to affect the tumour growth.

We conclude that thromboxane may be a potentially important prognostic factor for early recurrence of a local or distant tumour, independently of a number of other prognostic variables.

ACKNOWLEDGEMENTS

This study was generously supported by the Association for International Cancer Research, UK. Authors wish to thank Ms. Barbara Steiger, Gabrielle Beyer and Monika Bielesch for their expert technical assistance.

REFERENCES

1. Haybittle, J.L., Rev. Endo Relat. Cancer, 14:13, 1983.
2. Burstein, N.A. In: Carcinoma of the Breast: Diagnosis and Treatment, (Dorsi, C.J., Willson, R.E., eds). Little Brown & Co., Boston/Toronto, 1983, p. 59.
3. Powles, T.J., et al., Lancet II. 1977, 138.
4. Caro, J.F., et al., Am J. Med. 1979, 66:337.
5. Stamford, I.F., et al., In: Adv. Prost. Thr. Res. (Samuelsson, B., Ramwell, P.W., Paoletti, R., eds.), Raven Press, New York, Vol. 6, 1980, p. 571.
6. Malachi, T., et al., J. Cancer Res. Clin. Oncol. 1981, 102:71.
7. Honn, K.V., et al., Science. 1981, 212:1270.
8. Honn, K.V., et al., Biochem. Pharmacol. 1983, 32:1.
9. Nigam, S., et al., Prostaglandins, 1985, 29(4): 513.
10. Nigam, S. and Averdunk, R., In: Leukotrienes and Prostanoids in Health and Disease. New Trends Lipid Mediator Res. (Zor, U., Naor, Z., Danon, A., eds.), Basel, Karger, 1989, Vol. 3, p. 319.
11. Nigam, S. and Zakrzewicz, A., In: Adv. Prostagl. Thr. & Leukotr. Res. (Samuelsson, B., Ramwell, P.W., Paoletti, R., eds.), Raven Press, New York, 1991, Vol. 21B, 925-928.

12. Chiabrando, C., et al., Cancer Res. 1987, 47:1988.
13. Granstrom, E., and Kumlin, M., In:Prostaglandins and Related Substances: a Practical Approach (Benedetto, C., McDonald-Gibson, R.G., Nigam, S., Slater, T.F., eds.), IRL Press, Oxford, 1987, p. 5.
14. Nigam, S., In: Prostaglandins and Related Substances: a Practical Approach (Benedetto, C., McDonald-Gibson, R.G., Nigam, S. Slater, T.F., eds), IRL Press, Oxford, 1987, p. 45.
15. Catella, D., et al., Proc. Nat. Acad. Sci. USA, 1986, 83:5861.
16. Nussing, R. and Ullrich, V., Eicosanoids, 1990, 3(3):175.

CHRONIC NONSTEROIDAL ANTIINFLAMMATORY DRUG USE IN A COHORT OF PATIENTS WITH ADVANCED LUNG AND COLON CANCER

L.R. ZACHARSKI*, V. COSTANTINI*, T.E. MORITZ, and C.M. HAAKENSON

*Dartmouth Medical School and the Veterans Administration Medical School, White River Jct., Vermont 05001

INTRODUCTION

Studies in experimental tumor systems attest to the importance of abnormal prostaglandin metabolism in the pathogenesis of malignancy. The extensive literature on this subject has been reviewed (1-4) which has shown that inhibition of prostaglandin synthesis by nonsteroidal antiinflammatory drugs (NSAIDs) is capable of inhibiting carcinogenesis, tumor cell proliferation, and metastatic dissemination; and also restoration of depressed cellular immune function that is a feature of the tumor-bearing host. Relationships, presented schematically in simplified form in Figure 1, have been relatively well worked out in experimental models of colon carcinogenesis (3,5,7). Evidence indicates that deoxycholate (DOC) serves as a tumor promoter. DOC induces synthesis of the enzyme, ornithine decarboxylase (ODC). This enzyme induction requires the presence of prostaglandin E_2 (PGE_2). ODC is a rate-limiting enzyme in polyamine synthesis and polyamines stimulate tumor cell proliferation. NSAIDs inhibit PGE_2 production and thereby inhibit induction of ODC. ODC may be a marker for human, as well as animal, colon carcinogenesis (2,8).

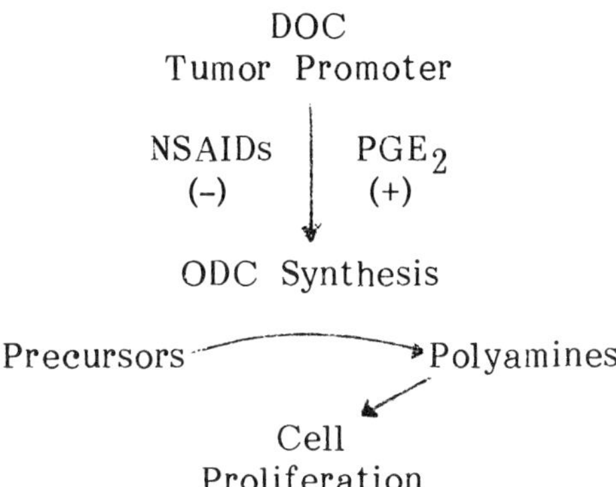

Figure 1. Simplified scheme of role of prostaglandin E_2 (PGE_2) in colon carcinogenesis. DOC = deoxycholate. ODC = ornithine decarboxylase. (+) and (-) = enhancing and inhibiting functions, respectively.

The scant information available on possible effects of NSAIDs in human malignancy has also been reviewed recently (2). A summary of uncontrolled clinical trials is presented in Table 1 and of controlled clinical trials in Table 2. Considering the abundant literature in experimental malignancies (1-4) and their relative ease of administration, the paucity of existing data on effects of NSAIDs on humans seems surprising.

Table 1. Summary of uncontrolled clinical trials of NSAIDs.

Agent	Tumor	Reference	Comment
1. Indomethacin, sulindac	desmoid tumors	9,10	Regression in some cases
2. Sulindac	colonic polyposis	11, 12	Polyp regression
3. Indomethacin + prednisolone	skin cancers	13	Regression of tumor
4. Piroxicam	various	14	Prolonged tumor doubling time
5. Aspirin	renal cell carcinoma	15	Increased (34%) response rate when used with interferon
6. Indomethacin	head and neck cancer	16	Tumor stabilization and regression in some patients

Table 2. Summary of controlled clinical trials of NSAIDs.

Agent	Tumor	Reference	Comment
1. Benorylate	breast	17	No effect
2. Aspirin	resected colorectal cancer	18	No effect
3. Aspirin + dipyridamole	resected colorectal cancer	19	No effect
4. Aspirin	small cell carcinoma	20	No effect
5. Aspirin + dipyridamole	polycythemia vera	21	No effect
6. Oxyphen-butazone	squamous cell	22	Statistically significant prolongation of survival at 5 and 10 years followup

In an attempt to obtain further information on such possible effects, a recently completed large clinical trial, VA Cooperative Study #188 (5,6), was designed to permit surveillance prospectively of drugs, including NSAIDs ingested by previously untreated patients with advanced carcinoma of the lung and colon. The results of this surveillance will be reported in detail elsewhere (2) and are summarized briefly here.

MATERIALS AND METHODS

The rationale, experimental design (including definitions of tumor categories and standard treatment given) and primary outcome data for this study has been published (23,24). Clinical data collected at entry to the study and at specified followup intervals included performance status, TN M stage, disease sites, prior weight loss, tumor response, time to disease progression, organ sites of new disease, symptoms, and survival. Extensive laboratory data were also collected. While defined exclusion criteria prevented entry of patients with various severe diseases other than malignancy, the study design permitted the attending physician to use any drugs that were indicated following entry to the study. An exception was aspirin, the administration of which was prohibited by the protocol. All other drugs ingested by patients entered to this study were recorded on the study data sheets. This compilation permitted identification of patients who ingested an NSAID while under observation as well as the duration of drug ingestion. Certain characteristics of patients who took versus did not take an NSAID were compared.

RESULTS

A total of 719 patients with carcinoma of the lung, that was catagorized as either limited to one hemithorax or disseminated, and disseminated (Duke's D) colon cancer were entered. Lung cancer patients were catagorized as having either non-small cell lung cancer (N-SCLC) or small cell carcinoma of the lung (SCCL). Of this total, 582 were found not to have taken an NSAID and 137 to have taken an NSAID. While a variety of NSAIDs were ingested, ibuprofen was used over twice as often as the next most commonly used drug, indomethacin. The average duration of NSAID administration was 4.1 months. Approximately 50% of NSAID users reported such use at the time of entry to the study. The remainder were found to have used NSAIDs at some time during followup.

The two treatment groups were comparable for most characteristics determined at the time of entry to the study. However, NSAID users had lower baseline total leukocyte counts and greater body weight. NSAID users with lung cancer had lower "N" (lymphnode) stage than non-users. Certain symptoms; including dizziness, flushing, diarrhea, and fatigue, were reported more frequently in NSAID users than non-users. However, it could not be determined whether such symptoms were related to the drug itself or the condition for which the drug was given. There was no increase in bleeding episodes in NSAID users. In general, NSAIDs appeared to be reasonably well tolerated in these patients with advanced malignancy. No difference between groups was noted in the incidence or organ distribution of disease in new sites that appeared during followup. Trends toward increased response rates and survival were not susceptible to definitive evaluation.

DISCUSSION

The limited information currently available in the literature (see Tables 1 and 2) highlights both the complexities involved and the potential for further studies of therapeutic effects of NSAIDs in human malignancy. The pilot data on a cohort of 137 patients with advanced lung and colon cancer reported here suggests that such studies are feasible. Unfortunatly, evaluation of endpoints of greatest interest (e.g. tumor response and survival) could not be carried out based on data from this study for several reasons. For example, NSAID use prior to entry to the study was neither recorded on the data sheets nor an exclusion criteria for entry to this study. Such prior use might have influenced outcome while under observation in this study in an unpredictable manner. More importantly, there was no common baseline for NSAID users versus non-users. Only about 50% of users reported NSAID ingestion at entry to the study. Increased longevity might have increased the chance of receiving an NSAID during followup and thus falsely created the impression of a causal relationship.

Conclusions on cause-and-effect relationships between abnormal prostaglandin production and the pathogenesis of human malignancy can only be drawn from well-designed intervention studies. The ability of NSAIDs to normalize certain cellular immune defects in cancer patients (2) may provide a means for evaluating the relative merits of various drugs and doses in anticipation of controlled (and preferably blinded) clinical trials. The design of such studies should take into consideration the likelihood that mechanisms will differ between tumor types and stages of the disease. However, appropriately conducted clinical trials shouild permit distinction between effects on carcinogenesis, cell proliferation, and tumor dissemination such that these relatively inexpensive and nontoxic agents can be prescribed rationally.

Finally, we have noted that NSAIDs are commonly given to ameliorate the toxic side effects of other forms of experimental cancer therapy, such as interleukin-2 (8). It is possible that at least a portion of the beneficial effect attributed to such experimental treatment may be a result of NSAIDs administered concomitantly (8).

REFERENCES

1. Honn, K.V., Busse, W.D. and Sloane, B.F. Biochem. Pharmacol. 32:111, 1983.
2. Costantini, V., Zacharski, L.R., Moritz, T.E. and Haakenson, C.M. Submitted for publication, 1989.
3. Nigro, N.D., Bull, A.W. and Boyd, M.E. J. Natl. Cancer Inst. 77:1309-1313, 1986.
4. Brockman, R.S. Cancer Invest. 1:485-493, 1983.
5. Narisawa, T., Takahashi, M., Niwa, M., Fukaura, Y., Wakizaka, A. Jpn. J. Cancer Res. 78:791-798, 1987.
6. Pollard, M., Lukert, P.H. J. Natl. Cancer Inst. 70:1103-1105, 1983.
7. Goldin, B.R. Prog. Clin. Biol. Res. 279:319-333, 1988.
8. Luk, G.D., Moshier, J.A., Ehrinpreis, M.N. Prog. Clin. Biol. Res. 279:227-239, 1988.
9. Belliveau, P., Graham, A.M. Dis. Colon Rectum 27:53-54, 1984.
10. Klein, W.A., Miller, H.H., Anderson, M., DeCoss, J.J. Cancer 60:2863-2868, 1987.

11. Gonzaga, R.A.F., Lima, F.R., Carniero, S., Maciel, J., Junior, M.A. Lancet 1:751, 1985.
12. Waddell, W.R., Loughry, R.W. J. Surg. Oncol. 24:83-87, 1983.
13. Al-Saleem, T., Ali, Z.S., Qassab, M. Lancet 2:264-265, 1980.
14. Breaw, J.L., Morere, J.F., Israel, L. Bull. Cancer 76:321-328, 1989.
15. Greagan, E.T., Buckner, J.C., Kahn, R.G., Richardson, R.R., Schaid, D.J., Kovach, J.S. Cancer 61:1787-1791, 1988.
16. Panje, W.R. Arch. Otolaryngol. 107:658-663, 1981.
17. Powles, T.J., Dady, P.J., Williams, J., Easty, G.C., Coombes, R.C. Adv. Prostaglandin Thromboxane Res. 6:511-516, 1980.
18. Lipton, A., Scialla, S., Harvey, H., Dixon, R., Gordon, R., Hamilton, R., Ramsey, H., Weltz, M., Heckard, R., White, D. J. Med. 13:419-429, 1982.
19. Lipton, A., Harvey, H., Dixon, R., Walker, B., Gordon, R., Street, T., Heckard, R., Antle, C., Ranhosky, A. Cancer Therapy Control 1:81-86, 1989.
20. Lebeau, B., Chastang, C. Bull. Europ. Physiopat. Resp. 22 (Suppl 8):1595, 1986.
21. Tartaglia, A., Goldberg, J.D., Berk, P.D., Wasserman, L.R. Semin. Hematol. 23:172-176, 1986.
22. Weppelmann, B., Monkemeier, D. Gynecol. Oncol. 17:196-199, 1984.
23. Zacharski, L.R., Henderson, W.G., Rickles, F., Forman, W.B., Van Eeckhout, J.P., Cornell, C.J., Jr., Forcier, R.J. and Martin, J.F. Am. J. Clin. Oncol. 5:593-609, 1982.
24. Zacharski, L.R., Moritz, T.E., Baczek, L.A., Rickles, F.R., Edwards, R.L., Forman, W.B., Forcier, R.J., Cornell, C.J., Haakenson, C.M., Ballard, H.S., Crum, E.D., Johnson, G.J., Levine, J., Hong, W.K., O'Donnell, J.F., Schilsky, R.L., Ringenberg, Q.S., Robert, F., Spaulding, M.B., Tornyos, K., William, C., Zucker, S., Faulkner, C.S. II, Eaton, W.L. and Hoppel, C.L. J. Natl. Cancer Inst. 80:90-97, 1988.
25. Lala, P.K. and Parhar, R.S. Cancer Res. 48:1072-1078, 1988.

Index